ENCYCLOPEDIA OF
PHARMACEUTICAL
TECHNOLOGY

VOLUME 16

ENCYCLOPEDIA OF PHARMACEUTICAL TECHNOLOGY

Editors

JAMES SWARBRICK
Vice President
Research and Development
AAI, Inc.
Wilmington, North Carolina

JAMES C. BOYLAN
Director
Pharmaceutical Technology
Hospital Products Division
Abbott Laboratories
Abbott Park, Illinois

VOLUME 16

UNIT PROCESSES IN PHARMACY:
THE OPERATIONS TO ZETA POTENTIAL

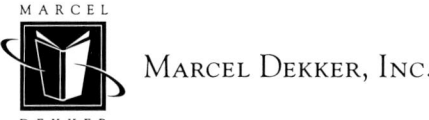 Marcel Dekker, Inc.   New York · Basel · Hong Kong

Library of Congress Cataloging in Publication Data
Main entry under title:

Encyclopedia of Pharmaceutical Technology.
editors: James Swarbrick, James C. Boylan.

Includes index.
1. Pharmaceutical technology—Dictionaries. I. Swarbrick, James.
II. Boylan, James C.
[DNLM: 1. Chemistry, Pharmaceutical-encyclopedias. 2. Drugs—encyclopedias. 3. Technology, Pharmaceutical-encyclopedias. QV 13 E565].
RS192.E53 1988   615'.1'0321-dc19

COPYRIGHT © 1997 BY MARCEL DEKKER, INC. ALL RIGHTS RESERVED.

Neither this book nor any part may be reproduced or transmitted in any form or by any means, electronic or mechanical, including photocopying, microfilming, and recording, or by any information storage and retrieval system, without permission in writing from the publisher.

MARCEL DEKKER, INC.
270 Madison Avenue, New York, New York 10016

LIBRARY OF CONGRESS CATALOG CARD NUMBER 88-25664
ISBN: 0-8247-2815-7

Current printing (last digit):
10 9 8 7 6 5 4 3 2 1

PRINTED IN THE UNITED STATES OF AMERICA

CONTENTS OF VOLUME 16

Contributors to Volume 16	v
Contents of Other Volumes	vii
Unit Processes in Pharmacy: The Operations David Ganderton and Anthony J. Hickey	1
Vaccines and Other Immunological Products Terry L. Bowersock and Kinam Park	115
Vaginal Delivery and Absorption of Drugs Karen Yu and Yie W. Chien	153
Validation of Pharmaceutical Processes Robert A. Nash	187
Validation of Pharmaceutical Water System Theodore H. Meltzer	211
Veterinary Uses of Drugs Joy B. Reighard	251
Water for Pharmaceutical Use Rostyslaw O. Slabicky	293
Water Sorption of Drugs and Dosage Forms Mark J. Kontny	307
Waxes Roland Bodmeier and Joachim Herrmann	335
Wet Granulation Ana I. Torres-Suárez and Maria Esther Gil-Alegre	363
Xenobiotic Metabolism Mohamadi A. Sarkar and William H. Soine	403
Zeta Potential Luk Chiu Li and Youquin Tian	429
Index to Volume 16	459

CONTRIBUTORS TO VOLUME 16

Roland Bodmeier, Ph.D. Professor, College of Pharmacy, Freie Universität Berlin, Berlin, Germany: *Waxes*

Terry L. Bowersock, D.V.M., Ph.D. Senior Research Scientist, Department of Infectious Disease Research, Pharmacia & Upjohn, Kalamazoo, Michigan: *Vaccines and Other Immunological Products*

Yie W. Chien, Ph.D. Professor of Pharmaceutics and Director, Controlled Drug-Delivery Research Center, Rutgers University, College of Pharmacy, Piscataway, New Jersey: *Vaginal Delivery and Absorption of Drugs*

David Ganderton Department of Pharmacy, King's College London, University of London, London, England: *Unit Processes in Pharmacy: The Operations*

Maria Esther Gil-Alegre, Ph.D. Assistant Professor, Department of Pharmacy and Pharmaceutical Technology, Complutense University, Madrid, Spain: *Wet Granulation*

Joachim Herrmann, Ph.D. Dr. Willmar Schwabe Arzneimittel, Karlsruhe, Germany: *Waxes*

Anthony J. Hickey Associate Professor of Pharmaceutics, School of Pharmacy, The University of North Carolina at Chapel Hill, Chapel Hill, North Carolina: *Unit Processes in Pharmacy: The Operations*

Mark J. Kontny, Ph.D. Associate Director, Pharmaceutical Development, G. D. Searle & Company, Skokie, Illinois: *Water Sorption of Drugs and Dosage Forms*

Luk Chiu Li, Ph.D. Associate Research Fellow, Advanced Drug Delivery, Hospital Products Division, Abbott Laboratories, Abbott Park, Illinois: *Zeta Potential*

Theodore H. Meltzer, Ph.D. Capitola Consulting Company, Arlington, Virginia: *Validation of Pharmaceutical Water System*

Robert A. Nash, Ph.D. Consultant, Professor of Industrial Pharmacy, Mahwah, New Jersey: *Validation of Pharmaceutical Processes*

Kinam Park, Ph.D. Professor, Department of Pharmaceutics, School of Pharmacy, Purdue University, West Lafayette, Indiana: *Vaccines and Other Immunological Products*

Joy B. Reighard, Ph.D. Associate Professor of Pharmacognosy, Temple University School of Pharmacy, Philadelphia, Pennsylvania: *Veterinary Uses of Drugs*

Mohamadi A. Sarkar, Ph.D. West Virginia University, School of Pharmacy Morgantown, West Virginia: *Xenobiotic Metabolism*

Rostyslaw O. Slabicky Manager, Systems Validation, Boehringer Ingelheim Pharmaceuticals Inc., Ridgefield, Connecticut: *Water for Pharmaceutical Use*

William H. Soine, Ph.D.   Virginia Commonwealth University, MCV Campus, School of Pharmacy, Richmond, Virginia: *Xenobiotic Metabolism*

Youquin Tian, Ph.D.   Senior Research Scientist, Advanced Drug Delivery, Hospital Products Division, Abbott Laboratories, Abbott Park, Illinois: *Zeta Potential*

Ana I. Torres-Suárez, Ph.D.   Professor, Department of Pharmacy and Pharmaceutical Technology, Complutense University, Madrid, Spain: *Wet Granulation*

Karen Yu, Ph.D.   Scientist, Cibus Pharmaceutical, Inc., Burlingame, California: *Vaginal Delivery and Absorption of Drugs*

CONTENTS OF OTHER VOLUMES

CONTENTS OF VOLUME 1

Contributors to Volume 1	v
Preface	vii
Absorption of Drugs Peter G. Welling	1
Abuse of Drugs Ahmad Rezvani and E. Leong Way	33
Adsorption at Solid Surfaces Herbert Rupprecht and Geoffrey Lee	73
Adulteration of Drugs and Drug Products Raymond E. Hamilton	115
Adverse Drug Reactions Therese I. Poirier	121
Advertising and Promotion of Prescription Drug Products Lloyd G. Millstein	147
Air Suspension Coating David M. Jones	189
Analysis and Assay of Drugs Robert V. Smith	217
Analysis of Biologic Fluids Stephen G. Schulman and Stephen H. Curry	233
Analysis of Recombinant Biologicals Robert L. Garnick, Michael J. Ross, and Charles P. du Mée	253
Animals in Drug Development Farrel L. Fort	315

Aqueous Film Coating
James A. Seitz   337

Aseptic Processing Operations, Validation of
William R. Frieben   351

Atomic Absorption Spectrophotometry
John P. Oberdier   371

Auditing of Pharmaceutical Processing
William J. Mead   383

Autoclaves and Autoclaving
Edward J. Leuthner   393

Autoxidation and Antioxidants
David M. Johnson and Leo C. Gu   415

Binders
Henning G. Kristensen   451

Bioabsorbable Polymers
Shalaby W. Shalaby   465

Bioavailability of Drugs and Bioequivalence
Marvin C. Meyer   477

CONTENTS OF VOLUME 2

Contributors to Volume 2   v

Biodegradable Polyester Polymers as Drug Carriers
M. Regina Brophy and Patrick B. Deasy   1

Biological Indicators
Peter Lancy and Karl Kereluk   27

Biopharmaceutics
Leon Shargel   33

Biopolymers for Controlled Drug Delivery
Avinash G. Thombre and John R. Cardinal   61

CONTENTS OF OTHER VOLUMES

Biosynthesis of Drugs
Christopher W. W. Beecher and Geoffrey A. Cordell   89

Biotechnology and Biologic Preparations
Hollis G. Schoepke   117

Biotransformation of Drugs
L. F. Chasseaud and D. R. Hawkins   129

Blenders and Blending Operations
M. S. Spring   159

Buccal Absorption of Drugs
James C. McElnay   189

Buffers and Buffering Agents
Lydia C. Kaus   213

Calorimetry in Pharmaceutical Research and Development
Siegfried Lindenbaum   233

Capsules, Hard
Brian E. Jones   251

Capsules, Soft
Robert F. Jimerson and F. S. Hom   269

Carcinogenicity Testing
Joseph L. Ciminera and Henry L. Allen   285

Cellulose Derivatives and Natural Products Utilized in Pharmaceutics
Jesse W. Wallace   319

Centrifugation
Graham C. Cole   339

Chemical Kinetics and Drug Stability
Jens T. Carstensen   355

Chewable Tablets
Robert W. Mendes and Aloysius O. Anaebonam   397

Chromatographic Analysis
Gary M. Pollack   419

Cleaning of Equipment
Samuel W. Harder   447

Clinical Evaluation of Drugs
Allen Cato, Allen Lai, and Robert Sutton   457

Clinical Pharmacokinetics and Pharmacodynamics
Margareta Hammarlund-Udenaes and Leslie Z. Benet   483

CONTENTS OF VOLUME 3

Contributors to Volume 3   v

Clinical Supplies
Michael McNear and Robert E. Shaffer   1

Coacervation/Phase Separation
Joseph A. Bakan and Anil M. Doshi   21

Colloids and Colloid Drug Delvery Systems
Diane J. Burgess   31

Coloring Agents for Use in Pharmaceuticals
Edward J. Woznicki and David R. Schoneker   65

Comminution
Eugene L. Parrott   101

Compendial Specifications
Lee T. Grady   123

Compression of Solids and Compressed Dosage Forms
Edward G. Rippie   149

Computer-Aided Drug Design
J. Phillip Bowen and Michael Cory   167

Computers in Pharmaceutical Technology
Onkaram Basavapathruni   201

Contamination Control
Richard G. Johnson   237

Continuous Processing of Pharmaceuticals
Kunio Kawamura   253

CONTENTS OF OTHER VOLUMES

Controlled- and Modulated-Release Drug-Delivery Systems
Yie W. Chien — 281

Cooling Processes and Congealing
James W. McGinity and Mark D. Coffin — 315

Coprecipitates and Melts
Madhu K. Vadnere — 337

Corrosion in Pharmaceutical Processing
Arvind N. Narurkar and Pai-Chang Sheen — 353

Cosmetics and Their Relation to Drugs
Martin M. Rieger — 361

Cosolvents and Cosolvency
Joseph T. Rubino — 375

Crystallization and the Properties of Crystals
Nair Rodríguez-Hornedo — 399

Dental Products
Sebastian G. Ciancio — 435

Dermal Diffusion and Delivery Principles
Gordon L. Flynn — 457

CONTENTS OF VOLUME 4

Contributors to Volume 4 — v

Design of Drugs: Basic Concepts and Applications
Jacques H. Poupaert — 1

Diffuse Reflectance Spectroscopy
Michael Bornstein — 23

Diluents
Jeffrey L. Czeisler and Karl P. Perlman — 37

Direct Compression Tabletting
Ralph F. Shangraw — 85

Disperse Systems
J. Graham Nairn   **107**

Dissolution and Dissolution Testing
James L. Ford   **121**

Dissolution of Pharmaceutical Suspensions
Paula Jo Stout, Stephen A. Howard, and John W. Mauger   **169**

Dosage Form Design: A Physicochemical Approach
Michael B. Maurin, Anwar A. Hussain, and Lewis W. Dittert   **193**

Dosage Forms: Non-Parenteral
Paul Zanowiak   **209**

Dosage Forms: Parenteral
Salvatore J. Turco   **231**

Dosing of Drugs: Dosage Regimens and Dose-Response
Chyung S. Cook and Aziz Karim   **249**

Dressings in Wound Management
Terence D. Turner   **283**

Drug Delivery and Therapeutic Systems
Felix Theeuwes, Patrick S. L. Wong, and Su Il Yum   **303**

Drug Information Systems
John M. Fischer   **349**

Drug Interactions
Daniel A. Hussar   **357**

Drug Product Selection by the Pharmacist
Robert P. Rapp   **377**

Drug Safety Evaluation
Farrel L. Fort   **389**

Dry Granulation
Kozo Kurihara   **423**

Dry Heat Sterilization and Depyrogenation
Frances M. Groves and Michael J. Groves   **447**

Drying and Driers
Kurt G. Van Scoik, Michael A. Zoglio, and Jens T. Carstensen   **485**

CONTENTS OF VOLUME 5

Contributors to Volume 5	v
Contents of Other Volumes	vii
Economic Characteristics of the R&D-Intensive Pharmaceutical Industry Douglas L. Cocks	1
Effervescent Pharmaceuticals Nils-Olof Lindberg, Hans Engfors, and Thomas Ericsson	45
Elastomeric Parenteral Closures Kenneth E. Avis and Edward J. Smith	73
Electrochemical Methods of Analysis Barbara J. Norris	89
Electron Beam Sterilization Marshall R. Cleland and Jeffrey A. Beck	105
Emulsions Gillian M. Eccleston	137
Enteric Coatings Walter G. Chambliss	189
Enzyme Immunoassay Hsin-Hsiung Tai	201
Enzymes Ingrid M. A. Verhamme and Albert R. Lauwers	235
Equipment Selection and Evaluation Bhoghi B. Sheth and Fred J. Bandelin	263
Ethics of Drug Making Michael Montagne	301
Ethylene Oxide Sterilization Robert R. Reich and Daniel J. Burgess	315
Evaporation and Evaporators David P. Kessler	337

Expert Systems as Applied to Pharmaceutical Technology
Felix Lai   361

Expiration Dating
Mark VanArendonk and G. R. Dukes   379

Extrusion and Extruders
K. E. Fielden and J. M. Newton   395

Fermentation Processes
Peter F. Stanbury   443

Cumulative Index to Volumes 1–5   475

CONTENTS OF VOLUME 6

Contributors to Volume 6	v
Contents of Other Volumes	vii
Film Coatings and Film-Forming Materials: Evaluation Galen W. Radebaugh	1
Films and Sheets for Packaging Shalaby W. Shalaby and Bernard L. Williams	29
Filters and Filtration Theodore H. Meltzer	51
Flame Photometry Thomas M. Nowak	93
Flavors and Flavor Modifiers Akwete L. Adjei, Richard Doyle, and Thomas Reiland	101
Flow Properties of Solids Stephen A. Howard and Jin-Wang Lai	141
Fluid-Bed Dryers, Granulators, and Coaters Leo K. Mathur	171
Fluorescence Spectroscopy Victoria Saldajeno de Leon and Stephen G. Schulman	197

CONTENTS OF OTHER VOLUMES

Food and Drug Administration: Role in Drug Regulation
James C. Morrison — 231

Foods and "Health Foods" as Drugs
Ara H. DerMarderosian — 251

Freeze Drying
Michael J. Pikal — 275

Gamma Radiation Sterilization
Geoffrey P. Jacobs — 305

Gas Chromatography
Isadore Kanfer — 333

Gastrointestinal Absorption of Drugs
Alice E. Loper and Colin R. Gardner — 385

Gels and Jellies
Cathy M. Klech — 415

Generic Drugs and Generic Equivalency
Arthur H. Kibbe and Lawrence C. Weaver — 441

Index to Volume 6 — 469

CONTENTS OF VOLUME 7

Contributors to Volume 7 — v

Contents of Other Volumes — vii

Genetic Engineering
Donald E. Frail — 1

Genetic Factors in Drug Use
David W. J. Clark — 37

Geriatric Drug Use
Sandra Knowles and Susan K. Bowles — 55

Glass as a Packaging Material for Pharmaceuticals
R. Paul Abendroth — 79

Good Laboratory Practice Regulations
Allen F. Hirsch   101

Good Manufacturing Practices: An Overview
Harriet Vickory and Laura Nally   109

Granulations
Henning Gjelstrup Kristensen and Torben Schaefer   121

Halohydrocarbons, Pharmaceutical Uses
Richard N. Dalby   161

Health Care Systems: The United States
Henri R. Manasse, Jr.   181

Health Care Systems: Outside the United States
Albert I. Wertheimer and Joaquima Serradell   201

Heat Transfer in Process Vessels
Richard E. Markovitz   213

Heating, Ventilation, and Air Conditioning
John W. Sutter   229

High-Performance Liquid Chromatography
R. Raghavan and Jose C. Joseph   249

History of Dosage Forms and Basic Preparations
Robert A. Buerki and Gregory J. Higby   299

Home Parenteral Therapy
Hetty A. Lima   341

Homogenization and Homogenizers
Graham C. Cole   361

Hospital Pharmacy
David S. Adler and Michael L. Kleinberg   373

Hydrates
Kenneth R. Morris and Nair Rodríguez-Hornedo   393

Hydrogels
Joke A. Bouwstra and Hans E. Junginger   441

Index to Volume 7   467

CONTENTS OF VOLUME 8

Contributors to Volume 8	v
Contents of Other Volumes	vii
Hydrolysis of Drugs Kenneth A. Connors	1
Immunoassay H. Thomas Karnes, Mohamadi A. Sarkar, Guenther Hochhaus, and Stephen G. Schulman	31
Implants and Implantation Therapy Hitesh R. Bhagat and Robert S. Langer	53
Infrared Spectroscopy Shuyen L. Huang	83
Instrumentation of Equipment Mika Vidgrén and Petteri Paronen	107
Interfacial Phenomena Tetsurou Handa, Yoshie Maitani, Koichiro Miyazima, and Masayuki Nakagaki	131
Intranasal Drug Delivery Kenneth S. E. Su	175
Ion Exchange Resins and Sustained Release Saul S. Borodkin	203
Iontophoresis Burton H. Sage	217
Irrigation Solutions Steven B. Moody	249
Isomerism J. DeRuiter, Thomas N. Riley, W. R. Ravis, and C. Randall Clark	259
Laminar Airflow Equipment: Engineering Control of Aseptic Processing Gregory F. Peters	317

Lens Care Products
Kiran J. Randeri, Ronald P. Quintana, and Masood Chowhan   361

Liability Aspects of Drugs and Devices
Gaile L. McMann   403

Lipids in Pharmaceutical Dosage Forms
Alan L. Weiner   417

Index to Volume 8   477

CONTENTS OF VOLUME 9

Contributors to Volume 9   v

Contents of Other Volumes   vii

Liposomes as Pharmaceutical Dosage Forms
Yechezkel Barenholz and Daan J. A. Crommelin   1

Liquid Oral Preparations
Jagdish Parasrampuria   41

Lozenges
Hridaya N. Bhargava and Robert W. Mendes   65

Lubrication in Solid Dosage Form Design and Manufacture
Paul Zanowiak   87

Management of Drug Development
Donald C. Monkhouse, Ralph A. Blackmer, and Wendy A. Valinski   113

Manufacture of Pharmaceuticals
John C. Griffin   133

Marketing of Pharmaceuticals
Mickey C. Smith   151

Mass Spectrometry
David M. Higton and Janet M. Oxford   171

Mass Transfer in Unit Operations
J. Graham Nairn   205

CONTENTS OF OTHER VOLUMES	xix
Mathematical Modeling of Pharmaceutical Data David W. A. Bourne	237
Medical Devices Michael Szycher	263
Metered-Dose Inhalers: Nonpressurized Systems Paul J. Atkins	287
Metered-Dose Inhalers: Pressurized Systems Gerald W. Hallworth	299
Microbial Control of Pharmaceuticals Nigel A. Halls	331
Microemulsions Gillian M. Eccleston	375
Microencapsulation Joseph A. Bakan	423
Index to Volume 9	443

CONTENTS OF VOLUME 10

Contributors to Volume 10	v
Contents of Other Volumes	vii
Microsphere Technology and Applications Diane J. Burgess and Anthony J. Hickey	1
Moisture in Pharmaceutical Products R. Gary Hollenbeck	31
Moisture-Solid Dosage Forms Jens T. Carstensen	67
Monoclonal Antibodies for Drug Delvery John B. Cannon, Pramod K. Gupta, and Ho-Wah Hui	83
Mouthwashes and Periodontal Disease Daniel A. Greenberg	121

Mucosal Adhesive Preparations Kalpana R. Kamath and Kinam Park	133
Nanoparticles Jörg Kreuter	165
Nasal Drug Delivery: Trends and Perspectives Frans W. H. M. Merkus and J. Coos Verhoef	191
New Drug Applications Dhiren N. Shah and Sidney Goldstein	223
Nonisothermal Kinetic Methods Luk Chiu Li	261
Nonprescription Drugs Clive Edwards	283
Nuclear Imaging in Pharmaceutical Research Raymond E. Gibson and H. Donald Burns	303
Nuclear Magnetic Resonance in Pharmaceutical Technology James S. Bernstein	335
Index to Volumes 1–10	353

CONTENTS OF VOLUME 11

Contributors to Volume 11	v
Contents of Other Volumes	vii
Nuclear Medicine and Pharmacy Richard J. Kowalsky and Alan F. Parr	1
Ocular Drug Formulation and Delivery Suketu D. Desai and James Blanchard	43
Optimization Techniques in Formulation and Processing Durk A. Doornbos and Pieter de Haan	77
Orphan Drugs Carolyn H. Asbury	161

CONTENTS OF OTHER VOLUMES — xxi

Otic Preparations — 185
William H. Slattery III and Richard E. Brownlee

Parenterals: Large Volume — 201
Salvatore J. Turco

Parenterals: Small Volume — 217
Michael J. Akers

Particle-Size Characterization — 237
Brian H. Kaye

Particulate Matter in Parenteral Products — 263
Michael J. Groves

Partition Coefficients — 293
Eric J. Lien

Patents in the Pharmaceutical Industry — 309
Stuart R. Suter

Pediatric Dosing and Dosage Forms — 329
Rosalie Sagraves

Pelletization Techniques — 369
Isaac Ghebre-Sellassie and Axel Knoch

Peptide and Protein Drug Delivery — 395
Lorraine L. Wearley and Ajay K. Banga

Percutaneous Absorption — 413
Thomas J. Franz and Paul A. Lehman

Permeation Enhancement through Skin — 449
Adrian C. Williams and Brian W. Barry

Index to Volume 11 — 495

CONTENTS OF VOLUME 12

Contributors to Volume 12 — v

Contents of Other Volumes — vii

Pharmaceutical Packaging
Donald C. Liebe   **1**

Pharmacokinetics and Pharmacodynamics
John J. Lima   **29**

Pharmacopeial Standards: European Pharmacopeia
Agnès F. Artiges   **53**

Pharmacopeial Standards: Japanese Pharmacopeia
Mitsuru Uchiyama   **73**

Pharmacopeial Standards: United Staes Pharmacopeia
Jerome A. Halperin and Lee T. Grady   **81**

Photodecomposition of Drugs
John V. Greenhill   **105**

Physiological Factors Affecting Drug Delivery and Availability
Neena Washington and Clive G. Wilson   **137**

Pilot Plant Design
Robert M. Franz, Robert D. Copeland, Lawrence D. Lewis, and William C. Stagner   **171**

Pilot Plant Operation
Leonard A. Amico, Ralph B. Caricofe, James D. English, Gary W. Goodson, Lawrence D. Lewis, and Robert M. Franz   **187**

Plant Products as Drugs
D. A. Lewis   **209**

Polarography and Voltammetry
A. David Woolfson   **237**

Polymers: Medicinal and Pharmaceutical
Julian H. Braybrook   **265**

Polymorphism: Pharmaceutical Aspects
Makoto Otsuka and Yoshihisa Matsuda   **305**

Post-Marketing Surveillance
Win M. Castle and Suzanne F. Cook   **327**

Potentiometry
Karel Vytřas   **347**

Powders as Dosage Forms
Jean-Marc Aiache and Erick Beyssac   **389**

CONTENTS OF OTHER VOLUMES	xxiii

Preformulation Studies on Drugs
Shigeru Goto, Nak-Seo Kim, and Yoshiyuki Hirakawa   **421**

Prescribing of Drugs
Michael C. Gerald   **443**

Index to Volume 12   **465**

CONTENTS OF VOLUME 13

Contributors to Volume 13   v

Contents of Other Volumes   vii

Preservation of Pharmaceutical Products
Sally F. Bloomfield and Fiona C. Sheppard   **1**

Preservative Testing
Norman A. Hodges and Stephen P. Denyer   **21**

Prodrugs
Lona L. Christrup, Judi Moss, and Bente Steffansen   **39**

Product License Applications (PLAs) and Establishment License Applications (ELAs) for Biological Products
Dhiren N. Shah and James G. Kenimer   **71**

Project Management
Jerome J. Groen   **121**

Protein Binding of Drugs
Sylvie Laganière and Iain J. McGilveray   **151**

Pyrogens and Pyrogen Testing
Marlys E. Weary   **179**

Quality Assurance of Drug Products
Richard Kaplan   **207**

Radiation Sterilization of Drugs
Stephen G. Schulman and Phillip M. Achey   **233**

Radiochemical Methods of Analysis
Kumaril Bhargava, Jie Du, Rajagopalan Raghavan, and Jose Joseph   **255**

Receptors for Drugs
Jeffrey M. Herz, William J. Thomsen, Richard Mitchell, and George G. Yarbrough   **283**

Rectal Administration and Absorption of Drugs
Joseph A. Fix and J. Howard Rytting   335

Registration of Drugs
William J. C. Currie and Richard W. J. Currie   353

Rheology of Pharmaceutical Systems
Brian Warburton   371

Robotics in the Pharmaceutical and Biomedical Laboratory
J. Wieling   409

Salt Forms of Drugs and Absorption
Lyle D. Bighley, Stephen M. Berge, and Donald C. Monkhouse   453

Index to Volume 13   501

CONTENTS OF VOLUME 14

Contributors to Volume 14   v

Contents of Other Volumes   vii

Self-Medication
Andrea Mant and Susan D. Whicker   1

Semisolid Preparations
Fred J. Bandelin and Bhogi B. Sheth   31

Sieving of Pharmaceuticals
John W. Mullin   63

Sintering of Pharmaceutics
Luk Chiu Li and Jane H. Li   87

Sonophoresis: Enhanced Transdermal Drug Delivery by Application of Ultrasound
Samir Mitragotri, Daniel Blankschtein, and Robert Langer   103

Spectroscopy, Emission
János Mink and Gábor Keresztury   123

Spheronization
J. Michael Newton   181

CONTENTS OF OTHER VOLUMES   xxv

Spray Drying and Spray Congealing of Pharmaceuticals
Michael J. Killeen   207

Starches and Starch Derivatives
Ann W. Newman, Imre M. Vitez, Chris Kiesnowski, and Ronald L. Mueller   223

Statistical Methods
Sanford Bolton   249

Surfactants in Pharmaceutical Products and Systems
Owen I. Corrigan and Anne Marie Healy   295

Suspensions
Robert A. Nash   333

Tablet Coating
Klaus Lehmann and Bianca Brögmann   355

Tablet Formulation
Larry L. Augsburger and Mark J. Zellhofer   385

Tablet Testing
James I. Wells   401

Technology Transfer Considerations for Pharmaceuticals
Karl F. Popp   419

Index to Volume 14   433

CONTENTS OF VOLUME 15

Contributors to Volume 15   v

Contents of Other Volumes   vii

Thermal Analysis of Drugs and Drug Products
Danièle Giron   1

Thin-Layer Chromatography
Joseph Sherma   81

Titrimetry
Vesa Virtanen   107

Tonicity
Jaymin C. Shah **141**

Tooling for Pharmaceutical Processes
Dale Natoli **163**

Topical Preparations
J. Graham Nairn **213**

Training of Personnel in the Pharaceutical Industry
Tara V. Sams **243**

Transdermal Drug Delivery Systems
Kenneth A. Walters **253**

Ultraviolet and Visible Spectrometry in Pharmaceutical Analysis
R. Raghavan and Jose C. Joseph **293**

Unit Processes in Pharmacy: Fundamentals
David Ganderton and Anthony J. Hickey **341**

Index to Volume 15 **399**

Unit Processes in Pharmacy: The Operations

Introduction

Unit operations in pharmaceutical manufacturing involve a number of well-defined processes. They may be applied in a variety of settings but may be considered in general terms. This article describes the major processes involved in the production of pharmaceuticals. Certain fundamental principles find their application in the following processes [1]. These fundamentals, notably heat and mass transfer, fluid flow, and particulates behavior can be seen individually and in combination in the crucial processes of pharmaceutical manufacturing [1,2].

Solution, solid state, colloid and surface chemistry may be employed to establish the physico-chemical nature of the product prior to and during manufacturing. Each of these topics has been dealt with in great detail elsewhere. Further information regarding these concepts can be found in previous volumes of this encyclopedia and in traditional pharmaceutics text books [3–6].

Emphasis has been placed on the general process. Pharmaceutical processes that are specific to certain prominent dosage forms or products are briefly described. A monograph of this nature must be restricted to some extent. There is, therefore, no discussion of the many alternative dosage forms to the traditional oral and parenteral products. These will necessarily involve unique processes which are beyond the scope of the present review.

Evaporation and Distillation

Evaporation

Evaporation may be defined as the removal of a solvent from a solution by vaporization, but is usually restricted to the concentration of solutions by boiling. Crystallization and drying, which may also utilize the vaporization of a liquid, are considered in subsequent sections.

Evaporation in the pharmaceutical industry is primarily associated with the removal of water and other solvents by boiling in batch processes. The principles that govern such processes apply more generally and are derived from a study of the transfer of heat to the boiling liquid, the relevant physical properties of the liquid, and the thermal stability of its components.

Heat Transfer to Boiling Liquids in an Evaporator

The heat required to boil a liquid in an evaporator is usually transferred from a heating fluid, such as steam or hot water, across the wall of a jacket or tube in or around which the liquid boils. A qualitative discussion of the methods used to secure high rates of heat flow can be based on Eq. (1),

$$Q = UA\Delta T \tag{1}$$

where Q is the rate of heat flow, U is the overall heat transfer coefficient, A is the area over which heat is transferred, and ΔT is the difference in temperature between the fluids.

The overall heat transfer coefficient is derived from a series of individual coefficients which characterize the thermal barriers that oppose heat transfer. Thus, for the heating fluid, the film coefficient for a condensing vapor, such as steam, is high, provided that permanent gases and condensates are removed by venting and draining. With liquid heating media, the velocity of flow over the heat transfer surface should be as high as is practicable. If the solid barrier consists of a thin metal wall, the resistance to heat flow is small. Resistance, however, is significantly increased by chemical scale which may be deposited on either side. The accumulation of scale should be prevented. A glass wall may provide the highest thermal resistance. Neglecting the thermal stability of the boiling liquid, circulation of the liquid should be rapid and, because of its influence on viscosity, the temperature of boiling should be as high as possible. Both factors promote high film coefficients on the product side of the wall.

Other factors described by Eq. (1) are the area of the heat transfer surfaces, which should be as large as possible, and the temperature difference between the heating surface and the boiling liquid. As long as the critical heat flux is not exceeded, the latter should also be large.

The Physical Properties of Solution and Liquids

A number of physical factors, which are interrelated in a complex way, are relevant to a study of evaporation. For a given heating fluid, the temperature difference across the wall of an evaporator is determined by the temperature of boiling, a variable controlled by the external pressure and the concentration of the solute in the solution. Both the boiling temperature and the solute concentration influence the viscosity of the solution, a factor which greatly affects the heat transfer coefficient. The temperature of boiling also determines the solubility of dissolved constituents and the degree of concentration which can be carried out without separation of solids.

The Relation Between Boiling Temperature and Solute Concentration. When a solute is dissolved in a solvent, the vapor pressure is depressed and the boiling point rises. Since it increases as the solute concentration increases, the temperature difference between the boiling liquid and the heating surface decreases. For dilute solutions, the expected rise in boiling point can be calculated from Raoult's law. However, this procedure is not applicable to concentrated solutions or to solutions of uncertain composition. For aqueous, concentrated solutions, Duhring's rule may be used to obtain the boiling point rise of a solution at any pressure. It states that the boiling point of a given solution is a linear function of the boiling point of water at the same pressure. A family of lines is required to cover a range of concentrations as shown in Fig. 1.

The Relation of Boiling Temperature and External Pressure. The temperature at which a solution of given composition boils is determined by the external pressure. The va-

Unit Processes in Pharmacy: The Operations

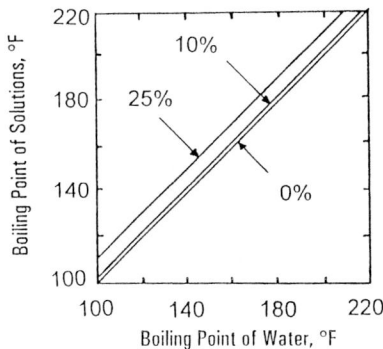

FIG. 1. Duhring chart for sodium chloride.

por pressure of a pure solvent at any temperature can usually be obtained from published tables. Alternatively, if the vapor pressure at two temperatures is known, the plot of the logarithm of the vapor pressure against the reciprocal of the absolute temperature yields an approximately straight line. For intermediate pressures, the temperature at which the solvent boils can be found by interpolation. If dissolved substances are present, the boiling point must be adjusted using Duhring's rule. This value permits an accurate estimate of the temperature differences in the evaporator.

Reduction in the external pressure lowers the boiling temperature and, if the associated increase in viscosity is not too great, increases the rate of evaporation. On large installations, a moderate vacuum is widely used to increases the capacity of an evaporator. The imposition of low pressures and low boiling temperatures is also necessary for the processing of thermolabile materials.

Boiling in tubes is commonly used in evaporators. Under these circumstances, the hydrostatic head developed by a column of liquid or the friction head imposed by its movement can create a local increase in pressure which suppresses boiling and reduces the evaporating capacity of the system.

The Relation of Viscosity to Temperature and Solute Concentration. The viscosity of a solution is modified by changes in temperature and solute concentration. Since a low viscosity promotes a high heat transfer coefficient, the exponential decrease of viscosity with increase in temperature is of great importance and indicates a high boiling temperature.

In general, the addition of a nonvolatile solute increases the viscosity of a solution at any temperature. Consequently, the viscosity of the solution increases as the evaporation proceeds. These effects, however, cannot be calculated.

If, at the operating temperatures and concentrations, the viscosity of a solution is high, satisfactory heat transfer coefficients may only be obtained by driving the liquid over the heating surface. In other systems, movement of a viscous liquid is assisted by gravity or the liquid in contact with the heating surface is disrupted mechanically by scrapers.

The Effect of Temperature on Solubility. The solubility of the components of a solution depends upon the temperature. Most commonly, solubility increases with increasing temperature, so that a higher concentration is possible at higher temperatures without the separation of solids. The reverse is true of liquids containing scale-forming solids with inverse solubility characteristics, such as calcium or magnesium sulfate, or materials that decompose and deposit, such as coagulable protein.

The Effect of Heat on the Active Constituents of a Solution. The thermal stability of components of a solution may determine the type of evaporator to be used and the conditions of its operation. If a simple solution contains a hydrolyzable material and the rate of its degradation during evaporation depends upon its concentration at any time, an exponential relation between the remaining fraction, F, and the time, t, characteristic of a first-order reaction, is obtained, as shown in Eq. (2).

$$F = e^{-kt} \qquad (2)$$

The dependence of the reaction velocity constant, k, on the absolute temperature, T, is expressed by Eq. (3),

$$k = Ae^{-\frac{B}{T}} \qquad (3)$$

where A and B are constants characteristic of the reaction. Thus, at temperatures T_1, T_2, and T_3, where $T_1 > T_2 > T_3$, the relation between the remaining fraction and the time of heating, shown in Fig. 2, emerges. This indicates the importance of the temperature and time of heating. If the latter can be shortened, the temperature of evaporation can be greatly increased without increasing the fraction which is degraded. If, therefore, the effect of temperature on the rate of evaporation is known, it is possible to define the conditions of time and temperature at which decomposition is a minimum.

In practice, the kinetics of degradation and the relation of evaporation rate and temperature are usually not known. This is particularly true when the criteria by which the product is judged are color, taste, or smell. In addition, the analysis above neglects the temperature variation in the evaporating liquid and the degradation in boundary films where temperatures are higher. Often, therefore, experiments are necessary to determine the suitability of an evaporation process.

In batch processes, the time of exposure to heat is well defined. This is also true of continuous processes in which the liquid to be evaporated is passed only once through the heater. In continuous processes, is where the liquid is recirculated through the heater, the average residence time, a, is given by the ratio:

$$\frac{\text{Working volume of evaporation}}{\text{Volumetric discharge}}$$

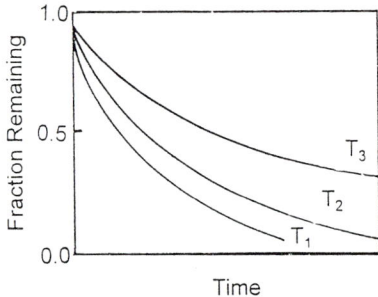

FIG. 2. The effect of time and temperature on degradation.

Unit Processes in Pharmacy: The Operations

The volumetric discharge is only an indication of the damage which prolonged heating may cause. If perfect mixing occurs in the evaporator, the fraction, f, which is in the unit for time t or less, is given by Eq. (4).

$$f = 1 - e^{-\frac{t}{a}} \qquad (4)$$

This relation shows, for example, that an evaporator with an average residence time of 1 h holds 13.5% of active principles for 2 h and about 2% for 4 h.

Evaporators

It is convenient to classify evaporators into natural circulation evaporators, forced-circulation evaporators, and film evaporators.

Natural Circulation Evaporators

Small-scale evaporators consist of a simple pan heated by jacket, a coil, or by both. Admission of the heating fluid to the jacket induces the liquid in the vessel to boil. Very small evaporators may be open, the vapor escaping to atmosphere or into a vented hood. Larger pan evaporators are closed, the vapor escaping through a pipe. Small jacketed pans are efficient and easy to clean and may be fitted for the vacuum evaporation of thermolabile materials. However, because the ratio of heating area to volume decreases as the capacity increases, their size is limited. Larger vessels must employ a heating coil which increases their evaporating capacity but makes cleaning more difficult.

The large heating area of a tube bundle is utilized widely in large-scale evaporators. Horizontal mounting, with the heating fluid inside the tube, is limited by poor circulation to the evaporation of nonviscous liquids in which the bundle is immersed. Normally, the tube bundle is mounted vertically; this configuration is known as a calandria. The boiling of liquids in a vertical tube and the earlier regimes of this process operate in a calandria. The length of tubes and the liquid level allow boiling to occur in the tubes, and the mixture of vapor and liquid rises until the entire calandria is just submerged. A typical evaporator is shown in Fig. 3a. The tubes are 4 to 6 feet (1.2–1.8 m) long and 2 to 3 in. (5–7.5 cm) in diameter. The low density of the boiling liquid and vapor creates an upward movement in the tubes. Vapor and liquid separate in the space above the calandria and the liquid is returned to the pool at the base of the tubes by a large central downcomer or through an annular space between the heating element and the evaporator shell. Feed is added and concentrate is withdrawn from the pool, as shown in Fig. 3a. As long as the viscosity of the liquid is low, good circulation and high heat transfer coefficients are obtained. In some evaporators, the calandria is inclined and the tubes are lengthened.

Forced-Circulation Evaporators

On the smallest scale, forced-circulation evaporators are similar to the pan evaporators described above, modified only by the inclusion of an agitator. Vigorous agitation increases the boiling film coefficient, the degree depending on the type and speed of the agitator. An agitator should be used for the evaporation of viscous materials to prevent degradation of material at the heated surfaces.

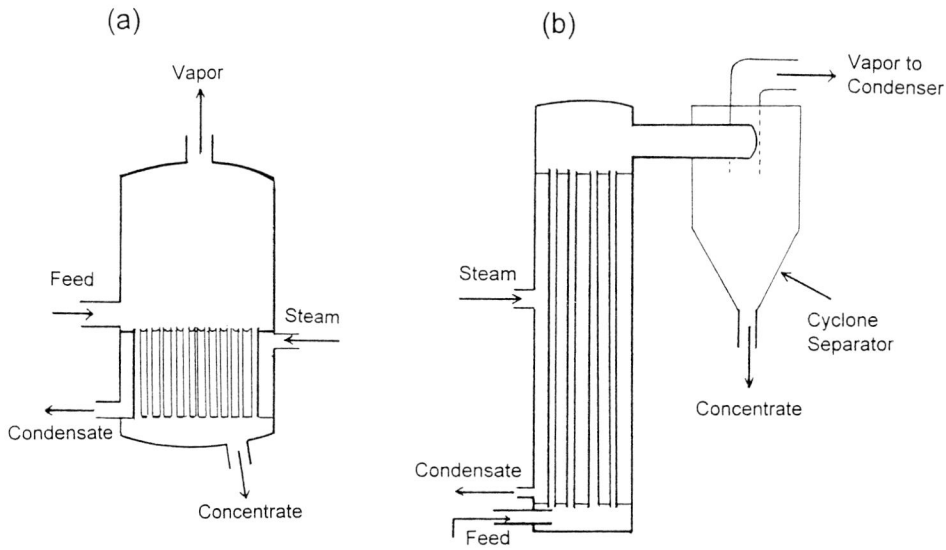

FIG. 3. (a) Evaporator with calandria; (b) climbing film evaporator.

Some large-scale continuous units are similar to the natural circulation evaporators already described. The natural circulation induced by boiling in a vertical tube may be supplemented by an axial impeller mounted in the downcomer of the calandria. This modification is used when viscous liquids or liquids containing suspended solids are evaporated. Such units are employed in evaporative crystallization. In other forced-circulation evaporators, the tube bundle becomes, in effect, a simple heat exchanger through the tubes of which the liquid is pumped. Commonly, the opposing head suppresses boiling in the tubes. Superheating occurs and the liquid flashes into a mixture of liquid and vapor as it enters the body of the evaporator.

Film Evaporators

In the short tubes of the calandria, an intimate mixture of vapor and liquid is discharged at the top. If the length of the tube is greatly increased, progressive phase separation occurs until a high velocity core of vapor is formed which propels an annular film of liquid along the tube. This phenomenon, which is one stage of flow when a liquid and a gas pass in the same direction along a tube, is employed in film evaporators. The turbulence of the film gives very high heat transfer coefficients, and the bubbles and vapor evolved are rapidly swept into the vapor stream. Although recirculation may be adopted, it is possible with the high evaporation rates found in long tubes to concentrate the liquid sufficiently in a single pass. Since a very short residence time is obtained, very thermolabile materials may be concentrated at relatively high temperatures. Film evaporators are also suitable for materials which foam strongly. Various types have been developed, but all are essentially continuous in operation, their capacity ranging from a few liters per hour upward.

The climbing film evaporator, which is the most common film evaporator, consists of tubes 15 to 30 feet (4.5–13.6 m) long and 1 to 2 in. (2.5–5 cm) in diameter mounted

Unit Processes in Pharmacy: The Operations

in a steam chest (Fig. 3b). The feed liquid enters the bottom of the tubes and flows upward for a short distance before boiling begins. The length of this section, which is characterized by low heat transfer coefficients, may be minimized by preheating the feed to its boiling point. The pattern of boiling and phase separation follows and a mixture of liquid and vapor emerges from the top of the tube to be separated by baffles or by a cyclone separator. Climbing film evaporators are not suitable for the evaporation of viscous liquids.

In the falling film evaporator, the liquid is fed to the top of a number of long heated tubes. Since gravity assists the flow down the tube, this arrangement is better suited to the evaporation of moderately viscous liquids. The vapor evolved is usually carried downward and the mixture of liquid and vapor emerges from the bottom for separation. Even distribution of liquid must be secured during feeding. A tendency to channel in some tubes leads to drying in others.

The rising-falling film evaporator concentrates a liquid in a climbing film section and leads the emerging liquid and vapor into a second tube section which forms a falling film evaporator. Good distribution in the falling film section is claimed and the evaporator is particularly suitable for liquids which increase greatly in viscosity during evaporation.

In mechanically aided film evaporators, a thin film of material is maintained on the heat transfer surface irrespective of the viscosity. This is usually achieved by means of a rotor, concentric with the tube, which carries blades that either scrape the tube or ride with low clearance in the film. Mechanical agitation permits the evaporation of highly viscous materials or those that have a low thermal conductivity. Since temperature variations in the film are reduced and residence times are shortened, the vacuum evaporation of viscous thermolabile materials becomes possible.

The Efficiency of Evaporators

In the pharmaceutical industry, economic use of steam may not be of overriding importance because the small scale of the operation and the high value of the product would not justify the additional capital costs of improved heating efficiency. In other industries, heating costs impose more efficient use of heat by utilizing the heat content of the vapor emerging from the evaporator, assumed, until now, to be lost in condensation. The two methods commonly used are multiple effect evaporation and vapor recompression.

In multiple-effect evaporation, the vapor from one evaporator is led as the heating medium to the calandria of a second evaporator, which, therefore, must operate at a lower temperature than the first. This principle can be extended to a number of evaporators, some stages working under vacuum. The limit is set by the relation of the cost of the plant and the vacuum services to the cost of the steam which is saved.

In evaporators employing vapor recompression, the vapor emerging is compressed by mechanical pumps or steam jet ejectors to increase its temperature. The compressed vapor is returned to the steam chest.

Vapor Removal and Liquid Entrainment

Vapor must be removed from the evaporator with as little entrained liquid as possible. The two determining factors are the vapor velocity at the surface of the liquid and the velocity of the vapor leaving the evaporator. On a small scale, surface vapor velocities are low but with increase in scale, the adverse ratio of surface area to volume creates higher velocities. Droplets formed by the bursting of bubbles at the boiling surface may be projected from the surface and foam may form. Various devices may be used to control entrainment at or near the surface. A high vapor space is provided above the boiling liquid to allow large droplets to fall and foam to collapse. Baffles may be used in the vapor space to arrest entrained droplets. When allowable, antifoaming agents, such as silicone oils, can be used to impede foaming.

Stokes' law shows that vapor of particular characteristics carries droplets upward against the force of gravity. Any entrained liquid not intercepted in the body of the evaporator is, therefore, carried forward in the higher velocity stream of the vapor uptake. Some droplets are caught there, the quantity depending on the geometry of the duct and the velocity of the vapor. At atmospheric pressure, the latter might be 50 ft/s (15 m/s). In vacuum evaporation, much higher velocities may be used. When the quantity of entrained liquid is high, the vapor is commonly led to a cyclone separator. This is employed with frothing materials and the vapor-liquid mixtures leaving a climbing film evaporator. In the separator, the entrained liquid is flung to the walls by centrifugal force and may be collected or returned to the evaporator. The vapor is led to a condenser.

Evaporation without Boiling

During heating, some evaporation takes place at the surface of a batch of liquid before boiling begins. Similarly, liquids that are very viscous or froth excessively may be concentrated without boiling. The diffusion of vapor from the surface is described by Eq. (5),

$$N_A = \frac{k_g}{RT}(P_{Ai} - P_{Ag}) \tag{5}$$

where N_A is the number of moles evaporating from unit area in unit time, k_g is the mass transfer coefficient across the boundary layer, R is the gas constant, T is the absolute temperature, P_{Ai} is the vapor pressure of the liquid, and P_{Ag} is the partial pressure of the vapor in the gas stream; k_g is proportional to the gas velocity.

Distillation

Distillation is a process in which a liquid mixture is separated into its component parts by vaporization. The vapor evolved from a boiling liquid mixture is normally richer in the more volatile components than the liquid with which it is in equilibrium. Distillation rests upon this fact. Although multicomponent mixtures are most common in distillation processes, an understanding of the operation can be based on the vapor pressure characteristics of two component or binary mixtures.

Binary Mixtures of Immiscible Liquids, Steam Distillation

If the two components of a binary mixture are immiscible, the vapor pressure of the mixture is the sum of the vapor pressures of the two components, each exerted inde-

Unit Processes in Pharmacy: The Operations

pendently and not as a function of their relative concentrations in the liquid. This property is employed in steam distillation, a process particularly applicable to the separation of high boiling substances from nonvolatile impurities. The steam forms a cheap and inert carrier. The principles of the process apply to other immiscible systems.

If a mixture of water and a high boiling liquid, such as nitrobenzene, is heated, the total vapor pressure increases and ultimately reaches the external pressure. The mixture boils and the vapors evolved are condensed to give a liquid mixture which separates under gravity. In practice, the vapors are produced by blowing steam into the liquid in a manner which gives intimate contact between the phases. Since both components contribute to the total pressure, the boiling temperature must be lower than the boiling point of either component. In the case of nitrobenzene and water, the boiling point at atmospheric pressure is about 99°C. To distil nitrobenzene alone at this temperature, a pressure of 20 mm Hg (2.66 kPa) must be imposed. Steam distillation, therefore, permits the distillation of water-immiscible materials of high boiling point without the use of a high vacuum or high temperatures, which might cause decomposition. This method, however, only separates such materials from nonvolatile constituents. Volatile impurities appear in the distillate.

The composition of the distillate is calculated in the following way. For two components, A and B, the total vapor pressure, P, is the sum of the vapor pressures of the components, P_A and P_B. Since the partial pressure of a component in a gaseous mixture is proportional to its molar concentration, the composition of the vapor is given by Eq. (6),

$$\frac{n_A}{n_B} = \frac{P_A}{P_B} \tag{6}$$

where n_A and n_B are the number of moles of A and B in the vapor, respectively. If W_A and W_B are the weights of A and B in the vapor, Eq. (7) holds,

$$\frac{W_A}{M_A} \cdot \frac{M_B}{W_B} = \frac{P_A}{P_B} \tag{7}$$

where M_A and M_B are the respective molecular weights. The distillate obtained from the vapor is $W_A + W_B$, and the percentage of A in the distillate is expressed by Eq. (8).

$$\frac{W_A}{M_A + W_B} \times 100 = \frac{P_A M_A}{P_A M_A + P_B M_B} \times 100 \tag{8}$$

The ratio of immiscible organic liquid to water in the distillate is increased if the former has a high molecular weight or a high vapor pressure.

Steam distillation under vacuum may be employed when the thermal stability of the material prohibits temperatures of about 100°C. A further variant is the introduction of unsaturated steam under conditions in which no condensation to water takes place. Only two phases, the liquid being distilled and the mixing vapors, are then present. The external pressure no longer fixes the temperature, as in a three-phase system, and any convenient value can be chosen.

The chief uses of steam distillation are the purification and isolation of liquids of high boiling point, such as aniline, nitrobenzene, or o-dichlorbenzene, and in the preparation of fatty acids and volatile oils. Many of the latter are prepared by introducing steam into a mixture of the comminuted drug and water. The method is also used to remove odoriferous elements, such as aldehydes and ketones, from edible oils. The dehydration of a material by adding a volatile, water-immiscible solvent, such as toluene, and distilling the mixture is a form of steam distillation. The solvent separates in the condensate and may be returned to the still.

Binary Mixtures of Miscible Liquids

The Relation of Vapor Pressure and Mixture Composition. In a binary mixture of two completely miscible components, the vapor pressure is a function of the mixture composition as well as of the vapor pressures of the two pure components. If the liquids are ideal, the relation of vapor pressure and composition is given by Raoult's law. At a constant temperature, the partial vapor pressure of a constituent of an ideal mixture is proportional to its mole fraction in the liquid. Thus, for a mixture of A and B, the partial vapor pressure of A is given by Eq. (9),

$$P_A = P_A^0 \cdot x_A \tag{9}$$

where P_A^0 is the vapor pressure of pure A and x_A is its mole fraction. Similarly, the partial vapor pressure of B is expressed by Eq. (10).

$$P_B = P_B^0 \cdot x_B \tag{10}$$

The total pressure of the system, P, is simply $P_A + P_B$.

These relations can be expressed graphically (Fig. 4). If the vapor pressure at a given temperature of each pure component is marked on a graph of vapor pressure versus mole fraction, the total vapor pressure at the same temperature of a liquid mixture of any composition falls on the straight line joining the vapor pressures of the two components.

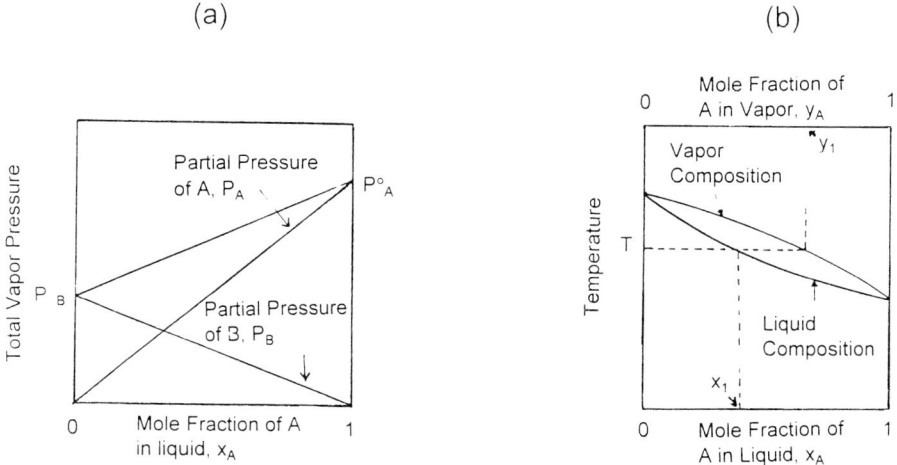

FIG. 4. (a) The vapor pressure of an ideal binary mixture expressed in terms of relative concentration; (b) temperature–composition diagram for a binary mixture.

The partial pressure of each component is indicated by the diagonals of Fig. 4a. A separate relation must be constructed for each temperature.

Very few liquid mixtures rigidly obey Raoult's law. Consequently, the vapor pressure data must be determined experimentally. Mixtures that deviate positively from this law give a total vapor pressure curve which lies above the theoretical straight line. Negative deviations fall below the line. In extreme cases, deviations are so large that a range of mixtures exhibits a higher or lower vapor pressure than either of the pure components.

Returning to ideal systems, the partial pressure of a component in the vapor is proportional to its mole fraction, as shown in Eq. (11) for component A,

$$P_A = y_A P \qquad (11)$$

where P_A is the partial pressure of A in the vapor and y_A is its mole fraction. Since $P_A = P_A^0 \cdot x_A$, Eqs. (12) and (13) can be written.

$$y_A = \frac{x_A P_B^0}{P} \qquad (12)$$

Similarly,

$$y_B = \frac{x_B P_B^0}{P} \qquad (13)$$

If A is the more volatile component, P_A^0 is greater than P. Therefore y_A is greater than x_A, that is, the vapor is richer in the more volatile component than the liquid with which it is in equilibrium.

The Relation of Boiling Point and Mixture Composition. For the purposes of distillation, curves relating vapor pressure and composition are usually replaced by boiling point curves. These are determined by experiments at the given pressure. If the system shows a steady increase in boiling point as the concentration of the less volatile component increases, the diagram given in Fig. 4b is obtained. The upper curve represents the composition of the vapor in equilibrium with the boiling liquid. A liquid of composition x_1 boils at temperature T and initially yields a vapor y_1 which is richer in the more volatile component. Ideal mixtures, and mixtures with small deviations from ideality, give curves of this type. If, however, deviations are sufficiently large, curves of the form shown in Fig. 5 are obtained. Figure 5a represents a system in which the vapor pressure of some mixtures is higher than the vapor pressure of the pure, more volatile component. This system exhibits a minimum boiling point and the composition of the liquid at this point is given by Z. This mixture, which is a constant boiling or azeotropic mixture, evolves on boiling a vapor of the same composition. In the binary system described in Fig. 5b, mixtures are formed with a vapor pressure which is lower than that of the less volatile component. The maximum boiling point is given by the azeotropic mixture, Z.

Systems that form minimum boiling mixtures are common. Ethyl alcohol and water provide an example, the azeotrope containing 4.5% by weight of water. The boiling point at atmospheric pressure is 78.15°C, 0.25°C lower than the boiling point of pure alcohol. Maximum boiling mixtures are less common. The most familiar example is

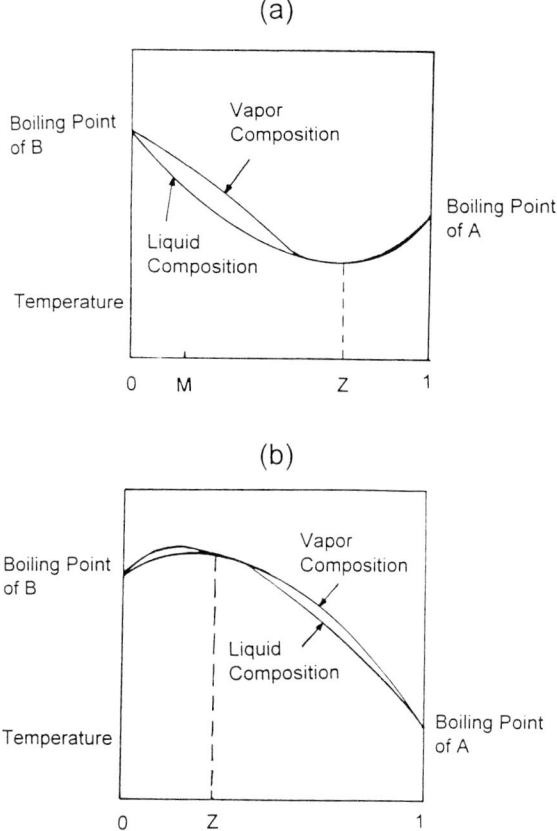

FIG. 5. Vapor–liquid equilibrium diagrams. The composition of the vapor is expressed as a function of liquid composition. The formation of an azeotrope is expressed by the point Z.

hydrochloric acid which forms an azeotrope boiling at 108.6°C containing 20.2% by weight of hydrochloric acid.

Mixtures that form azeotropes cannot be separated into the pure components by normal distillation methods. However, separation into the azeotrope and one pure component is possible. Efficient fractionation of the mixture M of Fig. 5a would give the azeotrope Z as distillate and pure *B* as the residue.

The composition of the azeotropic mixture of a system is a function of the total pressure, and it is possible in some cases to eliminate the constant boiling mixture by altering the pressure at which the distillation is performed. For example, at pressures less than 100 mm Hg (13 kPa) ethyl alcohol and water do not form an azeotrope but can be completely separated.

Vapor–liquid equilibrium diagrams of the form shown in Fig. 6 provide an alternative and convenient method of recording distillation data. They consist of a conventional graph relating the mole fraction of the more volatile component in the liquid, designated X, to the mole fraction of the more volatile component in the vapor, designated Y. An ideal binary system is shown in Fig. 6a. The temperature varies along each of

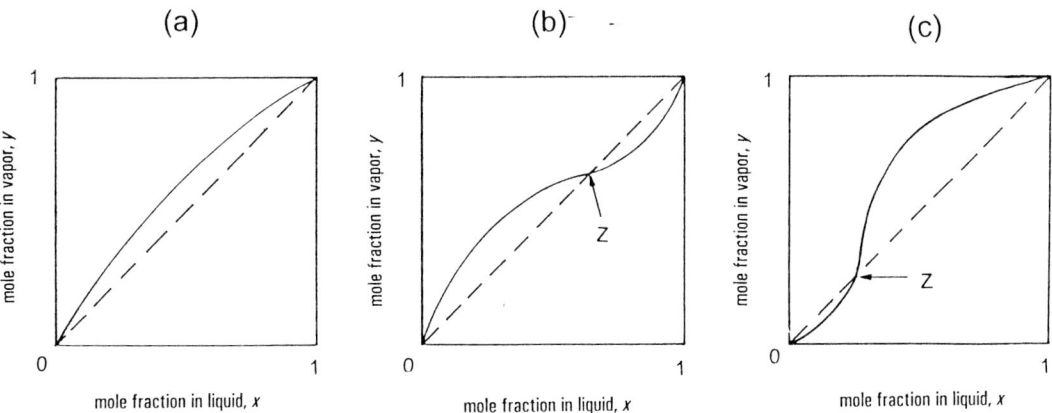

FIG. 6. Temperature–composition diagrams for binary mixtures which form azeotropes.

the curves and the diagram is only applicable to the pressure at which the variables were measured. Curves of minimum boiling mixtures and maximum boiling mixtures are drawn in Figs. 6b and 6c, respectively.

Simple or Differential Distillation

In simple or differential distillation, the vapor evolved from the boiling mixture is immediately removed and condensed. For the system shown in Fig. 4b, the liquid of composition x_1 evolves a vapor of composition y_1. Its removal impoverishes the liquid in the more volatile component. The composition of the liquid moves toward pure B and its boiling point increases. There is, therefore, a progressive change in the composition of the vapor, the mole fraction of the more volatile component steadily decreasing. Unless the boiling points of the two pure components differ widely, a reasonable degree of separation is not possible. The method may be used to remove low boiling solvents from aqueous solutions.

Rectification or Fractionation

In simple distillation, vapor enrichment is small. In fractionation, a term synonymous with rectification, the vapor leaving the boiling liquid is led up a column to meet a liquid stream or reflux which originates higher in the column as part of the condensate. In a series of partial condensations and vaporizations, the rising vapor becomes richer in the more volatile component at the expense of the falling liquid and high degrees of separation become possible. The columns, called fractionating columns, are of two basic types: packed columns and plate columns.

Packed Columns. These are used for laboratory and small-scale industrial distillation and are usually operated as a batch process. The column consists of a vertical, hollow, cylindrical shell containing a packing designed to offer a large interfacial contact area between liquid and vapor. The form of the packing varies but Raschig rings, which consist of small metallic or ceramic cylinders, are the most commonly used. Other shapes consist of saddles, Pall rings, Lessing rings, and meshes of woven wire or expanded metal. In a packed column, countercurrent interaction between the rising vapor and the falling liquid occurs throughout its length. The distillation rate and the size and shape of the packing must be chosen to give efficient support for the liquid phase, phase movement, and phase interaction. High rates of vapor flow may arrest or reverse the downward movement of liquid. This ultimately causes flooding of the column and determines the upper end of the operating range. The efficiency of the column is also decreased if the falling liquid fails to wet all the available surface of the packing, a condition which determines the lower limit of column operation. In general, packed columns operate under widely varying conditions without serious loss of efficiency.

Plate Columns. A plate column consists of a series of plates or trays on which the liquid is retained for some period during its movement down the column. The rising vapor is bubbled through this liquid, providing intimate contact between the phases. Liquid in reflux moves downward between plates and is usually carried by a downcomer. Contact between the vapor and liquid takes place in stages.

Plate columns operate efficiently over a limited range of conditions. They are mainly used in large-scale, continuous installations in which the conditions of distillation can be closely maintained.

Continuous and Batch Fractionation. Figure 7a shows the boiling point curve of a binary mixture. If a mixture of composition x_1 boils, a vapor of composition y_1 is evolved, and condensation gives a liquid of composition x_2. This is an ideal distillation stage. A second stage gives a liquid composition x_3 and, in this example, a further stage would give the more volatile component in an almost pure form.

These conditions are approached in continuously operated fractionating columns. In such a column, operating with continuous feed and product withdrawal, the composition of the liquid and vapor at any point does not vary with time. The process is examined with reference to the plate column shown in Fig. 7b, where the composition of the liquid on Plate 3 is assumed to be x_1. The vapor received at this plate from the plate below is bubbled through the liquid of the plate. Some of the less volatile component is condensed, increasing the mole fraction of the more volatile component in the

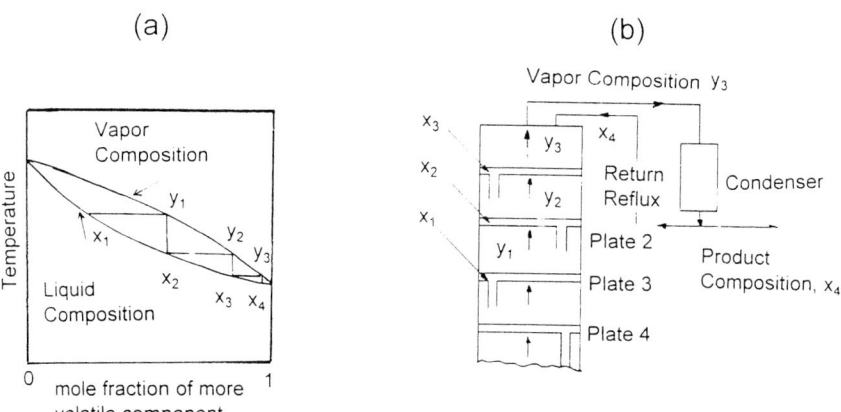

FIG. 7. (a) Three ideal stages; (b) the plate column associated with fractional distillation.

bubbles. The latent heat evolved by this condensation vaporizes some of the liquid on the plate. This vapor is richer in the more volatile component than the liquid. By these two mechanisms, the vapor leaving the plate moves toward equilibrium with the liquid on the plate. If equilibrium could be achieved, maximum enrichment of the vapor would occur corresponding to the appropriate horizontal line linking vapor-liquid equilibrium concentration on the boiling point curve. For the system shown in Figure 7b, this is the line $x_1 y_1$. Two more ideal distillation stages at plates 2 and 1 would complete the separation of this mixture. In practice, equilibrium is not achieved at the plates due to limited contact between the phases. Enrichment is set therefore less than that at an ideal stage and the discrepancy is a measure of plate efficiency.

Under steady column conditions, the concentration of the more volatile component in the liquid on any plate is maintained by the overflow or reflux of liquid richer in the more volatile component than the plate above. This is true of all parts except the top plate. Here, the mole fraction of the more volatile component must be maintained by returning part of the condensate from the last stage to the top plate. This is known as reflux return, and the reflux ratio is the ratio of the condensate returned to the column and the amount withdrawn as product. This ratio markedly affects the degree of separation which occurs in a given column. If the proportion of the condensate which is to be returned to the column is increased, the mole fraction of the more volatile component in the liquid on the top plate is increased. The mole fraction of this component in the emerging vapor is also increased and a purer product is obtained. Due to the increased overflow of liquid from plate to plate down the column, this is also true of all plates. Thus, by increasing the reflux ratio, the enrichment obtained with a given number of plates is increased. The amount of product, however, is decreased. A column operating at total reflux, in which the whole distillate is returned to the column, achieves a given enrichment with the minimum number of plates. This column, however, gives no product at all and an economic compromise is sought between a short column with a small number of plates operating with high reflux ratio and a long column of many plates operating with a low reflux ratio. Algebraic and graphical methods are used to calculate the theoretical number of plates required to separate a mixture in a column operating with a known reflux ratio.

In a packed column, enrichment of the vapor takes place continuously as the column is ascended. The enrichment taking place over a certain length of the column corresponds to the enrichment secured at a plate that behaves ideally. This is expressed as the height equivalent of a theoretical or ideal plate (HETP). This concept allows the account given for plate columns to be directly applied to packed columns. The height of packing required for a separation is simply the product of the HETP and the number of ideal stages required. The HETP is not constant for a given packing. It depends on the physical properties of the liquid and the vapor, such as density and viscosity, and upon the distillation rate.

In batch distillation, steady-state conditions are never achieved and the concentration of the more volatile component in the still or at any point in the column falls as the rich product is withdrawn from the top. The concentration of the more volatile component in the product also falls. To maintain a given product specification, it may be necessary to increase the reflux ratio from time to time. Alternatively, the reflux ratio could be so chosen that the average composition of the product complies with the specification, the first distillate being richer and the last poorer in the more volatile component.

Most distillations, whether operated as batch or continuous processes, are applied to mixtures of more than two components. If the boiling points of the components differ widely, the process may be treated as successive distillation of two component mixtures. If a mixture of three components, *A, B,* and *C,* is batch distilled, a column with sufficient plates initially separates the most volatile component, *A*, with a high purity. As the distillation progresses, the concentration of *A* in the distillate falls, and ultimately the column fails to produce a distillate of the required quality. An intermediate fraction is then distilled, consisting of *A* and *B*, until the distillate contains the required amount of *B*. After collection of this fraction, a second intermediate fraction is distilled to leave component *C* in the still. Intermediate fractions can be distilled with subsequent batches. A similar separation could be accomplished with two continuous columns, one separating *A* from *B* and *C* and another separation *B* from *C*.

To avoid thermal decomposition of a component in a mixture, distillation may be performed at a reduced pressure. In addition to the general principles described above, the following factors may be of importance. The pressure drop associated with the flow of vapor up the column, which is relatively small in atmospheric distillation, may become significant, producing a damaging increase in the temperature of the liquid in the still. Secondly, in packed columns, flooding occurs at lower distillation rates due to the high velocity of the rising vapor.

Separation of Azeotropes and Liquids of Similar Volatility

Systems that form azeotropes cannot be separated by fractional distillation, although in some cases the formation of the azeotrope can be precluded by changing the distillation pressure. Problems of separation are also found with mixtures of liquids with similar volatility. Separation of these systems can be facilitated by adding a third component. If this component forms one or more azeotropes with the original components of the mixture, the process is called azeotropic distillation. The addition of a relatively nonvolatile component, which alters the relative volatility of the original components, gives a process known as extractive distillation.

In the azeotropic distillation of minimum-boiling binary mixtures, the third component either forms a new binary azeotrope of lower boiling point or a ternary azeotrope of lower boiling point containing the original components in different proportions. The newly formed azeotrope must be easily separated after distillation. The process is illustrated by the dehydration of alcohol with benzene. The binary azeotrope of ethyl alcohol and water boils at 78.15°C, whereas the ternary azeotrope of benzene, water, and alcohol boils at 64.8°C, and the binary azeotrope of benzene and alcohol boils at 68°C. Distillation of the alcohol–water azeotrope with benzene yields the ternary azeotrope which separates on condensation to give two layers, one of which contains almost all the water. In a batch process, the column would give the benzene–alcohol azeotrope, leaving anhydrous alcohol in the still. In a continuous process, the various stages would each be performed on a different column.

Extractive distillation is illustrated by the separation of benzene and cyclohexane by adding phenol. The relative volatility of the original components is modified in such a way that cyclohexane is recovered as the distillate leaving a mixture of phenol and benzene, which is passed to a second column for separation. The phenol, which is added to the top of the column, appears to aid separation by preferentially dissolving benzene during its passage downward; this leads to the term extractive distillation.

Unit Processes in Pharmacy: The Operations

Molecular Distillation

Molecular distillation is carried out without boiling at very low pressures of the order 0.001 mm Hg (0.133 Pa). At these pressures, collision of molecules in the evolving vapor and reflection back to the liquid surface is greatly decreased and the mean free path of the molecules is of the same order as the distance between the evaporating surface and a condenser placed a short distance away. It then becomes possible to distil liquids of very high boiling point although the degree of separation cannot exceed one theoretical plate. The process is therefore used primarily to concentrate nonvolatile components in a high boiling medium. The vitamins in cod liver oil can be concentrated in this way. For the separation of liquids of comparable volatility, several separate distillation stages are necessary.

Since agitation due to boiling is absent, an alternative method of maintaining the more volatile component at the evaporating surface must be adopted. In the industrial molecular still shown in Fig. 8, the feed is introduced at the bottom of a heated conical rotor and flows upward as a thin liquid layer under the action of centrifugal force. The residue is caught in a gutter at the top. The vapor is condensed on a concentric, water-cooled condenser a short distance away and discharged.

Air Conditioning and Humidification

Air conditioning for comfort means the provision of heated or cooled filtered air. High moisture content or humidity is oppressive and a low humidity may cause irritation by

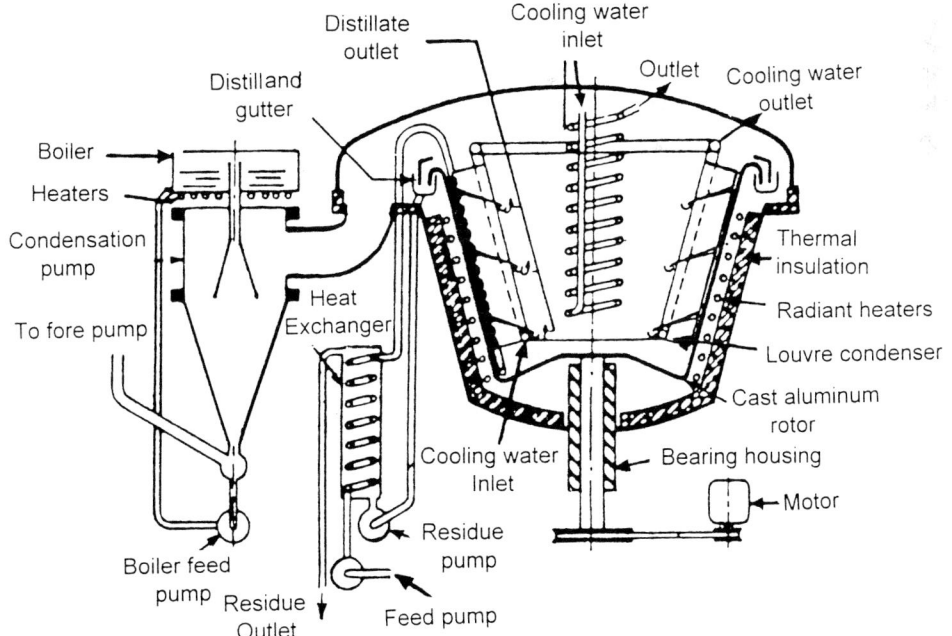

FIG. 8. Large-scale molecular still. (From Ref. 7.)

excessive loss of moisture from the skin. In some climates steps may be taken to add or remove water vapor. The air is simply cleaned, usually by passage through a fabric filter which may be dry or moistened with a viscous liquid, and heated electrically or by banks of finned tubes supplied with steam or hot water over which the air is blown. Electrostatic precipitation provides an alternative method of air cleaning. The fine particles entrained in the air are charged by the absorption of electrons as they pass between two electrodes. The charged particle then migrates in the electrical field and is finally arrested on one electrode.

The same general principles apply to the supply of air in some pharmaceutical processes. The control of its quality, however, may be more stringent. In areas where sterile materials are made and handled, for example, the cleaning process must remove bacteria. In other situations, it may be necessary to remove water vapor. The flow of powders is a sensitive function of moisture content, and the equilibrium moisture content of a material is determined by the humidity. Some tableting processes break down if the humidity is too high. In such processes, the scale of the air conditioning varies. It may be necessary to supply a whole room with air of a certain quality. Alternatively, conditioning may be restricted to a small area surrounding a particular piece of equipment.

Vapor and Gas Mixtures

The humidity of a vapor-gas mixture is defined as the mass of vapor associated with the unit mass of the gas. This principle is generally applicable to any vapor present in any non-condensable gas. In this section, however, only water vapor in air is considered. The percentage humidity is the ratio of humidity to the humidity of the saturated gas at the same temperature, expressed as a percentage. These terms should be carefully distinguished from the relative humidity with which they are somewhat distantly related. The relative humidity is the ratio of the partial pressure of the vapor in the gas to the partial pressure of the saturated gas. This is also usually expressed as a percentage. The relative humidity of a given vapor-gas mixture changes with temperature; the humidity does not.

The study of the properties of the air-water vapor mixture is called psychometry, and data are presented in various forms of psychometric charts presenting various data. In Fig. 9, humidity is plotted as ordinate and temperatures as abscissa. Percentage relative humidity is plotted as curves running across the chart. The use of this simplified chart is demonstrated later.

Hygrometry, the Measurement of Humidity

The accurate determination of the humidity of air is carried out gravimetrically. The water vapor present in a known volume of air is chemically absorbed with a suitable reagent and weighed. In less laborious methods, the humidity is derived from the dew point or the wet-bulb depression of a water-vapor mixture.

The dew point is the temperature at which a vapor-gas mixture becomes saturated when cooled at constant pressure. If air of the condition denoted by point A in Fig. 9 is cooled, the relative humidity increases until the mixture is fully saturated. This condition is given by point B; the temperature coordinate is the dew point, which can be measured rapidly by evaporating ether in a silvered bulb. The temperature at which dew

Unit Processes in Pharmacy: The Operations

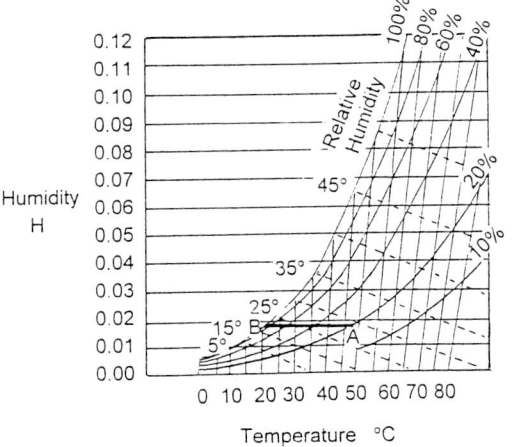

FIG. 9. A psychometric chart.

deposits from the surrounding air is noted and the humidity is read directly from a psychometric chart.

The derivation of the humidity from the wet-bulb depression requires a preliminary study of the transfer of mass and heat at a boundary between air and water. Since this process is also of importance in the study of drying, a detailed explanation is given below. If a small quantity of water evaporates into a large volume of air, conditions that make the change in humidity negligible, the latent heat of evaporation is supplied from the sensible heat of the water. As the latter cools, the temperature gradient between water and air promotes the flow of heat from the surrounding air to the surface. The rate of heat flow increases as the temperature falls until it equals the rate at which heat is required for evaporation. The temperature at the surface remains constant at what is known as the wet-bulb temperature. The difference between the air temperature and the wet-bulb temperature is the wet-bulb depression. If these temperatures are denoted by T_a and T_{wb}, the rate of heat transfer, Q, is given by Eq. (14),

$$Q = hA(T_a - T_{wb}) \tag{14}$$

where A is the area over which heat is transferred and h is the heat transfer coefficient. Mass transfer of water vapor from the water surface to the air is described by Eq. (15)

$$N = \frac{k_g}{RT}(P_{wi} - P_{wa}) \tag{15}$$

where P_{wi} is the partial pressure of water vapor at the surface, P_{wa} is the partial pressure of water vapor in the air, k_g is a mass transfer coefficient, and N is the number of moles transferred from the unit area in unit time. Rewriting Eq. (15) in terms of the mass, W, transferred at the whole surface in unit time gives Eq. (16),

$$W = \frac{M_w A}{RT} k_g (P_{wi} - P_{wa}) \tag{16}$$

where M_w is the molecular weight of water vapor and A is the area of the surface. If the partial pressure of water vapor in a system has the value P_w then, from the general gas equation, the mass of vapor in unit volume is

$$\frac{P_w}{RT} M_w$$

Similarly, if the total pressure is P, the mass of air in unit volume is

$$\frac{P - P_w}{RT} M_a$$

where M_a is the "molecular weight" of the air. The humidity, H, the ratio of these two quantities, is given in Eq. (17).

$$H = \frac{P_w}{P - P_w} \cdot \frac{M_w}{M_a} \tag{17}$$

If P is very much higher than P_w,

$$H = \frac{P_w}{P} \cdot \frac{M_w}{M_a}$$

Rearrangement and the substitution of humidity for partial pressure in Eq. (16) gives Eq. (18),

$$W = \frac{PM_a}{RT} k_g A (H_i - H_a) \tag{18}$$

where H_a is the humidity of the air and H_i is the humidity of the surface. The latter is known from the vapor pressure of water at the wet-bulb temperature. Since

$$\frac{PM_a}{RT} = \rho$$

Eq. (18) can be written as Eq. (19),

$$W = \rho k_g A (H_i - H_a) \tag{19}$$

where ρ is the density of the air. If the latent heat of evaporation is λ, the heat transfer rate necessary to promote this evaporation is given by Eq. (20).

$$Q = \rho k_g A (H_i - H_a) \tag{20}$$

Equating Eqs. (14) and (20) gives Eq. (21).

$$H_i - H_a = \frac{h}{\rho k_g \lambda} (T_a - T_{wb}) \tag{21}$$

Unit Processes in Pharmacy: The Operations

Both the heat and mass transfer coefficients are functions of air velocity. However, at air speeds greater than about 15 ft/s (4.5 m/s), the ratio h/k_g is approximately constant. The wet-bulb depression is directly proportional to the difference between the humidity at the surface and the humidity in the bulk of the air. In the wet- and dry-bulb hygrometer, the wet-bulb depression is measured by two thermometers, one of which is fitted with a fabric sleeve wetted with water. These thermometers are mounted side by side and shielded from radiation, an effect neglected in the derivation above. Air is drawn over the thermometers by means of a small fan. The derivation of the humidity from the wet-bulb depression and a psychometric chart are discussed later.

Many wet- and dry-bulb hygrometers operate without any form of induced air velocity at the wet bulb. This may be explained by examining another air–water system. If a limited quantity of air and water is allowed to equilibrate under conditions in which heat is neither gained nor lost by the system, the air becomes saturated and the latent heat required for evaporation is drawn from both fluids which cool to the same temperature. This temperature is the adiabatic saturation temperature, T_3. It is a peculiarity of the air–water system that the adiabatic saturation temperature and the wet-bulb temperature are the same. If water at this temperature is recycled in a system through which air is passing, the incoming air is cooled until it reaches the adiabatic saturation temperature at which point it is saturated. The temperature of the water, on the other hand, remains constant and all the latent heat required for evaporation is drawn from the sensible heat of the air. Equilibrium is expressed by Eq. (22),

$$(T_a - T_\infty)S = (H_\infty - H_a)\lambda \tag{22}$$

where T_a is the temperature of the incoming air and S is its specific heat, H_a and H_∞ are the humidities of the incoming air and the saturated air, and λ is the latent heat of evaporation for water.

The process of adiabatic saturation in which the humidity progressively rises and the temperature progressively falls is described on a humidity chart by adiabatic cooling lines which run diagonally to the saturation curve. Charts are specially constructed in such a way that these lines become parallel.

If a wet- and dry-bulb hygrometer is exposed to still air, the region adjacent to the wet bulb closely resembles the system described above. After a considerable period, equilibrium is attained and the wet bulb records the adiabatic saturation temperature.

When both wet- and dry-bulb temperatures have been found, the humidity is read from the psychometric chart in the following way. The point on the saturation curve corresponding to the wet-bulb temperature is found first. An adiabatic cooling line is then interpolated and followed until the coordinate corresponding to the dry-bulb temperature is reached. The humidity is read from the other axis.

The change in the physical properties of a hair or fiber with a change in humidity is utilized in many instruments. After calibration, they are suitable for use over a limited range of humidity.

Humidification and Dehumidification

Most commonly, air is humidified by passage through a spray of water. The humidity diagrams in Fig. 10 illustrate three methods: In the first, air at a temperature T_1 is heated to T_2. The latter is chosen in such a way that adiabatic cooling and saturation followed by heating to T_4 gives a humidity rise from H_1 to H_2. The humidification stage is per-

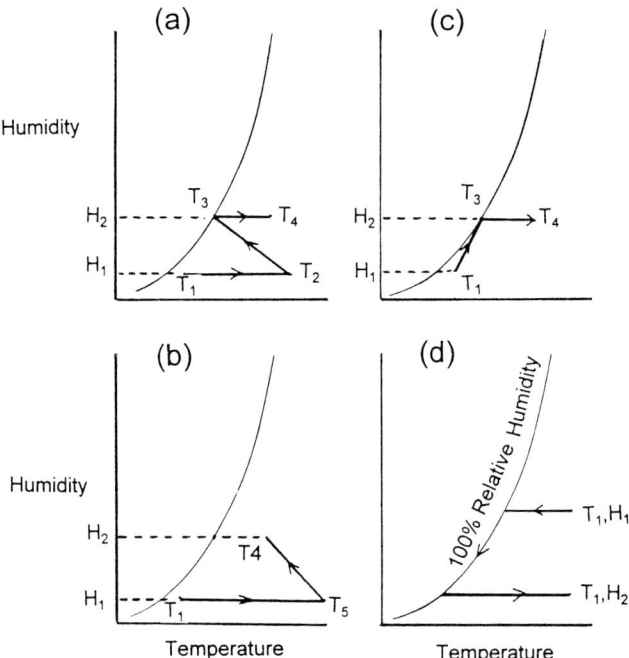

FIG. 10. The humidification of air, (a), (b), and (c); the dehumidification of the air, (d).

formed by passing the air through water sprays at the adiabatic saturation temperature, T_3. Alternatively in the second method, the incoming air could be heated to T_5 air of the correct humidity emerging when it is adiabatically cooled to T_4 with water. In neither of these methods is control of the water temperature necessary. In the third method, air of humidity H_1 and the temperature T_1 is passed through and saturated by a water spray maintained at T_3. On leaving the chamber, it is heated to T_4.

Small quantities of air are easily dehumidified by adsorbing the water vapor with alumina or silica gel arranged in columns. These are mounted in pairs so that one can be regenerated while the other is in use. Alternatively, the air can be cooled below the dew point. Excess water vapor condenses and the cold saturated air is reheated. For well-mixed gases, the process is described in Fig. 10.

Crystallization

As a unit operation, the term crystallization describes the production of a solid, single-component, crystalline phase from a multicomponent fluid phase. It may be applied to the production of crystalline solids from vapors, melts, or solutions. Crystallization from solution is most important. To complete the preparation of a pure dry solid, it is also necessary to separate the solid from the fluid phase, usually by centrifugation or filtration and by drying. The importance of crystallization lies primarily in the purification achieved during the process and in the physical properties of the product. A crystal-

Unit Processes in Pharmacy: The Operations

line powder is easily handled, is stable, and often possesses good flow properties and an attractive appearance.

Crystallization from a vapor, which occurs naturally, for example, in the formation of hoar frost, is employed in sublimation processes and for the condensation of water vapor during freeze-drying. Equipment may be regarded as specialized condensers in which the principal problems are the removal of the latent heat of crystallization and the discharge of the solid condensate. Condensers are commonly mounted in parallel in such a way that one can be shut down and emptied manually, by conveyor or by melting and draining, without interrupting sublimation.

In the pharmaceutical industry, crystallization is usually performed on a small scale from solutions, often in jacketed or agitated vessels. The conditions of crystallization, necessary for suitable purity, yield, and crystal form, are usually established by experiment. Nevertheless, a study of the principal factors which control crystallization is important. Much information is derived from the behavior of carefully prepared melts, which reveal more clearly than solutions the two stages of crystallization: nucleation and crystal growth. Nucleation describes the formation of small nuclei around which crystals grow. Without the formation of nuclei, crystal growth cannot occur.

Crystallization in Melts

A melt may be defined as the liquid form of a single material or the homogeneous liquid form of two or more materials which solidify on cooling. Crystallization in such a system passes through the following stages: supercooling, nuclei formation, and crystal growth.

If a single-component liquid is cooled, some degree, often high, of supercooling must be established before crystal nuclei form and growth begins. A metastable liquid region exists below the melting point which can only be entered by cooling. In this metastable, supercooled region, the absence of nucleation precludes the formation and growth of crystals. If, however, a crystal seed is added, growth occurs. The deliberate seeding of a metastable system is commonly employed in industrial crystallization. With further cooling, spontaneous nucleation usually takes place and the released heat of crystallization raises the temperature of the melt to its true melting point. With some materials, lower temperatures increase the viscosity and prevent nucleation. The liquid solidifies into a mass without crystallizing. This is known as vitrification and the products are called glasses. Many organic materials can be obtained in this form and, as with glass itself, devitrification may suddenly occur, particularly after heating.

Nucleation

In certain single-component systems, such as piperine, nucleation and crystal growth are independent and can be separately studied. The rate of nucleation as a function of supercooling is studied by maintaining the melt for a certain time at the given temperature and then quickly raising the temperature to the metastable region where further nucleation is negligible but the already formed nuclei can grow. Figure 11a illustrates the results of such an experiment. At low degrees of supercooling, little or no nucleation takes place. With further cooling, the rate of nucleation rises to a maximum and then falls. The relation, therefore, indicates that excessive cooling may depress the rate of crystallization by limiting the number of nuclei formed.

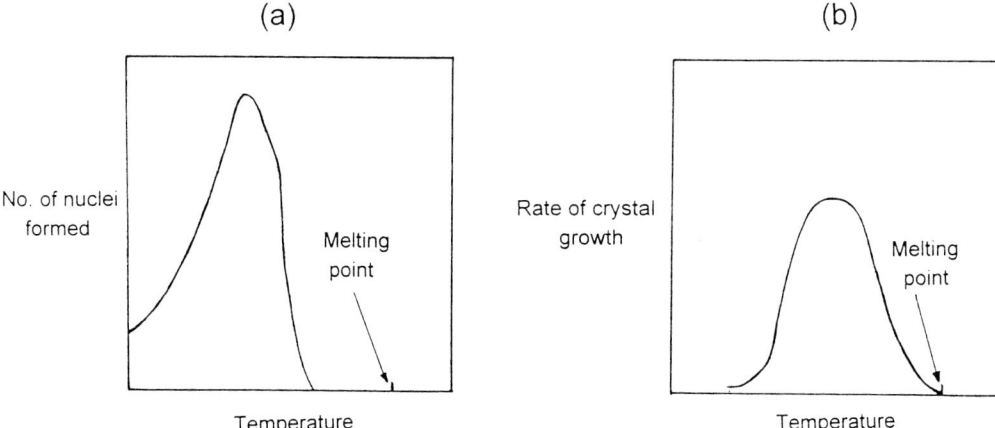

FIG. 11. (a) Change in nucleation with the degree of supercooling; (b) change in the rate of crystal growth with degree of supercooling.

Spontaneous nucleation occurs when sufficient molecules of low kinetic energy come together in such a way that the attraction between them is sufficient to overcome their momentum. The growth of a nucleus probably takes place over a very short period of time in a region of high local concentration. Once a certain size is reached, the nucleus becomes stable in the prevailing conditions. As the temperature falls, more molecules with low energy are present and the rate of nucleation rises. The decrease in nucleation rate at lower temperature is due to the increase in the melt viscosity.

Crystal Growth

If nucleation and crystal growth are independent, the latter can be studied by seeding a melt with small crystals under conditions of little or no natural nucleation. The rate of growth can then be measured. The relation between growth rate and temperature, shown in Fig. 11b, exhibits an optimum degree of supercooling, although the maximum growth temperature is normally higher than the temperature of maximum nucleation. The form of the crystal growth curve is again explained by the kinetics of the molecules. At temperatures just below the melting point, molecules have too much energy to remain in the crystal lattice. As the temperature falls, more molecules are retained and the growth rate increases. Ultimately, however, diffusion to and orientation at the crystal surface is depressed.

For crystal growth in a single component melt, the molecules at the crystal surface must reach the correct position at the lattice and become suitably orientated, losing kinetic energy. These energy changes appear as heat of crystallization which must be transferred from the surface to the bulk of the melt. The rate of crystal growth is influenced by both the rate of heat transfer and the changes taking place at the surface. Agitation of the system increases heat transfer by reducing the thermal resistance of the liquid layers adjacent to the crystal until the changes at the crystal face become the controlling effect.

Unit Processes in Pharmacy: The Operations

In multicomponent melts and solutions, deposition of material at the crystal face depletes the adjacent liquid layers and a concentration gradient is set up with saturation at the face and supersaturation in the liquid. Diffusion of molecules to the crystal face is discussed in the next section.

The account above describes the behavior of certain carefully prepared melts from which all extraneous matter is rigidly excluded. Dust and other insoluble matter may increase the nucleation rate by acting as centers of crystallization. Soluble impurities may increase or decrease the rates of both nucleation and crystal growth. The latter is probably due to adsorption of the impurity on the crystal face. Impurities may also affect the shape in which the material crystallizes.

Crystallization from Solutions

When a material crystallizes from a solution, nucleation and crystal growth occur simultaneously over a wide intermediate temperature range, making a study of these processes more difficult. In general, however, they are thought to be similar to nucleation and crystal growth in melts. The three basic steps, induction of supersaturation, formation of nuclei, and the growth of crystals, are explained with reference to the solubility curve shown in Fig. 12.

A solution at temperature and concentration indicated by point A may be saturated by either cooling to point B or by removing solvent (point C). With further cooling or concentration, the supersaturated metastable region is entered. If the degree of supersaturation is low, the spontaneous formation of crystal nuclei is highly improbable. Crystal growth, however, can be initiated by adding seeds. With increased supersaturation, spontaneous nucleation becomes more probable, and the metastable region is limited approximately by the line B'C'. If the solution is cooled to B' or concentrated by solvent removal to C', spontaneous nucleation is virtually certain. Crystal growth occurs also under these conditions. The rate of growth, however, is depressed at low temperatures.

During crystal growth, deposition on the faces of the crystal causes depletion of molecules in the immediate vicinity. The driving force is provided by the concentration gradient set-up, from supersaturation in the solution to lower concentrations at the crystal face. A high degree of supersaturation therefore promotes a high growth rate.

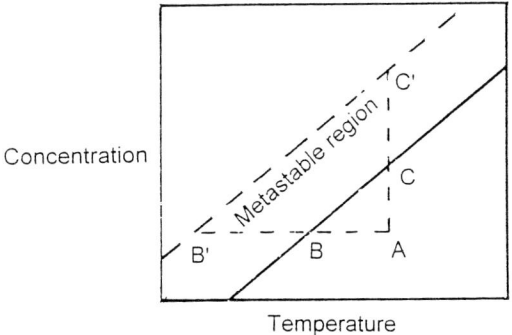

FIG. 12. The solubility–supersolubility diagram. The line BC is part of the solubility curve. Nucleation is unlikely to occur unless the degree of supersaturation indicated by the line C'B' is reached.

A reaction at the surface in which solute molecules become correctly orientated in the crystal lattice provides a second resistance to the growth of the crystal. Simultaneously, the heat of crystallization must be conducted away.

For given conditions of temperature and saturation, agitation modifies the rate of crystal growth. Initially, agitation quickly increases the growth rate by decreasing the thickness of the boundary layer and the diffusional resistance. However, as agitation is intensified, a limiting value is reached which is determined by the kinetics of the surface reaction. Figure 13 describes the effect of agitation on the rate of crystal growth in solutions of sodium thiosulfate of differing degrees of supersaturation.

As with melts, soluble impurities may increase or reduce nucleation rate. Insoluble materials may act as nuclei and promote crystallization. Impurities may also affect crystal form and, in some cases, are deliberately added to secure a product with good appearance, absence of caking, or suitable flow properties.

The temperature at which crystallization is performed may be determined by the crystal form or the degree of hydration required of the products. Reference to the solubility curves given in Fig. 14 shows that crystallization at 50°C yields $FeSO_4 \cdot 7H_2O$, at 60°C, $FeSO_4 \cdot 4H_2O$, and at 70°C, $FeSO_4$. Most materials, however, have one or possibly two forms. The degree of supersaturation of solution 1 is 5 g/L, of solution 2 10 g/L, and of solution 3 15 g/L.

The Design and Operation of Crystallizers

The purpose of crystallization is to produce, as far as possible, crystals of the required shape, size distribution, purity, and yield. This is achieved by maintaining a degree of supersaturation at which nucleation and crystal growth proceed at appropriate rates. Control of the number of nuclei formed controls the size of the crystals deposited from a given quantity of solution. Alternatively, crystal number and size can be controlled by adding the correct amount of artificial nuclei or seeds to a system in which little or no natural nucleation is taking place.

In most cases, the mode of operation is determined by the relation between the solubility of the solute and the temperature, (Fig. 14) which, in turn, determines how supersaturation is to be achieved. Other factors of importance are the thermal stability of the solute, the impurities which may be present, and the degree of hydration required.

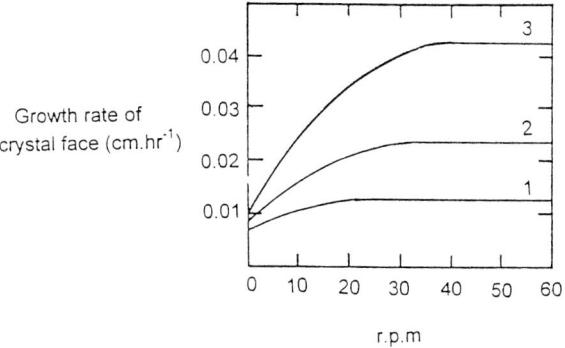

FIG. 13. The effect of agitation on the growth rate of a crystal of sodium thiosulfate (degree of supersaturation: 1 = 5 g/L, 2 = 10 g/L, and 3 = 15 g/L).

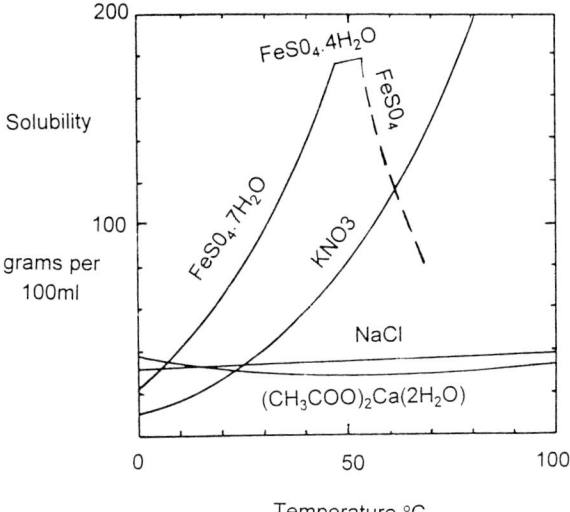

FIG. 14. Solubility curves. (From Ref. 8.)

If the solubility of the solute increases greatly with temperature, supersaturation and the deposition of a large proportion of the solute is brought about by cooling a hot concentrated solution. Sodium nitrate provides an example. Sodium chloride and calcium acetate, on the other hand, exemplify materials with a small or negative temperature coefficient of solubility. Here, supersaturation can best be achieved by evaporating a part of the solvent. In some cases, both evaporation and cooling are employed. The mother liquors following evaporative crystallization can be cooled to yield a further crop of crystals, provided there is a suitable change in solubility and that impurities present do not impede the process. In other crystallizers, flash cooling is used. A hot solution is passed into a vacuum chamber in which both evaporation and cooling take place.

Supersaturation can also be induced by the addition of a third substance which reduces the solubility of a solute in a solvent. These precipitation processes, which are important in the processing of thermolabile materials, are controlled by the temperature of mixing, the agitation, and the rate at which the third substance is added. Water-insoluble materials dissolved in water-miscible organic solvents can be precipitated by adding water. Alternatively, the aqueous solubility of many materials can be reduced by a change of pH or the addition of a common ion. Proteins can be salted out of solution by the addition of ammonium chloride and adjustment of the pH. Finally, the precipitation of a crystalline solid may be the result of a chemical reaction.

Crystallizers should produce crystals of even size. This facilitates the removal of the mother liquor and washing. If large quantities of the liquor are occluded in the mass of crystals, drying yields an impure product. In addition, crystals of even size are less likely to cake on storage.

Production of Very Fine Crystals

Fine powders are important components in pharmaceutical operations. If a substance has a steep solubility curve, fine crystals are produced by quickly cooling the solution through the metastable region to conditions under which the rate of nucleation is high and the rate of crystal growth is low. This method is not always possible, and the precipitation methods described above may be adopted.

Production of Large Crystals

Batch production of large, uniform crystals may be carried out in agitated reaction vessels by slowly controlled or natural cooling. Spontaneous nucleation is improbable to occur until solution A is cooled to X (Fig. 15). Crystallization follows the path XB. Better control is gained if the solution is artificially seeded; seeding is shown at X'. Crystallization follows the broken line $X'B$, the aim being to maintain the solution in the metastable region where the growth rate is high and natural nucleation is low. The course of the crystallization is clearly shown in Fig. 15. Initially, spontaneous nucleation may be allowed by cooling from A to X. As crystallization takes place, the degree of supersaturation and the concentration of the solute fall, ultimately reaching saturation at B when growth ceases. Closer control is secured by artificially seeding the supersaturated solution in the absence of natural nucleation. Seeding is indicated by the point, X'. The course of the crystallization is indicated by the broken line $X'B$.

An important principle for the continuous production of large even crystals is used in Oslo or Krystal crystallizers. A metastable, supersaturated solution is released into the bottom of a mass of growing crystals on which the solute is deposited. The crystals are fluidized by the circulation of the solution and classification in this zone allows the withdrawal of sufficiently large crystals from the bottom.

Crystallizers

Although other methods may be adopted, crystallizers can be conveniently classified by the way in which a solution is supersaturated. This leads to the self-explanatory terms, cooling crystallizer and evaporate crystallizer. In vacuum crystallizers, both evaporation and cooling takes place.

Cooling Crystallizers

Open or closed tanks, agitated by stirrers, are used for batch crystallization. The specific heat of the solution and the heat of crystallization are removed by means of jackets or coils through which cooling water can be circulated. Agitation destroys temperature gradients in the tanks, opposes sedimentation and the irregular growth of crystals

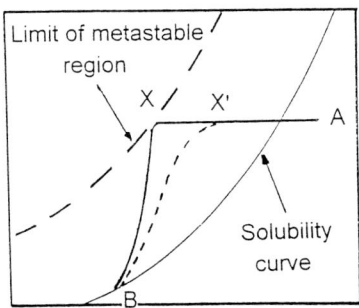

FIG. 15. The production of large crystals and the conditions of supersaturation.

Unit Processes in Pharmacy: The Operations

at the bottom of the vessel, and, as described above, facilitates growth. Similar equipment is used for crystallization or precipitation by the addition of a third substance.

Crystallizers for continuous processes often take the form of a trough cooled naturally or by a jacket. The solution enters at one end and crystals and liquid are discharged at the other. In one type of crystallizer, a slow moving worm works in the solution and lifts crystals off the cooling surface to distribute them through the solution and slowly convey them through the trough. In another crystallizer, the trough is agitated by rocking. Baffles are used to increase the residence time of the solution. Both types of crystallizers are characterized by low heat transfer coefficients. An alternative arrangement consists essentially of a double-pipe heat exchanger. The crystallizing fluid is carried in the central pipe with the countercurrent flow of the coolant in the annulus between the pipes. A shaft rotates in the central tube carrying blades which scrape the heat transfer surface. High heat transfer coefficients are obtained. An Oslo crystallizer, in which supersaturation is created by cooling, is described in Fig. 16a. The principles underlying this plant have already been described.

Evaporative Crystallizers

On a small scale, simple pans and stirred reaction vessels can be used for evaporative crystallization. Larger units may employ calandria heating, as shown in Fig. 16b. The downcomer, which must be large enough to accommodate the flow of the suspension, commonly houses an impeller, with forced circulation increasing the heat transfer to the boiling liquid. These units may be adapted for either batch or continuous processes in which crystal size is not of great importance. For continuous processes demanding close control of product size, an Oslo crystallizer, which saturates the solution by evaporation, may be employed.

Vacuum Crystallizers

Vacuum crystallizers produce supersaturated conditions by solvent removal and cooling (Fig. 16c). A hot concentrated solution is fed to an agitated crystallization chamber maintained at low pressure. The solution boils and cools adiabatically to the boil-

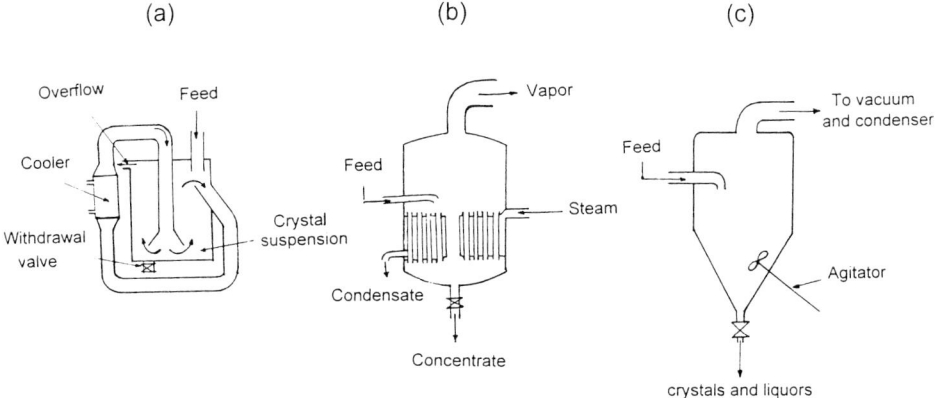

FIG. 16. (a) Cooling crystallizer; (b) evaporative crystallizer; (c) batch vacuum crystallizer.

ing point corresponding to the operating pressure. Crystallization follows concentration and the product is removed from the bottom of the vessel. The principles of the Oslo crystallizer are also employed in vacuum crystallization.

Filtration

The student of pharmacy will have used filtration extensively in the collection of precipitates in chemical analyses or in the preparation of parenteral fluids and will, therefore, anticipate the definition of filtration as the removal of solids suspended in a liquid or gas by passage through a pervious medium on which the solids are retained. The pervious medium or septum is normally supported on a base and these, together with a suitable housing providing free access of fluid to and from the septum, comprise the filter. The applications of filtration are diverse. They may he classified as clarification or cake filtration.

Methods

Clarification

Very high standards of clarity are imposed during the production of pharmaceutical solutions. The aim may be simply the presentation of an elegant product, although complete freedom from particulate matter is obviously necessary in the manufacture of most parenteral solutions. The solids are unwanted and are normally present in very small concentrations. Clarification may be carried out with the help of thick media which allow the penetration and arrest of particles by entrapment, impingement, and electrostatic effects. This leads to the concept of depth filtration in which particles, perhaps a hundred times smaller than the dimensions of the passages through the medium, are removed. Because of this, such filters are not absolute and must be designed with sufficient depth so that the probability of the smallest particle under consideration passing right through the filter is extremely small.

Depth filtration differs fundamentally from the use of media in which pore size determines the size of particle retained. Such filters may be said to be "absolute" at a particle diameter closely related to the size of the pore, so that there is a relatively sharp division between particles which pass the filter and those that are retained. An analogy with sieving may be drawn for this mechanism. The life of such filters depends on the number of pores available for the passage of fluid. Once a particle is trapped at the entrance to the pore, the contribution of the latter to the overall flow of liquid is very much reduced. Coarse straining with a wire mesh and membrane filter employ this mechanism.

Sterilization of liquids by filtration could be regarded as an extreme application of clarification in which the complete removal of particles as small as 0.3 µm must be ensured.

Cake Filtration

The most common industrial application is the filtration of slurries containing a relatively large amount of suspended solids, usually 3 to 20%. The septum acts only as a

Unit Processes in Pharmacy: The Operations

support in this operation, the actual filtration being carried out by the solids deposited as a cake. In such cases, solids may completely penetrate the septum until the deposition of an effective cake occurs. Until this time, cloudy filtrate may be recycled. The physical properties of the cake largely determine the method employed. Washing and partial drying or dewatering are often integral parts of the process. Effective discharge of the cake completes the process. The solids, the filtrate, or both may be wanted.

The Theories of Filtration

Filtration theory has two important aspects. The first describes the flow of fluids through porous media and is applicable to both clarification and cake filtration. The second, which is of primary importance only in clarification, concerns the retention of particles on a depth filter.

Flow of Fluids through Porous Media

The concept of a channel with a hydraulic diameter equivalent to the complex interstitial network which exists in a powder bed leads to Eq. (23),

$$Q = \frac{KA\Delta P}{\eta L} \qquad (23)$$

where Q is the volumetric flow rate, A is the area of the bed and L its thickness, ΔP is the pressure difference, and η is the viscosity of the fluid. The permeability coefficient, K, is given by

$$\frac{\varepsilon^3}{5(1-\varepsilon)^2 S_0^2}$$

where ε is the porosity of the bed and S_0 its specific surface area (cm²/cm³).

Factors Affecting the Rate of Filtration

Equation 23 may be used as a basis for the discussion of the factors which determine the rate of filtration.

Pressure. The rate of filtration at any instant of time is directly proportional to the pressure difference across the bed.

In cake filtration, deposition of solids over a finite period increases the bed depth. If, therefore, the pressure remains constant, the rate of filtration falls. Alternatively, the pressure can be progressively increased to maintain the filtration rate.

Conditions in which the pressure is substantially constant are found in vacuum filtration. In pressure filtration, a low constant pressure is usually employed in the early stages of filtration for reasons given below. The pressure is then stepped up as the operation proceeds.

This analysis neglects the additional resistance derived from the supporting septum and the thin layer of particles associated with it. At the beginning of the operation, some particles penetrate the septum and are retained in the capillaries in the manner of depth filtration, while others bridge the pores at the surface to begin the formation of the cake. The effect of penetration, which is analogous to the binding of a sieve, is to confer a resistance on the cake–septum junction which is much higher than the resistance of the clean septum with a small associated layer of cake. This layer may contribute heavily to the total resistance. Since penetration is not reversible, the initial period of cake filtration is highly critical and is usually carried out at a low pressure. The amount of penetration depends on the structure of the septum, the size and shape of the solid particles, their concentration, and the filtration rate.

When clarifying at constant pressure, a slow decrease in filtration rate occurs because material is deposited within the bed.

Viscosity. The inverse relation between flow rate and viscosity indicates that, as expected, higher pressures are required to maintain a given flow rate for thick liquids than are necessary for filtering thin liquids. The decrease in viscosity with increase in temperature may suggest the use of hot filtration. Some installations (e.g., the filter press) can be equipped so that the temperature of hot slurries can be maintained.

Filter Area. In cake filtration, a suitable filter area must be employed for a particular slurry. If this is too small, the excessively thick cakes produced require high pressure differentials to maintain a reasonable flow rate. This is of great importance in the filtration of slurries giving compressible cakes. In clarification, the relation is simpler. The filtration rate can be doubled by simply doubling the filter area.

Permeability Coefficient. The permeability coefficient may be examined in terms of porosity and surface area. Evaluation of the term

$$\frac{\varepsilon^3}{(1-\varepsilon)^2}$$

shows that the permeability coefficient is a sensitive function of porosity. When filtering a slurry, the porosity of the cake depends upon the way in which particles are deposited and packed. A porosity or void fraction from 0.27 to 0.47 is possible in the regular arrangement of spheres of equal size. Intermediate values are normally obtained in the random deposition of deflocculated particles of fairly regular shape. A fast rate of deposition, given by concentrated slurries or high flow rates, may give a higher porosity because of the greater possibility of bridging and arching in the cake. Although theoretically the particle size has no effect on porosity (assuming that the bed is large compared with the particles), a broad particle size distribution may lead to a reduction of porosity if small particles pack in the interstices created by larger particles.

Surface area, unlike porosity, is markedly affected by particle size and is inversely proportional to the particle diameter. Hence, as commonly observed in the laboratory, a coarse precipitate is easier to filter than a fine precipitate, even though both may pack with the same porosity. Where possible, a previous operation may be modified to facilitate filtration. For example, a suitable particle size may be obtained in a crystallization process by control of nucleation, or the proportion of fines in milling may be reduced by carefully controlling residence times. In most cases, however, control of this type is not possible and, with materials which filter only with difficulty, much may be gained by conditioning the slurry, an operation which modifies both the porosity and the specific surface of the depositing cake.

In clarification, high permeability and filtration rate oppose good particle retention. In the formation of clarifying media from sintered or loose particles, accurate control of particle size, specific surface and porosity is possible, and a medium can be designed which offers the best compromise between permeability and particle retention. The analysis of permeability given above can be accurately applied to these systems. Because of extremes of shape, this is not so with the fibrous media used for clarification. Here it is possible to develop a material of high permeability and high retentive capacity. Such a material is, however, intrinsically weak and must be adequately supported.

The Retention of Particles in a Depth Filter

Theoretical studies of particle retention have been restricted to granular media of a type used in the purification of municipal water. The aim is to predict the variation of filtrate quality with influent quality or time and then estimate the effect of removed solids on the permeability of the bed. Such studies have some bearing on the use of granular, sintered, or fibrous beds used for clarifying pharmaceuticals.

The path followed by the liquid through a bed is extremely tortuous. Violent changes of direction and velocity occur as the system of pores and waists (strictures) is traversed. Deflection of particles by gravity or, in the case of very fine particles, by Brownian motion brings the particles within the range of the attractive forces between particles and the medium and causes arrest. Inertial effects, that is, the movement of a particle across streamlines by virtue of its momentum, are considered to be of importance only in the removal of particles from gases. In liquid–solid systems, density differences are much smaller.

Opportunity for contact and arrest depends upon the surface area of the bed, the tortuosity of the void space, and the interstitial speed of the liquid. Since the inertial mechanism is ineffective, increase in interstitial velocity decreases the opportunity for contact and retention of particles by the medium. The efficiency of a filter therefore decreases as the flow rate increases. Efficiency, however, increases as the density or size of the influent particles increase and decreases as the particle size in the bed decreases. Each layer of clean filter is considered to remove the same proportion of the particles in the influent. Mathematically this is expressed by Eq. (24),

$$\frac{dC}{dx} = -KC \tag{24}$$

where C is the concentration of the particles which enter an element of depth dx. The value of K, which is a clarifying coefficient expressing the fraction of particles that deposit in unit depth of the bed, changes with time. Initially, the rate of removal increases and the efficiency of filtration improves. The reason for this may be that the deposition of particles in the bed is at first localized and the surface area and tortuosity increase. Later, the efficiency of removal decreases because deposition narrows the pores, reduces convolutions and surface area, and increases the interstitial liquid velocity. The failure of the medium to adequately retain particles, or the decrease in permeability and filtration rate eventually limit the life of the filter. If deposition is reversible, the permeability and retentive capacity can be restored by vigorous backwashing; the medium should be cheap and expendable.

A mathematical account of the theories of clarification with depth filters is found in the work of Ives [9,10] and Maroudas and Eisenklam [11].

The Conditioning of Slurries

The permeability of an ideal filter bed, such as that formed by a filter aid, is about 7×10^{-9} particles per cm^2. This is more than ten thousand times the permeability of a precipitate of aluminum hydroxide. The modification of the physical properties of the slurry can, therefore, be a powerful tool in the hands of the filtration engineer. This is called slurry conditioning and two methods, flocculation and the addition of filter aids, will be discussed here.

Flocculation of slurries is a common procedure where the addition of flocculating agents is permissible. The aggregates or flocs, which are characterized by a high sedimentation rate and volume, form cakes with a porosity as high as 0.9. Since this is also associated with a decrease in specific surface, flocculation markedly increases permeability. Such coagulates are, however, highly compressible and are therefore filtered at low pressures.

Filter aids are added in concentrations up to 5% to slurries which filter only with difficulty. The filter aid forms a rigid cake of high porosity and permeability due to favorable shape characteristics, a low surface area, and a narrow particle size distribution, properties that can be varied for different operations. This structure mechanically supports the fine particles originally present in the slurry. Diatomite, in the form of a purified, fractionated powder, is most commonly used. Other filter aids include a volcanic glass, called Perlite, and cellulose derivatives.

Filter aids cannot easily be used when the solids are wanted. Their excellent characteristics, however, leads to their use as a "precoat" mounted on a suitable support so that the filter aid itself forms the effective filtering medium. This prevents blinding of the septum. Precoat methods take several forms and are discussed below. A practical account of the properties and uses of filter aids has been given by Wheeler [12].

The Compressibility of Cakes

In the theory of cake filtration described above, the permeability coefficient was considered constant. The observation that a cake may be hard and firm at the septum junction and sloppy at its outer face suggests that the porosity may be varying throughout the depth of the cake. This could be due to a decrease in hydrostatic pressure from a maximum at the cake face to zero at the back of the supporting septum. It must be balanced by a thrust, originating in the viscous drag of the fluid as it passes through the cake, transmitted through the cake skeleton, and varying from zero at the cake face to a maximum at the back of the septum equal to the pressure difference. The relation between this compressive stress and the pressure applied across the cake is shown in Fig. 17.

So far it has been assumed that no deformation occurs under this stress, the cake is perfectly rigid. No cake, in fact, behaves in this way, although some, such as those composed of filter aids or of coarse, isodiametric particles, approximate closely to it. Others, such as cakes deposited from slurries of heavily hydrated colloidal particles,

Unit Processes in Pharmacy: The Operations

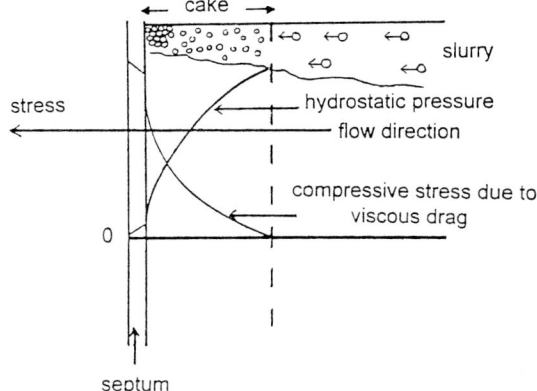

FIG. 17. Stress distribution in a filter cake.

are easily deformed, and the permeability coefficient, until now assumed constant, is itself a function of pressure, therefore Eq. (23) no longer applies. This effect can be so marked that an increase in pressure actually decreases the rate of filtration. Most slurries behave in a manner intermediate between these two extremes.

Cake Washing and Dewatering

Cake washing is of great importance in many filtration operations because the filtrate retained in the cake can be displaced by pure liquids. Filtration equipment varies in its washing efficiency and this may influence its choice. If the wash liquids follow the same course as the filtrate, the wash rate is the same as the final rate of filtration, assuming that the viscosity of the two liquids is the same and that the cake structure is not altered by, for example, peptization following the removal of flocculating electrolytes. Washing takes place in two stages. The first involves the removal of most of the filtrate retained in the cake by simple displacement. In the second, longer stage, the filtrate is removed from the less accessible pores by a diffusive mechanism. These stages are shown in Fig. 18.

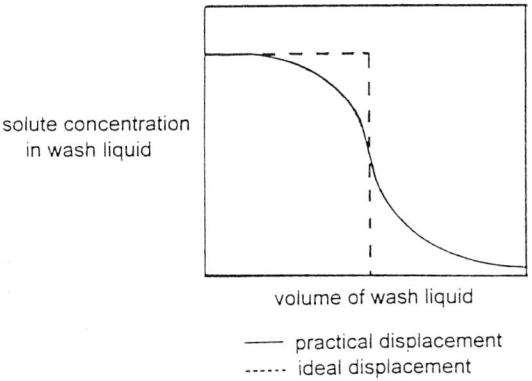

FIG. 18. Displacement of a filtrate by displacement washing.

Efficient washing requires a fairly cohesive cake which resists the formation of cracks and channels that offer a preferential course to the wash liquid. For this reason, cakes should have even thickness and permeability.

Subsequent operations, such as drying and handling, are facilitated by removing the liquid retained in the cake after washing which occupies 40-80% of the total cake volume. This is achieved by blowing or drawing air through the washed cake, leaving liquid retained only as a film around the particles and as annuli at the points of contact. Since both surface area and the number of point contacts per unit volume increase as the particle size decreases, the effectiveness of washing decreases with cakes composed of fine particles.

Filters

The method by which the filtrate is driven through the filter medium and cake, if present, may be used to classify filters into :

- Gravity filters
- Vacuum filters
- Pressure filters

Each group may be further subdivided into filters employed in continuous or batch processes although, due to technical difficulties, continuous pressure filters are uncommon and expensive. Centrifugation is another means of removing filtrate. Extensive surveys can be found in the literature [13,14].

Gravity Filters

Gravity filters, employing thick, granular beds, are widely used in municipal water filtration. However, the low operating pressures, usually less than 1.5 psi (10.3 kPa), give low rates of filtration unless very large areas are used. Their use in pharmacy is very limited. Gravity filters, using suspended media composed of thick felts, are sometimes employed for clarification on a small scale. On a somewhat larger scale, a wooden or stone tank, known as a nutsche, is used. The nutsche has a false bottom, which may act as the filter medium, although, more commonly, the bottom is dressed with a cloth. The slurry is added and the material filters under its own hydrostatic head. The filtrate is collected in the sump beneath the filter. Thorough washing is possible by simple displacement and diffusion or by resuspending the solids in a wash liquid and refiltering. The nutsche is comparatively difficult to empty and labor costs are high.

Vacuum Filters

Vacuum filters operate at higher pressure differentials than gravity filters. The pressure is limited naturally to about 12 psi (82.75 kPa), which confines their use to the deposition of fairly thin cakes of freely filtering materials. Despite this limitation, the principle has been successfully applied to continuous and completely automatic cake filtration for which the rotary drum filter is most extensively used.

The rotary drum (Fig. 19) in a typical construction, may be regarded as two concentric, horizontal cylinders, the outer cylinder being the septum with a suitable per-

Unit Processes in Pharmacy: The Operations

forated metal support. The annular space between the cylinders is divided by radial partitions producing a number of peripheral compartments running the length of the drum. Each compartment is connected by a line to a port in a rotary valve which permits the intermittent application of vacuum or compressed air, as dictated by the different parts of the filtration cycle. The drum is partially immersed in a bath to which the slurry is fed. The complete cycle of filtration, washing, partial drying, and discharge is completed with each revolution of the drum and usually takes from 1 to 10 min. The relative lengths of each part of the cycle, indicated by the segments superimposed on Fig. 19, depends on the cake-forming characteristics of the slurry and the importance of the associated operations of washing and drying. They may be varied by the depth of immersion and the speed of rotation in such a way that each compartment remains submerged for sufficient time for the formation of an adequate cake. Washing and dewatering can be carried out to the standard required during the remaining part of the cycle. The slurry must be effectively agitated during operation, or sedimentation will cause the preferential deposition of the finer particles, giving a cake of low permeability. Agitation must not, of course, erode the deposited cake. Maintaining a suspension of very coarse particles therefore becomes difficult or impossible and other methods of feeding must be adopted.

Filtration may be followed by a brief period of draining in which air is drawn through the cake, displacing retained filtrate. Sprays are used for washing, and devices that flood the cake have also been used. Dewatering, again achieved by drawing air through the cake, is followed by discharge. A scraper knife, assisted by compressed air which causes the septum to belly against the cutting edge, is commonly used. Highly cohesive cakes, such as those encountered in the removal of mycelial growth from antibiotic cultures, may be removed by means of a string discharge. A series of closely spaced, parallel strings run on the cloth around the drum. At the discharge section, the strings lift the cake away from the cloth and over a discharge roller after which the strings are led back to the drum.

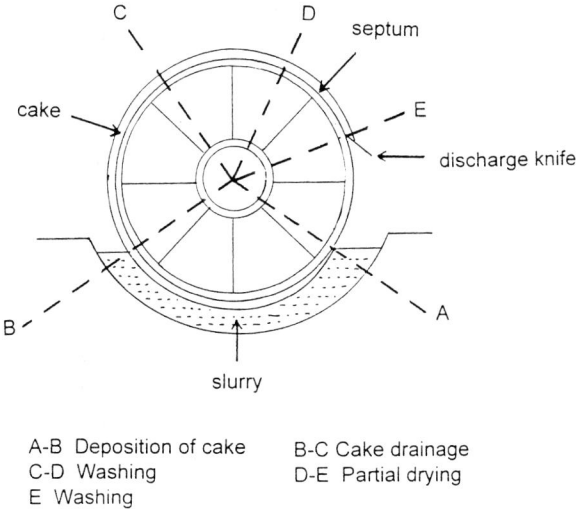

A-B Deposition of cake   B-C Cake drainage
C-D Washing   D-E Partial drying
E Washing

FIG. 19. Rotary vacuum filter.

Other variants of rotary drum filtration include top feed filtration and precoat filtration. As already mentioned, slurries containing coarse particles cannot be effectively suspended by the method described above. Such materials, which give rapid cake formation and fast dewatering, may be filtered by applying the slurry to the top of the drum with the help of a feed box and suitable dams. Sedimentation in this case assists filtration.

Precoat filtration, using a rotary drum, is applied to slurries that contain a small amount of fine or gelatinous material which plugs and blinds the filter cloth. Filtration is preceded by the deposition of a filter aid on the drum to a depth of up to 4 in. (10 cm). During filtration blinding of the surface layers occurs which are removed at the discharge section by a slowly advancing knife so that a clean filtering surface is continually presented to the slurry. The depth of the cut depends on the penetration of the precoat by the slurry solids and is usually of the order of a thousandth of an inch. This method has allowed the filtration of slurries which could not previously be filtered or which demanded the addition of large quantities of a filter aid.

For filtration on a smaller scale the nutsche is used. A vacuum is drawn on the sump of the tank giving a much faster filtration rate than in a gravity-operated process.

Pressure Filters

Due to the formation of cakes of low permeability, many slurries require higher pressure differentials for effective filtration than can be applied by vacuum techniques. For such operations pressure filters are used. They may also be used when the scale of the operation does not justify the installation of continuous rotary filters. Usually, operational pressure of from 10 to 100 psi (69–690 kPa) are applied across stationary filter surfaces. This arrangement prohibits continuous operation because of the difficulty of discharging the cake while the filter is under pressure. The higher labor costs of batch operation are offset by lower capital costs.

The most commonly used pressure filter is the plate-and-frame press (Fig. 20). It consists of a series of alternating plates and frames mounted in line on bars which

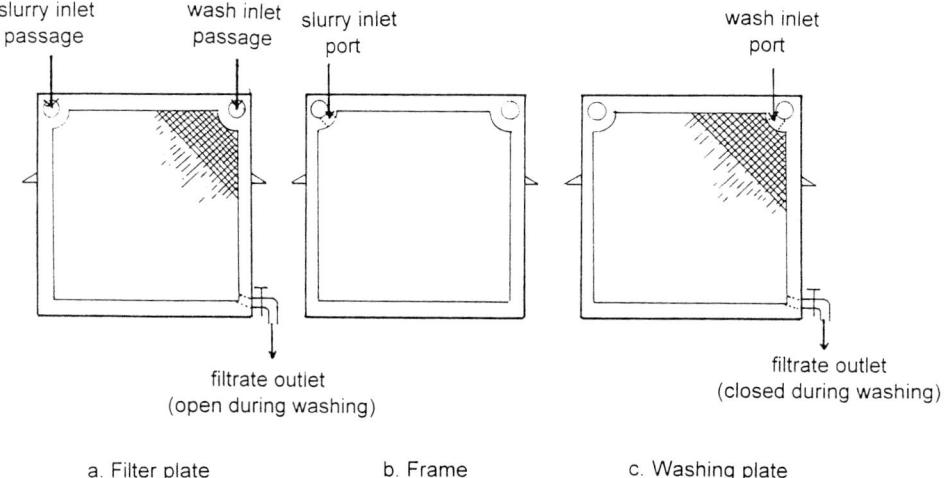

FIG. 20. The filter press, plates and frame.

Unit Processes in Pharmacy: The Operations

provide support and facilitate assembly and cake discharge. The filter cloth is mounted on the two faces of each plate and the press assembled (Fig. 21a) by moving the plates and frames together with a hand screw or hydraulic ram. This provides a series of compartments, the peripheries of which are sealed by the machined edges of the plates and frames uniting on the filter cloth which acts as a gasket. Dripping often occurs at this point, and therefore the press is less suitable for noxious materials. The dimensions of each compartment are determined by the area of the plates and the thickness of the intervening frame. These dimensions and the number of compartments used depend primarily on the volume of slurry to be handled and its solids content. The plate faces are corrugated by grooves or ribs which effectively support the cloth, preventing distortion under pressure and allowing free discharge of the filtrate from behind the cloth.

Coincident holes, shown in the top left corner of both plates and frames, provide, on assembly, a channel for the slurry (Fig. 21a) and simultaneous entry into each compartment through an entry port in each frame (Fig. 20b). All compartments therefore behave in the same way with the formation of two cakes on the opposing plate faces. Discharge of filtrate after passage through cake, cloth, and corrugations takes place through an outlet in the plate shown diametrically opposite the frame entry port (Figs. 20a,c). Filtration may be continued until the cake entirely fills the compartments or the accumulation of cake gives unsatisfactory rates of filtration.

Washing may be carried out by simply replacing the slurry by wash liquids and providing for its separate collection. This method, however, is inefficient due to erosion and channeling of the cake. Where efficient washing is required, special washing plates alternate with the plates described above. These contain an additional inlet which leads the wash liquid in behind the filter cloth. During washing, the filtrate outlet on

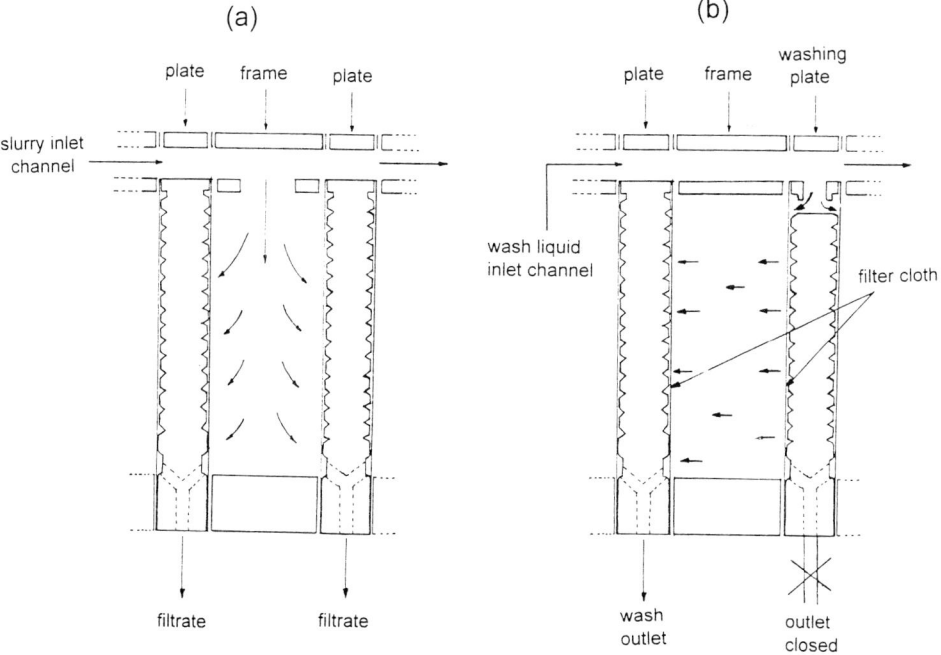

FIG. 21. The assembled filter press with a frame and two plates. Movement of liquid during (a) filtration, (b) washing.

the washing plate is closed so that the wash liquid flows through the cloth and the first cake in a direction opposite to that taken by the filtrate. The wash liquid then follows the course of the filtrate through the cake and cloth of the opposite plate. A diagrammatic representation of the flow of liquids during washing is given in Fig. 21b.

The development of filter media in sheet form with high wet strength and the ability to retain extremely fine particles extends the application of the plate-and-frame filter to clarification. Filter media are available in various grades and, when used in apparatus similar to that described above, may be used to clarify or sterilize liquids containing a very low proportion of solids. In sterilization by sheet filtration, the operation is carried out in two stages. The solution is first clarified, and the very clean filtrate is passed through the sterilizing sheet under a relatively low pressure. Before the operation, the assembled filter is sterilized by steam. The washing apparatus, assembled with suitable sheets, may also be used for air filtration.

Other filters widely used for clarification are the Metafilter and the Streamline filter. The former consists of a large number of closely spaced rings, usually made of stainless steel, mounted on a rod. The rod is fluted to provide channels for the discharge of filtrate. The passage of filtrate between the rings is provided by scallops stamped on one side of each ring maintaining a ring spacing between one and eight thousands of an inch. This construction provides a robust support for the actual filtering medium. It is mounted in a suitable pressure vessel, and large filters consist of a number of such units. For clarification, the filter is first coated by circulating filter aid of the correct grade. The finest materials are suitable for the removal of bacteria. The coat acts as a depth filter. Filter aids may also be added to the liquid to be clarified.

The "streamline" filter employs paper disks compressed to form a filter pack. The filtrate passes through the minute interstices between the disks, leaving any solids at the edge. This is the principle of edge filtration. Other filters, composed of metal plates or wires, operate on the same principle and are used for coarse clarification.

Many small-scale filters consist simply of a fixed, rigid medium, robust enough to withstand limited pressures, mounted in a suitable housing. These filters, which are also vacuum operated, are used to clarify by depth filtration. Media are composed of sintered metals, ceramics, plastics, or glass. Filters prepared from closely graded and sintered chemical powders are suitable for the sterilization of solutions by filtration on a manufacturing scale.

Filter Media

The choice of a filter medium for a particular operation demands considerable experience. In clarification, high filtration rates and the retention of fine particles are opposing requirements. Permeability and retentive capacity can be determined and used to supply small-scale experiments with the materials to be filtered. The necessary facilities are often made available by filter manufacturers. Other relevant factors are the contamination of the filtrate by the medium and associated housing, the adsorption of materials from solutions and, where necessary, the ability of the medium to withstand repeated sterilization.

In cake filtration, the medium must oppose excessive penetration and promote the formation of a junction with the cake to high permeability. The medium should also give free discharge of cake after washing and dewatering.

Rigid Media

Rigid media may be loose or fixed. The former is exemplified by the deposition of a filter aid on a suitable support. Filtration characteristics are governed mainly by particle size, size distribution, and shape in a manner described earlier. These factors may be varied for different filtering requirements.

Fixed media vary from perforated metals used for coarse straining to the removal of very fine particles with a sintered aggregate of metal, ceramic, plastic, or glass powder. The size, size distribution, and shape of the powder particles together with the sintering conditions control the size and distribution of the pores in the final product. The permeability may be expressed in terms of the coefficient given in Eq. (23). Alternatively, the medium may be characterized by air permeability. The maximum pore size, which is important in the selection of filters for sterilization, may be determined by measuring the pressure difference required to blow a bubble of air through the medium while it supports a column of liquid with a known surface tension. Full details of methods used for the measurement of air permeability and maximum pore diameter are given in *British Standard*, BS 1752, 1963.

Flexible Media

Flexible media may be woven or unwoven. Filter media woven from cotton, wool, synthetic and regenerated fibers, and glass and metal fibers are used as septa in cake filtration. Cotton is the most widely used natural fiber, nylon is predominant among synthetic fibers. Terylene is a useful medium for acid filtration. Penetration and cake discharge are influenced by twisting and plying of fibers and by the adoption of various weaves such as duck and twill. The choice of a particular cloth often depends on the chemical nature of the slurry.

Nonwoven media, in the form of felts and compressed cellulose pulps, are used for clarification by depth filtration. Unless carefully prepared, they have the disadvantage of losing fibrous material from the downstream side of the filter. The application of sheet media has already been discussed. High wet strength is conferred on paper sheets by resin impregnation. An alternative technique employs asbestos fibers supported in a cellulose framework.

Air Filtration

Removal of particulate matter from air, together with the control of humidity, temperature, and distribution, comprise air-conditioning. Solid and liquid particles are most commonly removed by filtration, although other methods, such as electrostatic precipitation, cyclones, and scrubbers, are used under some circumstances. The objective may be simply the provision of comfortable, healthy work conditions or may be dictated by the operations proceeding in the area. Some industrial processes demand large volumes of clean air.

The objective of air filtration is the reduction in number or complete removal of bacteria. It is applied, with varying stringency, to several operations associated with pharmacy. Where sterilization is the objective and the presence of inanimate particles is of secondary importance, other methods, such as ultraviolet (UV) radiation and heating must be added.

Bacteria rarely exist singly in the atmosphere but are usually associated with much larger particles. For example, it has been shown that 78% of particles carrying *C. welchii* were greater than 4.2 μm [15], with the average diameter exceeding 10 μm. On this basis, it has been suggested that air filters which are 99.9% efficient at 5 μm are adequate for filtration of air supplied to operating theaters and dressing wards [16]. On the other hand, filters used to clean air supplied to large-scale aerobic fermentation cultures must offer a very low probability that any organism will penetrate during the process. This became important in the deep-culture production of penicillin, where the ingress of a single penicillinase-producing organism could be disastrous. Similarly, stringent conditions are laid down for the supply of air to areas where sterile products are prepared and handled.

Mechanism of Air Filtration

A theoretical foundation for the filtration of air by passage through fibrous media was laid in the early 1930s by studies of the flow of suspended particles around various obstacles. In studies of the filtration of smokes [17,18] it has been shown that the following factors operate simultaneously in the arrest of a particle during its passage through a filter, although their relative importance varies with the type of filter and the conditions under which it is operated.

- Diffusion effects due to Brownian movement
- Electrostatic attraction between particles and fibers
- Direct interception of a particle by a fiber
- Interception as a result of inertial effects acting on a particle and causing it to collide with a fiber
- Settling and gravitational effects

Air filters operate under conditions of streamline flow as indicated by the streamlines drawn around a cylindrical fiber, shown in cross section in Fig. 22. It was assumed that capture of a particle takes place if any contact is made during its movement around the fiber. Once captured, the particle is not reentrained in the air stream and deposited deeper in the bed. Support for this assumption has been found by using an atomized suspension of *Staph. albus* and spores of *B. subtilis* [19]. Nevertheless, some fiber filters are treated with viscous oils, presumably to make capture more positive and to reduce reentrainment.

If a particle remains in a streamline during passage around the fiber, it is captured only if the radius of the particle exceeds the distance between the streamline and the fiber, a dimension dependent on the diameters of the particle and the fiber. This mechanism, termed "capture by direct interception," is independent of the air velocity, except insofar as the streamlines are modified by changes in air velocity.

Deviation of particles from streamlines can occur in a number of ways [18,20]. The chance of capture increases if Brownian movement causes appreciable migration across streamlines, an effect only important for small particles (less than 0.5 μm) and low air speeds, when the time span spent in the vicinity of a fiber is relatively long. These conditions also apply to capture which is the result of electrostatic attraction.

The inertial mechanism depends on the mass of the particle, the fiber diameter, and the velocity of approach. The particle deviates from the streamline and follows the

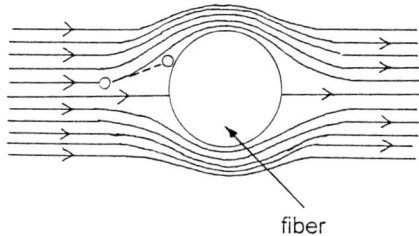

FIG. 22. Inertial capture of a particle by a fiber.

broken line shown in Fig. 22. Capture occurs if the deviation, which increases as the mass and velocity of the particle increase, brings the particle into contact with the fiber.

The simultaneous operation of mechanisms, at least one of which demands low air speeds and fine particles for effectiveness and another which requires large particles traveling at high speeds, suggests that maximum penetration could occur at an intermediate air speed. Conversely, there is, for any given condition, an optimal particle size for which the combined filtration effects are a minimum and penetration is a maximum. The former was confirmed with the help of various inanimate aerosols. A diagrammatic representation of the interaction of mechanisms is shown in Fig. 23.

Similar effects were demonstrated for bacterial aerosols [22] in a study of the efficiency with which a glass fiber mat collected *B. subtilis* spores atomized as particles just over a micrometer in radius (Fig. 24). A theoretical approach to the removal of industrial dusts has been developed [23–25].

Design, Operation, and Testing of Air Filters

Granular beds, fibrous media, and "absolute filters" prepared from cellulose and asbestos are used for high-efficiency air filtration. With fibrous and granular filters, the fractional reduction in particle content is assumed to be the same through successive incremental thicknesses of the filter, expressed by Eq. (25),

$$\frac{dC}{dx} = -kC \qquad (25)$$

where C represents the number of particles entering a section of thickness dx. The constant, k, is a measure of the filter's ability to retain a particle. It is a complex func-

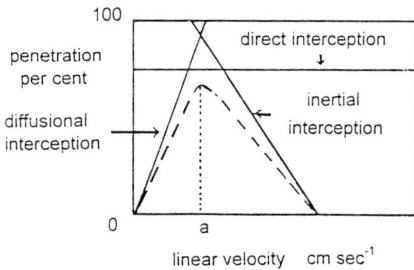

FIG. 23. Interaction of the mechanisms of particle arrest.

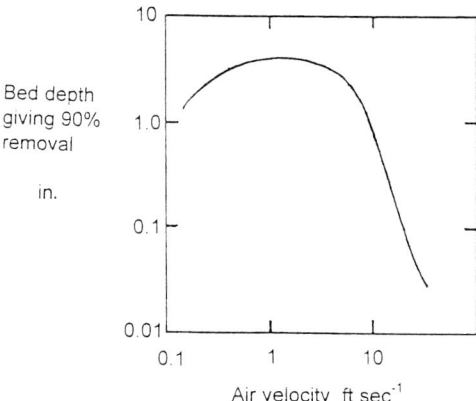

FIG. 24. Effect of airstream velocity on the removal of bacterial spores by a filter.

tion of fiber diameter, interfiber distance, and the operational air velocity. Integration between inlet and outlet conditions gives Eq. (26).

$$\log \frac{C_{\text{out}}}{C_{\text{in}}} = -kx \qquad (26)$$

The use of this log penetration effect in filter design has been described elsewhere [27]. If a certain filter thickness is capable of retaining 90% of the entering particles and 10^6 particles enter, 10^5 penetrate. If six thicknesses are used, Eq. (26) predicts that only one particle penetrates. The log-penetration effect has been confirmed for fibrous filters [22] and granular beds [28]. It must be stressed, however, that both fibrous and granular filters present passages very much greater than the fine particles they remove. Absolute sterility or absolute filtration at a certain particle size cannot be achieved. However, design variables, such as fiber diameter, the density with which fibers are packed, the thickness of the filter, and the air speed may be varied to give, for example, air which for a given input contamination is, with a high statistical probability, sterile.

In an earlier study, Terjesen and Cherryl [19] used a bacterial aerosol and a Bourdillon slit sampler to test the suitability of filters for air sterilization. They showed that 3-in. slabs of slag wool, composed of fibers most of which were less than 6 μm in diameter and compressed to a suitable density, gave sterile air when operated for 15 days at a face velocity of 0.5 ft/s. A similar efficiency was found for filters composed of glass fibers of similar diameters [28]. Resin-bonded filter mats composed of glass fibers, 12–13 μm in diameter, have also been described. A number of these mats, assembled to give a filter 12 in. deep, were effective in the removal of bacteria.

Bacteria may be effectively removed by passing air through deep granular beds of activated carbon, alumina, and other materials. Table 1 gives data on the efficiency of alumina in a bed 15 in. deep for the removal of *Serratia marcescens* from air [29]. The effect of two design variables, granule size and air speed is illustrated.

The extremely hazardous nature of radioactive dusts has promoted the design of high-efficiency air filters for establishments where such materials are handled. These filters may be used for any application requiring extremely pure air. The evolution of filters

TABLE 1 Removal of *Seratia marcescens* by a 15-in. (38 cm) Bed of Alumina Granules[a]

Air Velocity ft/min (m/s)	Efficiency, Percent Removal	
	8–16 Mesh[b]	16–32 Mesh[c]
80 (0.4)	—	92
240 (1.2)	88	99.4
480 (2.4)	98.7	99.9
720 (3.6)	99.86	—

[a]From Ref. 29.
[b]1–2 mm.
[c]0.5–1 mm.

which remove 99.995% of particles in the range of 0.1 to 0.5 μm has been described by White and Smith [30]. A medium in paper form was constructed from cellulose and asbestos. This could be pleated around corrugated spacers to give a large filtering area in a relatively small space. A paper, composed of very fine glass fibers, was later developed which resisted temperatures of up to 500°C and could, therefore, be sterilized.

The general object of design in all filters is the virtual certainty of removing the particles under consideration with a medium offering minimal resistance to the flow of air. Unlike liquid clarifiers, air filters become more efficient with time because accumulation of particles restricts the passages through the medium. This deposition causes an increase in the pressure differential required to maintain a given flow rate. When the filter has become laden with the certain amount of dust, it must be cleaned or replaced. The life of high-efficiency air filters may be lengthened by passing the air first through a coarse or "roughing" filter which removes the larger particles.

The use of bacterial aerosols as tracer organisms to test the efficiency of filters has already been described. Other tests with inanimate dusts are more generally used for the evaluation of filter performance. For general ventilation purposes, two tests are specified. The first determines gravimetrically the capacity of the filter to hold dust and still function satisfactorily. A standard dust of 5 or 20 μm is passed into the filter until a specified increase in air flow resistance occurs. The second test, which is also applicable to high-efficiency filters, determines the fraction of a methylene blue aerosol which passes through the filter under given conditions. The aerosol is generated by atomizing a 1% aqueous solution of methylene blue. The droplets dry to give a cloud of particles, 90% of which are below 0.2 μm. The test is therefore extremely stringent. The cloud is passed through the filter at a constant rate (30 L/min) and then through a strip of porous paper which collects any methylene blue particles that have penetrated. The stain due to the dye, after intensification in steam, is compared to a series of similar stains which correspond to known volumes of unfiltered air. Thus, if 60 L of filtered air give a stain which matches that produced by 12 mL of unfiltered air, the penetration is 0.02% [31]. Both tests are fully described in *British Standard*, BS 2831, 1957. An alternative method of evaluation penetration employs a cloud produced by the atomization of a solution of sodium chloride. After passage through the filter, part of the air is passed through a hydrogen flame. The intensity of the sodium flame produced is estimated with a photoelectric cell.

Centrifugal Operations

An object moving in a circular path is subjected to an outward centrifugal force which balances the centripetal force moving the object toward the center of rotation. This principle is used in the mechanical separations called centrifugal filtration and centrifugal sedimentation. In the former, a material is placed in a rotating perforated basket which is lined by a filter cloth used to separate a solid, which is retained at the cloth, from a liquid. It is essentially a filtration process in which the driving force is of centrifugal origin. In no way does it depend upon a difference in the density of the two phases.

In centrifugal sedimentation, the separation is due to the difference in the density of two or more phases. This is the more important process, where both solid–liquid mixtures and liquid–liquid mixtures can be completely separated. If, however, the separation is incomplete, there is a gradient in the size of the dispersed phase within the centrifuge due to the faster radial velocity of the larger particles. Operated in this way, the centrifuge becomes a classifier.

Centrifugal Filtration

The principles of filtration discussed previously can be directly applied to this process, although theoretical predictions of filtration rate and spinning time are uncertain. Centrifugal filtration is widely used for the separation of crystals and granular products from liquors but it is less effective if the slurry contains a high proportion of particles less than 100 μm. The advantages of the process are effective washing and drying. Residual moisture after centrifugation is far less than in cakes produced by pressure or vacuum filtration. By this method, the moisture content of a cake of coarse crystals can be reduced to as low as 3%. This facilitates the drying operation which normally follows. Enclosure of the centrifuge is easy, allowing toxic and volatile materials to be processed.

A typical batch filter is shown in Fig. 25a. It consists of a perforated metal basket mounted on a vertical axis. The cloth used to retain solids is often supported on a metal

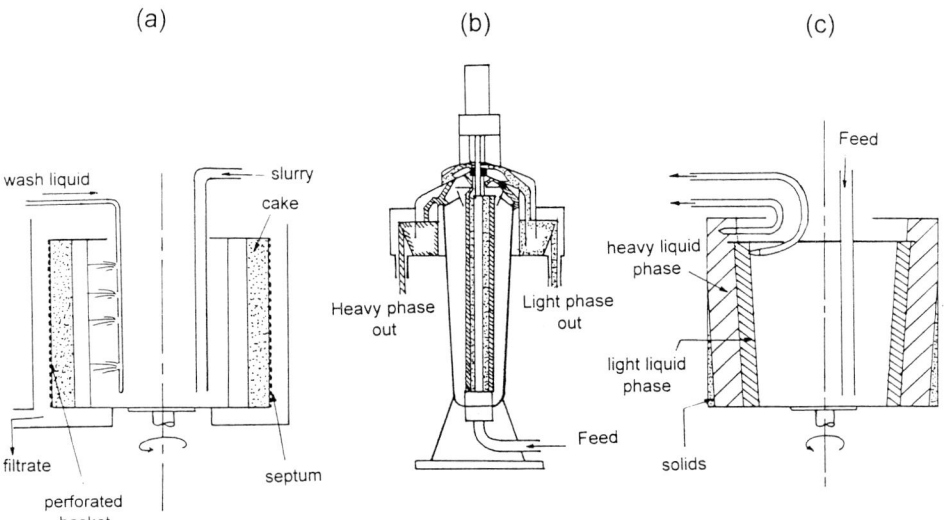

FIG. 25. (a) Batch centrifugal filter; (b) the Sharples supercentrifuge (Courtesy, Pennsalt Ltd.); (c) solid bowl batch centrifuge.

screen. Baskets mounted in the manner shown are emptied by shoveling the cake. If, however, top suspension is used, the cake can be more easily withdrawn through traps in the base of the basket. In batch operation, considerable time is lost during the acceleration and deceleration of the machine. Machines operating with continuous discharge of solids are used for separation of coarse solids for large-scale operations. Such machines are commonly constructed with a horizontal axis of rotation.

Centrifugal Sedimentation

The motion of a particle in a liquid is described by Stokes' equation. If its diameter is d, the rate u at which it settles by gravity in a liquid of viscosity η and density ρ is given by Eq. (27),

$$u = \frac{1}{18} d^2 \frac{\rho_s - \rho}{\eta} g \qquad (27)$$

where g is the acceleration due to gravity, and ρ_s is the density of the particle. In the centrifuge, the gravitational force causing separation is replaced by a centrifugal force. If the particle has a mass m and moves at an angular velocity ω in a circle of radius r, the centrifugal force is $\omega^2 r \cdot (m - m_1)$, where m_1 is the mass of the displaced ligand. The expression

$$\frac{\omega^2 r}{g}$$

is, therefore, the ratio of the centrifugal and gravitational forces in the example described above. Its value can exceed 10,000. The separation is quicker, more complete, and effective in systems containing very fine particles which do not settle by gravity because of Brownian movement.

Expressing the mass of the particle in terms of its volume and effective density, the centrifugal force can be written as in expression (28).

$$\frac{\pi}{6} d^2 (\rho_s - \rho) \omega^2 r \qquad (28)$$

In streamline conditions, the opposing viscous force is $3\pi d \eta u$, where u is the terminal velocity of the particle. Equating these expressions gives Eq. (29).

$$u = \frac{1}{18} d^2 \left(\frac{\rho_s - \rho}{\eta} \right) \omega^2 r \qquad (29)$$

The rate of sedimentation is proportional to the radius of the basket and the square of the speed at which it rotates. Centrifugal sedimentors can be divided into a number of types. For operations at very high speeds, the centrifuge bowl is tubular with a length/diameter ratio from 4 to 8. An example is the Sharples supercentrifuge illustrated in Fig. 25b. It operates up to 15,000 rpm or, in turbine-driven laboratory models, up to 50,000 rpm. The machine, which gives continuous discharge of two separated liquids, is widely used for the separation of emulsions. It is also an effective clarifier when the concentration of solids is very low. The solids are periodically discharged by scraping the walls of the centrifuge tube. Uses include the cleaning of fats and waxes, the fractionation of blood, and the recovery of viruses.

In disk-type centrifuges, baffles are introduced into the bowl in order to decrease the distance which particles travel before settling at the wall. These baffles split the liquid into a number of layers in which separation occurs. The length-to-diameter ratio is usually much lower than in tubular-bowl centrifuges, and operational speeds are also lower. In batch processes, the machine is discharged manually at intervals. Larger machines continuously or intermittently discharge the solids as a thick slurry through nozzles or valves at the periphery of the basket.

A solid-bowl batch basket is shown in Fig. 25c, where liquids are discharged by weirs or skimmers, two of which are shown, each taking off a liquid phase. Solids are discharged manually at the end of the process. In continuous models, a conveying scroll, operating at a slightly different speed from the basket, ploughs the solids to one end, discharging the material as a damp powder.

Drying

Drying may be defined as the vaporization and removal of water or other liquid from a solution, suspension, or other solid–liquid mixture to form a dry solid. The change of phase from liquid to vapor distinguishes drying from the mechanical methods of separating solids from liquids such as filtration. The latter often precede drying since, where applicable, they offer a cheaper method for removing a large part of the liquid.

Drying, as defined above, may still be confused with evaporation because the division of the two operations is, to some extent, arbitrary. Drying is normally associated with the removal of relatively small quantities of liquid to give a dry product. Evaporation is more often applied to the concentration of solutions. However, exceptions to these generalizations occur.

Adjustment and control of moisture levels by drying is important in the manufacture and development of pharmaceutical products. Apart from the obvious requirement of dry solids for many operations, drying may be carried out in order to:

- Improve handling characteristics, as in bulk powder filling and other operations involving powder flow, and
- Stabilize moisture-sensitive materials, such as aspirin and ascorbic acid.

A wide range of drying equipment is available to meet these ends, but in practice the choice is limited by the scale of the operation and may be determined partly or completely by the thermal stability of the material and the physical form in which it is required. In the pharmaceutical industry, batch sizes are frequently small and of high value, and the same drier may be used for different materials. These factors limit the application of continuous driers and promote the use of batch driers which give low product retention and are easily cleaned. Recovery of solvents, where economically justified, may be another factor affecting the choice of equipment.

Unit Processes in Pharmacy: The Operations

Theory

Theories of drying are limited in application inasmuch as drying times are normally experimentally determined. Nevertheless, an appreciation of the scope and limitations of the different drying methods is given here. The following terms are employed in discussing drying: humidity and humidity of saturated air, relative humidity, wet-bulb temperature, and adiabatic cooling line. Other terms may be defined as follows:

- Moisture Content. It is usually expressed as weight per unit weight of dry solids.
- Equilibrium Moisture Content. If a material is exposed to air at a given temperature and humidity, it will gain or lose moisture until equilibrium is reached. The moisture present at this point is defined as the equilibrium moisture content for the given exposure conditions. At a given temperature, it will vary with the partial pressure of the water vapor in the surrounding atmosphere. This is shown for a hypothetical hygroscopic material in Fig. 26 in which the equilibrium moisture content is plotted against the relative humidity. Any moisture present in excess of the equilibrium moisture content is called "free water."

Equilibrium moisture content curves vary greatly with the type of material examined. Insoluble, nonporous materials, such as talc or zinc oxide, have equilibrium moisture contents of almost zero over a wide humidity range. A moisture content between 10 and 15% may be expected for cotton fabrics under normal atmospheric conditions. Drying below the equilibrium moisture content for room conditions may be deliberately undertaken, particularly if the material is unstable in the presence of moisture; subsequent storage becomes important.

The equilibrium moisture content at 100% relative humidity represents the minimum amount of water associated with the solid which still exerts a vapor pressure equal to a separate water surface. If the humidity is reduced, only part of the water evaporates before a new equilibrium is established. The water retained at less than 100% relative humidity must, therefore, exert a vapor pressure less than that of a dissociated water

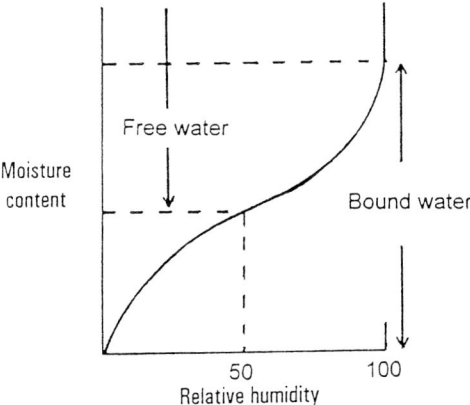

FIG. 26. The relation between equilibrium moisture content (EMC) and relative humidity for a hygroscopic solid. The broken line indicates the EMC at 50% relative humidity. If more water is present it is termed free water. The free water would be 50% removed if the material was dried with air at a relative humidity of 50%.

surface. Such water is called "bound water." Unlike the equilibrium moisture content, bound water is a function of the solid only and not of the surroundings. Bound water is usually held in small pores, confined within highly curved menisci, or it is present as a solution or adsorbed on the surface of the solid.

The value of equilibrium moisture content curves is illustrated by the examples given in Fig. 27. The equilibrium moisture content of the antacid granules, composed of magnesium trisilicate granulated with syrup, is a sensitive function of relative humidity. If it is to be dried to a moisture content of 3%, air at a relative humidity of less than 35% must be used. With a knowledge of the humidity of the circulating air, psychometric charts may be used to determine the minimum air temperature which will dry the material to the required standard. (In fact, the temperature has an effect on the equilibrium moisture content which is independent of the humidity, but this can be neglected to a first approximation.) The lactose granulation, on the other hand, has a low sensitivity to relative humidity. Drying at low relative humidities derived from high air temperatures causes only a marginal decrease in the final moisture content, and the stability of the active ingredients associated with the lactose filler could be impaired. This argument is only concerned with the final moisture content. It is not related to the rate of drying which would, of course, be higher at higher temperatures and lower humidities.

The effects of storage after drying may also be assessed from the equilibrium moisture content curves. Storage conditions are not critical for the lactose granulation [32,33]. If the antacid formulation is stored at a relative humidity of only 65% it would, given sufficient time, absorb moisture until the content was 9%. This could be associated with poor flow characteristics and its attendant difficulties during compression.

Evaporation of Water into an Air Stream

The evaporation of moisture into a warm air stream, with the latter providing the latent heat of evaporation, is a common drying mechanism although it is not easily adapted to the recovery of the liquid. In the evaporation from a liquid surface which, with the passage of air, falls to the wet bulb temperature corresponding to the temperature and

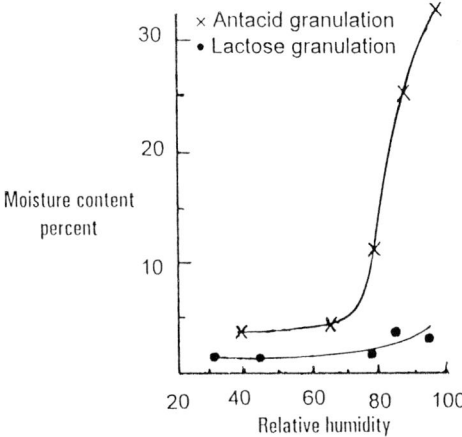

FIG. 27. Equilibrium moisture content curves for two tablet granulations, antacid and lactose.

Unit Processes in Pharmacy: The Operations

humidity of the air, the rate at which water vapor is transferred from the saturated layer at the surface to the drying stream is described by Eq. (15),

$$N = \frac{k_g}{RT}(P_{wi} - P_{wa})$$

where P_{wi} is the partial pressure of the water vapor at the surface, P_{wa} is the partial pressure of water vapor in the air, k_g is a mass transfer coefficient, and N the number of moles vapor transferred from unit area in unit time. Rewriting this in terms of the total mass, W, transferred in unit time from the entire drying surface A gives Eq. (16),

$$W = \frac{M_w A}{RT} k_g (P_{wi} - P_{wa})$$

where M_w is the molecular weight of water vapor, R is the gas constant, and T the absolute temperature. The mass transfer coefficient, k_g, is a function of the temperature, the air velocity, and the angle of air incidence. A high velocity or angle of incidence diminishes the thickness of the stationary air layer in contact with the liquid surface and therefore lowers the diffusional resistance.

The rate of evaporation may also be expressed in terms of the heat transferred across the laminar film from the drying gases to the surface, as shown in Eq. (14),

$$Q = hA(T_a - T_s)$$

where Q is the rate of heat transfer, A is the area of the surface, T_a and T_s are the temperatures of the drying air and the surface, respectively, and h is the heat transfer coefficient. The last is also a function of air velocity and the angle of impingement. If the latent heat of evaporation is λ, this affords a mass transfer rate, W, which is given by Eq. (30).

$$W = \frac{hA}{\lambda}(T_a - T_g) \tag{30}$$

Equilibrium drying conditions are represented by the equality of Eqs. (16) and (30). When these conditions pertain to drying, the surface temperature, T_s, which is the wet-bulb temperature, is normally much lower than the temperature of the drying gases. This is of great importance in the drying of thermolabile materials. If solids are present in the surface, the rate of evaporation is modified, the overall effect depending on the structure of the solids and the moisture content.

Static Beds of Nonporous Solids

The drying of wet granular beds containing nonporous particles which are insoluble in the wetting liquid, has been extensively studied. The operation is presented as the relation of moisture content and time of drying in Fig. 28a. It should be noted that the equilibrium moisture content is approached slowly. A protracted period may be required for the removal of water just above the equilibrium value. This is not justified if a small amount of water can be tolerated in further processing and indicates the importance of establishing realistic drying requirements. The stability of the solids, maintained, as shown later, at a temperature close to that of the drying air, may result in unnecessary deterioration.

The data have been converted to a curve relating the rate of drying to moisture content in Fig. 28b. The initial heating period during which equilibrium is established is short and has been omitted from both figures. Assuming that sufficient moisture is initially present, the drying-rate curve exhibits three distinct sections limited by the points A, B, C, and D. In section A-B, called the constant-rate period, moisture is evaporating from a saturated surface at a rate governed by the diffusion from the surface through the stationary air film in contact with it. An analogy with evaporation from a plain water surface can therefore be drawn and Eqs. (16) and (18) apply. The rate of drying during this period depends upon the air temperature, humidity, and speed, which, in turn, determine the temperature of the saturated surface. Assuming that these are constant, all variables in the drying equations given above are fixed, and a constant rate of drying is established which is largely independent of the material being dried. The drying rate is somewhat lower than for a free-water surface and depends to some extent on the particle size of the solids. During the constant-rate period, liquid must be transported to the surface at a rate sufficiently high to maintain saturation. The mechanism of transport is discussed later.

At the end of the constant-rate period, B, a break in the drying curve occurs. This point is called the critical moisture content, and a linear fall in the drying rate occurs with further drying. This section, B-C, is called the first falling-rate period. At and below the critical moisture contel, the movement of moisture from the interior is no longer sufficient to saturate the surface. As drying proceeds, moisture reaches the surface at a decreasing rate and the mechanism which controls its transfer influences the rate of drying. Since the surface is no longer saturated, it tends to rise above the wet bulb temperature.

For any material, the critical moisture content decreases as the particle size decreases. Eventually, moisture ceases to reach the surface which becomes dry. The plane of evaporation recedes into the solid, the vapor reaching the surface by diffusion through

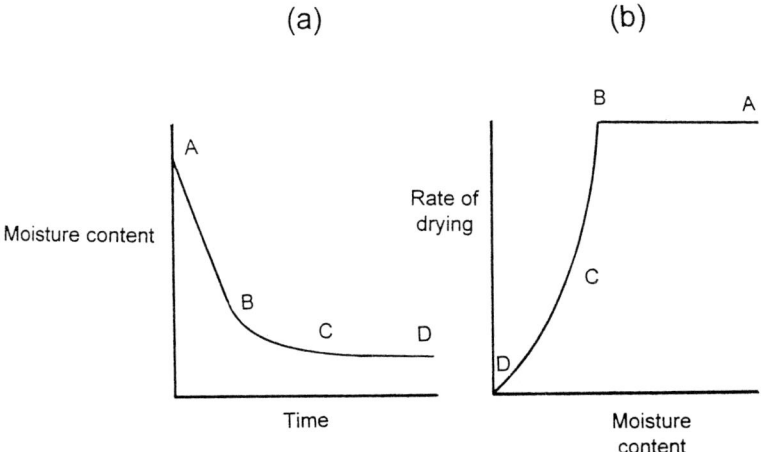

FIG. 28. (a) Relation of moisture content and time of drying; (b) rate of drying and moisture content.

Unit Processes in Pharmacy: The Operations

the pores of the bed. This section is called the second falling-rate period and is controlled by vapor diffusion, a factor which is largely independent of the conditions outside the bed but markedly affected by the particle size due to its influence on the dimensions of pores and channels. During this period, the surface temperature approaches the temperature of the drying air.

Considerable migration of liquid occurs during the constant-rate and first falling-rate periods. Associated with the liquid is any soluble constituent which forms a concentrating solution in the surface layers as drying proceeds. Deposition of these materials takes place when the surface dries. Considerable segregation of soluble elements in the cake can occur, therefore, during drying. These effects have been fully investigated [34].

If the soluble matter forms a skin or gel on drying rather than a crystalline deposit, a different drying curve (Fig. 29) is obtained. The constant-rate period is followed by a continuous fall in the drying rate in which no differentiation of first and second falling-rate periods can be made. During this period, drying is controlled by diffusion through the skin which is continually increasing in thickness. Soap and gelatin behave in this way.

The Internal Mechanism of Drying

Extensive studies have been made to determine the nature of the forces which initially convey moisture to the surface at a rate sufficient to maintain saturation and their subsequent failure. Movement of liquid may occur by diffusion under the concentration gradient created by depletion of water at the surface by evaporation, as the result of capillary forces, through a cycle of vaporization and condensation, or by osmotic effects. Of these, capillary forces offer a coherent explanation for the drying periods of many materials.

If a tapered capillary is filled with water and exposed to a current of air, the meniscus at the smaller end remains stationary while the tube empties from the wider end. A similar situation exists in a wet particulate bed and the phenomenon is explained by the concept of suction potential. A negative pressure exists below the meniscus of a curved liquid surface which is proportional to the surface tension, γ, and inversely proportional to the radius of curvature, r. (The meniscus is assumed to be a part of a

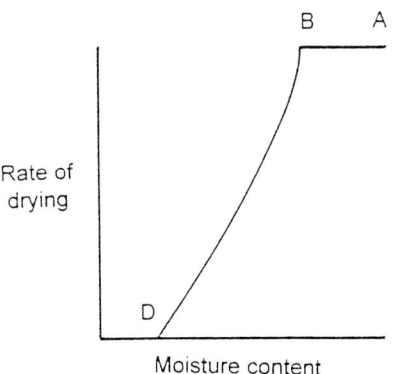

FIG. 29. Drying curve for a skin-forming material.

hemisphere.) This negative pressure or suction potential may be expressed as the height of liquid, expressed by Eq. (31),

$$h = \frac{2\gamma}{\rho g r} \qquad (31)$$

where ρ is the density of the liquid.

The suction potential, h_x, acting at a depth x below the meniscus is given by Eq. (32).

$$h_x = h - x \qquad (32)$$

The particles of the bed enclose spaces called pores connected by passages, the narrowest part of which is called the waist. The dimensions of the latter are determined by the size of the surrounding particles and the manner in which they are packed. In a randomly packed bed, pores and waists of varying sizes are found. Thus, the radius of a capillary running through the bed varies continuously. The depletion of water in this network is controlled by the waists because the radii of curvature are smaller and the suction potentials are greater than for the pores. Depletion occurs in the following way. As evaporation proceeds, the water surface recedes into the waists of the top layer of particles and a suction potential develops. The maximum suction potential a waist can develop is called its "entry" suction potential. This is exceeded for the larger waists by the suction potential developed by the smaller waists and transmitted through the continuous, connecting thread of liquid. The menisci in the larger waists collapse and the pores they protect are emptied, that is, a surface waist developing a suction potential, h_s, will, assuming an interconnecting thread of liquid, cause the collapse of an interior waist developing a suction potential h_i and distance x below the surface if $h_s > (h_i + x)$. The liquid in the exposed pores is lost at the surface by evaporation. This effect continues until a waist provides an opposing suction potential which is equal to or greater than the suction potential provided at that depth by the fine surface waist meniscus. The latter collapses and the pore it protects is emptied.

By this mechanism, a meniscus in a fine surface waist holds it position and depletes the interior of moisture. If sufficient full surface waists are present, the constant-rate period is maintained since the stationary air film in contact with the bed can be saturated. The first falling-rate period indicates that insufficient full-surface waists are present. Eventually, the collapse of all surface waists takes place, giving a breakdown of the capillary network supplying moisture to the surface, and the second falling-rate period ensues. The application of this mechanism has been describe fully eslewhere [35,36].

Static Beds of Porous Solids

The drying curve, obtained when the particles that compose the beds are themselves porous, is shown in Fig. 30. It differs from the curve obtained with nonporous materials inasmuch as the constant-rate period is shorter. The drying rate may be higher and is almost independent of particle size. The critical moisture content is a function of both pore size and particle size. During the first falling-rate period (Fig. 30a), the rate of drying falls steeply due, it is thought, to the drying of the surface granules. The sec-

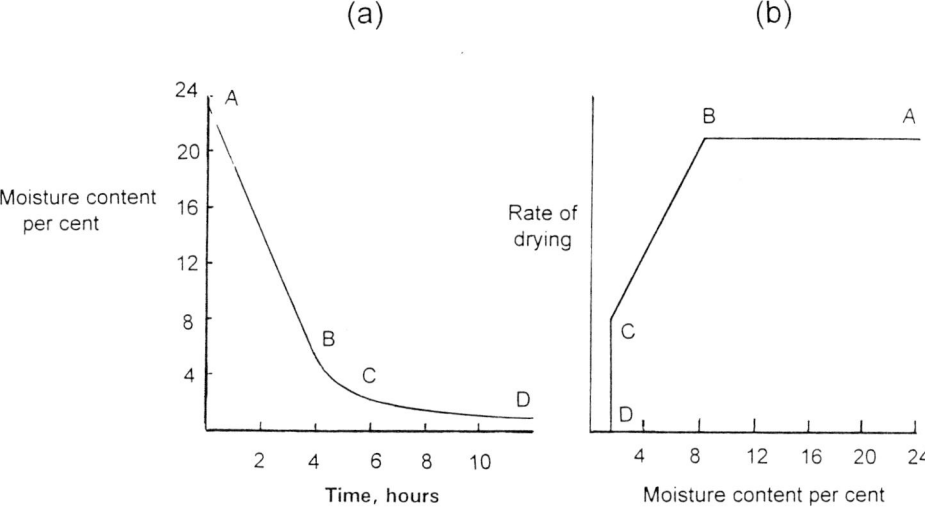

FIG. 30. Drying curves for a tablet granulation dried in a tray drier. (a) Moisture content vs. time; (b) drying rate vs. moisture content.

ond falling-rate period (Fig. 30b) is influenced by the diffusion of moisture from within the particles. The internal mechanism of drying beds of porous particles has been discussed by Corben and Newitt [37].

Through Air-Circulation Drying

If the particles are in a suitable granular form, it is often possible to pass the air stream downward through the bed of solids. Drying follows the pattern described previously, except that each particle or agglomerate behaves as a drying bed. The surface area exposed to the drying gases is greatly increased, and the drying rates are 10 to 20 times higher than those encountered when air is passed over a free surface.

Methods Involving Movement of the Solid

As an extension of drying by passing the air stream through a static bed of solids, it is possible to project air upward through the bed at a velocity high enough to fluidize the particles. Alternatively, the material may be mechanically subdivided and introduced into the drying stream. Both methods give high drying rates due to high interfacial contact between the drying surfaces and the air stream. Fluidized bed driers and spray driers, respectively, are based on these principles.

Other Methods of Drying

Apart from specialized driers using infrared or dielectric heating, the chief method of passing heat into a drying solid, other than from a hot air stream, is by conduction from a heated surface. When a wet solid is placed in contact with a hot surface, subsequent events depend on the temperature of the surface relative to the boiling point of the liquid, the nature of the solid, and the method of heating the surface. It is assumed here that the temperature of the surface is not hot enough for convective boiling to take place.

Considering a cake of finely divided solids saturated with water, a temperature gradient is established through the cake and evaporation from the free surface takes place at a rate governed entirely by the rate of heat input. During this period, the rate of evaporation and the temperature of a particular layer of cake are approximately constant. This continues until capillary forces are unable to transfer liquid to the free surface at the required rate. The temperature gradients during this period are given in Figs. 31a and 31b for conditions in which the shelf temperature is below and above the boiling point of the liquid, respectively.

With a heat flux so low that the partially dried cake can conduct heat away from the hot surface at the required rate, the free surface dries and a fictitious drying line recedes slowly into the cake, the vapor diffusing through the dry cake to the free surface. The temperature gradient during this falling rate period is shown in Fig. 31c. If the heat flux is high, the point at which mobile water can no longer reach the surface is marked by the onset of drying in a layer adjacent to the hot surface and vapor is forced through the wet cake above. As the solid dries, its temperature increases and a temperature gradient is established through the dry solids to the drying line which is receding upward (Fig. 31d). The free surface of the solid appears wet and is at a con-

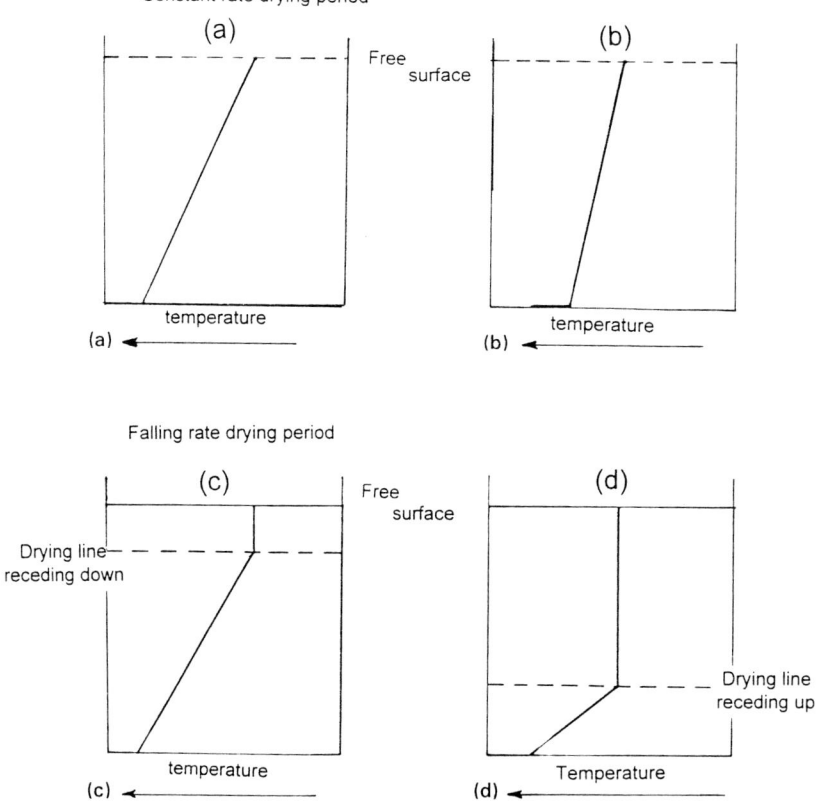

FIG. 31. Drying by conduction of heat from a heated surface.

stant temperature. These conditions are destroyed when the drying line reaches the surface.

In either case, a low and falling rate of drying persists as the absorbed water is removed. In this form of drying, the heat treatment received by the solid is not uniform but depends on its position in the cake.

A hot surface may also be used to dry solutions, such as milk or plant extracts, which do not readily give porous, crystalline solids on concentration. Apart from an initial constant-rate period, when heat transfer is mainly convective, drying periods are ill defined. As concentration proceeds, the liquor becomes more viscous and heat transfer is mainly by conduction. Large volume changes occur between initial and final stages. It is possible to dry thin films of solution to a solid film, but if deeper layers are taken, a skin is frequently formed at the free surface which is almost impervious to the vapor and frothing, and drying to a porous, friable structures occur. This may also happen if, during the upward recession of the drying line, the material above is too viscous to allow the escape of vapor.

Solids Moving Over a Hot Surface

Conditions in which the solids move over a heated surface are employed in tumbling and agitated driers. Drying rates are higher than those obtained in static beds because fresh solids are continually exposed to the hot surface. The heat treatment received by the solid is more uniform.

Batch Driers

Hot Air Ovens

Ovens operating by passing hot air over the surface of a wet solid which is spread over trays arranged in racks, provide the simplest and cheapest drier. In small installations, the air is passed over electrically heated elements and once through the oven. Larger units may employ steam-heated, finned tubes, and thermal efficiency is improved by recirculating the air. This is controlled by manually set dampers, and a common operating position gives 90% recirculation and 10% bleed-off. The heater blank is placed in such a position that the solids do not receive radiant heat and incoming air may be filtered. A typical hot air oven is illustrated in Fig. 32a.

The temperature–humidity sequence of the circulating drying air is shown in Fig. 32b. The incoming air, at a temperature and humidity given by point A, is heated at constant humidity to point B and passed over the wet solid. The humidity rises and the temperature falls as the adidabatic cooling line is followed until the air leaves the tray in condition C. It is then recirculated to the heater; two further cycles are shown in Fig. 32b.

It has been assumed here that all heat is drawn from the air and transmitted across the stationary air layer in contact with the drying surface, as described earlier. Surface temperatures are, in fact, modified by heat absorbed and conducted from unwetted surfaces, such as the underside of the tray, and by radiation.

The chief advantage of the hot air oven, apart from its low initial cost, is its versatility. With the exception of dusty solids, materials of almost any physical form may be dried. Thermostatically controlled air temperatures between 40 and 120°C permit

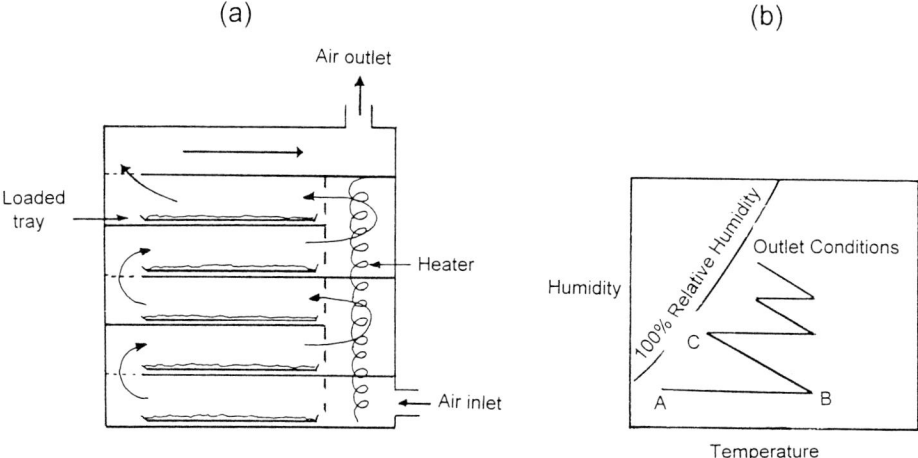

FIG. 32. Hot air oven. (a) A tray drier; (b) changes in the humidity and temperature of air circulating in an idealized tray drier.

heat-sensitive materials to be dried. For small batches, a hot air oven is, therefore, often the equipment of choice. However, the following inherent limitations have led to the development of other small driers:

- A large floor space is required for the oven and tray loading facilities.
- Labor costs for loading and unloading the oven are high.
- Long drying times, usually of the order of 24 h, are necessary.
- Solvents can be recovered from the air only with difficulty.
- Unless carefully designed, nonuniform distribution of air over the trays results in variations in temperature and drying times within the oven. Variations of ± 7°C in temperature have been found from location to location during the drying of tablet granules [38]. Poor air circulation may permit local saturation and the cessation of drying.

An extensive analysis of tray drying and the effect of operational variables has been given by Shepherd et al. [39].

If the material is of suitable granular form, drying times may be reduced to 1 h or less by passing the air downward through the material laid on mesh trays. The oven in this form is called a batch through-circulation drier.

Vacuum Tray Driers

Vacuum tray driers, as shown in Fig. 33a differing only in size from the familiar laboratory vacuum oven, offer an alternative method for drying small quantities of material. When scaled up, construction becomes massive to withstand the applied vacuum and cost is further increased by the associated vacuum equipment. Vacuum tray driers are, therefore, only used when a definite advantage over the hot air oven is secured, such as low temperature drying of thermolabile materials or the recovery of solvents from the bed. The exclusion of oxygen may also be advantageous or necessary in some operations.

Unit Processes in Pharmacy: The Operations

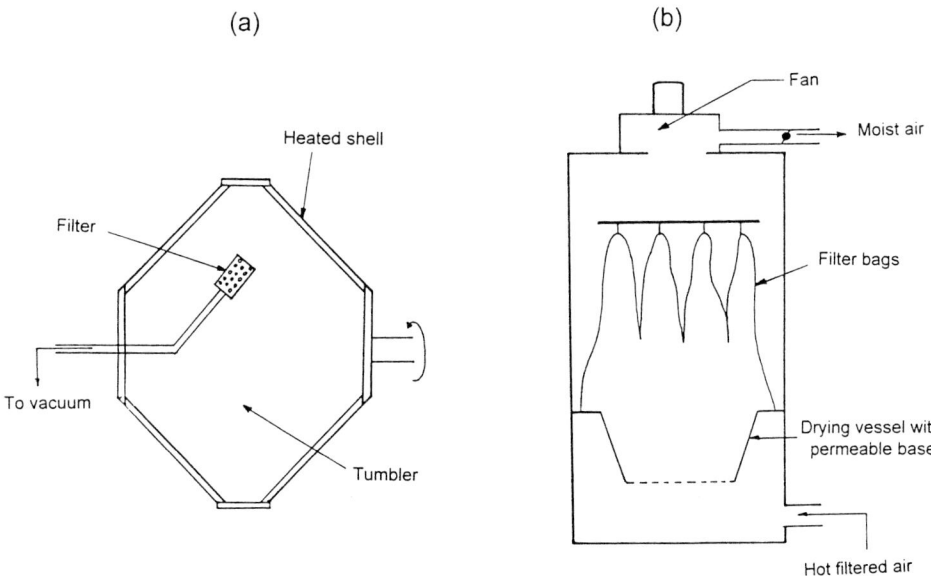

FIG. 33. Vacuum tray driers. (a) Rotary vacuum drier; (b) fluidized-bed drier.

Heat is usually supplied by passing steam or hot water through hollow shelves. Drying temperatures can be carefully controlled and, for most of the drying cycle, the material remains at the boiling point of the wetting liquid under the operating vacuum. Radiation from the shelf above may cause a significant increase in temperature at the surface of the material if high drying temperatures are used. Drying times are long, usually of the order of 12 to 48 h.

Tumbling Driers

The limitations of ovens, particularly with respect to the long drying times, has, where possible, promoted the design and application of other batch driers. The simplest of these is the tumbler drier; its most common shape, the double cone, is shown in Fig. 33a [40]. Operating under vacuum, it provides controlled low temperature drying, the possibility of solvent recovery, and increased drying rates. Heat is supplied to the tumbling charge by contact with the heated shell and heat transfer through the vapor. Optimum conditions are established experimentally by varying the vacuum, the temperature and, if the material passes through a sticky stage, the speed of rotation. With correct operation, a uniform powder should be obtained as distinct from the cakes produced when static beds are dried. Some materials, such as waxy solids, cannot be dried by this method because the tumbling action causes the material to aggregate into balls [40].

A normal charge would be about 60% of the total volume and, for driers 2–7 ft (0.6–2 m) in diameter, drying times of 2 to 12 h may be expected. In studying the application of tumbler driers to drying tablet granules, periods of 2–3.5 h were sufficient instead of 18 h required by hot air ovens [41]. The mixing and granulating capacity of the tumbling action has suggested that these operations could precede drying in the same apparatus.

Fluidized-Bed Driers

The term "fluidization" is applied to processes in which a loose, porous bed of solids is converted to a fluid system, having the properties of surface leveling, flow, and pressure-depth relationships, by passing the fluid up through the bed.

Fluidized-bed techniques, employing air as the fluidizing medium, have been successfully applied to the drying of solids of the suitable physical form. The high interfacial contact between drying air and solids gives drying rates 10 to 20 times higher than those obtained during tray drying. Drying curves for this method are shown in Fig. 34.

The drier, illustrated in Fig. 33b, consists of a basket of plastic or stainless steel with a perforated bottom which is mounted in the body of the drier and into which the material to be dried is placed. Heated air may be blown or sucked through the bed. The air leaving the basket passes through an air filter and may be recirculated. Particle properties, such as shape and size distribution, affect fluidization and a unit must have a variable air flow, adjusted in such a way that the material is fluidized but not carried into the filters. For this reason, the material must have a fairly close size range to avoid elutriation of fine particles into the filters.

Fluidized-bed driers are particularly suitable for granulated materials and are being increasingly used for tablet granulations, providing that product changeover is not too frequent. It may be advantageous to preform other materials, such as a dewatered filter cake, into granules solely in order to employ fluidized-bed drying. If the conditions are ideal for fluidizing, the granulation does not require further grinding. Tray driers, on the other hand, produce a caked product which may require mild comminution. Variation in temperature, which may be quite marked in tray driers, is virtually eliminated in fluidized-bed driers by the intense mixing action. The floor space for a given capacity is small compared with that for a tray drier. Machines vary in size, handling up to 250 kg. Drying times, maximum, minimum, and optimum air velocities, air temperature, and the tendency to cake and channel are established experimentally as those

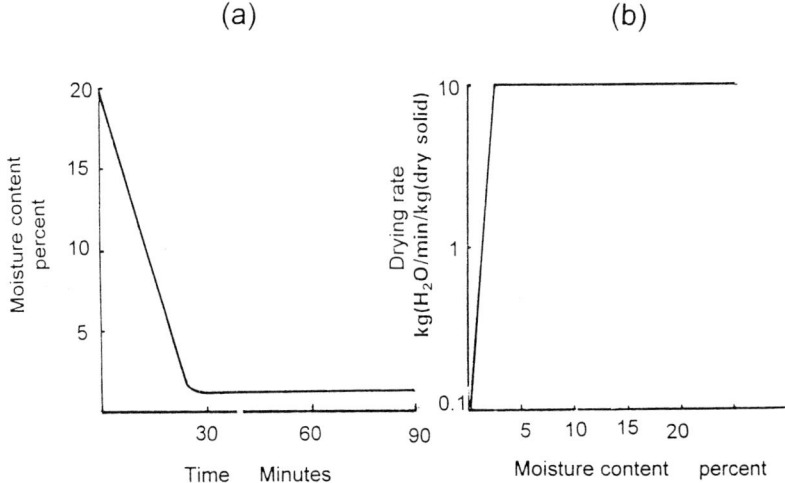

FIG. 34. Drying curves obtained during fluidized-bed drying of a tablet granulation. (a) Moisture content vs. time; (b) drying rate vs. moisture content.

cannot be predicted accurately at present.

Erosion and the production of large amounts of fines might be expected from the intense turbulent movement, but experience shows that the opposite occurs. The particles are to some extent "padded" by the surrounding fluid in such a way that there is little contact between particles or that the impact energy is low.

Agitated Batch Dryers

Agitated batch driers consist of a jacketed cylindrical vessel with agitator blades designed to scrape the bottom and walls. They may operate at atmospheric pressure or under vacuum. Pasty materials that could not be handled in tumbling or fluidized-bed driers, may be successfully dried at rates higher than can be achieved in an oven.

Freeze Drying

Freeze drying is an extreme form of vacuum drying in which the solid is frozen and drying takes place by subliming the solid phase [42–46] at low temperatures and pressures. Establishing and maintaining these conditions, together with the low drying rates obtained, constitutes the most expensive method of drying which is only used on a large scale when other methods are inadequate.

Freeze drying is extensively used when rapid decomposition occurs during normal drying. Another application concerns substances that can be dried at high temperatures but are thereby changed in some way. Fruit juices, for example, are reputed to lose subtle elements of flavor and odor, and proteinaceous materials are partly denatured by the concentration and higher temperatures associated with conventional drying. Drying of blood plasma and some antibiotics are important large-scale applications of freeze drying. On a smaller scale, it is widely used for the dehydration of bacteria, vaccines, blood fractions, and tissues.

Freeze drying is theoretically a simple technique. Pure ice exhibits an equilibrium vapor pressure of 4.6 mm Hg (611 Pa) at 0°C and 0.1 mm Hg (13.3 Pa) at –40°C. The vapor pressure of ice containing dissolved substances is, of course, lower. If, however, the pressure above the frozen solution is less than its equilibrium vapor pressure, the ice sublimes, eventually leaving the solute as a sponge-like residue equal in apparent volume to the original solid and, therefore, of low bulk density. The latter is readily dissolved by adding water, and therefore freeze drying has been called "lyophilic drying" or "lyophilization." No concentration in the normal sense of the word occurs and structural changes in, for example, protein solutions, are minimized.

In practice, many difficulties are encountered. Under conditions of high vacuum, water vapor must be trapped or eliminated. To maintain drying, heat must be supplied to the frozen solid to balance the latent heat of sublimation without melting the frozen solid. Difficulties become acute if a product like blood plasma is dried in the final container under aseptic conditions.

In the first stage of the process, the material is cooled and frozen. If the temperature of a dilute solution of a salt is slowly reduced, leveling occurs in the time–temperature curve just below 0°C due to the liberation of the latent heat of fusion of ice, and pure ice separates. With further cooling, the solution becomes concentrated until the eutectic mixture is formed which freezes, resulting in a plateau in the cooling curve. This is a clear indication of complete freezing. If the concentration of the liquid eutectic mixture is low, the material may appear to be completely frozen at higher temperatures. Under these conditions, some drying from a liquid phase occurs, possibly with damaging results. This can be detected by measuring the electrical resistance of the ice which becomes infinitely high at the freezing point of the eutectic mixture. Conversely, thawing markedly reduces resistance, an effect that can be used to automatically control the state of the drying solid. Protein solutions do not give clearly defined eutectic points and are usually frozen to below −25°C before drying. Freezing is carried out quickly to prevent concentration of the solution and produce fine ice crystals. Some degree of supercooling may be induced followed by a very quick freeze. Freezing may or may not be carried out in the drying chamber. If drying in final containers is necessary, small-scale operations may employ immersion in a coolant such as liquid air or isopentane. For larger-scale installations a blast of very cold air may be used. Alternatively, evaporative freezing, in which the liquid is cooled to near its freezing point and the system rapidly evacuated, is employed. The evaporating liquid cools and freezes rapidly. This technique may be complicated by frothing caused by the evolution of dissolved gases. For bulk drying, the liquid is placed in shallow trays on refrigerated shelves in the drying cabinet.

A suitable surface area-to-depth of solid ratio must be provided to facilitate drying. Thin layers of frozen liquid are used in bulk drying. The surface area of bottle-dried plasma may be increased by spinning in a vertical axis during freezing to give a frozen shell about 2 cm thick around the inside periphery of the bottle. Spinning also prevents frothing during evaporative freezing by inhibiting bubble formation.

In plasma processing, freezing, drying, and subsequent handling must be carried out aseptically. This condition is maintained by a filter at the neck of the bottle which allows the passage of water vapor but prevents the ingress of bacteria. Similar precautions are taken during the drying of antibiotics.

An effective drying vacuum from 0.05 to 0.2 mm Hg (6.6–26.6 Pa) may be provided by directly pumping water vapor and permanent gases, originally present or derived from the drying material and from leaks, out of the system. Normal practice, however, favors installing a refrigerated condenser between the drying surface and the pump. This arrangement allows a smaller pump, handling mainly permanent gases, to be used but demands a low condenser temperature, such as −50°C, to remove water vapor at the low operating pressure. A system for freeze drying bulk liquids in trays is shown in Fig. 35a.

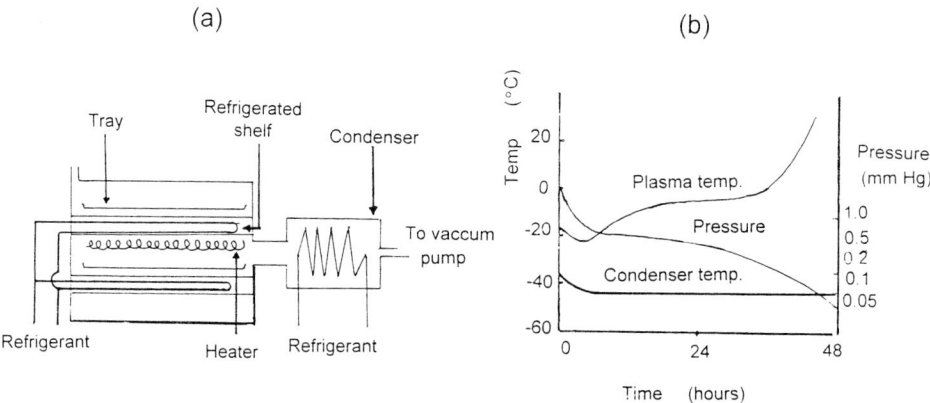

FIG. 35. (a) Equipment for freeze drying bulk liquids in trays; (b) variations in temperature and pressure during the freeze-drying cycle for blood plasma.

Unit Processes in Pharmacy: The Operations

During drying, heat must be supplied to the drying surface. When drying a material such as plasma in a final container, a temperature gradient is established across the container wall and through the ice to the drying surface by means of a heater suitably mounted in relation to the container. The power dissipated by the heater must be carefully controlled in order to prevent melting at the ice–container junction, the point nearest the heat source at the highest temperature. At any time, the conditions prevailing are such that the rate of evaporation is approximately constant, and temperatures and pressure adjust so that there is a temperature and pressure gradient from the drying surface to the condenser. As evaporation proceeds, a drying line recedes into the solid. With the thinning of the ice layer, the temperature gradient through the ice is modified by the decreasing resistance to heat flow. An increase in the drying rate due to an increase in temperature and vapor pressure of the drying surface might, therefore, be expected. In practice, this is modified by the layer of dried plasma which offers considerable resistance to the flow of vapor. In addition, the bacterial filter causes a large, constant pressure drop. Evaporation of pure ice without the filter and plasma layer would be 300 times faster. When the plasma is nearly dry, its temperature is allowed to rise to about 30°C to facilitate final drying; total drying time is about 48 h. The temperatures and pressure in the system during this period are shown, as a function of time, in Fig. 35b.

If the product is not being dried in its final container, radiant heat may be used to provide the latent heat of sublimation. If the dried solid can be removed continuously, high drying rates are possible. Not only is heat provided directly to the drying surface but there is little danger of melting the ice at the container wall.

Continuous Driers

Although many types of continuous driers are available, the scale of the operation for which they are designed is rarely appropriate to pharmaceutical manufacture. As with most continuous operations, the cost is disproportionately high for small units. Spray and drum driers provide an exception, because residence times in the driers are short and thermal degradation is minimized. Under some conditions, freeze drying may be the only practicable alternative.

Spray Driers

The solution or suspension to be dried is sprayed into a hot air stream and circulated through a chamber. The dried product may be carried out to cyclone or bag separators or may fall to the bottom of the drying chamber and be expelled through a valve. The chambers are normally cylindrical with a conical bottom although proportions vary widely. A typical spray drier is illustrated in Fig. 36. The process can be divided into four sections: atomization of the fluid, mixing of the droplets, drying, and finally removal and collection of the dry particles.

Atomization may be achieved by means of single-fluid or two-fluid nozzles or by spinning-disk atomizers. The single-fluid nozzle (Fig. 37a) operates by forcing the solution under pressure through a fine hole into the air stream. An intense swirl is conferred on the liquid before it emerges from the orifice, causing the jet to break up. In the two-fluid nozzle (Fig. 37b), a jet of air simultaneously emerges from an annular aperture concentric with the liquid orifice. Both types are subject to clogging and se-

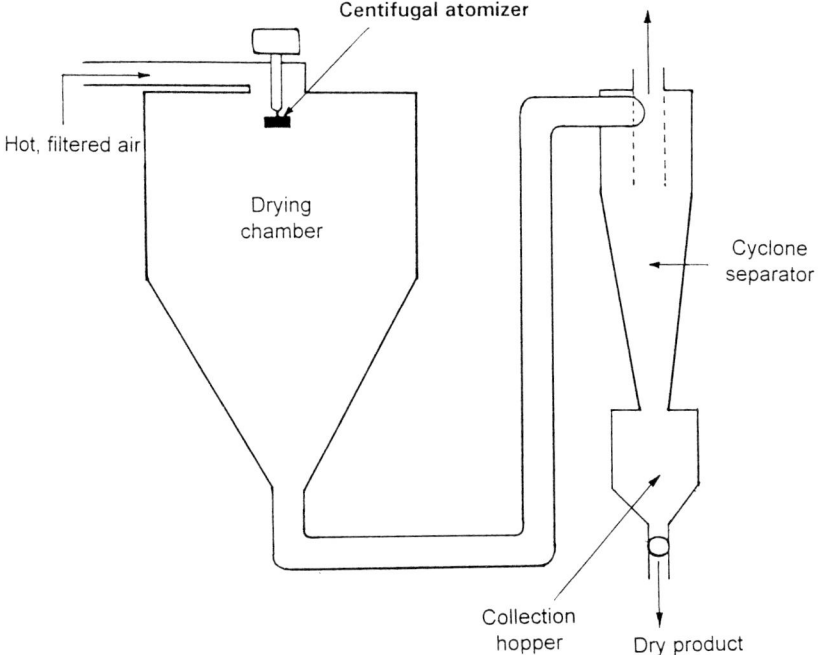

FIG. 36. Spray drier.

vere erosion, and therefore neither is well suited to spraying suspensions. The spinning disks (Fig. 37c) are most versatile and consist, in their simplest form, of a mushroom-shaped disk spinning at 5,000 to 30,000 rpm. Other designs include the slotted disk (Fig. 37d) which sprays thick suspensions and, if special feeding arrangements are used, pastes. The main factors determining the size of the droplets are the viscosity and surface tension of the liquid, the fluid pressure in the nozzles or, for spinning disks, size and speed of rotation. A reasonably uniform and controllable size within the range of 10–500 μm is desirable.

In vertical spray driers, the flow of the drying gas may be concurrent or countercurrent with respect to the movement of droplets. The movement of the gas is, however, complex and highly turbulent. Good mixing of droplets and gas occurs, and the heat and mass transfer rates are high. In conjunction with the large interfacial area conferred by atomization, these factors give very high evaporation rates. The residence time of a droplet in the drier is only a few seconds (5–30 s). Since the material is at wet-bulb temperature for much of this time, high gas temperatures of 150–200°C may be used even with thermolabile materials. Although the temperature of the material rises above the wet-bulb temperature at the end of the process, the drying gas is cooler and the material is almost dry, a condition in which many materials are thermally less sensitive. For these reasons it is possible to dry complex vegetable extracts, such as coffee or digitalis, milk products, spore suspensions, and other labile materials without significant loss of potency or flavor.

Drying is considered to take place by simple evaporation rather than by boiling and it has been observed that a droplet reaches a terminal velocity within about one foot of the atomizer. Beyond this, there is no relative velocity between the droplet and the drying

Unit Processes in Pharmacy: The Operations

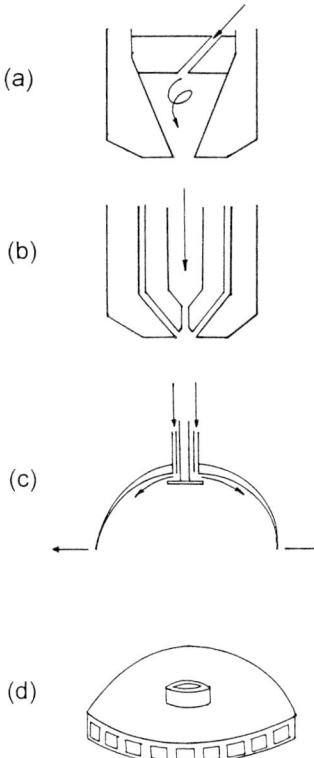

FIG. 37. Atomizers. (a) Single-fluid nozzle; (b) two-fluid nozzle; (c) spinning disk; (d) slotted disk.

gas unless the former is very large. The droplets may dry to form a solid, spherical particle. If, however, the emerging solids form a skin, internal pressure may inflate the particle and the final dry form will consist of hollow spheres which may or may not have a blow hole. These xenospheres may also fragment, resulting in a final product of agglomerates of finely divided solids. It has been found experimentally that the product bulk density, which is lowest for xenospheres and highest for fragmented solids, increases as the inlet air temperature is lowered and the drop size increases. A higher feed concentration increases the bulk density because drops of the same size give spheres with thicker walls.

These attractive physical characteristics provide further advantages to spray drying. The product often has excellent flow and packing properties which greatly facilitate handling and transport. As an example, spray-dried lactose is a widely used tablet excipient which flows, packs, and compacts without prior granulation. Similarly, a slurry of fillers and other excipients could be granulated by spraying and drying. After adding an active principle, the mix could be compressed without further processing.

The capital and running costs of spray driers are high, but if the scale is sufficiently large, it may provide the cheapest method. When thermolabile materials are dried on a small scale, costs will be 10 to 20 times higher than for oven drying. Air used to dry fine chemicals or food products is heated indirectly, thus reducing thermal efficiency and increasing costs. In some other installations, hot gases from combustion may be used directly.

Drum Driers

The drum drier consists of one or two slowly rotating, steam-heated cylinders. These are coated with solution or slurry by means of a dip feed, as illustrated in Fig. 38a and Fig. 38b, in which the lower portion of the drum is immersed in an agitated trough of feed material or, in the case of some double-drum driers, by feeding the liquor into the gap between the cylinders as shown in Fig. 38c. Spray and splash feeds are also used. In dip feeding, the hot drum must not boil the liquid in the trough. Drying takes place by simple evaporation rather than by boiling. The dried material is scraped from the drum by a knife at a suitable point.

Drying capacity is influenced by the speed of the drum and the temperature of the feed, which may be preheated. With the double-drum drier, the gap between the cylinders determines the thickness of the film.

Drum driers, like spray driers, are relatively expensive in small sizes and their use in the pharmaceutical industry is largely confined to drying thermolabile materials where the short contact time is advantageous. Drums are normally fabricated from stainless or chrome-plated steel to reduce contamination. The heat treatment to which the solid is subjected is more intense than in spray drying and the physical form of the product is often less attractive. During drying, the liquid approaches its boiling point and the dry solids attain the temperature of the drum surface.

Size Reduction and Classification

The Importance of Fine Particles in Pharmacy

Although fine particles can be produced directly by controlled precipitation, crystallization, or by drying a fine spray of solution, in many cases the material is powdered in some kind of mill. From the authors' point of view, the most important result of this operation is the increase in the surface area of a given weight of the powder and its influence on diffusional processes. A cube of 1 cm edge has a surface area of 6 cm^2.

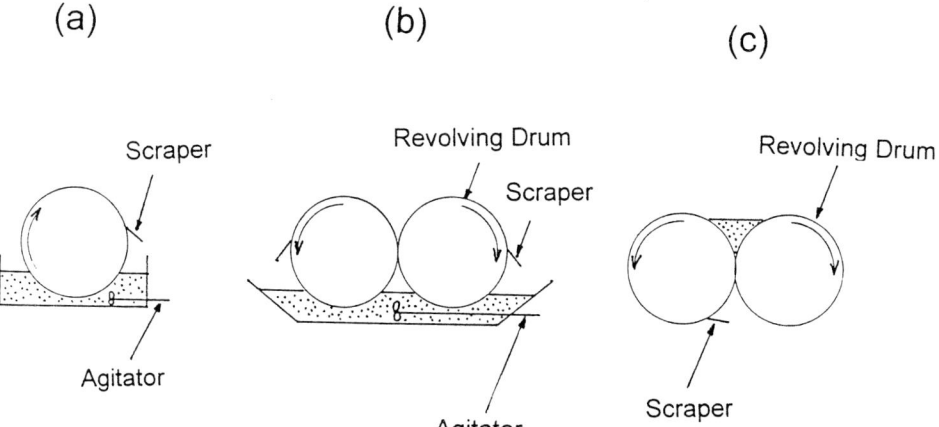

FIG. 38. Drum driers. (a) Dip feed; (b) immersion feed; (c) gap feed.

Unit Processes in Pharmacy: The Operations

An ideal size-reduction process would divide this cube into cubes of 0.1 cm edge, producing 1000 particles, each with a surface area of 0.06 cm^2 and a total surface area of 60 cm^2. A tenfold increase in surface area has been provided by a tenfold decrease in particle size. In general terms, the surface area is inversely proportional to the particle size, assuming that the shape of the particles remains the same.

The rate of most chemical and physical reactions involving solids and liquids is greatly influenced by the area of interfacial contact. In chemical reactions, a reagent must diffuse toward the surface of the solid, whereas the reaction products diffuse away from the surface, a procedure that depends, among other parameters, on the area between the solid and liquid. The effect of particle size on dissolution rate exemplifies another aspect of diffusion which is of importance to the pharmacist. Most commonly, drugs are taken orally in the form of solid particles, and absorption, which is usually rapid, must be preceded by dissolution. A full discussion of the role of particle size in oral, parenteral, and topical therapy may be found in reviews [47–49].

The rate at which fine chemicals or drugs are extracted from a vegetable source is increased by an increase in surface area. Reduction of particle size increases the area available for transfer of materials and decreases the distance over which solvent and solute must diffuse to have a marked effect on the drying of porous materials.

Other effects, not based on diffusion and its dependence on surface area, are found in mixing and various formulation requirements. If a sample is withdrawn from a mixture of powders, it is unlikely to contain exactly the correct proportion of ingredients. However, the larger the number of particles in the sample, the closer the sample will represent the overall proportions of the mixture. Therefore the accuracy of the sample can be increased by increasing the number of particles it contains, that is, reduce the particle size of the components of the mix. Eventually the sample might form a tablet or capsule. Since difference of particle size promotes segregation, the components should be produced with a similar particle-size distribution.

Formulation requirements often dictate the use of fine particles. Impalpability and spreading are required of dusting and cosmetic powders. Particles of 35–40 μm can be detected as single particles when applied to the skin and may give the impression of grittiness. Such powders should, in general, be finer than 30 μm. When powders are tinted, the particle size of powder and pigment affect the final color. In tableting, careful size reduction of imperfect tablets provides a material suitable for compression. The flow properties of suspensions of high disperse phase concentration is affected by particle size and size distribution. At a given disperse phase concentration, a decrease of particle size gives an increase in viscosity, whereas a broadening of particle size distribution yields a decrease in viscosity. Sedimentation is a function of particle size.

Numerous examples have been quoted to stress the importance of fine particles in pharmacy. Milling or grinding offers a method by which these may be produced. Size classification is a means, where applicable, of selecting a desired fraction or of removing oversize or undersize particles, and size analysis provides the analytical tool by which these operations may be assessed and controlled.

Fundamental Aspects of Crushing and Grinding

A basic study of crushing and grinding considers the physical properties of the material, the crushing mechanism itself, and its relation to the mechanism of failure. When a stress, which may be compressive, tensile, or shear, is applied to a solid, the latter deforms. Initially, the deformation or strain is the distortion of the crystal lattice by relative displacement of its components without change of structure. Complete recovery follows the removal of the stress and behavior is elastic. Figure 39 illustrates the deformation of a solid under a tensile stress; elastic behavior is shown over section AB. Below the elastic limit B, stress is proportional to strain and is related to it by various moduli. Beyond the yield point C, permanent or plastic deformation occurs and, as shown by release of stress at point D, all strain is not recoverable. Sliding along natural cleavage planes is occurring in this region. Plastic deformation is terminated by failure or fracture which is normally a gradual and reproducible process preceded by thinning of the material. The stress at point E is a measure of the strength of the material. The area under the curve at any point represents the strain energy per unit volume absorbed by the specimen up to that strain. The limiting strain energy per unit volume is the energy absorbed up to the point of failure.

An extensive period of plastic deformation is shown in Fig. 39 and the material would be classified as ductile. For the brittle materials normally encountered in grinding, little plastic deformation takes place and points C and E almost coincide. Fracture is here explained in terms of cracks and flaws naturally present in the material. It occurs suddenly and with shattering. The energy employed in stressing the particle to the point of failure reappears mainly as heat on release of strain in a manner analogous to the sudden release of a stressed spring.

The theoretical strength of crystalline materials can be calculated from interatomic attractive and repulsive forces. The strength of real materials, however, is found to be many times smaller than the theoretical value. The discrepancy is explained in terms of flaws of various kinds, such as minute fissures or irregularities of lattice structure known as dislocations. These have the capacity to concentrate the stress in the vicinity of the flaw. Failure may occur at a much lower overall stress than is predicted from the theoretical considerations. Failure occurs with the development of a crack tip which propagates rapidly through the material, penetrating other flaws which may, in turn, produce secondary cracks. The strength of the material depends therefore on the random distribution of flaws and is a statistical quantity varying within fairly wide limits. This concept explains why a material becomes progressively more difficult to grind. Since the probability of containing an effective flaw decreases as the particle size decreases, the strength increases until, with the achievement of faultless domains, the strength of the material equals the theoretical strength. This position is not realized in practice due to complicating factors such as aggregation.

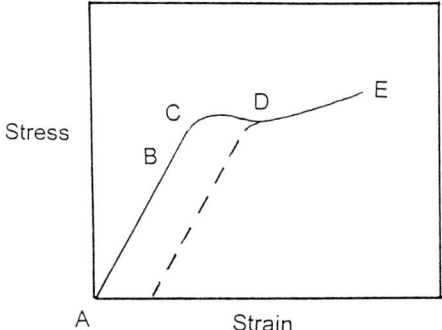

FIG. 39. The tensile deformation of a ductile material.

The strength of most materials is greater in compression than in tension. It is therefore unfortunate that technical difficulties prevent the direct application of tensile stresses. The compressive stresses commonly used in comminution equipment do not cause failure directly but generate by distortion sufficient tensile or shear stress to form a crack tip in a region away from the point of primary stress application. This is an inefficient but unavoidable mechanism. Impact and attrition are the other basic modes of stress application. The distinction between impact and compression is referred to below. Attrition, which is commonly employed, is difficult to classify but is probably primarily a shear mechanism.

In any machine, one mode of stress application usually predominates. It must be correctly chosen with respect to the mechanical properties of the material. Compression, for example, is useless for the comminution of fibrous or waxy solids. Attrition is generally necessary for all fine grinding.

The deformation and subsequent failure of a brittle material is not only a function of stress but also of the rate at which the stress is applied. Different results may be obtained from slow compressive breaking and impact breaking at the same energy level. Particle shape, size, and size distribution may be affected. In impact breaking, the rate of stress application is so high that the limiting strain energy may be exceeded several times by the suddenness of the operation. The reason is that fracture is time dependent, a lag occurring between the application of maximum stress and failure.

Stress application is further complicated by "free crushing" and "packed crushing" mechanisms. In free crushing, the stress is applied to an unconstrained particle and released when failure occurs. In packed crushing, the application of stress continues on the crushed bed of particles. Although further size reduction occurs, the process is less efficient due to vitiation of energy by the effects of interparticulate friction and stress transmission via particles which do not themselves fracture. This is easily demonstrated when a crystalline material is ground in a pestle and mortar. The fine powder initially produced protects coarser particles. If the material is sieved and oversize particles are returned, the operation may be completed with far less effort.

Free crushing is most nearly approached in the roller mill, which explains the high efficiency of the machine, and, to a lesser extent, in other continuous processes in which individual particles are presented to the grinding media. Packed crushing occurs in ball mills.

The Efficiency of Grinding

The relation between the energy supplied to a mill and the size reduction achieved has been extensively investigated. The efficiency of the process reflected by such a relation is of small importance in pharmacy because the applications are limited. For completeness, however, they are considered below.

Most of the energy supplied to the mill is ultimately dissipated as heat due to mechanical inefficiency. Most of the remainder or net grinding energy also appears as heat produced on the release of strain energy, a small part being added to the internal energy of the system as, for example, surface energy.

Various hypotheses relate the net grinding energy applied to a process and the size reduction achieved. The first, proposed by Karl von Rittinger in 1867, states in Eq. (33) that the energy necessary for size reduction is directly proportional to the increase in surface area,

$$E = k(S_p - S_f) \tag{33}$$

where E is the energy consumed, and S_p and S_f are the surface area of the product and feed materials, respectively. The constant, k, depends on the grinding unit employed and represents the energy consumed in enlarging the surface area by one unit. The relation between surface area and particle size has already been derived, and Eq. (34) may therefore be written,

$$E = k'\left(\frac{1}{d_p} - \frac{1}{d_f}\right) \tag{34}$$

where d_f and d_p are the particle sizes of feed and product particles, respectively.

The hypothesis indicates that energy consumption per unit area of new surface produced increases faster than the linear ratio of feed and product dimensions, a phenomenon already noted and explained. The proportionality of net energy input and new surface produced has been confirmed in some grinding operations.

Although Rittinger's law is concerned with surfaces and not with the energy associated with those surfaces, it is rational to relate the crushing energy consumed and the surface energy gained by increase of surface area, thereby arriving at a measure of efficiency. In experiments in which single particles are crushed, up to 30% of the applied energy appears as surface energy. In practical systems, where application of stress is less ideal, the net grinding energy is 100 to 1000 times greater than that associated with the new surface, that is, the efficiency of the process, on this basis, is between 0.1 and 1%.

The relation of energy to surface area provides little information on the grinding process and does not influence mill design. It provides, however, the basis of some grindability tests in which a known amount of energy is supplied to a mill and the increase in surface measured. This application is restricted to fine grinding.

Conversion of grinding energy to surface energy is neglected in Kick's law, promulgated in 1885. It is based on the deformation and brittle failure of elastic bodies and states that the energy required to produce analogous changes of configuration of geometrically similar bodies is proportional to the weight or volume of those bodies. The energy requirements are independent of the initial particle size and depend only on the size reduction ratio. Kick's law predicts lower energies than the relation proposed by Rittinger. The theory, however, demands that the resistance to crushing does not change with particle size. The role of flaws present in real materials is not considered, with the result that the energy required for fine grinding, when the apparent strength may have greatly risen, is underestimated.

A third theory of comminution gives results intermediate between the predictions of the laws of Kick and Rittinger [50]. It rests upon three principles: the first states that any divided material must have a positive energy register. This can only be zero when the particle size becomes infinite. The input energy, E, for any size reduction process then equals the product energy register minus the feed energy register. The energy associated with a powder increases as the particle size decreases, and it may be assumed that the energy register is inversely proportional to the particle size to an exponent, n. Hence, Eq. (35) is valid.

Unit Processes in Pharmacy: The Operations

$$E = E_p - E_f = \frac{K}{d_p^n} - \frac{K}{d_f^n} \tag{35}$$

The second principle of this theory [50] assigns to n a value of i, stating that "the total work useful in breaking, which has been applied to a stated weight of an homogeneous material, is inversely proportional to the square root of the diameter of the product particles."

The third principle states that breakage of the material is determined by the flaw structure. This aspect of size reduction has already been discussed.

A modification to Kick's law, sometimes known as the fourth law of comminution, has also been proposed [51]. For its discussion, the reader is referred to the original paper.

An empirical, but realistic approach to mill efficiency is gained through experiments in which the energy consumed and size reduction achieved are compared with values obtained in a laboratory test operating under free crushing conditions. All energy supplied in the latter is available for crushing and the test is assumed to be 100% efficient. Both slow crushing and impact tests are used. A large number of single particles may be simultaneously crushed and the work done is measured [52]. The latter is related to the size reduction. Similar measurements can be made during practical milling, expressing the efficiency of the process as a percentage of the free crushing value. On this basis, the approximate efficiency of the roll crusher is 80%, of the swing hammer mill 40%, of the ball mill 10%, and of the fluid energy mill only 1%.

The Operation of Mills

In some operations, such as those in which ores are processed, size reduction may constitute a major proportion of total process costs. The efficiency with which energy is utilized is, therefore, of great importance. Drugs, on the other hand, fall into a high cost class of materials processed in relatively small quantities. The contribution of grinding to total costs is, therefore, smaller and the choice of machine can usually be made on technological rather than economic grounds. Generally, drugs are easy to grind. The operation is classified as fine grinding if the bulk of the product passes a 200 mesh screen (76 μm) or as superfine grinding if a powder of a few microns or less is required. Most pharmaceutical grinding falls into these classes, although coarser grinding is applied to vegetable drugs before extraction.

Heywood [53] has stated that any type of crushing or grinding machine exhibits optimal comminution conditions for which the ratio of the energy to new surface is minimal. If finer grinding is attempted in such a machine, the ratio is increased. Mills may thus become grossly inefficient if called upon to grind at a size for which they were not designed. A limited size reduction ratio is imposed upon a single operation, larger ratios being obtained by the adoption of several stages, each employing a suitable mill. The fluid energy mill, which presents a size reduction ratio of up to 400, is exceptional.

A low retention time is inherent in free crushing machines. Little overgrinding takes place and the production of excessive undersize material or fines is avoided. Protracted milling times are found with many low-speed mills, with the result that considerable overgrinding takes place. Accumulation of product particles within the mill reduces the effectiveness of breaking stresses and the efficiency of milling progressively decreases.

This is typical of "open-circuit" grinding, in which the material is passed only once through the mill, remaining until virtually all has reached the required product size. An overall increase in efficiency is secured in "closed-circuit" grinding. Product particles are removed from the mill by means of a current of air or liquid or, alternatively, by screens. The removed product may be classified and any oversize material returned to the mill. Adoption of closed-circuit grinding techniques is only possible on a relatively large scale. On a smaller scale, the effect can be simulated by periodic classification of the entire mill contents and the removal of material which has reached the required size.

Dry and Wet Grinding

Between the approximate limits of 5 and 50% moisture, materials cake and do not flow. Both factors oppose effective grinding. Dry grinding is carried out at low moisture contents, the upper limit depending on the nature of the material. Although 5% or more moisture may be permissible for vegetable drugs, it would prove excessive during the milling of a coarse, impervious solid.

Wet grinding is a common procedure when a fluid suspension is required and drying, which would provide a significant drawback, is unnecessary. An excellent dispersion can be produced simultaneously, which in some operations provides the primary objective, size reduction being of secondary importance. Wet grinding may also be adopted when the size reduction achieved during dry grinding is prematurely linked by aggregation.

Certain general advantages are secured during wet grinding, including increased mill capacity, a lower energy consumption, the elimination of hazards from dust, and easier handling of materials. The principal disadvantage, apart from the possible inclusion of a drying stage, is the increased wear of the grinding medium.

Contamination

Wear of grinding elements, which occurs in all mills, results in the contamination of the product. This factor influences the choice of constructional materials such as ceramics and stainless steel, the most commonly used. Contamination is normally slight. However, in the protracted periods often associated with the production of very fine powders, it may become serious. This is illustrated by the data presented in Fig. 40 which shows a progressive increase in a sulfated ash value of the material due to wear of the ceramic mill.

Closed mills, preventing the ingress of bacteria, must be used for grinding sterile materials.

Temperature Sensitivity

Care must be exercised during the milling of temperature-sensitive materials, especially for a very fine product; caking results if the softening point is exceeded. Materials may be chilled before grinding or facilities provided for cooling the mill during grinding. Waxy solids can be successfully ground with dry ice, the low temperatures conferring brittle characteristics on the material. Chemical degradation may occur at high grind-

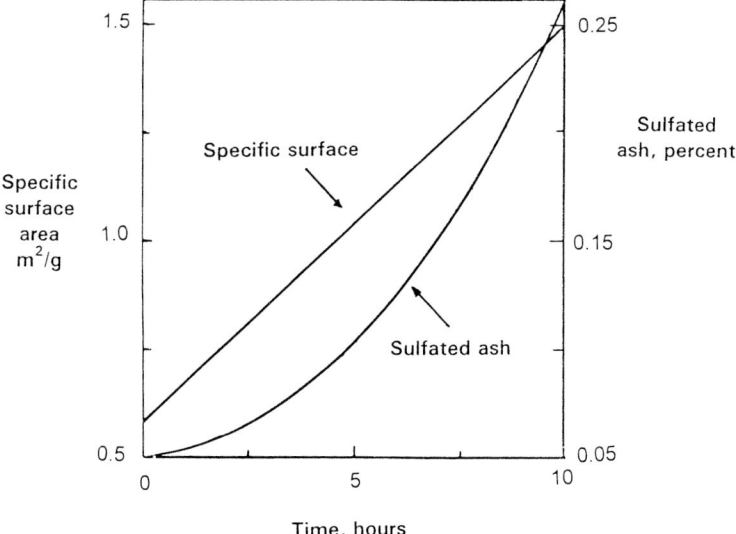

FIG. 40. Contamination of griseofulvin during milling.

ing temperatures. Oxidative changes can be prevented by grinding in an inert atmosphere such as nitrogen.

Structural Changes

Several examples of change of physical structure during very fine grinding have been reported, for example, changes in the crystal form of calcium carbonate after ball milling [54], distortion of the kaolinite lattice [55], and formation of various barbiturate polymorphs [56]. Changes such as these could affect solubility and other physical characteristics which, in turn, might influence formulation and therapeutic value.

Dust Hazards

Hazards from dust may become acute during dry grinding. Extremely potent materials require dust proofing of machines and dust-proof clothing and masks for operators. Danger may also arise from the explosive nature of many dusts.

Grinding Equipment

The following equipment is in regular use for dry-grinding pharmaceutical materials: edge- and end-runner mills, hammer mills, pin mills, ball mills, vibratory mills, fluid energy mills, colloid mills, and roller mills.

The fluid energy mill is becoming widely used for the production of superfine powders. The ball mill and the colloid mill are used for wet grinding and the production of liquid dispersions. The end-runner mill and adaptations of the roll mill may be used to comminute and disperse powders in semisolid bases as, for example, in the production of ointments.

Edge- and End-Runner Mills

The edge-runner mill consists of one or two heavy granite or cast iron wheels or mullers mounted on a horizontal shaft and standing in a heavy pan. Either the muller or the pan is driven. The material is fed into the center of the pan and is worked outward by the action of the muller. While in the zone traversed by the muller, comminution occurs by compression due to the weight of the muller, and by shear. The origin of the shear forces is indicated in Fig. 41a. The linear velocity of the pan surface varies over the line of contact between muller and pan. For efficient grinding, this dimension is large compared with the diameter of the pan. Muller and pan speeds may only coincide on one hypothetical circle and at other positions a varying amount of slip must occur. A scraper continually moves material from the perimeter of the pan to the grinding zone.

The end-runner mill is similar in principle and consists of a rotating pan or mortar made of cast iron or porcelain. A heavy pestle is mounted vertically within the pan in an off-center position (Fig. 41b). The mechanism of size reduction is compression due to the weight of the pestle, and shear. The latter is developed by the relative movement

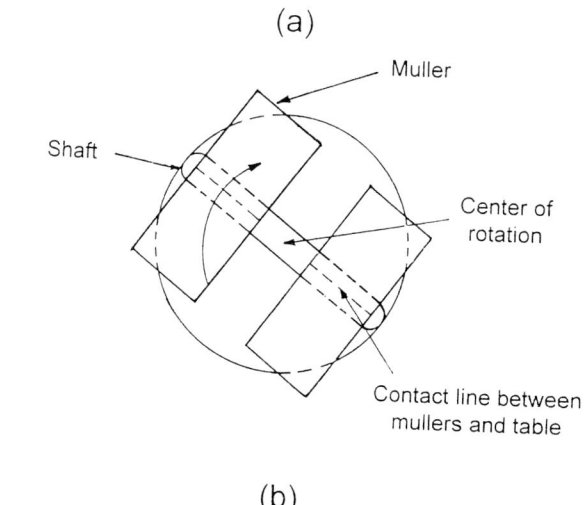

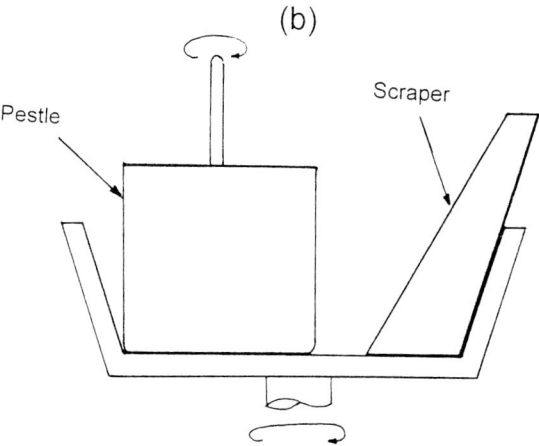

FIG. 41. (a) Edge-runner and (b) end-runner mill.

Unit Processes in Pharmacy: The Operations

of muller and pan which varies over the face of the muller. The muller is friction-driven by the pan through the ground material. A scraper is used to redirect the material into the grinding zone.

Both mills operate at slow speeds on a packed bed. Both produce moderately fine powders and operate successfully with fibrous materials. Wet grinding with very viscous materials, such as ointments and pastes, is also possible.

Hammer and Comminution Mills

The hammer mill typifies a group of machines operating at very high speeds and acting primarily by impact on a freely suspended particle. The term "disintegrator" is also used. High efficiency, which would be expected from the operation of a free crushing mechanism, is reduced because the blows delivered are in excess of the minimum required for breakage.

A typical machine (Fig. 42a) consists of a disk rotating at speeds up to 8000 rpm. The higher speeds are used for fine grinding in relatively small machines. A balanced number of hammers is fitted to the disk which may be fixed or pivoted, presenting flat, knife, or file edges to the material. The material is fed to the top or the center of the mill and broken by direct impact until fine enough to pass through the screen which forms the lower part of the mill casing. A range of screens is normally provided. Due to a tangential exit, the product size is considerably smaller than the screen apertures. The disk and hammers act as a centrifugal fan, drawing large volumes of air through the mill. Entrained dust must be separated with a bag filter or a cyclone separator.

The mill processes dry, crystalline materials which do not soften under milling conditions, and many crude drugs. Speed of rotation and the size and shape of the screen apertures are interrelated factors controlling the size of the product. A considerable amount of very fine powder is produced. The temperature can rise markedly during passage through the mill with consequent risk of fusion or decomposition of susceptible drugs.

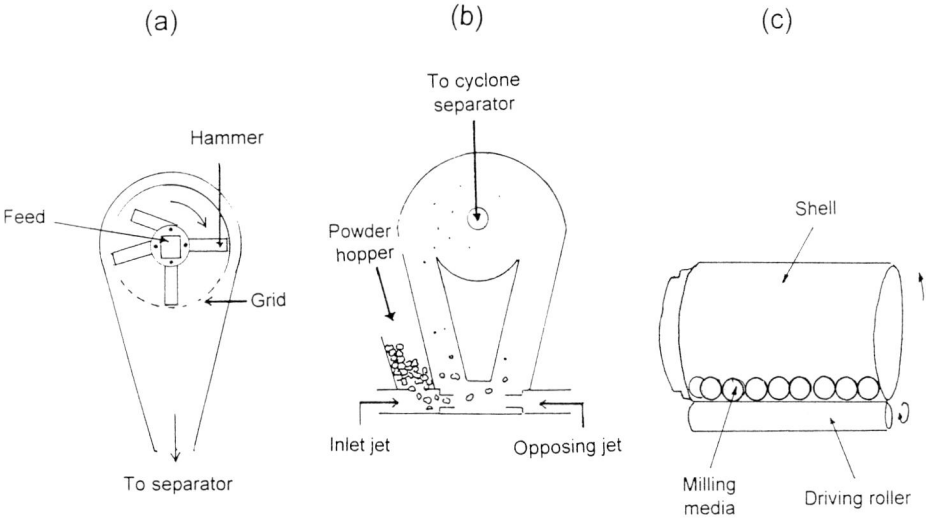

FIG. 42. (a) Impact mill with pivoted hammers; (b) comminution mill; (c) ball mill.

Great versatility, derived from simple variation of screen, rotor speed, and type of blade, is characteristic of the refined mills commonly used in the pharmaceutical industry. The Fitzmill (The Fitzpatrick Company of America and Manesty Machines Ltd) and the Apex Comminuting Mill (Apex Construction Co., London) are mobile machines constructed largely of stainless steel (Fig. 42b). Both offer a large screen area and operate at various speeds. A reversible rotor permits the use of blades presenting a flat, impact face or a cutting edge to the material. Materials are ground by high speed operation of the impact face. The knife edges may be used at lower speeds for wet granulation and the precision reduction of the imperfect tables produced during dry granulation. The mill may be jacketed to control temperatures. Mixing, wet grinding, and ointment milling may be performed.

Pin Mill

Pin mills consist of two horizontal steel plates with vertical projections arranged in concentric circles on opposing faces, more closely spaced toward the periphery. The projections of the two faces intermesh. The material is fed through the center of the stationary upper disk on to the lower revolving disk and propelled by centrifugal action toward the periphery. The passage between the pins provides size reduction by impact and attrition. The material is collected in the annular space surrounding the disks and passes to a separator. The large volumes of air drawn through the mill are discharged through the separator. Absence of screens and gratings provides an action free from clogging. The machine is suitable for grinding soft, nonabrasive powders, and low milling temperatures permit the processing of heat-sensitive materials. The fineness of the grind may be varied by using disks with different pin dispositions.

Ball Mill

The ball mill is widely used for fine grinding. Extremely fine powders may be produced although milling times are often protracted. Despite simple construction, the mill is extremely versatile. It can be used for wet or dry grinding in continuous or batch processes. The latter are usually imposed by the scale of pharmaceutical operations. Because the mill is a closed system, sterility can be maintained or an operation can be conducted in an inert atmosphere if necessary. Materials of widely differing mechanical properties can be ground by the combined effects of impact and attrition characteristic of the mill.

The ball mill, in its simplest form, is illustrated in Fig. 42c. It consists of a rotating, hollow cylinder containing balls, usually made of stainless steel or stoneware. During grinding, the balls slowly wear and are eventually replaced. For general purposes, the mill contains balls of different sizes which perform different functions. Loading varies, typically, the mill is half filled with balls and the material to be ground is added to overfill the interstices between the balls. The apparent volume of the total charge is commonly 60% of the mill volume. In operation, the distance the charge moves up the mill casing depends upon the centrifugal force, a function of the speed at which the mill rotates and the friction between charge and mill lining. These effects determine the pattern of movement within the mill. At low grinding speeds, the balls tumble, roll, and jump down the free face of the charge, a pattern described as "cascading." With increase in speed, the pattern progressively changes to "cataracting" where the balls are carried almost to the top of the mill and fall directly on to the charge below.

The grinding contributions of impact and attrition vary in these movement patterns. Attrition predominates in the cascading mill and depends to some extent on the surface area of the balls. The effect can, therefore, be enhanced by the use of small balls. Impact breaking becomes more important in the cataracting mill, the most effective action being derived from the high kinetic energy of the larger balls, a factor influenced by their density.

If there is sufficient friction between the mill lining and the charge, the latter will "key" to the mill at higher speeds and rotate with it. This is termed "centrifuging" and since there is no relative movement between the balls, no grinding occurs. The speed marking the onset of centrifuging is called the critical speed. Theoretically it represents conditions for which the centrifugal and gravitational forces acting on a ball at the top of the mill are balanced. If the mass of the ball is m, the gravitational force is given by mg and the centrifugal force by mv_c^2/r, where v_c is the critical speed and r is the distance of the ball from the axis of the mill, that is, the radius of the mill minus the radius of the ball, expressed by Eq. (36).

$$v_c = \sqrt{gr} \qquad (36)$$

In practice, centrifuging does not occur until well above the theoretical critical speed and varies with mill loading and the amount of slip between charge and lining. Mills usually operate at between 50 and 80% of the critical speed. The lower speeds are used for wet grinding and very fine dry grinding.

If a low coefficient of friction permits extensive slipping between mill and charge, centrifuging cannot occur even at very high mill speeds. Under these "super-critical" conditions, the grinding action differs from the pattern described above.

By correct choice of ball size, mill speed, and diameter, the ball mill may be used to grind material of widely different particle size. In coarse dry grinding, the energy associated with the largest ball falling the diameter of the mill must be sufficient to break the largest particle. Very fine grinding, on the other hand, is best effected by the attrition between a large number of small balls. The most important limiting factor in the production of very fine particles by milling is agglomeration. Ultimately, the reduction of new surface by rebonding may equal the increase in surface due to fracture. This is shown as point A in the relation of specific surface area and milling time given in Fig. 43. With further grinding, the effective particle size may actually increase. Agglomeration during fine dry grinding is usually more severe than in wet grinding. In both cases, however, additives can sometimes be used to limit its effect.

The ball mill also provides a simple mechanical means of producing dispersions of solids in liquids. Wet grinding depends on the attrition characteristic of the cascading mill, the effect being greater the smaller the balls and the higher the viscosity of the suspension. The latter should not prevent the correct movement of the charge. Where their use is permissible, the addition of surface-active agents may greatly accelerate the process of preventing reaggregation of the particles. Surface-active agents can also alter the physical properties of the solid, lowering the breaking strain and rendering the particle more brittle. A higher ratio of solids to liquid, which aids efficient milling, is possible if the system is deflocculated.

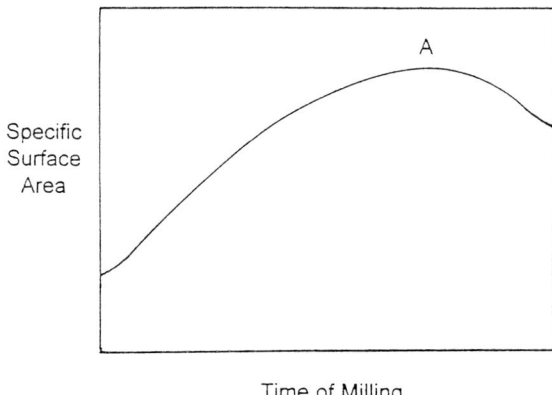

FIG. 43. The effect of particle agglomeration during milling.

In large-scale, continuous installations, the mill may be modified to apply grinding forces appropriate to the size of particle being ground. In the tube mill, the ratio of length to diameter is greatly increased, and the mill is divided into several compartments each containing balls of different average size. The coarse material first enters the compartment containing the largest balls. It is then conveyed to successive compartments containing smaller balls and capable of progressively finer grinding. In the Harding conical ball mill natural segregation is induced by the conical shape. The largest balls operate at the largest diameter and, through the kinetic energy acquired during the extensive fall, create high impact stresses suitable for breaking coarse particles. The material first passes through this region. With further progress through the mill, the greater surface presented by the smaller balls promotes finer grinding by attrition.

Vibratory Mill

In the ball mill, the energy for grinding is derived from the acceleration of the balls in a gravitational field. Under normal conditions, the latter limits the speed at which a mill of a given diameter can be run and therefore limits the rate at which energy can be applied to the process. Long milling times are characteristic of the ball mill. The advantage of vibratory milling is mainly based on this limitation since it is possible by this method to develop accelerations much greater than those induced by the earth's gravitational field. Grinding can be more energetic and milling times can be greatly reduced.

A simple vibratory mill consists of a mill body containing the grinding media, usually porcelain or stainless steel balls. The mill body is supported on springs which permit an oscillatory movement. This vibration is usually, but not necessarily, in a vertical plane. The suspended mass is maintained in a state of forced vibration by some means, such as the rotation of a shaft on which unbalanced weights are mounted. The charge is subjected to movements of high frequency and small amplitude. The resultant chattering of the mill gives comminution by attrition. Characterized by relatively high speed grinding, this mill is usually more flexible than the ball mill, charging and discharging and adaption to continuous processing being much easier. The more efficient use of the energy applied and the shorter grinding times usually result in lower milling temperatures than those in a ball mill. Construction, however, is more complex and the feed size of the material is limited to approximately 0.25 in. (6 mm) and less. The mill is not suitable for grinding resilient materials which cannot be ground by impact since the shear forces developed are less than those found in a ball mill.

A refined example of this principle is found in the Podmore-Boulto Vibro-Energy Mill, shown in Fig. 44a. It consists of an annular grinding chamber accommodating a medium of small cylinders. These align coaxially in a three-dimensional vibratory field to give close packing and line contact between moving surfaces. This mill, it is claimed, gives preferential grinding of coarse material leading to products with narrow particle size distributions.

The Fluid Energy Mill

The fluid energy mill offers an alternative method of producing very fine powders. The general term "micronizer" is a trade name coined by a company which originated a particular type of fluid energy mill. In all mills of this type, the grinding results mainly from attrition between the particles being ground, the energy inducing movement of the particles being supplied in the form of compressed fluids; air and steam are widely used.

A common type of fluid energy mill is illustrated in Fig. 44b. The material is blown into the grinding chamber through a venturi feed placed at its perimeter. The compressed fluid enters the chamber through nozzles tangential to a hypothetical circle within the

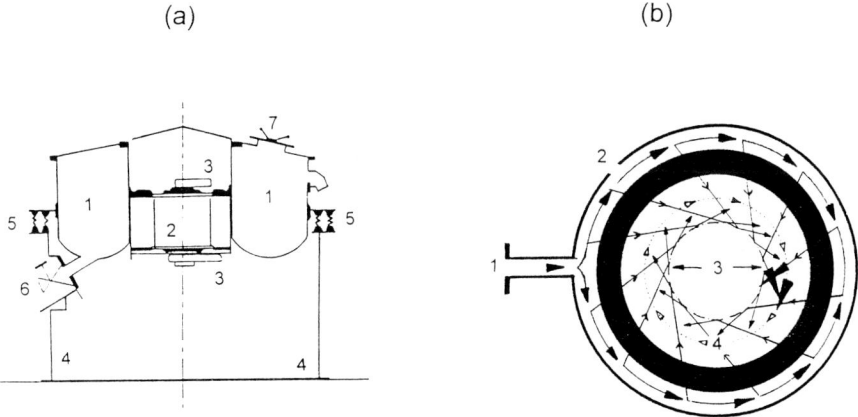

FIG. 44. (a) Vibro-energy mill. 1. Annular grinding chamber; 2. Motor; 3. Out-of-balance weights; 4. Mill base; 5. Spring circle; 6. Discharge valve; 7. Top cover. (b) Fluid energy mill. 1. Main inlet for compressed air or superheated steam; 2. Fluid energy supply manifold; 3. Pitch circle to which all jet axes are tangential; 4. Grinding jet axis; →Forces from grinding jets; ─► Tangential forces produced by cyclone; ---▻ Action of three simultaneous forces on material causing attrition and particle size reduction; ─► Rotational forces from jets creating cyclone.

grinding chamber. The particles are violently accelerated by the rotating fluids and are subjected to the influence of successive nozzles. Grinding results from impact between particles which are subjected to the intense classifying action of the circulating fluid. Oversize particles remain in the grinding zone while fine powder and spent grinding fluid spirals to the central outlet.

For a given machine, the size reduction depends upon the size of the feed, its rate of introduction to the grinding chamber, and the pressure of the grinding fluid. The most important factors are the geometry of the grinding chamber and the number and angle of the nozzles.

Powders with all particles below a few microns may be quickly produced by this method. The disadvantage of high capital and running costs may not be serious in the pharmaceutical industry because of the high value of the materials often processed. For grinding drugs, the mill is usually made of stainless steel. Large volumes of air compressed to about 100 psi (690 kPa) must be provided.

Colloid Mills

Colloid mills are used for wet grinding and dispersion. They operate by shearing relatively thin layers of material between two surfaces, one of which is moving at a high angular velocity relative to the other. Although very fine dispersions can be produced, they are not, as the name implies, of colloidal dimensions. Colloid mills are also widely used in the preparation of emulsions.

A typical colloid mill consists of a stator and rotor with flat working surfaces, often of stainless steel or carborundum. The clearance is adjustable from virtually zero upward. The rotor is rotated at several thousand rpm and the slurry of already fine material passes through the clearance under the action of centrifugal forces. Surface-active agents fulfill the same function in colloid mills as in ball milling.

Roller Mills

Roller mills may be used to grind pastes and plastic dispersions. They operate by inducing crushing and shearing forces in a thin layer of the paste as it passes through the narrow clearance between two rollers. Commonly, shear forces are intensified by the differing peripheral velocity of the rolls. The clearance between the rolls is variable and depends on the plasticity of the mass, the gap increasing as the stiffness of the material increases. With thin pastes, the milling action is similar to that of the colloid mill.

Classification or Size Separation

In the introduction to this article, the influence of particle size on several processes was described. The operation in which particles of a suitable size are selected and others rejected, because they are too small or too large, is called classification or size separation. This process is also important in closed-circuit grinding, the removal of fine powders to promote flow, and in the restriction of particle size distribution to prevent segregation or enhance appearance.

Although a number of particle properties can be used to classify a powder, only two are important. The first is based on the ability of a particle to pass through an aperture. This is sieving or screening. The second employs the drag forces on a particle moving through a fluid. The term "classification" is sometimes restricted to this method of separation but here the terms "elutriation" and "sedimentation" are used. In general, screening is applied to the separation of coarse particles and sedimentation to the separation of fine particles.

Sieving and Screening

Sieves and screens are widely used for the classification of relatively coarse materials. For very large particles (>0.5 in.) a robust plate perforated with holes is used. However, the pharmaceutical applications of screening are for much smaller particles and screens are in the form of woven meshes. Unless special methods are used to prevent clogging and powder aggregation, the lower useful limit is in a cloth woven with 200 mesh/in. (70–80 μm). Fine screens of this type are extremely fragile and must be used with great care.

A series of suitable sieve cloths is described in the Fine Mesh Series of *British Standard*, 410, 1962. It specifies the gauge of the wire and the permitted weaving tolerances. In successive meshes of this series, the mesh space changes by a factor of $4\sqrt{2}$. In the mesh series commonly chosen for size analysis, 16-22-30-44-60-85-120-170, alternate screens are selected so that the mesh spacing decreases by $\sqrt{2}$ and the area of the apertures is halved. For classification, one or more meshes of suitable weave can be chosen from this series and mounted in a frame.

In operation, the mesh should be lightly loaded in order that all particles capable of passing the mesh (undersize) have a chance to do so. The mesh must, therefore, be agitated both to ensure access of particles to the holes and to clear holes blocked by particles just unable to pass. Under these conditions, the rate of sieving is proportional to the number of undersize particles on the screen; it therefore decreases exponentially.

Most screening, particularly of coarse materials, is carried out under dry conditions. The wet screening of dilute slurries is adopted for powders that aggregate strongly, clog the mesh, or become electrostatically charged by the vibrations of the screen. Sieving errors arising from the cohesion of small and large particles and the retention of the former on a coarse mesh is avoided. Wet screening is particularly useful if the subsequent process is wet and drying is unnecessary.

For small-scale classifications, test sieves with meshes conforming to BS 410 can be used. The mesh is mounted on a circular brass frame (8, 12, or 18 in. in diameter), a rim on the lower edge enabling it to "nest" with the sieve below. When the chosen sieves are equipped with a lid and a receiving pan, the agitated assembly becomes an effective small-scale grading unit. Sieving is stopped when the rate at which particles pass the mesh has reached some low value or after some predetermined time at which the rate is known to be low.

As the scale of the operation increases it becomes, in general, less precise. For continuous screening, the feed material is made to move across the screen to a point of discharge. The residence time on the screen is usually short and many undersize particles traverse it without falling through. With an increase of sieving area, the meshes become more fragile and the finest meshes must be supported with a coarser wire. An example of a large-scale separator utilizes a circular screen, up to 5 ft (1.5 m) in diameter, vibrated in a horizontal plane, the gyratory movement being imparted by an out-of-balance fly wheel connected to the assembly. In other machines, the mesh is rectangular and inclined at a shallow angle (5–30°). A gyratory movement is developed and the material to be classified is fed to the top. These machines may bear more than one deck, thus allowing the separation of the powder into several fractions at one time.

Elutriation and Sedimentation

The balance of the drag force on the particle and the forces promoting movement occurs at the terminal velocity, which depends, among other parameters, on the size of the particle; this is the property on which several classifiers are based. The fluid is air or a liquid. The latter affords a higher precision because dispersion can be more thorough. In air, high shear forces cannot be developed and dispersing agents cannot be used.

The simplest classifier is a rising current of fluid in which the particles are suspended. In this case, the force opposing the upward drag is gravitational. If the opposition develops a terminal velocity higher than the current speed, the particle falls. This is the principle of elutriation; the particle size d at which the separation is made follows from a rearrangement of Eq. (35) for conditions in which Stokes' law is valid; it is given by Eq. (37),

$$d = \sqrt{\frac{18\eta u}{(\rho_s - \rho)g}} \qquad (37)$$

where $\rho_s - \rho$ is the density difference between solid and fluid, η is the viscosity of the fluid, and μ is the speed of the upward current.

The elutriator shown in Fig. 45a consists of three tubes. The first is smallest in diameter and offers the highest upward liquid velocity. Coarse particles with a high terminal velocity settle in this tube while the remainder is swept to the bottom of the second. The diameter of the second tube exceeds that of the first and elutriation speeds

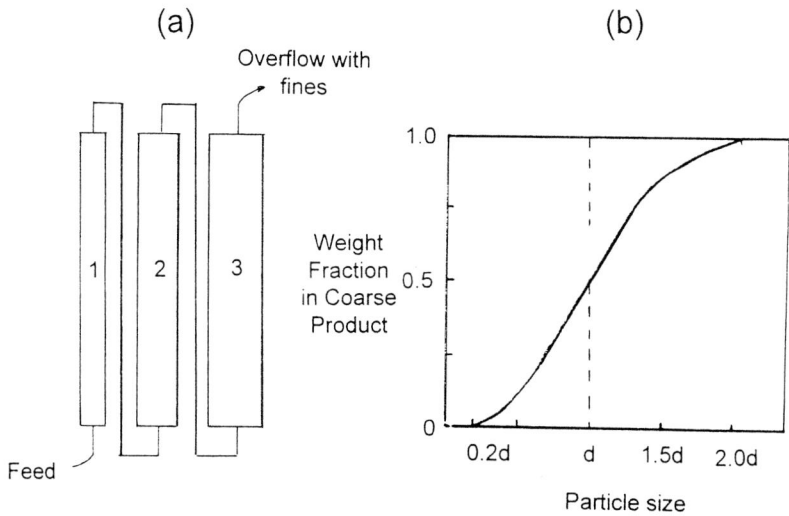

FIG. 45. (a) An elutriator; (b) grade efficiency curve.

Unit Processes in Pharmacy: The Operations

are lower. Only fine particles are swept into the third tube where the process is repeated at a finer size. In this way, the original slurry is divided into four fractions.

In practice, fluctuations in flow conditions due to natural convection and a violation of the conditions for which Stokes' law is valid blur the point of separation. The evaluation of the separation must, therefore, take account of the fine particles which fall with the coarse particles and the coarse particles which move to the fine fraction. This is best expressed by a grade efficiency curve (Fig. 45b). Returning to Eq. (37), a particle of size d should be stationary in the elutriation tube. Due to fluctuating conditions, it eventually resides with the coarse or the fine fractions, the chances being equal. The weight fraction in each is, therefore, 0.5 at this particular size. It is assumed here that of the particles which are twice this size ($2d$), virtually all appear in the coarse product.

The weight fraction here is one. Similarly, all particles of size $0.2d$ move to the fine product resulting in a weight fraction of zero in the coarse product. As shown in Fig. 45b, a sigmoid curve, passing through 0.5 at size d, links these extremes. The closer these extremes and the steeper the curve, the more efficient the separation. A grade efficiency curve of this type can be used as an appraisal of any sedimentor or elutriator.

Gravitational sedimentation is not of great importance in small-scale classification. Sedimentation in a spinning fluid stream is, however, widely used. The most common classifier of this type is the cyclone separator shown in Fig. 46. The fluid enters tan-

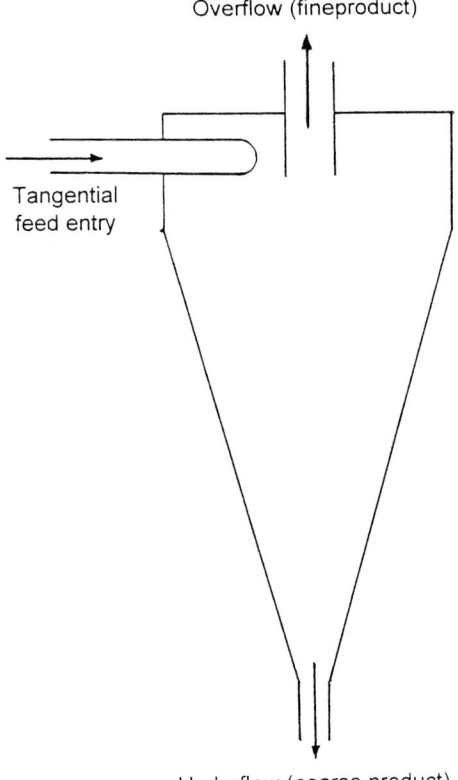

FIG. 46. A cyclone separator.

gentially and acquires an intense spinning motion, spiraling downward into the cone before rising to the outlet as a central core. The inlet speed is very high and large angular velocities are developed. Due to centrifugal force, particles move radially across the spinning stream to fall at the wall into the cone. Operated in this way, complete separation of solids occurs and the cyclone is, therefore, an effective air cleaner. Operated with lower centrifugal forces, the cyclone transports the finest particles to the exhaust, leaving the coarser particles to fall into the cone. Cyclone classifiers are designed for use with either liquid or air.

The centrifuge is normally operated to completely separate two phases. If, however, the rate at which the feed passes through does not allow all particles to settle, the action of a classifier is developed. This is illustrated by a solid-bowl centrifuge which consists of a steel shell in the form of a frustrum mounted horizontally. It contains a conveying screw at the wall which rotates at a slightly higher speed than the shell. Particles that settle at the wall are conveyed to the narrow end of the shell and discharged. Fine particles are entrained with the overflow to the other end. Further details of this and other centrifugal classifiers have been given by Treasure [57].

Mixing

Mixing has been defined [58] as an operation ". . . in which two or more ingredients in separate or roughly mixed condition are treated so that each particle of any one ingredient is as nearly as possible adjacent to a particle of each of the other ingredients." The term "blending" is synonymous and "segregation" or "demixing" is the opposite.

Mixing is a basic step in most process sequences. It is normally carried out to secure uniformity of composition, so that small samples withdrawn from a bulk material represent the overall composition of the mixture, and to promote physical or chemical reactions, such as dissolution, in which natural diffusion is supplemented by agitation. Mixing has been classified [59] as follows:

- *Positive mixing* which applies to systems that, given time, would spontaneously and completely mix. Examples are provided by two gases or two miscible liquids; mixing apparatus is used on such systems to accelerate mixing.
- *Negative mixing* is demonstrated by suspensions of solids in liquids. Any two-phase system in which the phases differ in density separates unless continuously agitated.
- *Neutral mixing* occurs when neither mixing nor demixing takes place unless the system is acted upon by a system of forces. Examples are found in the mixing of solids and of solids with liquids when the concentration of the former is high.

Mixing must embrace all combinations of the three states of matter. The theory of mixing should be able, when the system to be mixed has been defined, to dictate the type and design of the mixer, such as volume, shape, and type of impeller, and the process conditions, such as degree of agitation, and the time and power required. Theoretical knowledge is, however, insufficient to predict the performance of mixers.

More commonly, choice is based upon broad empirical principles which are supported by practical tests.

Scale of Scrutiny

Whether or not materials are satisfactorily mixed depends upon the subsequent operations in which the mixture plays a part. Any mixture, if examined on a small enough scale, shows regions of segregation. An acceptable degree of mixing is related to subsequent operations in a process sequence. The term "scale of scrutiny" has been introduced [59] to describe the minimum size of the regions of segregation in a particular mixture which would cause it to be regarded as insufficiently mixed. For example, if a tablet is to contain 100 mg of drug A and 100 mg of drug B, the powder from which the tablets are to be made must be sufficiently mixed that on drawing a sample of 200 mg from the mixture, the sample contains, within narrow limits, the correct amounts of A and B. The way in which A and B are dispersed within the sample may be of no importance so long as the tablet is not divided. The scale of scrutiny is here determined by the weight of the tablet. In general, a small scale of scrutiny is applied if the unit size of the product is small and if too much or too little of one component is very undesirable.

In addition, two further useful concepts may be introduced here to describe unmixedness: the scale of segregation and the intensity of segregation. The scale of segregation is a measure of the size of the regions of unmixed materials. In the example given above, the intensity of segregation shows the extent to which A has been diluted with B and vice versa. These two concepts are usually interrelated. A high intensity of segregation can be tolerated so long as the scale of segregation is small. Alternatively, a larger scale of segregation may be tolerated if the intensity of segregation is reduced.

Mixing of Solids

Pharmacy offers many important examples of the mixing of solids. In several forms of drug presentation, the attainment of accurate dosage depends on an adequate mixing operation at some stage in production. Since the dose unit may be small (e.g., 100 mg), a small scale of scrutiny is applied.

The mixing of all systems of matter involves a relative displacement of the particles, whether they are molecules, globules, or small crystals, until a state of maximum disorder is created and a completely random arrangement is achieved (Fig. 47b).

A perfect mixture, which, with a practical sample, would offer point uniformity, is shown in Fig. 47a. Such an arrangement is, however, virtually impossible, and no mixing equipment can do better than produce the random mixture shown in Fig. 47b. In such a mixture, the probability of finding one type of particle at any point in the mixture is equal to the proportion of that type of particle in the mixture.

The mixing of solids differs from the mixing of liquids in that the smallest practical sample withdrawn from a mixture of two miscible liquids contains many millions of particles. In the mixing of solids, a small sample contains relatively few particles, and examination of Fig. 47b should show that such samples show considerable variation with respect to the overall composition of the mixture and that this variation should be reduced as the number of particles in the sample is increased. Assessing the varia-

FIG. 47. Diagrammatic representation of (a) a perfect mix and (b) a random mix. The latter does not show point uniformity.

tion in, for example, drug content in a series of samples drawn from a mixture of powders is of great importance. The tablet machine may be regarded as a volumetric sampling device and the variation in drug content between one tablet and the next is largely controlled by the mixing stage which precedes it.

Properties of a Random Mixture

In 1953, Lacey [60] showed that the variation in the composition of samples drawn from a random mixture of two materials could be expressed by Eq. (38),

$$s = \sqrt{\frac{p(1-p)}{n}} \quad (38)$$

where s is the standard deviation of the samples, p is the proportion of one component, and n is the number of particles in the sample. The relation requires that the two components are alike in particle size, shape, and density and can only be distinguished by some neutral property, such as color. If very many samples, each containing a given number of particles, are withdrawn from a mixture of equal parts of two materials, the results of analysis can be presented in the form of a frequency curve in which the samples are normally distributed around the mean content of the mixture, and 99.7% of the samples will fall within the limits $p = 0.5 + 3\sigma$. The standard deviation of the samples is inversely proportional to the square root of the number of particles in a sample. If the particle size is reduced to the extent that the same weight of sample contains four times as many particles, the standard deviation is halved. The distribution of samples and the effect of size reduction is shown in Fig. 48.

In a critical examination of pharmaceutical mixing, Train [61] showed that samples of a random mixture of equal parts A and B must contain at least 800 particles if 997 out of every 1000 samples were to lie between ± 10% of the stated composition, that

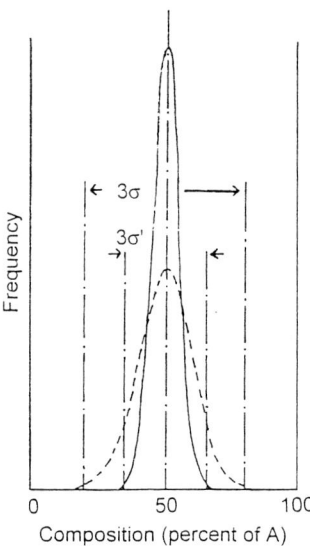

FIG. 48. Distribution of samples drawn from a mixture of equal parts A and B. The broken line represents data for the coarser powder.

is, the proportion, p, of A = 0.5 ± 0.05, where σ = 0.05/3. The effect of the number of particles in a sample on the percentage variation about the mean content of a mixture of equal parts A and B was summarized by Train in the diagram reported in Fig. 49. It may be used to show that if, in the above examples, limits of ± 1% were substituted, 90,000 particles must be present in each sample. The true standard deviation is given the symbol σ. The standard deviation estimated by the withdrawal of a number of samples is denoted s.

If, instead of equal parts A and B, the proportion of an active ingredient, A, in the mixture was 0.1 (10%), imposition of limits of ± 10% (in 997 cases out of 1000) requires that each sample shall contain over 8000 particles. If the proportion of active constituent is 0.01, or 1%, a figure of 90,000 particles per sample is obtained, and if

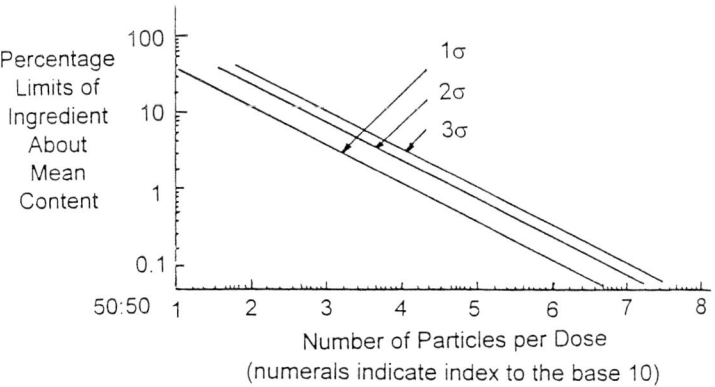

FIG. 49. General theoretical relationship between number of particles and percentage limit of ingredient for a 50:50 mix. (From Ref. 61.)

the limits are reduced to +1%, the active constituent is 0.01, or 1%, a figure of 90,000 particles per sample is obtained, and if the limits are reduced to ± 1%, the figure is 9×10^6.

The theoretical derivation of these results is based on component particles which are alike in size, shape, and density. This condition is not encountered in the practical mixing of solids and, as shown later, any of these factors may prevent the formation of a random mixture. The value of the number of particles per sample derived in any example must therefore be raised if the limits given are to be maintained.

As the proportion of an active ingredient in a mixture decreases, the number of particles in each sample or dose must increase and materials of smaller particle size must be used. This statement indicates the limitation of the mixing of solids. Production of very fine powders is difficult and often attended by severe aggregation, thus defeating the object of size reduction in the mixing process. Where the proportion of active constituent is very small and is finally presented in a small dose unit, dry mixing of solids may fail to produce an adequate dispersion of one component in another, and other methods, such as spraying a solution of one component on to another, must be adopted.

Another example of the relation of dose uniformity and number of particles in the dose is found with two components that are separately granulated before mixing. This procedure is sometimes adopted for reasons of stability during granulation. The variation in samples drawn from such a system is much greater than the variations in a mixture which was mixed before granulation because the effective number of particles in the sample is greatly reduced.

Degree of Mixing

A quantitative expression that defines the state of a mixture is necessary if a rational answer to the question; "Is this material well enough mixed?" is to be made. Such an expression would also allow the course of mixing to be followed and the performance of different mixers to be compared. The most useful method of expressing the degree of mixing is by measuring the statistical variation in composition of a number of samples drawn from the mix. The scale of scrutiny determines the size of the samples, and their number depends on the accuracy required of the assessment.

As already shown, a series of samples drawn from a random mix exhibits a standard deviation of s_r. An index of mixing, M, suggested by Lacey [62] is given by Eq. (39),

$$M = \frac{s_r}{s} \qquad (39)$$

where s is the standard deviation of samples drawn from the mixture under examination. This approaches unity as mixing is completed. Equation (40) has been suggested,

$$M' = \frac{s_0 - s}{s_0^2 - s_r} \qquad (40)$$

where s_0 is the standard deviation of samples drawn from the unmixed materials. It is equal to $p(1-p)$, where p is the proportion of the component in the mix. It has been modified [62] to Eq. (41), using the variance of the samples,

$$M'' = \frac{s^2 - s_r^2}{s_0^2 - s_r^2} \tag{41}$$

This is a fundamental equation for expressing the state of the mixture, the index M'' varying from zero to one.

The binomial and Poisson distributions have also been used to examine the state of a mixture. If the proportion of black particles in a random mixture of black and white particles is p, the probability, $P(x)$, of obtaining x black particles in a sample of n particles is given by Eq. (42).

$$P(x) = \binom{n}{x} p^x (1-p)^{n-x} \tag{42}$$

If p is small (< 0.15) and n is large, the Poisson distribution can be used, applying Eq. (43),

$$P(x) = e^{-m} \frac{m^x}{x!} \tag{43}$$

where $m = np$, the mean number of black particles in the samples of n particles. This relation may be used in an assessment of dry mixing equipment [63]. If m is greater than 20 and more than 10 samples are taken, then:

- About 10 of the samples have the number of black particles outside the limits $m \pm 1.7\sqrt{m}$,
- About 5% of the samples have the number of black particles outside the limits $m \pm 2.0\sqrt{m}$, and,
- About 1% of the samples has the number of black particles outside the limits $m \pm 2.6\sqrt{m}$.

The results of such tests, in which small cubes of polythene were mixed in a double-cone blender, are shown in Fig. 50a and b. The probability that the results plotted in Fig. 50a came from a random mixture is less than 0.01, with 19 out of 34 samples exceeding the 1-in-10 limits. The densities of the two components in this example were 0.92 and 1.2. The results given in Fig. 50b were obtained when the components were of the same density and the probability that the samples were drawn from a random mixture was 0.7.

Alternatively, satisfactory mixing may be established by imposing standards dictated by the operations in which the mixture is to take part. For example, Kaufman [64] measured the variance of ten samples drawn at random from a mixture of procaine penicillin and dihydrostreptomycin being mixed in a tumbler blender. The variance of the samples at different times during mixing is shown in Fig. 51. The samples, which in this case weighed 5 g, represent the ultimate subdivision of a production-size antibiotic mixture. An acceptable degree of homogeneity was set at a standard deviation of 5%, giving a variance of $(0.05)^2$, and this was achieved after just over 100 revolutions of the mixer. [The line around the experimental values of the variance in Fig. 51 defines the limits within which the true variance lies ($P = 0.9$)]. By this method, the suitability of the machine and operating characteristics were established.

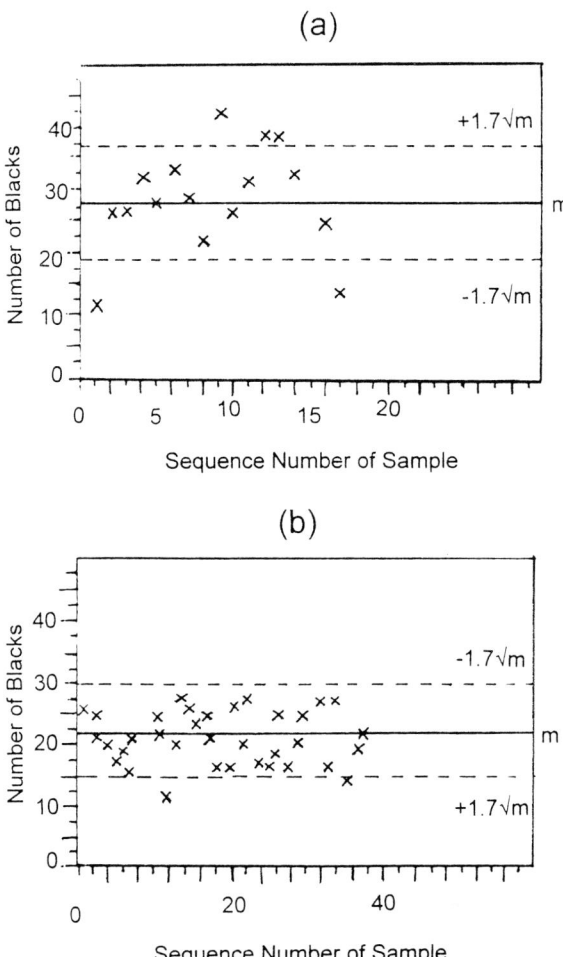

FIG. 50. Variation in the number of black particles in samples drawn from a tumbler blender; (a) $p < 0.01$; (b) $p = 0.7$.

Mechanism of Mixing and Demixing

The randomization of particles by relative movement, one to another, is achieved by the following mechanisms:

- *Convective mixing*, where groups of adjacent particles are transferred from one location in the mass to another,
- *Diffusive mixing*, where the particles are distributed over a freshly developing surface, and
- *Shear mixing*, where slip planes are set up within the mass.

All take place to some extent during mixing, but they vary in extent with the type of mixer used. In general, a large diffusional element is necessary if the scale of scrutiny is small. In addition, distortion of portions of the material by intense shear forces,

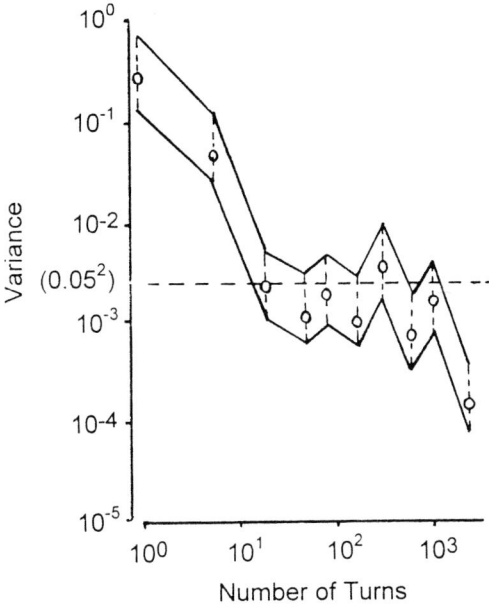

FIG. 51. Decrease in the variance of samples drawn from a mixture of penicillin (40%) and dihydrostreptomycin in a twin-shell blender.

as in mulling, and the scattering of individual particles by impact, processes normally associated with size reduction, are used for some mixing operations.

Convective mixing predominates in machines utilizing a mixing element moving in a stationary container, for example, the horizontal ribbon mixer. Groups of adjacent particles are moved from one position to another, steadily decreasing the scale of segregation.

Diffusive mixing predominates in tumbler mixers. The material is tumbled as it is lifted past its angle of repose. Mixing occurs when a particle changes its path of circulation through a collision or by being trapped in voids presented by another layer of particles.

Shear mixing occurs when forces acting on the particles induce the formation of a slip place, resulting in relative displacement of two regions. Shear mixing occurs, for example, in the rearrangement of shapes as the main charge falls from end to end in a double cone mixer. Train [61] has stressed the importance of expansion or dilation of the material so that shear forces may be effective. A practical corollary is that efficiency will be reduced if the machine is overfilled.

The mild forces involved in the examples given above may be insufficient to adequately disperse materials that tend to aggregate. The more energetic processes of mulling and impact milling may then be used. Size reduction and mixing are carried out simultaneously, although the former may be slight. An example is found in the incorporation of ferric oxide and basic zinc carbonate in the production of calamine. For mixing of this type the hammer mill, mullers, and ball mills charged with small balls are frequently used. The batch being processed at any time must contain the correct amount of materials. If the hold-up capacity of the mill is sufficiently large, this can be achieved by a correctly proportioned feed. Otherwise, the product will have to be mixed a second time by some other method to correct large-scale segregation of low intensity.

If all the particles in a mixture reacted equally to an applied force, all mixers would eventually produce a random mixture, although the time taken would vary, the more efficient mixer producing a random mix more quickly. The characteristics of real mixtures prevent this, and differences in particle size, shape, and density oppose randomization; of these, differences in particle size are most important. The role of these factors in opposing mixing and promoting demixing is demonstrated by the analysis of horizontal drum mixing [65]. Movement of material in a radial plane is shown in Fig. 52. The static mass of particles is lifted past its angle of repose and particles tumble down the free surface, accelerating to the center of the mixer and decelerating before entering the static bed. The zone in which this takes place is the mixing zone, and since it is in contact with the static bed in which no mixing takes place and which is moving in the opposite direction, a velocity gradient develops across the mixing zone, that is, a layer of particles is passing over the layer beneath, and so on. This zone is in an expanded state and particles are therefore passing over voids in the layer beneath. Mixing occurs when a particle is trapped by moving into a void, changing its path of circulation. This mechanism suggests an optimum running speed. If it is too slow, not enough events occur. If it is too fast, there is not sufficient time for capture.

As long as one type of particle is not preferentially caught, random mixing eventually occurs in the radial plane. If, however, one component is smaller, denser, or has certain shape characteristics, it is preferentially trapped and moves into the lower layers of the mixing zone until it finally concentrates as a central core running the length of the mixer. Similar effects occur in axial mixing, and the final shape of the segregated zone formed under the influence of axial and radial movement depends on the flow properties of the material. Similar effects have been reported with a double-cone blender [63]. Segregation also occurs with materials dumped from the mixer.

In general, one component concentrates at one position in the mixer when a simple, repetitive, and symmetric movement occurs. Modern design tends to the rotation of asymmetric shapes or to symmetric shapes rotated asymmetrically, often with an abrupt reversal in the movement of the charge. Even so, segregation may still occur after a long period of mixing. The variance of samples decreases during mixing to a minimum value. This is followed by a period of demixing, the variance finally achieving a higher equilibrium value. It is therefore possible to overmix.

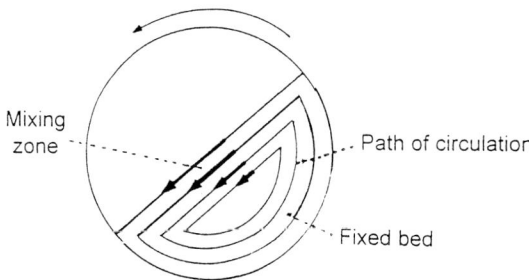

FIG. 52. The mechanism of radial mixing and demixing. The arrows describe the variations of velocity in the mixing zone.

Mixing Rate

Since mixing is a process of achieving uniform randomness, the rate of mixing is proportional to the amount of mixing still to be done. If, at the start a particle changes its path of circulation, it is most likely to find itself in a different environment. The mixing rate is therefore high. At the end of the process, the particle is less likely to find a different environment, and such a change gives no useful mixing. Fewer mixing events take place, and the mixing rate finally reaches zero. It can be represented for any mixing mechanism by Eq. (44),

$$\frac{dM}{dt} = k(1 - M) \tag{44}$$

where M, the index of mixing, has already been defined. Integration of this equation gives Eq. (45).

$$M = 1 - e^{-kt} \tag{45}$$

The rate constant, k, depends on the physical nature of the materials being mixed and on the geometry and operation of the mixer.

Mixing Machines

Mullers and impact millers have been discussed earlier in this article.

Trough, Ribbon, and Paddle Mixers

A simple trough mixer consists of a semicircular trough in which an impeller, such as a number of paddles mounted at diverse angles on a shaft running the length of the trough, rotates, lifting and distributing the material in an irregular manner. Convective and shear mixing occurs, as well as some fine-scale diffusive mixing when the impeller lifts material clear of the main charge.

The ribbon mixer employs a ribbon-like conveying scroll. The helix, which may be continuous or interrupted, is rotated in a semicircular trough and mixing again occurs through convection and shear, giving rapid coarse-scale dispersion. Two ribbons set to convey material in opposite directions are frequently fitted to the shaft. Although little axial mixing in the vicinity of the shaft occurs, mixtures with high homogeneity can be produced by prolonged mixing, even when components differ in particle size, shape, or density or tend to aggregate.

Tumbler Mixers

Tumbler mixers operate by a mainly diffusive mechanism; their use is confined to free-flowing and granular materials. The mild forces employed, which preclude the mixing of materials that aggregate strongly, allow friable materials to be handled satisfactorily. The more elaborate geometrical forms are most commonly used because movement of material in all planes, which is necessary for rapid overall mixing, is induced. Internal baffles and lifter blades may also be incorporated. For example, axial movement of material along the length of a simple drum mixer is slow and can be enhanced by these methods.

Mixing of Liquids

In the mixing of miscible liquids, any practical scale of scrutiny embraces a very large number of particles. If, therefore, a mixture of liquids is randomized by agitation, for all practical purposes it can be regarded as uniform. Miscible liquids are classified as positive mixtures and would, given time, mix completely without external help. The time required for mixing is reduced by agitation during which the scale of segregation is reduced, allowing a fast decay in the intensity of segregation by natural diffusion. In general, no great problems are encountered unless the scale of the operation is very large. Miscible liquids are most commonly mixed by impellers rotating in tanks, including paddles, propellers, and turbines.

In conjunction with the design of the containing vessel, these provide a region of intense shear in the vicinity of the impeller with the induction of high velocity gradients and turbulence within the liquid, and the projection of the disturbance as a flow pattern extending throughout the volume of the container. This pattern is dictated by the type and position of the impeller, the design of the tank, and the flow properties of the material.

All the material should pass through the impeller zone at frequent intervals of time, the design of the mixer preventing the formation of "dead" zones. The turbulent, high velocity flow of liquid from the impeller causes mixing by projecting eddies into, and entraining liquid from, the neighboring zones. The thin ribbons of one component in another rapidly become diffuse and finally disappear through molecular diffusion.

The flow pattern may be analyzed in terms of its three components of motion:

- Radial flow, in a direction perpendicular to the impeller shaft,
- Longitudinal or axial flow, in a direction parallel to the shaft, and
- Tangential flow, in which the liquid follows a circular path around the shaft.

A satisfactory flow pattern depends on the correct balance of these components. In a cylindrical tank, radial flow gives rise to axial flow by reaction at the wall of the tank. Tangential flow receives no such modification. Its predominance as laminar flow circulation supports stratification at various levels. Furthermore, a vortex is created at the surface of the liquid which may penetrate to the impeller, causing air to be dispersed in the liquid. In general, tangential flow should be minimized by moving the impeller to an off-center position, thus destroying the symmetry of the mixer, or by modification of the flow pattern by means of baffles. Tanks with vertical agitators may be baffled by one, two, or more strips mounted vertically on or just away from the vessel wall. These reduce but do not eliminate tangential flow, whereas little modification of radial and axial flow occurs. Baffles produce additional turbulence.

Additional factors must be applied to the mixing of two immiscible liquids. This operation, which is encountered, for example, in liquid–liquid extraction, involves the production and maintenance of a large interfacial contact area. In addition, separation of phases because of differences in density must be opposed by an adequate axial flow pattern. The high rates of shear induced by the rotation of a propeller or turbine cause globules of the disperse phase to be drawn into an unstable filament of liquid which breaks and reforms into smaller globules. Unless stabilized by surface-active agents, the reverse process, coalescence, occurs in zones where velocity gradients are small.

Paddle Mixers

Figure 53 shows four types of paddle mixers. The mixing element is large in relation to the vessel and rotates at low speeds (10–100 rpm). A simple paddle, with upper and lower blades, suitable for mixing miscible liquids of low viscosity, is shown in Fig. 53a. A tangential flow pattern predominates with zones of turbulence to the rear of the blades. The gate paddle, Fig. 53b, is suitable for mixing liquids of higher viscosity, and the anchor paddle, Fig. 53d, with low clearance between pan and blade is useful for working across a heat transfer surface. Stationary paddles intermeshing with the moving element suppress swirling in the mixer illustrated in Fig. 53c. In the other examples, baffles are also necessary. Unless paddle blades are pitched, poor axial turnover of the liquid occurs. Paddles are therefore not suitable for mixtures that separate.

Propeller Mixers

Propellers are commonly used for mixing miscible and immiscible liquids of low viscosity. The marine propeller is typical of the group. High speed rotation (400–1500 rpm) of the relatively small element provides high shear rates in the vicinity of the impeller and a flow pattern with mainly axial and tangential components. They may be used in unbaffled tanks when mounted in an off-center position or inclined from the vertical. In large-scale operations, horizontal mounting in the side of the vessel is frequently used.

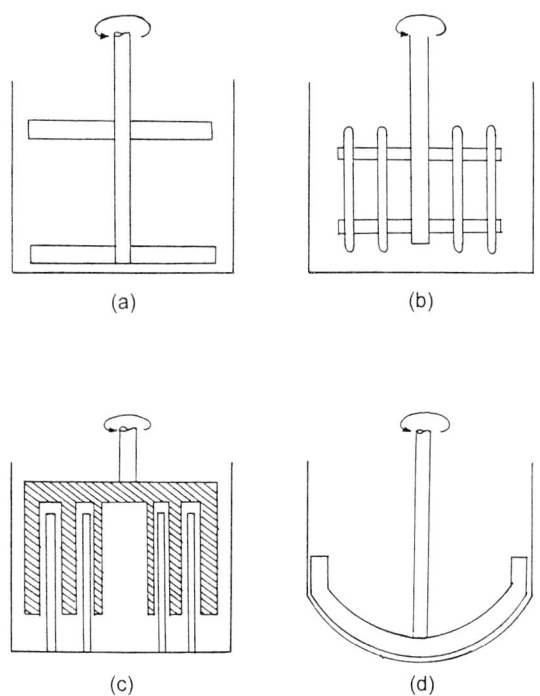

FIG. 53. Paddle mixers. (a) Simple; (b) gate; (c) stationary; (d) anchor.

Turbines

Turbine designs are intermediate between paddles and propellers. Turbines are effective mixers over a wide viscosity range and provide a very versatile mixing tool. The ratio of radial to tangential flow, the predominating parameters with this impeller, increases as the operating speed increases. Pitched-blade turbines are sometimes used to increase axial flow. Baffles must be used to limit swirling unless the turbine is shrouded. This impeller produces a discharge with no tangential component.

Mixing of Liquids and Solids

Examples of solid–liquid mixing are found in dissolution and crystallization and in the control of chemical reactions between solids and liquids. Randomization of materials for subdivision and presentation may also be the object, as, for example, in the production of toothpaste.

The flow properties of a liquid-solid mixture alter markedly with change in the ratio of the two phases. At low-solid disperse-phase concentrations, flow properties are Newtonian and mixing by impellers is satisfactory so long as the components of flow oppose settling. Under these conditions, it may be desirable to increase the size and decrease the speed of the impeller. For a given power input, flow patterns are improved at the expense of turbulence. Unless the difference in density between solid and liquid is small, paddles are ineffective for suspending solids. Otherwise, the discussion presented for the mixing of liquids may be applied.

Anomalous flow characteristics are exhibited at higher disperse-phase concentrations in which the apparent viscosity is a function of the shear rate. The apparent viscosity may increase or, more commonly, decrease as the speed of the impeller is increased. Mixing is achieved by suitable impellers, notably the turbine, as long as adequate flow patterns in the entire volume of the mixing vessel are created. Turbulence is less effective as a mechanism of mixing and regimes of laminar flow are extensive.

Further increase in apparent viscosity occurs at higher disperse-phase concentrations. This is often associated with the development of a yield value. Unlike with true liquids, shear forces must exceed a certain level before deformation occurs. Since the shear forces developed by particles suspended in liquids are small, sedimentation does not occur, and the mixture may be classified as neutral. Mixing by impellers is precluded if the apparent viscosity is very high because the projection of adequate flow patterns is impossible. Alternative methods must be used in which the mixing element passes all stations in the mixing vessel. For thin pastes, machines typified by the domestic food mixer are used. Imposition of planetary movement on the rotation of the mixing element causes all parts of the mix to be sheared at intervals. Very high shear rates are produced as the element sweeps out zones close to the wall of the container. In other machines, the containing vessel rotates.

For thicker pastes and plastics, a kneading, stretching, and folding action is employed. The sigma blade, mounted axially in a trough, is a commonly used mixing element. Intense shear is induced by the close clearance between element and container. Simultaneous transport around the trough occurs so that all portions of the mass are periodically deformed. Considerable variation in rheological properties may occur during mixing and robust construction of the mixer is essential.

The differential speed of mill rolls induces high shear rates in the material. This machine is suitable for paste mixing. With more fluid dispersions, the ball mill and the

Unit Processes in Pharmacy: The Operations

colloid mill may be used. Solids that aggregate may be successfully dispersed, although subsequent stability may require the addition of a deflocculating agent.

Blending solids with very small quantities of liquid, an operation commonly used for granulating powders, presents extreme problems of uniformity. If the material does not become plastic and pasty, it does not mix by shear deformation in the manner described above. Mixing is best achieved by spraying the liquid as fine droplets on to a highly mobile powder which is continually and rapidly developing new surfaces. In this way, all the particles can be exposed to the spray. A closed ribbon mixer, planetary mixer, or sigma blade mixer can be used. Alternatively, tumbler mixers can be fitted with a spray device. If the solid is itself a mixture, the material must be completely mixed before the liquid is added. Otherwise, homogeneity is difficult to achieve.

Sterilization

Sterilization processes do not result in a product that can be described as absolutely sterile or nonsterile inasmuch as the process is a statistical phenomenon. A variety of techniques are available [66], including heat, radiation, ethylene oxide sterilization, and sterile filtration.

Thermal Sterilization

The amount of heat required to sterilize depends upon the magnitude (T), duration (t), and amount of moisture present, $t \propto 1/T$.

For example, heat coagulates protein in the living cell. The temperature required for this phenomenon to occur is inversely proportional to the moisture present.

Dry Heat

Relatively stable substances that resist degradation at high temperatures ($> 140°C$) are suitable candidates for dry heat sterilization. A 2-h exposure at $180°C$ or 45 min at $260°C$ kills spores as well as vegetative forms of microorganisms. These exposure periods do not include the lag time from loading of the oven until sterilization temperature is reached. The lag time depends on the geometry and operating features of the oven and the characteristics of the load.

Both natural and forced-convection oven types can be employed; they have been described in the section on drying. The forced-convection oven offers the advantages of uniformity of heat distribution and reduction in lag time in comparison with the natural-convection system. The dry-heat method is reserved almost exclusively for glass or metal as other materials char (cellulose), oxidize (rubber), or melt (plastic) at these temperatures.

Moist Heat

Moist heat offers the advantage of greater effectiveness at low temperatures. The thermal capacity of steam is much greater than that of hot air. Spores and vegetative forms of bacteria may be effectively destroyed in an autoclave employing steam ($121°C$) under pressure (15 psig) for 20 min or (27 psig at 132°C) for 3 min. The lag time to complete exposure of the material to be sterilized is important.

Radiation

Ultraviolet light is frequently employed to reduce airborne microbial contamination. Surface sterilization is usually achieved by employing a mercury vapor lamp with an emitted light of 253.7 nm.

Radiation sterilization includes the use of the ionizing radiation of x rays and gamma rays. The former are derived from bombardment of a heavy metal target with electrons. Gamma rays are obtained from atomic nucleus decay from excited to ground state.

The energy evolved from radiation can be equated to photon behavior where $E = h\nu$ and $\nu = C/\lambda$ (E and ν are the energy and frequency of a photon, respectively), h is Planck's constant, and C and λ are the speed and wavelength of light, respectively. The energy absorbed from the radiation sources equates to the dose.

$$1 \text{ rad} = 100 \text{ erg/g of material absorbing}$$
$$= 6.24 \times 10^{13} \text{ eV/g}$$
$$= 2.4 \times 10^{-6} \text{ cal/g } (10 \times 10^{-6} \text{ J/g})$$

There are a variety of radiation sources. ^{60}Cobalt decays to ^{59}Co in the core of a nuclear reactor to emit two photons (1.17 and 1.33 MeV) and an electron (0.31 MeV). The half-time for decay is 5.3 years. ^{137}Cesium decays emitting one photon (0.661 MeV). Cesium has a 33-year half-life. An electron beam can be accelerated to an energy equivalent of 5–10 MeV. At energies below 5 MeV, penetration is insufficient for sterilization. Depth of penetration can be correlated with energy levels; for example, materials with density equivalent to water ($\rho = 1$ g/cm^3) are penetrated 0.5 cm/MeV. ^{60}Cobalt gives rise to radiation that penetrates 30 cm through water. Accelerating electrons have a high dose rate and exposure is only required for seconds. ^{60}Cobalt has a lower dose rate, and an exposure for hours is required.

Ionizing radiation arises from the photoelectric effect, the Compton effect, or ion pair production. Gamma radiation causes local and intense damage and may break chemical bonds. The primary target is the deoxyribonucleic acid (DNA) of the microorganism. In addition, free radicals may be formed, such as peroxides that result in intracellular and extracellular peroxides by a chain reaction that causes damage.

Resistance to Damage

Damage depends on the amount of energy absorbed relative to the number and resistance of the microorganisms being irradiated. Unicellular organisms have greater resistance than multicellular ones. Gram-positive bacteria have greater resistance than gram-negative bacteria. Finally, bacterial spores have greater resistance than vegetative forms. Viruses are more resistant than bacteria. The energy required to reduce the population of viruses by 90% (D value), is 0.5 Mrad (5 mGy). Fungi are equivalent to bacterial spores in their resistance.

In order to evaluate the dose, a number of parameters must be known. What magnitude of source (e.g., ^{60}Co) is available? A typical source ranges from 500,000 to 2×10^6 Curies (Ci) where 1 Ci is 3.7×10^{10} disintegrations per second. The product geometry and the speed of the conveyor carrying it to the source must be known. The dose can be evaluated by a variety of dosimetric techniques. In bulk or ampoules containing liquids, ferric ammonium sulfate and ceric sulfate can be used and the absorbance change evaluated by UV spectrophotometry; however, this is only accurate for ^{60}Co and ^{137}Cs.

Radiochromic solids can be utilized and evaluated by visible spectrophotometry. Amber and red polymethyl methacrylate are used to evaluate 0.1–1.0 or 0.5–5.0 Mrad, respectively. Nylon film is examined for opacity following exposure and may be used to evaluate exposures of 0.1–5.0 Mrad.

Validation requires the determination of the bioburden and the D value. These represent the dose required to achieve sterilization and the estimated dose. If low D values are obtained, the dose may be regarded as overkill. *Bacillus pumulis* exhibits inherently high resistance to gamma-ionization radiation (D values 0.15–0.22 Mrad). The FDA prefers a 12-log reduction in microorganisms. The dose required is approximately 2.6 Mrad.

Product Development

The product, container, and closure must be evaluated for physical and chemical stability. A number of radiation-induced changes can potentially occur. The product may change in color, odor, flavor, potency, biocompatibility, and toxicity. The container may lose rigidity and become brittle and leachable. The product and container may be assessed by exposure to multiple doses and single high doses of radiation. The long-term stability can be evaluated under ambient storage conditions, at elevated temperatures, and under worst-case shipping conditions.

Dose mapping can be performed by determining the minimum radiation point in the load. Multiple dosimeters can be used to view vertical quadrant through the lead. Dosimeters are routinely set to measure the minimum dose.

Ethylene Oxide

Ethylene oxide (bp, 10.8°C) is a gaseous alkylating agent. It alkylates proteins and ribonucleic and deoxyribonucleic acid in microorganisms. It replaces labile hydrogen with hydroxyethyl groups. Ethylene oxide is utilized as a surface sterilant. Bulk crystalline materials can occlude vegetative bacterial cells or spores with crystals. Consequently, ethylene oxide does not reach them. The final step prior to sterilization is an aseptic recrystallization step.

Ethylene oxide is a colorless gas with an aromatic odor. The threshold limit for the odor is 700 ppm. The OSHA specification for worker exposure is 10 ppm. The toxicity of ethylene oxide is similar to that of ammonia. It causes conjunctival and respiratory irritation, dizziness, headaches, and vomiting. It is known to be mutagenic and may be carcinogenic. By-products include ethylene glycol (bp, 198.9°C) and ethylene chlorhydrin (bp, 128.4°C). Pure ethylene oxide is flammable and explosive. It is generally mixed with propellant (88:12) or carbon dioxide (90:10). Ethylene oxide polymerizes in the liquid state in 90–120 days. In this form it may plug lines or deposit polymerized sludge.

Ethylene oxide inactivates all microorganisms. The sterilizing rate depends upon its concentration, the temperature, the duration of exposure, and the water content of the microorganism. Inactivation follows classical first-order kinetics and is irreversible. Relative humidity is synergistic, at 30–60% the microorganism hydrates. The water acts as a vehicle to transport the gas through polyethylene and polypropylene. Polystyrene traps ethylene oxide and dissipates it over years and thus is not appropriate for ethylene oxide sterilization. Temperatures of 40–60°C are suitable for heat-sensitive articles. Cycle times are longer at low temperatures, relative humidities, or ethylene oxide concentrations. Generally, concentrations of 350–700 mg/mL are employed; cycle times vary from 4 to 12 h.

Following sterilization the load is degassed by a dynamic process wherein filtered air is passed over the product for 12–72 h. Degassing usually takes place in the treatment chamber but may be moved to a sterile facility. The process is monitored using *Bacillus subtilis var. niger* as a biological indicator, commercially available as spore strips (10^6 spores per strip). In addition, the load is probed with thermocouples during validation. The gaseous mixture is sampled at different points in the sterilizer for gas chromatographic analysis.

Sterile Filtration

Several filter geometries are available for sterile filtration. They consist of flat membranes in a stainless steel press (< 293 mm), pleated membranes housed in stainless steel cartridges, and stacked plates in the form of flat segments of membrane filters.

Matrix filters consist of fibers with pores having a depth up to 120 μm. Cellulose nitrate may be dissolved in a highly volatile solvent, such as amyl acetate, ether, or dioxane. A gel-forming solvent, acetone, ethanol, or propanol, may be added. The mixture is poured on a flat plate and placed in a controlled-temperature environment to dry. Pore size is dependent on the concentration of the gel-forming solvent. A number of other substances may be used as filter material, including cellulose, acetate and butyrate, polyamides (nylon), polysulfones, fluorocarbons (Durapore membranes), polyvinylidene difluoride (hydrophobic), or surfaces modified with organic amides (hydrophilic), acrylic polymers, or polyvinyl chloride. To make some membranes hydrophilic, surfactants may be added including Tween 80, Triton X-100, hydroxypropyl cellulose, or glycerol. Sieve filters are made of polycarbonate (Nucleopore, 10 μm thick). Collimated uranium fission products form nucleation tracks in film. Exposure to chemical etching determines the pore size.

Adsorption and Screening

Most membrane filters, when wetted, have a negative charge. Bacteria have a similar negative charge and do not necessarily remain on the filter. Filters with other characteristics can be selected under these circumstances. Positively charged (AMF Zeta Plus Membrane) or protein- and peptide-adsorbing (Pall Posidyne Nylon 66) filters can be selected.

Unit Processes in Pharmacy: The Operations

Ionic strength, pH, pressure, and flow rate affect particle adsorption. The flow rate through a filter is expressed by Eq. (46),

$$Q = \frac{C_i \, A \, P}{V} \qquad (46)$$

where C_i is the inherent resistance of the filter to flow (a function of void volumes), A is the surface area, P is the pressure, and V is the viscosity.

Filters are rated according to nominal pore size and absolute pore size (the largest pore in the filter); this recognizes that a pore size distribution exists.

Filter Integrity

The filter integrity can be evaluated by a number of techniques. The destructive test involves filtering a suspension of bacterial cells (*Pseudomonas diminuta*, 0.3×1 µm), through a 0.2-µm filter. If 6 L of suspension containing 1×10^7 organisms per mL are passed through a 1-µm filter, there should be no microorganism and an 8-log reduction would have occurred. The bubble-point test assumes that pores can be characterized as capillaries. When totally wetted, all the capillaries should be full of water or solution. The pore length is generally much greater than the diameter. Pressure is applied to the wetted filter. The bubble-point pressure, P, may be described by Eq. (47),

$$P = \frac{4 \, \gamma \, \cos \theta}{D} \qquad (47)$$

where γ is the surface tension (72 dynes/cm² or 7.2 Pa), θ is the contact angle, and D is the diameter of capillary. The bubble-point test is performed before and after sterile filtration.

A specified area of filter must be soaked in a specified volume of product for a designated time. The accelerated stability of active ingredients at 40–60°C for 60 days must be established prior to the selection of a filter for a particular purpose. The extent of damage, and the nature and quantity of extractables and their potency have to be evaluated.

Extraction and Leaching

Leaching or solid–liquid extraction are terms that describe the extraction of soluble constituents from a solid or semisolid by means of suitable solvents. The process, which is used whenever tea or coffee is made, is an important stage in the production of many fine chemicals found naturally in animal and vegetable tissue. Examples are found in the extraction of fixed oils from seeds, offering an alternative to mechanical expression; in the preparation of alkaloids, such as strychnine from Nux vomica beans or quinine from Cinchona bark; and in the isolation of enzymes, such as rennin, and hormones, such as insulin, from animal sources. In the past, a wider importance attended the process because the products of simple extraction procedures, known as galenicals, formed the major part of the ingredients used to fulfill a doctor's prescription.

Methods

Leaching in the pharmaceutical and allied industries is operated as a batch process because high cost materials are processed in relatively small quantities. Frequent changes of material may be made, creating problems of cleaning and contamination. For these reasons, continuous extraction, which is characterized by a large throughput and the mechanical movement of the solid counter to the flow of solvent, is not applicable to pharmaceutical extraction and is not described here.

Whatever the scale of the extraction, leaching is performed in one of two ways. In the first, the raw material is placed in a vessel, forming a permeable bed through which the solvent or menstruum percolates. The wanted constituents are dissolved, and the solution issues from the bottom of the bed. This liquid is sometimes called the miscella and the exhausted solids the marc. The process is called leaching by percolation. The second process employs immersion and consists of immersing the solid in the solvent and stirring. After a suitable period of time, solid and liquid are separated.

The choice of extraction method depends primarily on the physical properties of the basic material and its particle size. A coarse, rigid powder forms beds of high permeability and percolation is suitable. The expense of finer grinding is avoided and the subsequent separation of solids and liquids is facilitated. The process can be conducted in such a way that a concentrated product is obtained. Other materials, such as fine powders of compressible animal tissues, do not form permeable beds and the immersion method must be chosen. Some compensation for the difficulties of separation and the dilution of the extract during washing may be found in a more rapid and more complete extraction, because of the use of finer powders, intimate contact between solids and liquid, and the absence of channeling.

The use of pressure extends the application of percolation to materials that form beds of low permeability. Alternatively, permeability may be increased by grinding the solids with a supporting material such as glass wool.

Percolation

Coarsely ground material is placed in the body of the extractor which may be jacketed for control of the extraction temperature. The packing must be even or the solvent flows preferentially through a limited volume of the bed and leaching is inefficient. In large extractors, channeling is prevented or reduced by horizontal, perforated plates placed at intervals in the bed; these redistribute the percolating liquid.

Solvent imbibition swells dried materials and reduces the permeability of the bed. This is most marked with aqueous solvents. If swelling occurs, it is necessary to moisten the material with water or with the solvent before it is packed into the extractor.

Once the extractor is packed, leaching may be conducted in a number of ways. The body of the extractor may be completely filled with the solvent. Liquid is withdrawn from the body through the false bottom and more solvent is added until the marc is exhausted. Alternatively, the solution issuing from the bottom may be returned to the top. After a period of recirculation, the liquid is completely withdrawn and fresh sol-

Unit Processes in Pharmacy: The Operations

vent admitted. In both processes, a period of steeping or soaking may precede the movement of liquid.

In beds of high permeability, adequate movement of liquid is obtained by simple gravity operation in an open vessel. If the material forms a dense bed, however, the liquid must be pumped through if suitable flow rates are to be secured. A closed extraction vessel must be used. Closed extraction vessels are also necessary for high-temperature extraction and extraction with volatile solvents. In other methods, the liquid is forced upward through the bed. Possible migration of fine material downward and the formation of a region of low permeability at the bottom of the bed is prevented in this way. In other processes, the bed may not be immersed in the solvent which is simply sprinkled on the upper surface and allowed to trickle through the bed, the voids of which are mainly filled with air.

Simple extractions of this type, if carried to completion, require large amounts of solvent and yield dilute extracts. These disadvantages can be overcome if the extraction is followed by evaporation. These operations are often integrated in an extraction plant. The leach liquids leaving the extractor enter an evaporator heated, for example, by a calandria. Since most materials encountered are heat sensitive, this equipment is operated at reduced pressure. The vapor leaving the evaporator is condensed and returned to the extractor. In extracts with water-immiscible solvents, any water derived from the feed material and present in the condensate is separated and rejected. The extraction is stopped when the leach liquid is free from wanted constituents; a concentrated extract remains in the evaporator.

Leaching by percolation provides a simple method of separating leach liquid and solid during the extraction. When this is completed, the permeable bed is largely drained, permitting extensive solvent recovery. Further recovery can be gained by mechanical expression.

Immersion

In pharmaceutical processes, leaching by immersion is carried out in simple tanks which may be agitated by a turbine or paddle. If the solids are adequately suspended, intimate contact between the phases promotes efficient extraction. Incomplete extraction due to channeling is avoided and difficulties due to swelling do not arise. Problems arise, however, in the subsequent separation of the phases. The materials to which leaching by immersion is applied are normally either finely divided or coarse and compressible. When agitation ceases, the solids settle and the leach liquid can be siphoned or pumped off by lines suitably placed in the tank. The sediment, however, contains a large volume of the leach liquid which must be recovered by resuspending the solids in fresh solvent, allowing the solids to sediment and decanting the supernatant liquid. Cake filtration provides an alternative method of separation. The leach liquid remaining in the cake is displaced by passing a wash liquid. In some cases, a filter press may be used for both extraction and separation.

Solvent

The ideal solvent is cheap, nontoxic, and nonflammable. It is highly selective, dissolving only the wanted constituents of the solid. It should have a low viscosity, allowing easy movement through a bed of solids, and, if the resulting solution is to be concentrated by evaporation, have a high vapor pressure. These factors greatly limit the number of solvents of commercial value. Water and alcohol, and mixtures of the two, are widely used. Both, however, are nonselective, leaching varying proportions of gums, mucilages, and other unwanted components. Most of the tinctures and liquid extracts used in pharmacy are simple, impure extracts made with water or mixtures of water and alcohol. Acidified or alkaline mixtures of water and alcohol are used to extract insulin from comminuted pancreas. A more selective extraction is given by petroleum solvents, benzene, and related solvents. In the preparation of many pure alkaloids, the powdered material is moistened with an alkaline solution, packed into a bed, and leached with petroleum. Subsequent purification by fractional crystallization is facilitated by the absence of gums. Acetone and chlorinated hydrocarbons also find applications in leaching. In some cases, specific properties of the wanted constituents may suggest a particular solvent. Eugenol, for example, can be readily extracted from cloves with a solution of potassium hydroxide.

Leaching Rate

Whatever method is adopted, leaching consists of a number of consecutive diffusional or mass transfer processes. The solvent first penetrates the raw material and dissolves the soluble elements. These diffuse in the opposite direction to the surface of the solid matrix and through the liquid layers at its surface to reach the bulk solution. These processes are under the influence of an overall concentration gradient, the concentration being lowest in the bulk solution. Any of these processes may be responsible for limiting the rate at which leaching proceeds. In pharmaceutical leaching, however, the solid matrix is usually cellular, a structure which normally offers the highest diffusional resistance. The complexity of such structures does not permit a strict analysis of the processes of mass transfer. Nevertheless, the simple diffusional concepts expressed in Fick's law suggest that the following factors influence the leaching rate:

- The size distribution of the leached particles,
- The temperature of leaching,
- The physical properties of solvent, and
- The relative movement imposed upon the solids and the liquid.

Size and Size Distribution of the Solid Particles

The particle size of the solids determines the distance which solvent and solute must diffuse within the solid matrix. Since this distance offers the major diffusional resistance, its reduction by comminution raises the rate of leaching, the concentration gradient being effectively increased. In addition, the inverse relationship between particle size and surface area requires an increase in the area of contact between the matrix and the surrounding liquid. Transfer of solute at this boundary is therefore facilitated. In leaching by immersion, a further advantage conferred by size reduction is the ease with which finer particles are suspended. Finally, extensive cell rupture occurs during grinding, allowing more direct contact between solvent and solute and more rapid dissolution and diffusion.

Other factors, however, operate against size reduction. Leaching by percolation demands the formation of a permeable bed. Low permeability gives low flow rates and low extraction rates. Permeability is a complex function of both particle size and porosity, the former determining how a given void space is to be disposed within the bed. The disposition of the void space consists of few channels of relatively large diameter, that is, a bed of high permeability, if the particle size is large. In leaching by immersion, the difficulties of separating solid and liquid increase as the particle size decreases.

The opposition of the factors suggests an optimum particle size for any particular extraction. This is determined to some extent by the physical nature of the solids. A dense, woody structure would be extracted as a fine powder. An example is given by the root of Ipecacuanha. A leafy structure, on the other hand, would be more satisfactorily leached as a coarse powder.

Both porosity and permeability are influenced by the particle size distribution. A high porosity is secured if the distribution is narrow. Small particles may otherwise fill the interstices created by the contact of larger particles. After grinding it is often necessary, therefore, to classify the product and remove undersize material. This material would then be bulked with the fines from other batches and extracted separately. A further advantage arising from a narrow size distribution is even packing and the creation of a regular system of pores and waists. This promotes even movement of solvent and solution through the bed.

In some cases, size reduction may take a particular form. Seeds and beans are often rolled or flaked to produce extensive cell rupture. In other processes, the cell wall, although depressing the rate of extraction, may make the extraction more selective by preventing the movement of unwanted materials of high molecular weight. Here, the size reduction must leave most cells intact.

Temperature

Within the limits imposed by the thermal stability of the wanted constituents, a high extraction temperature appears desirable. The solubility of most materials increases with increasing temperature, allowing higher solute concentrations and higher concentration gradients. Both this and the increased diffusivity result in higher extraction rates. In many cases, however, materials are susceptible to heat degradation and cold extraction must be used. In addition, the selectivity of a solvent may be impaired at high temperatures. An example of the use of moderately high temperatures is the extraction of Rauwolfia alkaloids with boiling methanol.

The Relative Movement Imposed Upon the Solids and the Liquid

The major and controlling resistance to the diffusion of the solute to the bulk solution is normally found in the cell matrix. Increase in the rate of movement of the solution past the surface does not, therefore, greatly affect the rate of extraction. This is in marked contrast to the processes of dissolution and crystallization. Nevertheless, movement is imposed upon the solvent in both general methods described above.

In the percolation of a liquid through a bed of solids, mass transfer of the solute from the surfaces of the solid to the liquid in the interstices of the bed takes place by molecular diffusion and by natural convection arising from the density changes created by dissolution. Although these processes are slow, they are much faster than mass transfer in the matrix under the same concentration differences. Concentration gradients in the liquid outside the particles are, therefore, very low. At any point in the bed, the introduction of dilute solution from above and the loss of concentrated solution to below decrease the interstitial concentration by dilution or displacement. This effect can be considered simply to reduce the solute concentration at the junction of solid and solution, thus imposing a favorable concentration gradient within the matrix.

Similarly, the agitation of the slurry in leaching by immersion is not primarily to decrease the thickness of the boundary layer at the surface and its diffusional resistance. Rather, agitation serves only to keep the particles in suspension and to equalize the solute concentration throughout the liquid. If the particles settle, the solute must diffuse through the stagnant fluid filling the interstices of the bed. High diffusional resistance is created and the rate of extraction is lowered. These conditions are characteristic of the maceration process of the *British Pharmacopoeia*.

Applications

The processes described here are integrated in order to facilitate the production of pharmaceutical dosage forms. The following examples are intended to illustrate the application of the processes in the dominant pharmaceutical settings. They have been selected to demonstrate the broad application of unit operations in pharmaceutical manufacturing. Unique processes are associated with each dosage form. This is no less the case for dermatologics, intranasal and inhalation products, and the range of alternative pharmaceuticals than for the examples given. Nevertheless, the majority of processes and their underlying principles [1] are similar from one dosage form to the next.

Parenteral Products

Parenteral products are intended for injection into a variety of subdermal and submucosal locations [67]. Their manufacture can be defined as a sequence of operations intended to be performed in certain environments or under specific conditions. Figure 54 illustrates the sequence in which these processes may be combined. This flow dia-

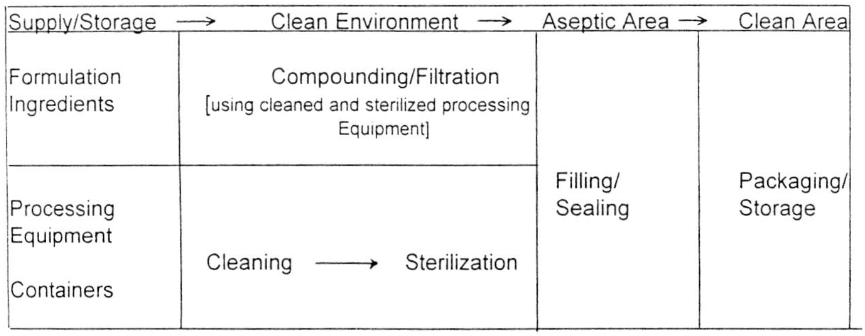

Supply/Storage →	Clean Environment →	Aseptic Area →	Clean Area
Formulation Ingredients	Compounding/Filtration [using cleaned and sterilized processing Equipment]		
Processing Equipment		Filling/ Sealing	Packaging/ Storage
Containers	Cleaning → Sterilization		

FIG. 54. Flow diagram illustrating the various processes in sterile parenterals production.

Solid Dosage Forms

The majority of solid dosage forms are intended for oral ingestion. The drug released from the dosage form is available at the site of absorption or action within the gastrointestinal tract. Table 2 illustrates the sequence in which processes may be combined to manufacture solid dosage forms.

Additional processes are required for the production of tablets beyond those described previously. As these processes are not ubiquitous in pharmaceutical manufacturing they are dealt with only briefly here.

Granulation

Following particle size reduction and blending the formulation may be granulated [68], which provides homogeneity of drug distribution in the blend. In addition, it may help flow properties and compression characteristics of the powder. Large granules can be prepared from primary particles by drying from a slurry (with techniques described above) or spraying with granulating solution. Figure 55a shows a top-spray granulator. An alternative method (Fig. 55b) employs an auger to force the blend between rollers, thereby forming a compressed solid which disintegrates into large aggregates [69].

The steps involved in granulation begin with transferring powders to a mixer and blending the product. The granulation solution can be added and coarse milling or wet granulation begun. Finally, the product is dried and milled to an appropriate size.

Compression

Compressed solids, tablets, or caplets, are prepared by placing the blend of component additives in a cylinder or die, above a moveable piston or punch. An upper punch is brought into the top of the piston, and pressure applied to the distal ends of the punches forces the powder into a compact (Fig. 56). The quality of the product depends upon

TABLE 2 Tableting Unit Processes in Sequence of Performance

Tableting Operation	Consequence of	
	Excess Activity	Insufficient Activity
Size reduction	Poor wetting	Poor availability
Mixing	Demixing	Nonuniformity
Granulation	Slow dissolution	Flow and compression problems
Drying	Compression problems	Slow dissolution
Sizing	Flow and compression problems	Nonuniformity
Blending	Slow dissolution	Nonuniformity
Compression	Slow dissolution	Friability problems
Coating	Slow dissolution	Inadequate protection
Printing	Defects	Defects

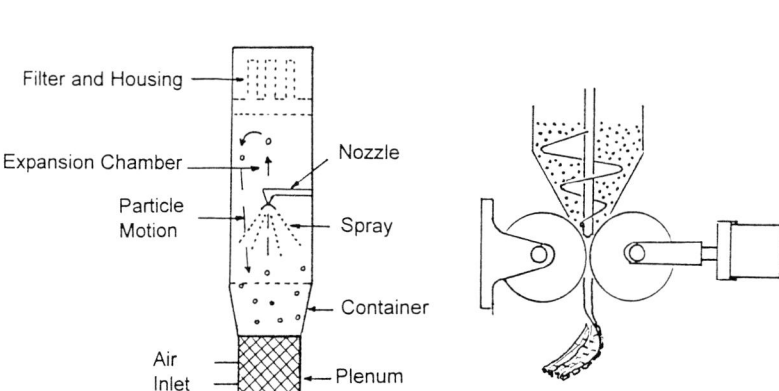

FIG. 55. (a) Top spray granulator; (b) chilsonator.

the cohesive forces acting on the powder upon compression. These cohesive forces are influenced by the selection of additives in the dosage formulation. One method of evaluating tablet manufacture considers the effect of the applied pressure on porosity of a compressed powder [70]. Data may be plotted as the negative natural logarithm of porosity against applied pressure in the form of a Heckel plot [71]. The slope of this plot is proportional to the yield value (ϕ, elastic limit) with a value of $1/3\phi$.

Bioprocessing

The use of biotechnology in the manufacture of pharmaceuticals is of increasing interest. Consequently, these techniques require attention in the planning of unit processes.

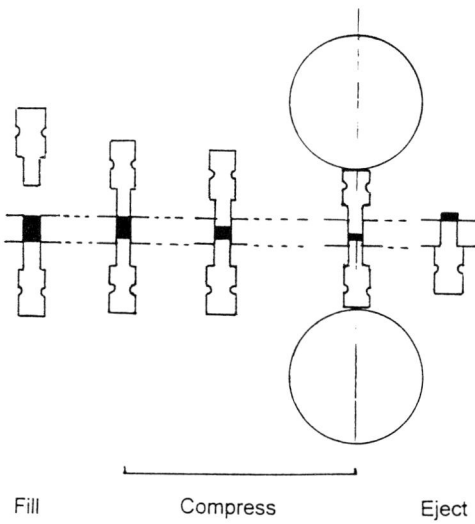

FIG. 56. Sequence of events in tablet press operation.

Unit Processes in Pharmacy: The Operations

Bioprocessing can be considered in terms of small-scale bioreactors, or fermenters, and the translation of such processes into large-scale economically viable production operations [72,73].

Bioprocessing is by no means a new field. The topicality of this subject is due to the increased interest in the use of isolated cells and micro-organisms as manufacturing tools. It might well be argued that this technology was developed millenia ago for the purposes of wine and beer production. More recently, the use of attenuated microorganisms or isolated antigenic materials for vaccination resulted in further developments. In the last decade, the interest in genetic engineering and manipulation of the genetic code of certain microorganisms has produced a revolution in the manufacturing of pharmaceuticals.

Bioreactors

The major difference between a biotechnological process and other pharmaceutical manufacturing operations is the need for a bioreactor (Fig. 57). These bioreactors may be required to produce expressed proteins utilizing bacteria, yeast, insect, or mammalian cells [73]. Table 3 illustrates the various processes [72]. It would be difficult to describe the various bioreactor elements and their permutations. Some of simplest examples of bioreactors are shown in Fig. 58.

Conclusion

Pharmaceutical manufacturing entails the combination of a number of unit processes. The major processes have been described in this article. Brief outlines of the applications of these processes to parenteral, solid dosage form, and biological materials production are given.

The efficiency, quality, and economy of manufacturing depends upon an understanding of the individual operations involved in processing. In many cases, unlike in other

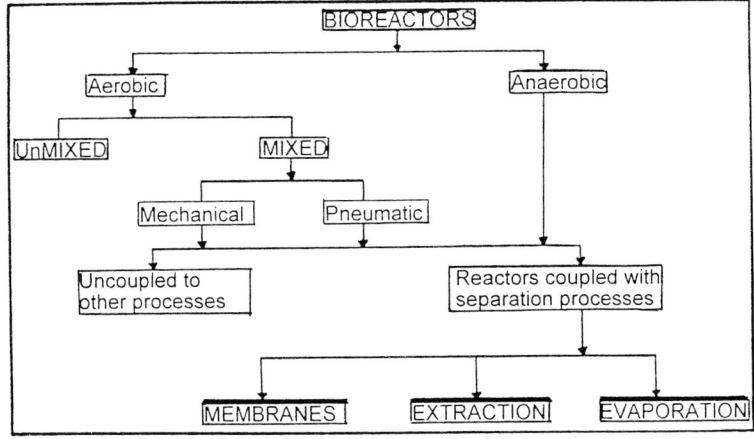

FIG. 57. Schematic of types of bioreactor.

TABLE 3 Biotechnological Processing

Stage	Activity	Impact
First	Reactions: catabolic, anabolic, enzymatic, degradation, and stoichiometric	Molecular
Second	Metabolite translocation; compartments differentiation; genetic changes	Individual cells
Third	Growth; dispersed, segregated, and mixed culture interactions	Populations of cells
Fourth[a]	Reaction mixers: mass and heat transfer; dynamics and control; coupled to processes	Bioreactor
Fifth[a]	Separation unit operations; process synthesis and integration; quantitative and qualitative evaluation for process design	Process design

[a]Traditional unit operations.

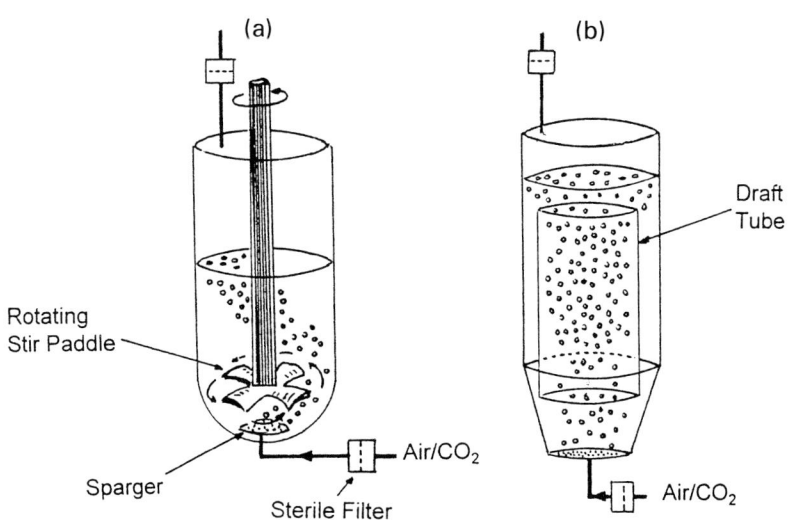

FIG. 58. Bioreactors: (a) stirred tank reactor; (b) airlift fermentor.

industrial processing, safety and efficacy of a therapeutic agent may be affected. A guide or introduction to the practical aspects of unit processes in pharmacy is provided here.

Acknowledgments

The authors are grateful to Ms. Valerie McNair-Purvis and Mr. Neville Concessio who assisted in technical aspects of the preparation of this manuscript.

Most of the text is based on a portion of the book entitled *Unit Processes in Pharmacy* by David Ganderton published in 1968 by Heineman Medical Books, Ltd., and

Unit Processes in Pharmacy: The Operations

now out of print. It is appropriate to acknowledge the contributions to that original volume. The following is a quotation from the book.

> The manuscript was originally the commission of Dr. D. M. Moulden. I [DG] acknowledge the considerable help given by his ideas, plans and drafts. In addition, I thank Mr. Ian Boyd and Dr. John Hersey who read and criticized the manuscripts.

Bibliography

T. Allen, *Particle Size Measurement*, 4th ed., Chapman and Hall, New York, 1990.

Andrews, G. A., Kniseley, R. M., and Wagner, H. N., *Radioactive Pharmaceuticals*, US Atomic Energy Commission, Washington, 1966.

Ansel, H. C., Popovich, N. G., and Allen, L., 6th ed., *Pharmaceutical Dosage Forms and Drug Delivery Systems*, Williams and Wilkins, Malvern, PA, 1995.

Avis, K. E., *Process Engineering Applications*, Interpharm Press, Inc., Buffalo Grove, IL, 1995.

Banker, G. S., and Rhodes, C. T., eds., *Modern Pharmaceutics*, 2nd ed., Marcel Dekker, Inc., 1990.

Carey, V. P., *Liquid-Vapor Phase-Change Phenomena*, Hemisphere Publishing Corporation, New York, 1992.

Carstensen, J. Y., *Pharmaceutical Principles of Solid Dosage Forms*, Technomic Publishing Co., Lancaster, PA, 1993.

Cheremisinoff, P. N., ed., *Air/Particulate Instrumentation and Analysis*, Ann Arbor Science, Ann Arbor, 1981.

Chulia, D., Deleuil, M., and Pourcelot, Y., *Powder Technology and Pharmaceutical Processes*, Elsevier Science B. V., Amsterdam, 1994.

Groves, M. J., *Parenteral Technology Manual*, 2nd ed., Interpharm Press, Buffalo Grove, IL, 1988.

Groves, M. J., Olson, W-P., and Anisfeld, M. H., *Sterile Pharmaceutical Manufacturing*, Interpharm Press, Buffalo Grove, IL, 1991.

Hesketh, H. E., and El-Shobokshy, M. S., *Predicting and Measuring Fugitive Dust*, Technomic Publishing Company, Lancaster, 1985.

Hyman, D., Mixing and Agitation. In: *Advances in Chemical Engineering*, Vol. 3, Academic Press, 1962.

Klegerman, M. E., and Groves, M. J., *Pharmaceutical Biotechnology Fundamentals and Essentials*, Interpharm Press, Buffalo Grove, IL, 1992.

Lachman, L., Lieberman, H. A., and Kanig, J. L., *The Theory and Practice of Industrial Pharmacy*, 3rd ed., Lea & Febiger, Philadelphia, 1986.

Lefebvre, A. H., *Atomization and Sprays*, Hemisphere Publishing Corporation, New York, 1989.

Little, A., and Mitchell, K. A., *Tablet Making*, 2nd ed., The Northern Publishing Co., Ltd., Liverpool, 1963.

Masters, K., *Spray Drying Handbook*, 5th ed., Longman Scientific and Technical, and John Wiley and Sons, Inc., New York, 1991.

Mullin, J. W., *Crystallization*, 3rd ed., Butterworth-Heinemann, London, 1993.

Wert, C. A., and Thomson, R. M., *Physics of Solids*, 2nd ed., McGraw Hill, Inc., New York, 1970.

Mullin, J. W., *Crystallization*, Butterworth, London, 1961.

Pietsch, W., *Size Enlargement by Agglomeration*, John Wiley and Sons, New York, 1991.

Prokop, A., Bajpai, R. K., and Ho, C., *Recombinant DNA Technology and Applications*, McGraw Hill, Inc., New York, 1991.

Tien, C., *Granulator Filtration of Aerosols ad Hydrosols*, Butterworths, Boston, 1989.
Van-Hook, A., *Crystallization: Theory and Practice*, A.C.S. Monograph No. 152, Chapman and Hall, London, 1961.
Weidenbaum, S. S., Mixing of Solids, *Advances in Chemical Engineering*, Vol. 2, Academic Press, New York, 1958.

References

1. Ganderton, D., and Hickey, A. J., Unit Process in Pharmacy: Fundamentals, In *Encyclopedia of Pharmaceutical Technology*, Vol 15 (J. Swarbrick and J. C. Boylan, eds.), Marcel Dekker, Inc., New York, 1996, pp. 341–398.
2. McCabe, W. L., Smith, J. C., and Harriott, P., *Unit Operations in Chemical Engineering*, 5th ed., McGraw Hill, Inc., New York, 1993.
3. Martin, A., *Physical Pharmacy*, 4th ed., Lea & Febiger, Philadelphia. 1993.
4. Ansel, H. C., Popovich, N. G., and Allen, L. V., *Pharmaceutical Dosage Forms and Drug Delivery Systems*, 6th ed., Williams and Wilkins, Malvern, PA, 1995.
5. Shotton, E., and Ridgway, K., *Physical Pharmaceutics*, Clarendon Press, Oxford, 1974.
6. Florence, A. T., and Atkins, D., *Physicochemical Principles of Pharmacy*, 2nd ed., MacMillan Press, Ltd., London, 1988.
7. Hickman, K. C. D., Commercial molecular distillation, *Industr. Eng. Chem.*, 39:686 (1947).
8. Coulson, J. M., and Richardson, J. F., *Engineering*, Vol. 2, Pergamon Press, New York, 1955.
9. Ives, K. J., *Proc. Inst. Civ. Engrs.*, 25:345 (1963).
10. Ives, K. J., Symposium: Interaction between fluids and particles, *Inst. Chem. Engr.*, p. 260 (1962).
11. Maroudas, A., and Eisenklam, P., *Chem.Eng. Sci.*, 20:867 (1965).
12. Wheeler, R. J., *Filtration*, 1:41 (1964).
13. Salter, K. C., and Hosking, A. P., *Chem. Eng. Pract.*, 6:487 (1958).
14. Dickey, G. D., *Filtration*, Reinhold, New York, 1961.
15. Noble, W. C., *J. Path. Bact.*, 81:523 (1961).
16. Williams, R. E. O., Blower, R., Garrod, L. P., and Shooter, R. A., *Hospital Infection—Causes and Prevention*, Lloyd-Luke, London, 1961, p. 167.
17. Suits, C. G., *The Collected Works of Irving Langmuir*, Vol. 10, Pergamon, New York, 1961, p. 394.
18. Hinds, W. C., *Aerosols Technology, Properties, Behavior and Measurement of Airborne Particles*, John Wiley and Sons, New York, 1982, pp. 164–186.
19. Terjsen, S. G., and Cherry, C. B., *Trans. Inst. Chem. Engrs.*, 25:89 (1947).
20. Reist, P. C., *Aerosol Science and Technology*, 2nd ed., McGraw Hill, Inc., New York, 1992.
21. Ramskill, E. A., and Anderson, W. L., *J. Coll. Sci.*, 6:416 (1951).
22. Humphrey, A. E., and Gaden, E. L., *Industr. Eng. Chem.*, 48:2172 (1956).
23. Stairmand, C. J., *Trans. Inst. Chem. Engrs.*, 28:130 (1950).
24. Hesketh, H. E., and El-Shobokshy, M. S., *Predicting and Measuring Fugitive Dust*, Technomic Publishing Co., Inc., Lancaster, PA, 1985, pp. 1–33.
25. Fuchs, N. A., *The Mechanics of Aerosols*, Dover Publications, Inc., New York, 1964.
26. Gaden, E. L., and Humphrey, A. E., *Industr. Eng. Chem.*, 48:2172 (1956).
27. Gaden, E. L., and Humphrey, A. E., *Industr. Eng. Chem.*, 47:924 (1955).
28. Cherry, G. B., McCann, E. P., and Parker, A., *J. Appl. Chem.*, 1:S103 (1951).

29. Sykes, G., and Carter, D. V., *J. Appl. Bacteriol.*, 17:286 (1954).
30. White, P. A. F., and Smith, S. E., *Research*, 13:228 (1960).
31. Green, H. L., and Lane, W. R., *Particulate Clouds: Dusts, Smokes, and Mists*, Spon, Ltd, London, 1957, p. 334.
32. Scott, M. W., Lieberman, H. A., and Chow, F. S., *J. Pharm. Sci.*, 52:284 (1963).
33. Scott, M. W., Lieberman, H. A., and Chow, F. S., *J. Pharm. Sci.*, 52:994 (1963).
34. Newitt, D. M., Na Nagara, P., and Papadopoulos, A. L., *Trans Inst. Chem. Engrs.*, 38:273 (1960).
35. Ceaglske, N. H., and Hougen, O. A., *Indust. Eng. Chem.*, 29:805 (1937).
36. Pearse, J. F., Oliver, T. R., and Newitt, D. M., *Trans. Inst. Chem. Engrs.*, 27:1 (1949).
37. Corben, R. W., and Newitt, D. M., *Trans. Inst. Chem. Engrs.*, 33:52 (1955).
38. Scott, M. W., Lieberman, H. A., Chow, F. S., Rankell, A. S., and Johnston, G. W., *J. Pharm. Sci.*, 52:284 (1963).
39. Shepherd, C. B., Hadlock, C., and Brewer, R. C., *Industr. Eng. Chem.*, 30:388 (1938).
40. Scott, M. W., *J. Pharm. Sci.*, 52:284 (1963).
41. Cooper, J., Swartz, C. J., and Suydam, W., *J. Pharm. Sci.*, 50:67 (1961).
42. Pikal, M. J., Roy, M. L., and Shah, S., *J. Pharm. Sci.*, 73:1224–1237 (1984).
43. Nail, S. N., *J. Parent. Drug Assoc.*, 34:358–368 (1980).
44. Jennings, T. A., *J. Parent. Sci. Techn.*, 42:118–121 (1988).
45. Dushman, S., and Lafferty, J. M., *Scientific Foundations of Vacuum Technique*, 2nd ed., John Wiley and Sons, New York, 1962, p. 48.
46. Ho, N. F. H., and Roseman, T. J., *J. Pharm. Sci.*, 68:1170–1174 (1979).
47. Newman, A. C. C., and Axon, A., *Soc. Chem. Ind. Monograph*, 14:291 (1961).
48. Lees, K. A., *J. Pharm. Pharmacol.*, 15:43T (1963).
49. Wagner, J. G., *J. Pharm. Sci.*, 50:359 (1961).
50. Bond, F. C., *Trans. Amer. Inst. Min. (Metall.). Engrs.*, 193:484 (1952).
51. Holmes, J. A., *Trans. Inst. Chem. Engrs.*, 3S:125 (1957).
52. Carey, W. F., and Stairmand, C. J., Recent advances in mineral dressing, *Inst. Min. Metall.*, p. 117 (1953).
53. Heywood, H., *Chem. Eng. Pract.* 3:8 (1957).
54. Gammage, R. D., and Glasson, D. R., *Chem. Ind.*, 1466 (1963).
55. Gregg, S. J., *Trans. Br. Ceram. Soc.*, 54:257 (1955).
56. Cleverley, H., and Williams, P. P., *Chem. Ind.*, 49 (1959).
57. Treasure, C. R. G., *Trans. Inst. Chem. Engrs.*, 43:T199 (1965).
58. Perry, R. H., and Chilton, C. H., *Chemical Engineer's Handbook*, 5th ed., McGraw Hill, New York, 1973.
59. Dankwerts, P. V., *Research*, 6:355 (1953).
60. Lacey, P. M. C., *Trans. Inst. Chem. Engrs.*, 21:53 (1953).
61. Train, D., *Pharm. J.*, 185:129 (1960).
62. Lacey, P. M. C., *J. Appl. Chem.*, 4:257 (1954).
63. Adams, J. F. E., and Baker, A. G., *Trans. Inst. Chem. Engrs.*, 34:91 (1956).
64. Kaufman, A., *Industr. Eng. Chem. (Fundamental)*, 1:104 (1962).
65. Donald, M. B., and Roseman, B., *Br. Chem. Engng.*, 7:749 (1962).
66. Avis, K. E., and Akers, M. J. In: *The Theory and Practice of Industrial Pharmacy*, 3rd ed. (L. Lachman, H. A. Lieberman, and J. L. Kanig, eds.), Lea & Febiger, Philadelphia, 1986, pp. 619–638.
67. Boylan, J. C., and Fites, A. L., *Modern Pharmaceutics*, 2nd ed., Marcel Dekker, Inc., New York, 1990, pp. 491–538.
68. Carstensen, J. T., *Theory of Pharmaceutical Systems*, Vol. 2, *Heterogenous Systems*, Academic Press, New York, 1973, p. 223.
69. Doelker, E. In: *Powder Technology and Pharmaceutical Processes* (D. Chulia, M. Deleuil, and Y. Pourcelot, eds.,), Elsevier, Amsterdam, 1994, pp. 403–471.

70. Carstensen, J. T., *Pharmaceutical Principles of Solid Dosage Form*, Technomic Publishing Company, Lancaster, PA, 1993, p. 73.
71. Heckel, R. W., *Trans. Metal. Soc. AIME,* 221:671 (1961).
72. Propkop, A., and Bajpai, R. K. In: *Recombinant DNA Technology and Applications* (A. Prokop, R. K. Bajpai, and C. Ho, eds.), McGraw Hill, Co., New York, 1991, pp. 415–459.
73. Hofmann, F. K. In: *Pharmaceutical Biotechnology, Fundamentals and Essentials* (M. E. Klegerman and M. J. Groves, eds.), Interpharm Press, Buffalo Grove, IL, 1992, pp. 138–164.

DAVID GANDERTON
ANTHONY J. HICKEY

Vaccines and Other Immunological Products

Introduction

Antigens and Vaccines

A vaccine is any preparation administered to an individual to produce or enhance immunity to a particular disease or condition. Vaccines can consist of whole bacteria, viruses, protozoa, or cells, either live or killed, or subunits of these organisms such as cell membranes or walls, or products elucidated by these organisms such as exotoxins that are not a structural component, or the DNA or RNA of such subunits cloned within a vector that then translates the substance within a host which recognizes the antigen. It has now been shown that for viruses and bacteria, DNA can itself induce an immune response in the host that can recognize the organism [1–3]. Antigens are substances that can bind to antibodies or specific receptors on B or T lymphocytes. Antigens are immunogenic if they are capable of inducing a specific immune response by antibody formation or T-cell recognition. All immunogens are therefore antigens because they are recognized by the immune response they induce. However, the reverse is not true. For example, haptens are small antigens that can be recognized by an immune response that they cannot induce alone. The efficacy of a vaccine depends on the immunogenicity of the component for which an enhanced immune response is intended. In most cases, this is an infectious agent but it can be other cells. For example, there is much interest in developing a fertility vaccine which would induce an immune response in females to sperm which would interfere with zygote formation. Cancer treatment is another area where vaccines are being developed. In general, the most potent immunogens are proteins followed by polysaccharides, especially in regard to the induction of humoral or antibody-based immunity. Protection depends on both humoral immunity which includes antibodies circulating in the blood or at mucosal surfaces. For cell-mediated immunity (CMI), or immunity dependent on T lymphocytes and other cell types, only proteins can perform as immunogens. For CMI, native proteins are not recognized by the immune system. Instead, they must be broken down and processed by antigen-presenting cells such as macrophages or dendritic cells and presented on the surface of these cells in association with the major histocompatibility molecule (MHC) in order to induce an immune response.

Design of Vaccines

The immune response to these subunits or whole organisms depends on the character of the components and the following factors:

1. Composition of antigens
   Molecular size
   Chemical make-up
      Protein, carbohydrate, nucleic acid, or lipid

Molecular structure of proteins
  Primary, secondary, and tertiary structures
  Structure of epitopes (B- or T-dependent)
Hydrophobicity/hydrophilicity
Foreignness to host and genetic make-up of host
2. Dose of antigen
3. Route of administration to host
4. Target
   Infectious agents, cancer cells, host tissues (fertility)

These factors determine how antigens interact with the cells in the immune system that initiate the immune response. Foreignness refers to a substance being different from host tissues. In general, an individual's immune system is developed not to recognize its own tissues as immunogens. Some bacteria or viruses mimic host tissues to avoid detection, for example, the M protein of *Streptococcus pyogenes* [4]. This allows the bacteria to replicate without inducing a host-immune response. When the host does recognize these microbes, there is danger that the immune response may also recognize self-antigens as well and induce disease. Molecular size is important. There is a correlation of size with immunogenicity; molecules in the range of 100,000 Daltons are good immunogens, whereas those less than 10,000 Daltons are poor immunogens [5]. Chemical composition also affects immunogenicity. Polymers of repeating units of one molecule, even an amino acid of a very large size, are poor immunogens.

The primary, secondary, tertiary, and quaternary structure of proteins affect the immunogenicity of a substance. Computer programs are available that can predict the most immunogenic sites of complex proteins if the amino acid sequence is known [6]. The hydrophobicity and hydrophilicity of amino acid sequences as well as the primary and tertiary structures are taken into consideration in these models. The more hydrophilic an area is, the more immunogenic it is. The surface exposure of sequences is also important. Structures folded in such a way that they are internal to a protein are less likely to be exposed and to initiate an immune response. These structures are more likely to induce a cell-mediated immune response following processing by antigen-presenting cells [7–9]. Externally oriented protein entities are also more immunogenic. X-ray crystallography can be used to visualize protein regions and predict more immunogenic epitopes [10].

Epitopes are regions of antigens that induce an immune response. Antigens are composed of multiple epitopes, each of which induces a clonal response by one lymphocyte. This means that most vaccines, even if composed of a pure subunit antigen, induce a polyclonal antibody response. In other words, several clones of lymphocytes, each specific to one epitope, are stimulated to expand and produce a response to one specific region (epitope) of the antigen. In this way, if an infectious organism changes its antigenic make-up due to mutation or loss of a virulence plasmid encoding for an antigen, the host immune response is still able to recognize other epitopes of the antigen and maintain an immune response. The degradability or solubility of antigens is important in the induction of an immune response. Antigens that are large or particulate are more immunogenic because they are more likely to be phagocytosed and processed by macrophages. Soluble antigens, or those not able to be degraded because the host lacks enzymes to break them down, are less immunogenic. The MHC genotypye of a host is important in determining the immune response. This is most common in mice strains where known haplotypes respond better to well characterized antigens than other haplotypes. This has also been shown to affect the response of purebred animals such as cattle and swine [5,11,12].

The dose of antigen used in a vaccine is important in stimulating an immune response. A dose too low results in too few lymphocytes being stimulated, or nonresponsiveness being induced, and an insufficient immune response. A dose too high induces a nonresponsive lymphocyte response or tolerance. Repeated exposures to antigen are better than one dose. Initial doses stimulate clonal expansion of antigen-specific lymphocytes as well as development of memory B and T cells. Upon subsequent exposure to an antigen, the clonal proliferation begins sooner, producing even more antibodies or a higher CMI. Repeated exposures can be accomplished by multiple individual inoculations, an attenuated live vaccine, or a vector that can replicate within the host, or by the use of controlled-release preparations or adjuvants that regulate the release of the antigen from the site of administration to the immune system. The repeated exposure stimulates the clonal expansion of antigen-specific lymphocytes, thereby increasing the immune response. The route of administration affects the quality and quantity of the immune response. Most vaccines are administered by intramuscular or subcutaneous injection. This enhances the circulating humoral immune response. Administration of antigen to a mucosal surface primarily induces a secretory IgA response. The role of route of administration will be discussed in more detail below.

The design of vaccines depends to some degree on the target for which immunity is desired. For infectious agents, some of the key immunogens and the role of the immune system in stimulating protective immunity to viruses, bacteria, and protozoa will be discussed here. An important consideration in inducing an immune response is that many infectious agents are capable to avoid detection and interaction with the immune response of the host. Outer membranes of microbes may be shed, leaving antibodies bound to them and therefore unable to attack the infectious agent. Microbes may express surface antigens that mimic host antigens or live within host cells to avoid detection. In some cases, microbes constantly change their surface antigens in such a way that as soon as an immune response is developed, it no longer binds to the intended antigen. Other microbes invade and disarm or kill cells of the immune system. Examples of these will be discussed later.

Types of Antigens
Whole Organisms
Inactivated Microorganisms

A growing number of antigens are used in vaccines, varying from entire organisms (live or inactivated) to purified subunits, recombinant derived subunits, and more recently, DNA encoding for antigens of the following types:

1. Whole organisms (viruses, bacteria, protozoa, helminths)
   Inactivated microorganisms
   Attenuated microorganisms
2. Subunit vaccines
   Proteins

    Purified components
    Recombinant derived components
Anti-idiotype vaccines
    Lipid antigens
    Polysaccharide antigens
Nucleic acids

Examples of these antigens and how they are used will be discussed below.

Vaccines can be composed of many different forms of infectious agents for which immunity is desired. Whole organisms can be used inactivated (killed) or attenuated live. In some cases, virulent organisms are administered by an abnormal route of infection. Organisms are inactivated in a variety of ways, the most common involving treatment with chemicals (formaldehyde) or γ-irradiation. The method of inactivation can enhance antigenicity of immunogens, in some cases by causing agglutination of smaller units into larger, and sometimes more easily recognizable clumps by the immune system. Care must be taken that inactivation does not denature antigens into immunogens that stimulate antibodies which no longer recognize native antigens, or totally destroy important antigens altogether. Vaccines of inactivated microbes are fairly simple and inexpensive to produce. Inactivated organisms stimulate good humoral immunity, but require multiple inoculations to induce a good antibody titer. These are very safe vaccines because the organisms used are not able to replicate or revert to virulence and cause disease in the host. However, in general inactivated vaccines do not induce very good cell-mediated immunity, which is important in resistance to intracellular infections caused by viruses, certain bacteria such as *Salmonella spp.*, or protozoa such as *Plasmodium*. Organisms that spend a considerable part of their time within host cells are not susceptible to antibody detection while in the host cells. Therefore, antibodies alone are not likely to induce immunity to allow the host to clear the infection.

Attenuated Microorganisms

Attenuation of organisms for vaccines usually involves growing the organism in vitro under abnormal conditions to select avirulent organisms. This includes cultivation in abnormal hosts, in vitro cell lines from the same host but from an organ not normally affected, at different pH and temperatures, or using an isolate from one host to vaccinate a different host species. When inoculated into a host in a vaccine, these organisms are able to replicate for a short period of time thereby inducing an immune response that recognizes the wild-type organism, but without causing disease in the host. It is important to note that the history of vaccines began with investigations of the use of unattenuated and attenuated organisms to prevent diseases. In fact, the name vaccine derives from these initial efforts when, in the early 19th century, Jenner discovered that smallpox could be prevented by inoculating individuals with cowpox or vaccinia virus. This was found to be safer than the original method used for hundreds of years prior to this time whereby smallpox was initially controlled by transferring pox material from infected humans to others. Measles virus was attenuated by adapting virus to replicate in monkey kidney cells and further attenuated in duck embryo and human tissue culture cell lines [13-15]. The Sabin polio vaccine viruses were attenuated by a combination of passages in monkeys and in vitro cultivation in monkey kidney epithelial cells [16]. A strain of *Mycobacterium tuberculosis* the Bacille Camet-Guerin (BCG) strain

Vaccines and Other Immunological Products

was attenuated by cultivating it for 231 passages over 13 years on media containing increasing amounts of bile, a component not usually added to culture medium for this organism.

Temperature-sensitive mutants have been selected for use in several viruses as well in bacteria. Isolates are selected that grow at temperatures slightly lower than the core temperature of the host. For example, a ts variant of influenza virus grows well at 32–34°C in the upper respiratory tract but not at 37–38°C in the lower respiratory tract. The vaccine virus can replicate in the upper airways and stimulate an immune response without causing pneumonia [17].

Another strategy to produce safer attenuated vaccines involves the production of a mutant that lacks the ability to cause disease but is similar enough to the wild-type organism to induce protective immunity. This has been accomplished with viruses and bacteria, for example, *Salmonella typhimurium*. Auxotrophic aroA, aroB, and aroC mutants are unable to replicate without the aromatic amino acids which are not available within the host. *S. typhimurium* or *typhi* can also be rendered avirulent by mutating regulatory genes that are needed for virulence but when altered, render the *Salmonella* avirulent. They are, however, capable of replication at least for short periods of time in the host [18]. The *Salmonella* survive for a short period of time within the host stimulating immunity but they cannot cause disease, revert to virulence, and survive in the environment where they could possibly pick up virulence attributes by conjugation or transfection from other gram-negative bacteria. The pseudorabies (herpes) virus has been altered to generate gene-deleted or altered mutants. The genes deleted include gC, gG, and gE genes (nonessential glycoproteins) involved in nucleocapsid assembly, and altered thymidine kinase gene. These altered viruse vaccines are in use and have been shown to reduce viral shedding by pigs and increase the infective dose needed for wild-type virus to infect pigs, but not to totally prevent infection. Gene-deleted vaccines have the advantage that they permit eradication of wild-type infected swine in the face of vaccination, since it is possible to differentiate isolated virus and virus antibodies of wild type from vaccine strain viruses [19,20].

Attenuated vaccines possess several advantages over inactivated vaccines. They require fewer inoculations because the organism replicates within the host. They also stimulate both a humoral and cell-mediated immunity since replication allows for endogenous as well as exogenous antigen processing. Stimulation of CMI requires endogenous processing of antigen. However, attenuated vaccines are less stable than inactivated vaccines and have a shorter shelf life. Refrigeration is more critical, which is rarely possible in developing countries. Another potential problem is that inactivated vaccines can revert to virulent form in the host, especially immunosuppressed or immature hosts, and cause disease.

Subunit Vaccines

Induction of Humoral and Cell-Mediated Immunity

Some of the shortcomings of inactivated and attenuated vaccines can be overcome by using purified subunit vaccines. Attenuated or inactivated vaccines require cultivation of microbes to generate fairly large amount of the required antigen. In some cases, organisms can be cultured in vitro and supernatants or sonicated organisms are used to isolate and purify one component (bacterial pili, flagella, or cell walls proteins) that can be employed for a subunit vaccine. Either native purified or sythesized polysaccharide vaccines can be used. For some subunit vaccines, less infectious agents need to be cultvated by recombinant technology. Recombinant subunit vaccines can be extremely useful for diseases in which the microbe responsible for the disease cannot be easily cultivated in vitro such as *Trepomena pallidum*, the cause of human syphilis. Exotoxins produced by bacteria can be purified in this way, inactivated, and used as toxoid vaccines. Outer membrane proteins, pili, flagella, cell-wall components of bacteria, protozoa, or helminths, fusion, "envelope" proteins or glycoproteins of viruses can be prepared and used to stimulate immunity to the infecting pathogen. Many of these components are proteins. Once a subunit has been identified, immunodominant epitopes or the entire sequence can be cloned into a bacterial, viral, or cellular vector and large quantities of the material made by recombinant nucleotide techniques. These vaccines usually induce very good humoral immunity which may be sufficient to induce protection in some diseases but not all. In the case of polysaccharides, a B-cell immune response, which is composed almost entirely of IgM, is induced.

Cell-mediated immunity is needed for the control of intracellular pathogens. For protein antigens, it can be induced by incorporation of the gene for the vaccine protein into a virus-like vaccinia, polio, or adenovirus, or an intracellular bacterial vector like *S. typhimurium*, or BCG [12,21,22]. The vector is administered orally or intranasally and colonizes the host. As it replicates, the protein of the cloned gene is transcribed and the protein expressed in a way that leads to presentation with MHC 1 or MHC 2 molecules, resulting in a CMI response that is not possible with the purified protein alone. A cell-mediated immune response to a subunit antigen can also be induced by the production of synthetic peptides that contain T-cell specific epitopes [23]. In this case, care must be taken that the resultant synthetic peptides stimulate an immune response and not immunosuppression. The responsiveness of T cells varies, and whereas one subpopulation may be stimulated by a synthetic peptide, another subpopulation may be suppressed. Yet another way to induce CMI is by combining both B and T epitopes synthetic peptides to a solid matrix coated with monoclonal antibodies to the epitopes with the MAB or antigen binding sites exposed outward to attach the epitopes. This creates a solid antibody–antigen complex that can stimulate both a humoral and CMI response [24]. Protein micelles, immunostimulating complexes (ISCOMS), polymeric microparticles, or liposomes are alternative ways to incorporate a mixture of B and T epitopes in a particulate manner to stimulate both a humoral and CMI immune response [25–27].

Protein Subunits

Subunit vaccines are continually sought as safer and more readily available immunogens. For highly infectious pathogens that present a risk in preparation as well as for organisms that cannot be easily cultivated in vitro, recombinant subunit antigens are the best method of preparation. The simplest design of a vaccine consists of one antigen to induce protective immunity. There are some examples of a single factor being sufficient to induce protective immunity such as tetanus toxoid. However, subunit vaccines based on an understanding of disease pathogenesis are not always successful. Vaccines containing the F protein of respiratory syncytial virus (RSV) were expected to induce solid immunity since fusion of the virus with the host cell requires this factor [28]. However, recombinant purified proteins, or recombinant vectors expressing the F protein, even in combination with the G and 22-kD proteins, have been disappointing in reducing experimental virus infections [29]. Bacteria are more complicated genetically and typically possess several virulence mechanisms. Therefore, it is not unexpected that subunit vaccines would need to contain multiple factors. For many yearrs a bacterin has been used to prevent infections caused by *Bordetella pertussis*, the etiological agent of whooping cough in children. This vaccine has been controversial as it has been associated with seizures and brain damage in vaccinates. Some countries have discontinued its usage with a subsequent rise in the respiratory disease. These reactions appear to be associated with some unknown factors found in the vaccine. There has been a concerted effort to develop an effective vaccine without these side effects. An acellular vaccine containing the pertussis toxin and filamentous hemagglutinin was the first to be introduced as a means of overcoming the neurological side effects of the bacterin [30]. Later it became clear that multiple antigens are necessary for adequate immunity [31]. Several recent studies compared two-to-five subunit components, including pertussin toxin, filamentous hemagglutinin, outer membrane protein (pertactin), and two other agglutinogens to the standard whole-cell vaccine. Results indicate better efficacy with the three-to-five component vaccines than with the two-subunit or whole-cell vaccines [32]. The subunit vaccines produced fewer injection-site reactions with fewer than 10% of patients developing inflammation compared to more than 50% for whole-cell vaccinates.

Lipid–Polysaccharide Subunits

Recombinant technology has made tremendous contributions toward the production of protein subunit vaccines. However, other approaches may be necessary to address how to deal with lipid or other nonprotein antigens. Synthesis of these antigens may not be practical. One method to induce subunit or epitope-specific immunity is with the help of anti-idiotype vaccines. Antibodies are very specific in their binding-site reactivity which is referred to as the idiotypic determinant located on the variable (V) region of the immunoglobulin. The paratope is the part of the antibody that binds to the antigen. Antibodies made to a specific paratope of an idiotype mimic the conformation and shape of the immunizing antigen. These are called anti-idiotypic antibodies. Because they are mirror images of the antigen, they can be used instead of the antigen to induce an immune response. Hybridomas producing monoclonal anti-idiotypes can be produced as a practical source of antigenic material. The sequence of the V region can be cloned and the gene sequenced, leading to the creation of synthetic anti-ids, or the gene can be inserted into a vector to produce the anti-id in vitro or inserted into an expression vector vaccine [33]. Anti-idiotype vaccines are useful in cases where antigen exhibits poor immunogenicity, the pathogen is dangerous to handle in the laboratory, or antigens are too similar to host antigens to be recognized. Certain carbohydrate tumor antigens are recognized as self with poor immunogenicity. Anti-idiotypes are sufficiently different from self that they can induce an immune respone. The carbohydrate moieties cannot be easily produced in vitro to make a subunit vaccine in this case [34]. *Schistosoma mansoni* carbohydrate surface antigen is a good vaccine candidate. However, *Schistosomes* cannot be easily cultivated in vitro, making purfication of this material very difficult. Anti-idiotype vaccines would provide a strategy to create a mimic antigen for the control of this disease [35]. Other examples of diseases for which anti-idiotype vaccines have been developed include *Streptococcus pneumoniae, Listeria monocytogenes, Trypanosoma rhodesiense,* hepatitis B, and Sendai viruses [36].

Infectious Agent Vaccines

Viral Vaccines

Immunity to viral infections involves both humoral and cell-mediated responses. Antibodies (especially secretory IgA present at mucosal surfaces) block the attachment and subsequent invasion of the host by viruses. Antibodies also bind to surface proteins of viruses that mediate fusion of the virus with host-cell membranes, an important step necessary for viruses to invade host cells. IgG and IgM can bind to viruses, and especially in the case of the pentavalent IgM, agglutinate viruses, thereby opsonizing them for uptake and degradation by macrophages. Binding of antibodies to viruses makes them susceptible to killing by complement when macrophages recognize the Fc receptors of bound antibodies. Viruses stimulate cell-mediated immunity through the endogenous or exogenous pathways of antigen processing. Exogenous processed antigens refer to interaction of virus outside the cell with T-helper (Th) cells. The type-1 Th cells produce cytokines, such as interferon gamma (IFN-γ), which directly enhance antiviral activity within a cell, and interleukin-2 (IL-2) which activates cytotoxic T lymphocytes (CTL). The two cytokines together activate natural killer cells, a leukocyte population that aids in killing virus-infected cells, especially early in infection. Tumor necrosis factor (TNF), a potent activator of macrophages, is also induced. The CTLs are induced by processing of viral antigens through the endogenous pathway after the viruses have invaded a cell. The virus particles are broken down and antigens are coexpressed with MHC 1 receptors on the surface of the cell. The coexpression with MHC 1 activates the CTLs which, in turn, kill the virus-infected cells that are the source of new viruses for spread of the infection. This CTL response is very specific for viruses as shown by passive transfer studies. The transfer of CTLs to a susceptible host confers protection against challenge by a homologous virus strain (influenza) but not against heterologous (rhino) viruses. In general, antibodies are important for the protection against infection by homologous virus in the future. However, for long-lasting cross-reactive immunity, CTL is very important for most viruses.

Subunit viral vaccines include those surface antigens needed for virus fusion to the host cell. Polio virus infections have been well controlled by an oral vaccine stimulating secretory IgA (sIgA). The sIgA effectively blocks viral attachment to mucosal epithelial cells in the gastrointestinal tract, the site of host invasion by polio. As another example, influenza vaccines are designed to induce an antibody response to the surface antigens hemagglutinin (HA), important for virus attachment to host cells and to neuraminidase (NA), which facilitates viral budding from the host cell by cleaving sialic acid residues from virus and host membrane glycoproteins. Influenza viruses are classifed by the HA and NA antigen type, for example, A/Puerto Rico/8/34 (H0N1). Antibodies to the HA and NA are effective in neutralizing virus and preventing infection. However, these antibodies are strain specific. Unfortunately, there are several strains of influenza virus with different HA and NA antigens. Over time, every 10–15 years in the past 60 years, there has been a major antigenic shift in which a considerable change has taken place in either the HA or NA antigenic type. Antibodies to heterologous strains of influenza with a different HA or NA are not protective. In addition to these major antigenic shifts, there are antigenic drifts (i.e., point mutations) in the HA or NA that occur gradually over time. These mutations commonly occur in the region of the HA antigen most intimately involved in binding to sialic acid receptors on host cells [37]. Therefore, antigenic drift can result in sufficient antigenic changes to allow the virus to avoid antibodies to this antigen necessary for attachment of the virus to the host cell. Although antibodies are important in preventing viral attachment and provide protection from reinfection by the same influenza strain, they also are of primary importance for recovery from infection.

Cell-mediated immunity involving CTLs can confer protection to a challenge by a lethal dose of virus. Even though the antibody response is strain specific, and passive transfer of virus neutralizing antibodies to HA and NA can confer protection in CTL-deficient mice, the CTL response can be cross-protective to other HA and NA strains [38]. Replication of virus within host cells results in the processing of internal viral proteins through the endogenous antigen pathway, those not expressed on the surface of the virus and therefore not likely to stimulate a protective antibody response. Influenza has six internal proteins including a nucleoprotein (NP) that is antigenically conserved between strains. The NP is recognized by a subset of CTLs that cross-react to all three of the major human strains of influenza (H1N1, H2N2, and H3N2). At present, nearly all vaccines used include either HA or inactivated influenza virus. However, the best induction of CTLs requires replication of virus within host cells although there is evidence that inactivated virus containing NP can induce CTLs [39]. Passive transfer of CTL cells can confer immunity [40], but is not required for recovery from influenza infection [41]. The role and best means of inducing CTL remain somewhat controversial. Some evidence suggests that although long-term virus-specific CTL is possible [42], other studies suggest that the presence of virus or viral antigen is necessary for protective CTL [43]. Overall, it appears that the long-term presence of antigen is needed for optimal immune stimulation [44].

The newest method of inducing CTL to influenza is by injecting DNA coding for NP into mice [2,45]. The DNA is expressed by host cells resulting in endogenous processing of antigens as they are produced. This method of inoculation is discussed more fully below. However, not all MHC 1 haplotypes react equally well with the nucleoprotein [46]. Therefore, a vaccine based on NP alone may not be effective for all individuals. The enhancement of the CMI to cross-reactive antigens as well as of humoral immunity to the HA and NA is now the challenge facing the development of more effective influenza vaccines.

Viruses have many ways to interfere with immune function. Influenza is one example of a virus in which surface antigens change to help the virus avoid neutralizing antibodies. Other viruses have also developed ways to avoid antibodies. Herpes simplex viruses produce a glycoprotein that inhibits activation of both the classical and alternative complement pathways. Vaccinia virus secretes a protein that inhibits activation of the classical complement pathway. Not only does influenza virus change surface antigens, rhinoviruses (the cause of the common cold), and human immunodeficiency virus (HIV) rapidly mutate, changing their antigenic components [47]. The immune system can be suppressed by invasion and lysis of lymphocytes or macrophages by paramyxovirus, measles virus, Epstein-Barr virus (EBV), cytomegalovirus, and HIV. This immunosuppression can be specific for one type of cells such as Th cells CD8+ which are selectively depleted by HIV. It can also depend on abnormal cytokine expression. The EBV produces a protein that suppresses Th-1 subset cytokine expression of IFN-γ, IL-2, and TNF necessary for CMI responses. Adenoviruses and cytomelalovirus interfere with MHC-1 expression with antigen [48–50].

Bacterial Vaccines

The simplest vaccines include the whole organisms. An example of an effective attenuated bacterial vaccine is the altered strain of *Mycobacterium bovis* called BCG (Bacille Camette Guerin). This vaccine is useful in the prevention of tuberculosis in humans caused by *M. tuberculosis* in sites outside the lungs. Efficacy can be as high as 80% in preventing the respiratory form of the disease. Since an estimated two billion people are infected wordwide at present, and antibiotic-resistant strains are rapidly developing, there is a great need for a much more effective vaccine. Inactivated vaccines are also used. Pertussis or whooping cough has been controlled by an formaldehyde-inactivated *Bordetella pertussis* vaccine. Epidemiological studies have shown that this vaccine reduces serious forms of pertussis (seizures, encephalitis, brain damage, and death) by 100- to 1000-fold. However, its risks include encephalitis-like reactions which emphasizes the efforts to develop a more effective vaccine with fewer side effects.

The advantages and disadvantages of whole attenuated and inactivated bacterial vaccines have been described above. Although there are some very effective bacterins, there are some problems that must be addressed. Many can be solved with the help of subunit vaccines, many of which are effective against bacteria pathogens. Lipopolysaccharide (LPS) is a major cell-wall component of gram-negative organisms. It is composed of a lipid A (nearest to cell wall), a core region, and most external, of O-polysaccharides of varying lengths, exhibiting heterogeneity in the side chains. The core region contains regions that are highly conserved between strains within a species as well as between bacterial species. The core LPS of *Escherichia coli* has been used to create a vaccine to prevent coliform mastitis, a low-morbidity, high-mortality disease of dairy cattle [51]. Similar vaccines, based on rough mutants of *S. typhimurium* as well as *E. coli* LPS core antigen vaccines, have been shown to induce immunity across gram-negative species [52]. The economic advantage of these types of vaccines appears to be the control of coliform mastitis in dairy cattle, where it causes severe endotoxemia, shock, and death. Applications to human diseases are not as advantageous at this time. Despite the increasing incidence of septicemia in humans in the past 50 years, cross-reactive anticore LPS vaccines have not demonstrated efficacy in this arena.

Polysaccharides present in bacterial capsules offer a challenge for inducing immunity. Antibodies to capsular polysaccharide antigens in bacteria such as *H. influenzae* are important, since these capsules are used in the attachment of bacteria to host cells. They interfere with phagocytosis and prevent antibodies to other bacterial components from reaching their target by acting as a shield. Capsular polysaccharides are an important antigen in *Haemophilus influenzae* type B infections in humans. This organism causes upper respiratory, CNS, and middle-ear infections, especially in infants. The polysaccharide antigens are strong B-cell activators but induce only a short-acting IgM response without T-cell memory. Conjugation of polysaccharide antigens to a protein carrier produces a much more effective vaccine that stimulates both IgG as well as IgM because T-helper cells are activated. There are four licensed vaccines of the *H. influenzae* type-B polysaccharide antigen, conjugated to diphtheria or mutant CRM_{197}, or tetanus toxoid as well as to the outer membrane proteins of *Neisseria meningitidis* [53]. Each of these vaccines induce an IgG response in children below 2 years of age. These children respond poorly to polysaccharide antigens in spite of the fact they are in the age group most susceptible to *H. influenzae* infection. To some extent, a B-cell memory response is also induced. These vaccines vary widely in their immunogenic profiles, age at which immunity is induced, length of protective immunity, and composition, including polysaccharide components [54]. Improvements continue to be made in the development of polysaccharide conjugate vaccines. There is also a group-B Streptococcus polysaccharide conjugate vaccine used for pregnant women. It induces IgG that crosses the placenta to protect the neonate from congenitally acquired Streptococcal meningitis [55].

Many bacteria produce a proteinaceous exotoxin that is involved in the pathogenesis of disease as well as of potent antigens. In many diseases, antibodies that neutralize the toxin confer protection from disease. Inactivated toxin or toxoid can be a good vaccine. It is important to inactivate the toxin (usually by chemicals such as formaldehyde or heat) in a way that eliminates the biological activity of the toxin without affecting its immunogenicity. Tetanus toxoid is an example of a bacterial toxin that is a major factor in causing disease initiated by *Clostridium tetani*. However, it is very effective in inducing antibodies that bind to the toxin, preventing its binding to the postsynaptic ganglia where it causes the characteristic contracture of opposing muscle groups that results in tetany. Yet tetanus is still very deadly to animals and humans, causing an estimated 1 million deaths worldwide in newborn infants. The availability of vaccine, the need for several inoculations in children to induce protective immunity, and the severity of disease in very young infants are crucial issues for the control of this disease.

Many toxins are composed of two units, one (the B subunit) mediates binding to host cells, and the other (the A subunit) interferes with cell function. The A subunit has no effect without the presence of the B subunit. In the case of *Vibrio cholerae*, the cause of cholera, a severe diarrheal disease in humans, the A subunit activates adenylate cyclase, resulting in ionic imbalance as sodium and chloride ions leave the cell, resulting in diarrhea. A vaccine consisting of the B subunit prevents binding of the toxin to the host cells. Without binding of the B subunit, the A subunit cannot induce disease. A vaccine containing inactivated *V. cholerae* and B subunit is very effective in controlling cholera [56].

Other surface antigens can be used in vaccines. Pili are used by many bacteria for the attachment necessary for colonization of the host. In many cases, there is wide genomic variation in pili making univalent vaccines ineffective. This is true for *Neisseria gonorrhoeae* in humans [57]. However, for enterotoxigenic *E. coli*, there are limited pili types associated with neonatal diarrhea in cattle and swine. The pili K88, K99, F41, and 987p are associated with diarrhea in piglets, wherease K99 and F41 are found in calves. Pili can be harvested in quantities to produce vaccines. Pili from a diarrhea-causing strain of *E. coli* induced antipili biliary IgA, reduced bacterial adherence to intestinal epithelium, and increased antipili lymphocyte proliferation in spleen cells in orally vaccinated rabbits [58]. Vaccine administered to dams produces colostral antibodies that effectively prevent attachment of piliated strains of *E. coli* in the neonates. A similar situation exists for colonization factor I (CFA), an adhesin produced by *E. coli* in humans. There are many CFA types, and the most common types can be used to produce vaccines to prevent diarrhea in infants. The CFA of *E. coli* stimulates immunity to prevent the colonization of the gut in rabbits [59]. Intraduodenal administration of CFA II, another colonization factor, enhanced proliferation by lymphocytes from both the spleen and Peyer's patches, and stimulated CFA II-specific antibody-secreting cells in spleen [60]. In a phase I clinical trial with CFA II administered orally to human volunteers, five of ten subjects developed antibody-secreting cells II in peripheral blood mononuclear cells to proteins contained in CFA. Three of these vaccinated subjects did not develop diarrhea when challenged with live enterotoxigenic *E. coli*, indicating a 30% protection for this oral vaccine [61].

Outer membrane proteins can be used in vaccines to induce opsonizing antibodies. In *P. haemolytica* the 40-kD outer membrane protein has been highly associated with protective immunity in cattle challenged with virulent organisms. For *P. haemolytica*, outer member proteins (OMPs) stimulate immunity equal to or better than vaccine based on the primary virulence mechanism, a leukocyte-specific toxoid [62]. Cattle vaccinated with OMPs had pulmonary lesions equal to or less severe than those in cattle vaccinated with leukotoxoid or with live virulent organisms. OMPs as well as iron regulated (IROMPs) produced under conditions of iron starvation, are in use or under investigation as putative subunit vaccines for a variety of bacterial infections at this time, including use in meningococci, and *Borrelia burgdorferi*. Unfortunately, the variability in antigenicity has precluded inclusion of OMPs from these organisms in any useful vaccine [57].

Protozoan and Metazoan (Helminth) Vaccines

Protozoa are unicellular eukaryotic organisms responsibe for serious human diseases, including malaria, sleeping sickness, and leshmaniasis. It is estimated that 1 billion people are infected with malaria or shistosomasis with 1-2 million deaths per year. Induction of immunity to protozoan and metazoan infectious agents may require stimulation of antibodies as well as CMI since the organisms spend part of their time in the blood and part of their time within cells. For example, malaria is caused by the protozoan *Plasmodium falciparum*. Mosquitoes carry the infective-stage sporozoites which enter the blood and rapidly travel to the liver where they quickly infect hepatocytes. The sporozoites are in the blood for only 30 min. Within the hepatocytes, the sporozoites replicate rapidly and mature into the next stage as merozoites which are released into the blood where they infect erythrocytes. The sporozoites are covered by a 45-kD protein, the circumsporozoite (CS) antigen that mediates attachment to hepatocytes [63,64]. Most adults exposed to irradiated sporozoites are fully protected from challenge by virulent organisms. Since the sporozoites must be irradiated within mosquitoes, this approach is impractical to pursue. However, subunit vaccines containing B and T epitopes of the CS antigen have evolved from these studies. These subunits are based on repeating sequences of the CS antigen. Individuals in endemic areas possess antibodies to this epitope, and mice challenged with virulent *P. falciparum* following treatment with monoclonal antibodies to this epitope were protected. However, trials in humans using the B-eptitope-repeating subunit were disappointing. In spite of having relatively high specific antibody titers, only one of three volunteers was protected when challenged by virulent organisms [65]. Coupling the B-cell epitope to a common T-cell epitope should improve the humoral immune response by also inducing a T-memory response.

Cell-mediated immunity is very important in controlling *Plasmodium* infections. Mice vaccinated with irradiated *Plasmodium* and depleted of CD8+ T (CTL) cells were susceptible to challenge with virulent *Plasmodium*, whereas CD4+ T-cell-depleted mice or untreated mice were resistant to infection [66]. Furthermore, adoptive transfer of T cells to susceptible nonvaccinated mice conferred protection to challenge. This represents CD8+ T cells induced by MHC 1 presentation of antigen or sporozoites on hepatocytes. There may also be some CD4+ T-cell delayed-type sensitivity (DTH) response following interaction of sporozoite antigens with MHC 2 molecules on liver Kupfer cells.

The CS of *P. falciparum* has been cloned into an avirulent *Salmonella typhi* vector. The Salmonella expresses the CS antigen when inoculated into humans. A third of the volunteers developed antibodies to CS and only one individual developed cytotoxic T cells [67]. Use of such a live vector can be an effective way to introduce antigens into the endogenous pathway of antigen processing to stimulate CMI. Although promising, better expression of the CS protein by the *Salmonella* is needed for a more predictable level of immunity. The major T epitopes of *Plasmodium* also happen to be sites of high variability in amino acid sequences [68]. It is difficult to stimulate a T-cell response with a subunit vaccine. In addition to this problem, the primary amphipathic (T epitopes) amino acid sequences were also found to be the most highly variable sequences. This would allow the *Plasmodium* to escape immune detection. Other proteins may need to be screened to find more conserved regions for epitope selection for more effective stimulation of immunity.

Vaccines effective against protoza must also deal with changing epitopes. The sleeping sickness *Trypanosomes* show considerable variation in the major antigen, variant surface glycoprotein (VSG). An individual *Trypanosome* carries up to 1000 VSG genes but only expresses one at a time [69]. As *Trypanosomes* replicate in the bloodstream, an effective antibody response is produced which eliminates most of the organisms from the host. However, a small number survive and shift VSG antigen type, allowing a new wave of rapid replication of *Trypanosomes* in the blood. This continual antigenic shift makes production of an effective vaccine very difficult.

Unlike protozoans that are unicellular and often intracellular pathogens, helminths are large multicellular worms that are extracellular pathogens. Although being extracellular makes helminths more accessible to the immune system, there are typically few involved in an infection, and the immune response is typically poor becaus of the limited exposure. Helminths can also limit antigen exposure by masking their surface proteins. For example, *Shistosomes,* the etiologic agents of Shistosomiasis, decrease expression of antigens on their external surfaces. They further avoid immunodetection by coating themselves with glycoprotein antigens derived from the host. Shistosomal infections induce primarily an IgE antibody response. This is regulated by a Th2-type response driven by IL-4 cytokine release to drive B cells to switch to IgE production. IgE binds to the worm surface and is bound by eosinophils. The eosinophils release granules that damage the parasite. Experimental studies in mice suggest that induction of IgE is not protective. When mice are vaccinated with an experimental *Shistosome* vaccine, a T-DTH response is characterized by IFN-γ secretion and macrophage attraction to the worms. Inbred IFN-γ or T-DTH-deficient mice are susceptible to Shistosomal infection, whereas IgE-deficient mice can develop protective immunity. Apparently, the *Shistosomes* stimulate a Th2-immune response that down regulates the Th1 response, thereby preventing the IFN-γ and T-DTH response from occurring [70].

Vaccines containing antigens of the infective stage (cercariae) and early adult phase (shistosomules) look most promising since these stages appear to be most susceptible to immune responses. Studies to identify immunogenic proteins have identifed several possible antigens for vaccine development. One of the more promising antigens is the 28-kD glutathione S-transferase (P28). Recombinant protein vaccines have been shown to protect mice from experimental challenge [71]. Major B and T epitopes have been identified in P28, including the 155–131 epitope which stimulates protective immunity in rats [72]. When multimers of this small peptide were expressed as fusions with a carrier protein such as a fragment of tetanus, good antibody production was induced [73]. It remains to be seen how effective this construct will be in protecting humans.

Arthropods carry many diseases and can cause disease themselves by sucking blood from the host. These parasites remain on the surface of the host where they do not come into direct contact with the host immune system except by their feeding activities. One approach to control these infections is the use of midgut antigens. Antibodies produced to midgut antigens would react to the internal organs of the biting arthropod following feeding. These antibodies can interfere with gut function, slowing down growth, egg laying capacity, or killing the arthropod in some cases [74]. Although too early to predict meaningful success, this novel approach to antigens that would not normally interact with the host immune system warrants further investigation.

Therapeutic Vaccines

Vaccination can be used as a therapeutic treatment. For example, in a mouse model of *Helicobacter* infection, oral immunization with recombinant *Helicobacter pylori* urease B subunit was shown to eradicate a preexisting *Helicobacter felis* infection [75]. In the mouse model *Helicobacter felis*, a bacterial strain closely related to *Helicobacter pylori*, colonized the gastric mucosa and induced gastric lesions similar to those found in humans [76]. The possibility of vaccination as a therapeutic treatment against *Helicobacter* infection is interesting, since current antibiotic-base chemotherapies are not optimal and may not prevent recurrence of *Helicobacter pylori* infection [75]. If the reinfection with *Helicobacter pylori* can be prevented in humans by oral vaccination, it would provide the best therapeutic treatment for chronic gastritis and peptic ulcer.

Another example of therapeutic vaccination is the use of DNA motifs as immunostimulators. Certain nucleotide motifs are potent B-cell activators, enhancing B-cell activity within a very short time (within 12 h). This suggests that vaccines could be given in the face of an outbreak or shortly after exposure and can quickly stimulate an immune response. Mice inoculated with a CpG motif showed a dramatic reduction in *Listeria monocytogenes* following challenge; this would not be possible using routine vaccination protocols [77]. Therapeutic vaccination is expected to not only cure an otherwise chronic disease but also provide protection from reinfection.

Fertility Vaccines

There is great interest in vaccines to control fertility. Ideally, such vaccines would induce a state of infertility that could be reversed at a later time. Vaccines to control fertility have utilized a variety of approaches, including directing the immune response to the egg surface (sperm-receptor proteins), sperm-surface antigens, or reproductive hormones. Experimental success has been attained in this regard using a purified surface protein of sperm. Guinea pigs vaccinated with this material regained fertility a year later [78]. More recently, a recombinant protein antigen of fox sperm was administered orally to rats. The number of antibody-secreting cells detected in the intestine of these rats was similar to that seen in rats in which the same antigen was first injected into Peyer's patches and then intraduodenally [79]. Conjugation of the human reproductive hormones, chorionic gonadotrophin and luteinizing hormone-releasing hormone to protein carriers or muramyl dipeptide has also been investigated. When injected into animals, antibodies to the hormones were produced that cause atrophy of spermatocytes and inhibited fertility [80,81]. The zona pellucida surrounding the egg contains glycoproteins that provide binding sites for sperm. In mice, three such molecules have been identified. One glycoprotein ZP3 is the primary binding site for sperm. Antibodies to a peptide sequence reduces fertility in mice [82]. A B-cell epitope was identified in this peptide sequence that was poorly immunogenic. Conjugation of a more immunogenic protein could have increased the immunogenicity of this contruct. Alternatively, these researchers created a chimera whereby the gene for the B-cell epitope was cloned with a virus coat protein known to be a good immunogen. This resulted in a chimeric protein when expressed in a recombinant vector. Chimeric constructs consisting of virus coat protein with a B cell epitope of ZP3 have been purified and shown to induce antibodies in mice that recognized both the synthetic and authentic ZP3 glycoprotein and to be associated with the zona pellucida in vaccinated mice [83].

Routes of Vaccine Administration
Parenteral Vaccination

Vaccines have been effectively used in protecting humans and livestock from contagious and deadly diseases [84]. One of the most important problems in vaccination is to find the best method of presenting the antigen to the host immune system. Antigens can be delivered by intravenous, intraperitoneal, intradermal, intranasal, and oral routes of administration. Despite the recent advances in mucosal immunization, parenteral vaccination is still the choice of immunization for most antigens. The main method of influenza prophylaxis is immunization with parenterally administered inactivated influenza vaccine. It was demonstrated that a rapid immune response occurred simultaneously in the blood and the upper respiratory tract of subjects vaccinated subcutaneously with inactivated influenza vaccine. The number of influenza virus-specific antibody-secreting cells (ASC) in peripheral blood and tonsils increased rapidly to a peak within one week, followed by a decline to low levels after two to three weeks [85]. It appears that in some cases the parenterally administered vaccine can elicit a local immune response in the tonsils. Although parenteral vaccination may induce mucosal immunity, it alone is known to be insufficient at inducing mucosal immune responses. This limits the usefulness of parenteral vaccination.

Although parenteral vaccine injection has produced most reliable results, it is not the most desirable mode of administration. Vaccination with hypodermic needles is a highly labor-intensive procedure and not practical for a large number of subjects, especially animals. For example, vaccines are used in the routine control of Newcastle disease in chickens. The application of vaccines by intramuscular injection requires individual handling of the birds which is impractical [86]. Recently, jet injector guns have been used for parenteral vaccination. Although this method may eliminate all the concerns and inconveniences associated with hypodermic needles, it may cause the spread of infectious diseases if used without proper maintenance and hygiene [87].

Mucosal Vaccination

In everyday life, humans are exposed to various exogenous agents, including potentially harmful microorganisms, through the mucosal surfaces in the gastrointestinal, respiratory, and urogenital tracts. Considering the huge area of the mucosal surfaces, one can postulate that there must be important protective mechanisms at these sites. In fact, the mucosal immune system produces 70% of the body's antibodies [88]. The mucosal tissues are interconnected in a common mucosal immune system (CMIS) which is essentially separated from systemic immunity [89]. In a common mucosal defense system, an antigen interacting with localized lymphoid tissue at one inductive site can stimulate IgA precursor cells which migrate and elicit an immune reaction at other mucosal sites (Fig. 1).

Since a mucosal surface is the first port of entry of many infectious pathogens, preventing infections at the mucosa provides an immunological first line of defense against diseases [90]. This makes priming of the mucosal-associated lymphoid tissue (MALT) by vaccination most desirable. Parenteral vaccination alone is insufficient for inducing mucosal immune responses. Stimulation of the MALT usually requires direct contact between the immunogen and inductive lymphoid tissue such as Peyer's patch in the intestine at a mucosal surface [91].

Recent progress in mucosal immunization, especially oral immunization, provides new avenues of vaccination offering a unique advantage which is lacking in parenteral vaccination. Delivery of numerous antigens by a variety of routes (oral, nasal, rectal, vaginal) elicits production of antigen-specific secretory IgA at mucosal surfaces. Of the various routes, oral vaccination (Fig. 2) is preferred because of its ease of administra-

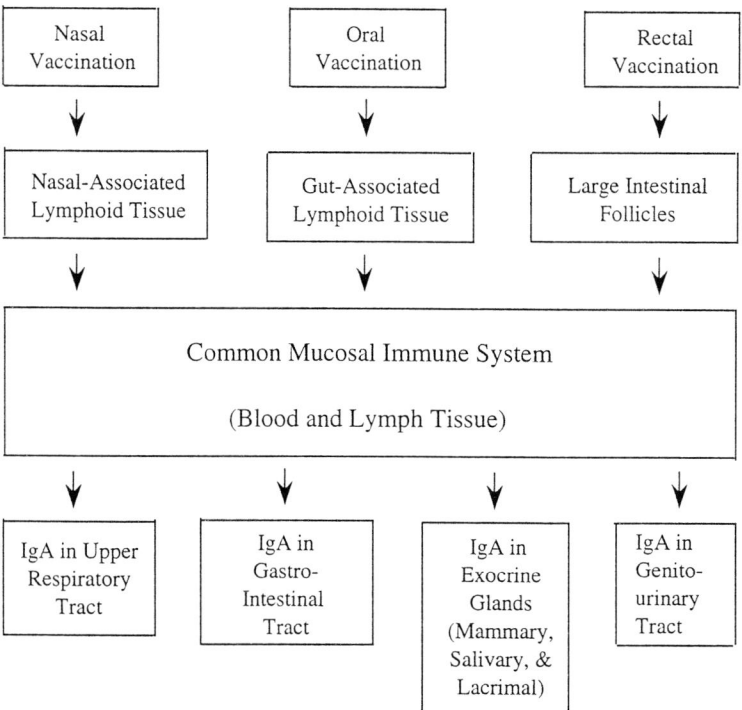

FIG. 1. Mucosal immunization and production of IgA antibodies in various mucosal surfaces via the common mucosal immunization system. Nasal and rectal vaccinations usually result in IgA production in the upper respiratory and genitourinary tracts, respectively, whereas sites effective for oral vaccination are expected to include many mucosal surfaces.

Vaccines and Other Immunological Products

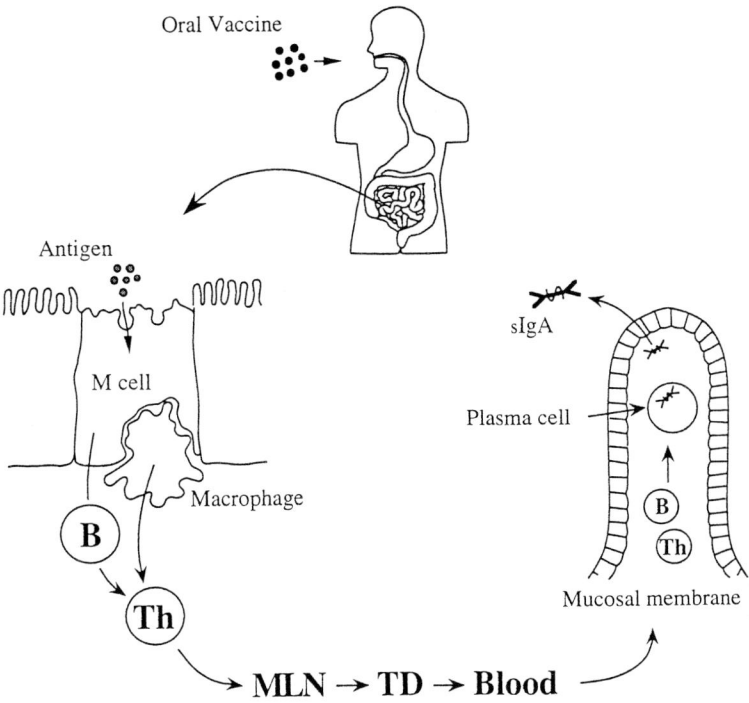

FIG. 2. Mucosal immunization by oral vaccination. After oral vaccination, an antigen is taken up by M cells in the Peyer's patch of the gut-associated lymphoid tissue. The antigen is passed to the macrophages and B cells (B) which present the antigen to T-helper (Th) lymphocytes. These cells migrate into the blood via the mesenteric lymph nodes (MLN) and the thoracic duct (TD). Subsequently, these cells localize in the effector sites, that is, the mucosal membranes of the gastrointestinal tract, upper respiratory tract, and genitourinary tract, and glandular tissue. At the effector sites, the migrating B cells develop into plasma cells which produce IgA antibodies. Polymeric IgA is then released as secretory IgA (sIgA) through epithelial cells.

tion and relatively low cost [92]. In addition, the gastrointestinal tract (GIT) is the largest inductive site in the common mucosal immune system. Other mucosal routes such as rectal and intravaginal routes are expected to be used less often because of unacceptability by a majority of population. In addition, the immunity induced at these sites is poorly characterized at this time. An example of the efficacy of oral vaccines is shown by the development of an orally administered polio vaccine. This vaccine not only circumvented many of the above-mentioned inconveniences and costs but, by avoiding injection, enhanced the acceptability to individuals of all ages.

Recently, it was suggested that oral vaccination can be used as a therapeutic treatment of gastric ulcers. The therapeutic efficacy of the recombinant *H. pylori* urease vaccine in mice was shown to be comparable with that achieved with the combined antibiotic–antacid treatment in humans. The oral vaccination is preferred to conventional treatment of ulcers, since it is a very simple and quick procedure compared with long-term conventional treatment. In addition, vaccines stimulate the defense mechanisms of the body to establish long-lasting immunity [75].

Although it offers many advantages over other methods of inoculation, oral vaccination does not always induce sufficient immunity. One of the reasons is that antigens can be degraded by enzymes in the GIT as well as by acids in the stomach [93]. Prevention of antigen degradation is the first step for successful oral vaccination. When gastric enzymes were inhibited by adding protease inhibitors before oral vaccination, complete immunity was obtained [94]. Another potential shortcoming of oral vaccination is that the uptake of antigens from the GIT is very poor. Even after ingestion of gram quantities of antigen, only nanogram amounts of antigenic material were found to pass the intestinal barrier [95]. It is also possible that for certain antigens oral vaccination may simply be less effective than parenteral vaccination in inducing systemic immunity [96]. The protection resulting from oral vaccination is known to last for a relatively short period of time, ranging from a few months to a year [88]. To obtain the desirable immunity equivalent to systemic immunization, oral vaccination requires much higher and more frequent doses [91]. Highly effective adjuvants may be needed in oral vaccine formulation to induce effective long-lasting immunity at mucosal tissues. Adjuvants in vaccines are discussed below.

Maternal immunization may be considered as one important application of oral vaccination. The digestive capacity of the stomach of newborn babies is not fully developed. This allows antibodies acquired in the colostrum from the mother to reach the gut in an active state. Maternal lymphocytes migrate from the intestine to the mammary gland, resulting in the transfer of the maternal immunologic profile to the offspring [97]. The lacteal secretion can contribute to both systemic and local immunity in the gut of the neonate. Studies on maternal immunization have provided a possibility that maternally derived antibodies may be used for immune-based protection in neonates, especially for intestinal diarrheal diseases that affect infants in the first weeks of life. In humans, breast feeding was shown to be associated with a substantial reduction of the risk of severe cholera in infants [98]. This raised a possibility that vaccination of mothers might provide protection to young children. The maternal immunization may find wider applications in animal vaccination. The feasibility of inducing long-term production and transfer of protective maternally derived antibodies to chicken hatchlings is currently being evaluated [99]. If successful, this approach would be extremely cost-effective since vaccination of a single breeding hen would lead to protection of over 100 broiler chicks [99].

Combination of Parenteral and Oral Vaccination

The combination of mucosal and systemic immunization routes (e.g., parenteral immunization followed by oral immunization or vice versa) generally induces mucosal immune responses that are superior to immunization by either route alone [96]. Pigs showed some protection after intramuscular inoculation with formalin-inactivated *Mycoplasma hyopneumoniae* vaccine in incomplete Freund's adjuvant. A booster inoculation with the same vaccine in microspheres injected intraduodenally onto the mucosal surface of Peyer's patches, increased the protection in pigs [93].

Adjuvants

Adjuvants are compounds that augment immune responses to a specific antigen. To augment immune responses by adjuvants is critical in the development of vaccines with weak immunogens, such as subunit vaccines [100]. A new generation of genetically engineered subunit vaccines are safer and better defined, but weaker immunogenically than inactivated or attenuated vaccines. The successful application of these subunit vaccines requires strong adjuvants to provide the desired immune response an antigen-specific protective immunity without side effects [84,101,102].

Adjuvants range from alum (aluminum phosphate, aluminum hydroxide, and aluminum sulfate) to complete Freund's adjuvant (killed mycobacteria in mineral oil). Alum is currently the only adjuvant approved by the FDA for human application. It is, however, not effective for all antigens and results mostly in humoral immunity [103]. Complete and incomplete Freund's adjuvants are highly effective, but are currently not used in humans due to toxicity and reactivity. The effects of adjuvants are not universal and depend on the immunogen and the delivery route. The mechanism of of their action is not clearly understood, and therefore their classification and selection remains an empirical process [100]. Adjuvants come in many different forms; although alum has been the standard adjuvant for human vaccines, there are many new adjuvants under investigation with many now in clinical trials. Adjuvants have been developed with a variety of effects from broad spectrum B- and T-cell effects, to specific activity for either B-cell activity or cytotoxic T-cell activity. These include modifications of existing adjuvants, such as monophosphoryl lipid-A, a less toxic LPS-modified adjuvant, muramyl dipeptide (a component of CFA) and its derivatives, saponins including extracts of *Quillaja saponaria*, cytokines (IL-1, IL-2, IL-6, γ-IFN), Schiff-base compounds [104], bacterial polynucleotides [77], and microparticles such as iscoms and liposomes. Many of these are covered in detail in a recent text [100]. In general adjuvant effects can be divided into the two major mechanisms, depot effect and immunostimulation [102].

Sustained-Release Effects

Adjuvants can provide sustained long-term release of antigens which results in increased immune response. Alum [101] and microparticles [105] deliver vaccine immunogens to the system more slowly than soluble immunogens. Antigens adsorb onto the surface of alum and are slowly released from the surface. Thus, the adjuvant effect of alum depends highly on the dose as well as the degree of antigen adsorption [106]. The release of antigens can be controlled more effectively by controlled-release technology which has been used extensively in the development of a new generation of drug delivery systems. The ultimate goal of controlled-release technology is to develop formulations that achieve the desired immune response by a single immunization [107]. The persistence of immunogen administered by controlled-release formulation is expected to result in an immune response equal to or better than that provided by multiple immunizations [87]. The single-immunization formulation solves the problems associated with the requirement for repeated visits for immunization. The more visits are required for complete immunization, the less likely it is that patients return for all inoculations. Single-dose inoculations would also reduce patient fears associated with the pain and adverse reactions to injections.

Most soluble antigens are not effective oral immunogens and require large and frequent dosing for mucosal immune responses. The superior practicality of oral immunization and its ability to induce mucosal immunity are compromised by the lack of powerful mucosal adjuvants that improve immunogenicity and thus facilitate the construction of effective oral vaccines [89].

A variety of compounds, ranging from polycations such as polyorinthin to vitamin A, have been shown to have adjuvant property when administered orally with antigen

[89,108]. The common aspect of these adjuvants is that they can influence the structural and/or functional integrity of the mucosal surface to which they are applied. The most potent mucosal adjuvant identified to date is cholera toxin, which is the primary enterotoxin produced by *Vibrio cholerae* bacteria. Cholera toxin and the analogous heat-labile enterotoxin from *E. coli* are both powerful mucosal immunogens and adjuvants. They are known to increase gut permeability and uptake of luminal antigens [89]. They provide specific binding to intestinal epithelium, including M cells of Peyer's patches, and increase the immune response to antigens administered with them. The adjuvant effect of these toxins is primarily contained in the B subunit. This was an important consideration since the toxic portion of this two-part toxin requires both the B subunit (for attachment) and the A subunit (which enters the cell to interfere with cell functions). The B subunit alone cannot cause diarrhea. It was suggested that the potential to exploit cholera toxin B subunit as an antigen carrier molecule for mucosal immunizations in humans should be explored more thoroughly [109]. Oral immunization with cholera toxin B subunit in humans resulted in a substantial specific IgA antibody-producing cell response not only in the gut mucosa but also in the blood, and most significantly, in a distant mucosal tissue such as the salivary glands [109].

As pointed out above, uptake of antigens in the intestines is a very inefficient. Methods of increasing uptake of antigens by Peyer's patches is of primary interest to improve the delivery and efficacy of oral vaccines. Cholera toxin B can be used as an adjuvant as well as an adhesion factor to enhance binding and antigen uptake. Other materials are under investigation for increasing antigen uptake. Plant lectins can be used to enhance the uptake from the gut, since they use surface carbohydrates of the brush border membrane as receptors and induce endocytotic uptake [97]. Lectins may not directly enhance the immune response, but may play an important role in increasing uptake of antigen which improves the immune response.

Immunostimulating Effects

Adjuvants provide immunostimulating effects. Immunostimulating components of adjuvants specifically activate portions of the immune system, increasing the immune response in several ways. The precipitated antigens are more readily taken up by macrophages which process antigens and present them to T-helper lymphocytes. This occurs with alum and both complete (CFA) and incomplete Freund's (IFA) adjuvants. In some cases granulomas form in response to antigens, thereby attracting an even larger number of macrophages. This may also enhance cytokine production, especially of interleukin-1 which, in turn, activates T-helper cells. Granulomas form especially in response to complete Freund's adjuvant. Another mechanism of action of adjuvants is to enhance expression of costimulatory signals required for activation of T-helper cells by macrophages. Adjuvants such as CFA and LPS increase the expression of the costimulatory molecules on macrophages. The B lymphocytes can bind to antigen directly. Some adjuvants (LPS, *Bordetella pertussis* toxin, and polynucleotides) specifically activate B-cell binding to antigen [110,111].

Safety

One of the most important factors to be considered in the selection of adjuvants is in safety (or toxicity). Although some adjuvants, such as complete and incomplete Freund's adjuvants, lipopolysaccharides, chloera toxin, and those containing bacterial products, are highly effective, they are too toxic to be used in humans and even in laboratory animals [102]. Adjuvanticity and safety have to be carefully balanced to obtain the desired immune responses with minimum side effects. In choosing adjuvants for parenteral vaccination, acute or subacute tissue damage at the site of injection as well as pyrogenicity need to be considered [112].

Liposomes have been identified as safe adjuvants. They are phospholipid vesicles made of single- or multicompartment bilayer structures. Liposomes are known to induce humoral and cellular immunity to a number of antigens and act as immunoadjuvants [113–115]. Since soluble antigens become particulates by being incorporated into liposomes, they become more effective in eliciting immune responses. The physiocochemical factors that influence the degree of the immunological responses are liposome size, surface charge and charge distribution, lipid composition, and the position of the antigens [116]. In general, negatively charged liposomes are taken up more extensively than neutral or positive charged liposomes [117]. Liposomes based on naturally occurring phospholipids are highly safe and nontoxic. Liposomes have the advantages that they can deliver both hydrophilic and hydrophobic antigens in a sustained-release profile. Since antigens are shielded by the lipid bilayer from the environment, their toxicity, if present at all, can be reduced or eliminated [118]. The extensive experience with liposomes as controlled drug delivery systems, knowledge about the adjuvant effect of liposomes, and lack of toxicity make the liposomes prime candidates in the development of new adjuvants [116].

Antigen Delivery Systems for Enhanced Response

Of the many variables affecting the outcome of immunization, the most crucial factor may be the selection of the antigen delivery system. Depending on how antigens are delivered, the immune response can be significantly different. Antigen delivery systems can be classified as live attenuated microorganisms and nonliving encapsulation (microparticulate) systems.

1. Live recombinant vectors
   Avirulent viruses (vaccinia, adenovirus, etc.)
   Avirulent bacteria (Mycobacterium, Salmonella, Shigella, etc.)
2. Nonliving encapsulation systems
   Polymeric microparticles
   Liposomes
   ISCOMS
   Protein aggregates

Live Attenuated Organisms

Since the success with live attenuated oral vaccines against tuberculosis and polio more than three decades ago, a number of live attenuated microorganisms have been used as antigen delivery systems. Live vaccines generally result in a better immune response of longer duration than those obtained by nonliving immunogens [90]. Attenuated strains of microorganisms can be spontaneously formed or induced by heat or chemical or ultraviolet mutagenesis. Recently, pathogenic microorganisms have been attenuated by genetic engineering, that is, mutating specific genes or removing some toxic genes. Attenuated recombinant *Salmonella* strains have successfully expressed genes from other organisms and thus been used as vectors in delivering heterologous antigens [90]. Other examples of live attenuated microorganism vaccines are BCG, adenovirus, and poliovirus.

Live attenuated vaccines can induce a broad and long-lasting immune response. They are relatively easy and cheap to manufacture, since they do not require purification of antigens or formulation with adjuvants [90]. Another advantage of the attenuated live vaccines is that they can be administered by the natural route of infection. Since much of the infection occurs through the mucosal surfaces, live attenuated vaccines are best suited for protecting against pathogens which enter the body through the mucosal surfaces [91]. Live attenuated oral vaccines are expected to provide the most convenient and effective means of vaccinating against enteric disease [119]. Orally administered attenuated *Salmonella* strains are known to colonize the mucosal associated lymphoid tissue in the GIT where they express and release cloned genes of subunit vaccines [90].

However, one of the drawbacks of live microorganisms is that attenuated pathogens may invoke the very disease they are designed to prevent if they are insufficiently attenuated [90]. Even if they are sufficiently attenuated, they still may cause severe infections in immunocompromised individuals. On the other hand, if pathogens are over-attenuated, they cannot replicate sufficiently and therefore fail to trigger a appropriate immune response. Thus, it is important to attain the right balance between minimal virulence and maximal immunogenicity. This can be achieved in a normal population, but may be difficult in a population with even minor defects in immune competence [112]. Another important consideration in the use of live vector-based vaccines is that the distribution requires refrigeration which may not be readily available in underdeveloped countries. This requirement may offset the advantages of live vector vaccines [87].

Recombinant Vaccines

New technologies are necessary to achieve several objectives in vaccine production:

- Increase the supply of vaccines for which the demand cannot be met. An example is the production of hepatitis B virus surface antigen vaccine purified from human serum which can now be made by recombinant expression in *Saccharomyces cerevesiae*.
- Increase product safety; acellular pertussis vaccines that are effective yet less reactogenic are being produced.
- Make vaccines that could previously not be produced (because of difficulties in cultivating organism in laboratories to produce antigens). Recombinant antigens of protozoa such as Schistosoma can be mass-produced by expression vectors in vitro.
- Design of delivery systems that would reduce the number of doses and avoid injections to induce long-lasting immunity from an early age on.
- Make adjuvants or techniques to eliminate the need for adjuvants (by direct administration of vaccine into a cell). Better adjuvants are more readily available and can be used to induce better, longer-lasting antibody titers and cell-mediated immu-

nity; DNA injection makes intracellular administration of antigen quick and efficient [120].

An approach to minimize the virulence and maximize the immunogenicity is to use subunit vaccines composed of antigenic components (usually proteins) free of pathogenic impurities [84]. However, the immune responses by subunit vaccines are not as broad (e.g., cell-mediated immunity, humoral immunity, and antibodies of wider specificity) as those of vector-administered immunogens [87]. Immunogens can be expressed by recombinant technologies using a variety of vectors such as vaccinia or other poxviruses, BCG, salmonella, and adenovirus. These vectors have been chosen because of their safety, ability to replicate in the host without inducing disease (adenoviruses are naturally nonpathogenic in humans, for example), and efficiency in expressing encoded genetic material within a host. Examples of viruses and bacterial vectors are described above. Most bacterial vectors have been gram-negative organisms that colonize the intestinal tract. An alternative approach is the use of commensal oral gram-positive organisms that colonize the nasal and gut surfaces. *Streptococcus gordonii* transfected with bacterial or viral protein genes was able to colonize and express the foreign genes for at least two months following colonization of mice [121]. Commensal organisms and food-grade bacteria have increased the range of possible bacterial vectors for vaccine delivery [122,123].

Antigen-encoding plasma DNAs have been shown to be effective immunogens following injection or applied directly to mucosal surfaces [1]. The DNA is taken up by host cells which express the protein antigen. This offers several advantages over subunit vaccines which must be purified. Recombinant-derived products depend on an appropriate expression vector for production. Purified subunit antigens primarily stimulate a humoral immune response. If presented in an expression vector into the host, the vector may cause disease or an immune response to the vector may lead to its elimination. The DNA vaccines overcome these problems and deliver the vaccine material to the cell where it is expressed. Absorption by antigen-presenting cells results both in a MHC-I CMI response and B-cell memory immune response. The method of inoculation determines the efficiency of transfection with intramuscular inoculation far superior in expression. However, comparable immune responses can be induced by intratracheal or intradermal administration, presumably due to the presence of efficient immune effector systems. Intradermal administration with a "gene gun" requires two to three powers of ten less of DNA to induce an immune response in spite of far lower efficiency of transfection.

Protective immunity mediated by cytotoxic T-lymphocyte activity and memory B-cell response has been induced to homologous strains of influenza in animals using DNA that codes for surface glycoproteins [1,2]. Protection to heterologous influenza strains could be induced using the antigenically conserved nucleoprotein DNA from influenza [45]. A similar approach using nucleoprotein DNA of lymphocytic choriomenigitis virus induced protective immunity as well [124]. The last two studies demonstrate the effectiveness of endogenously expressed and processed viral proteins to induce MHC I restricted cytotoxic lymphocytes. Oral administration of DNA for incorporation into intestinal sites has ben successful using attenuated Shigella to deliver plasmid DNA to colonic musosal cells [125]. This technique could be tried further to enhance and modulate mucosal immune responses. Bacterial DNA (hsp65) coding for the 65-kDa heat-shock protein of *Mycobacterium leprae*, an antigen conserved among mycobacterial species, stimulated surprisingly good protective immunity in mice challenged by *M. tuberculosis*. Good cytotoxic lymphoctye and delayed-type hypersensitivity responses were seen in mice vaccinated with the hsp65 DNA [3]. This technique shows great promise for intracellular pathogens, especially those such as *M. tuberculosis* which is increasing in prevalence and showing increasing antibiotic resistance; long-term antibiotic therapy is required, resulting in poor patient compliance.

Molecular applications of vaccines have spawned some interesting capabilities. *Vibrio cholerae* causes diarrhea in humans due to a two-component enterotoxin. The enterotoxin adhesion to host cells is mediated by the pentameric B subunit. Antibodies preventing the binding of the B subunit can eliminate the toxic activities and prevent diarrhea. The gene of the B subunit has been identified and sequenced. Plant vectors have been transfected with the B subunit gene of *V. cholerae* which has successfully transformed tobacco plants and potatoe tubers. The tubers express and concentrate the protein antigen up to 15–20 µg per 5 g of potato. Mice fed these transgenic tobacco leaf extracts or potato tubers developed serum and intestinal antibodies to the B subunit [126,127]. Hepatitis B surface antigen and Norwalk virus capsid proteins have been introduced into plants as well [126,128]. Besides potato, canola and banana are also being investigated as possible transgenic plant sources that could be used in vaccine foods for humans and animals. This provides an interesting cost-effective method to vaccinate individuals at a mucosal site where the infection occurs, and without the need for individuals to return to a medical center for booster vaccines. A chimeric peptide-virus coat protein, using a peptide of the ZP3 glycoprotein of the zona pelucida of mice and the outer coat protein of tobacco mosaic virus, has been produced in tobacco. The tobacco mosaic virus concentrated the chimeric protein to levels of 2.5 mg/g of leaf. Purified peptide chimeras induced antibodies that bound to the zona pellucida in inoculated mice. In vitro assays confirmed that the antibodies bound synthetic and authentic ZP3 glycoprotein. Although promising as a means of controlling fertility, use of ZP3 so far suggests that the vaccine may not be easily reversed. Significant inflammation of the ovaries has been seen in vaccines based on ZP3 in mice [83].

Nonliving Microparticulate Delivery Systems

Nonliving microparticulates that can be used as antigen delivery systems include polymeric microparticles, liposomes, and proteins or protein aggregates. Polymeric microparticles and liposomes have been used extensively as controlled-release dosage forms for many drugs including antigens [129,130]. Delivery of antigens by microparticulate delivery systems has the potential benefits of reducing the number of inoculations, enhancing the immune response via both parenteral and oral vaccination routes, and reducing the total antigen dose required to achieve immune protection [131]. The definition of microparticles depends on the applications; in the vaccine area, microparticles are defined as particles less than 50 µm [132].

For parenteral vaccination, biodegradable polymeric microparticles made of poly-(lactide-*co*-glycolide) (PLG) are commonly used as vaccine carriers. Microspheres less than about 100 µm in diameter can be easily administered by injection through standard-sized needles (22 gauge or smaller), eliminating the need for surgical implantation [133]. Sustained release of antigens from microparticles enhances immune responses in much the same way as the alum adjuvants. Microparticles can be taken up directly by macrophages, which may provide a route to evade neutralization of delivered antigens by maternal antibodies [98]. Alternative methods of microparticle production can also have an adjuvant effect. Recently it was shown that surface-modified diamond nanoparticles could dramatically increase the immune response to an antigen of low immunogenicity. When mussel adhesive protein (MAP), a material proposed as a surgical adhesive, is prepared with complete Freund's adjuvant, poor immune responses are induced. However, when MAP was prepared with the diamond nanoparticles, a strong specific immune response was induced in rabbits. Although general usage of diamonds in vaccines may not sound practical, the technology demonstrates the capability to dramatically enhance immunogenicity of weak antigens with the help of innovative nanoparticle materials [134].

Preparation of PLG microparticles requires high curing temperatures and organic solvents. These can damage or affect antigens and reduce their immunogenicity. In the preparation of microparticles for parenteral administration, the residual solvent used in the preparation of the polymeric microparticles should be carefully removed to avoid toxic effects in the host.

Polymeric microparticles can be used to deliver antigens by oral administration. The polymeric microparticles protect antigens from acidic and enzymatic degradation in the gastrointestinal tract, and thus serve as a stable vaccine vehicle with extended shelf life. Oral vaccination employing microparticles is an interesting technology which provides new avenues of vaccination. Since oral vaccination is most convenient and cost effective, the focus here will be on the use of microparticles in oral vaccination.

Microparticles

Delivery of peptide and protein drugs by oral administration is an important developing technology. Delivery of insulin by oral administration would be a breakthrough if it could be achieved at a clinically significant level. The main problem with the delivery of protein drugs is that they are degraded by strong acids in the stomach and enzymes in the GI tract. Furthermore, the efficiency of the uptake of macromolecules from the intestine is known to be very low. Microparticles, including aggregates of proteins and synthetic or natural polymers, are absorbed from the intestine by several mechanisms. Although microparticles can be absorbed by a mechanism called "persorption," it is not exploited for delivery of protein drugs since it is a passive process with very low efficiency [132]. Antigens are generally peptides and proteins and their oral delivery needs to be distinguished from the delivery of other protein drugs such as insulin. The delivery of protein drugs requires a rather large quantity for the long term, whereas the delivery of antigens requires only a small amount for a very short period of time. For this reason, oral vaccination is highly feasible. For example, oral administration of microencapsulated influenza A vaccine virus induced levels of serum antibody in mice comparable to parenterally administered microspheres [135].

The basis of oral vaccination using antigen-containing microparticles is that, following oral administration, the microparticles are taken up by the Peyer's patches. The M cells in the epithelium of Peyer's patches are capable to absorb the soluble macromolecular antigens and microparticles from the intestine [97]. A number of studies have shown that microparticles can be taken up by Peyer's patches, depending on the size, dose, and surface properties [136–139]. Microparticles used in the uptake by Peyer's patches have been made of polystyrene, polymethyl methacrylate, polybutyl cyanoacrylate, poly(lactide-*co*-glycolide), polyacyl starch, dextran, albumin, and alginic acid. More microparticles are taken up with increasing particle surface hydrophobicity. Hydrophobic polystyrene particles were taken up to the greater extent than hydrophilic cellulose particles, and microparticles smaller than 10 µm are preferentially taken up by the Peyer's patches. The future success of oral vaccination depends heavily on the design of antigen carriers which are specifically targeted to Peyer's patches and other lympohoid tissues that sample antigen.

A variety of different types of vaccine formulations under development or currently being used have been discussed. Examples are shown in Table 1 to emphasize the growing diversity of designs.

Evaluation, Production, and Safety

Clinical Trials

The need to regulate vaccine production is recognized worldwide to assure the quality of the licensed products. For example, in the United States the Center for Biologics Evaluation and Research of the Food and Drug Administration regulates vaccine production by licensed manufacturers. Guidelines for international vaccines promulgated by the World Health Organization have been adopted as national regulations by many countries around the world. The European Economic Community (EEC) has agreed to regulations that apply for all member countries. The primary objectives of these regulations is to assure the safety, potency, purity, and efficacy of vaccines [140]. Only vaccines produced by licensed manufacturers following Good Manufacturing Practices (GMPs) and abiding by regulations regarding plant, personnel, and production protocols can be licensed. Regulations are becoming increasingly more standardized to assure a uniform product quality in the United States, EEC, and Japan. Such standardization will increase the distribution of vaccines among these countries [141]. This more global approach to disease control should help alleviate the shortage of vaccines in developing nations and stabilize vaccine prices which now vary widely [142].

The safety and immunogenicity of new vaccines must be evaluated before widespread usage to determine efficacy and the risks of undesired side effects. Vaccines must also stand the test of challenge in field conditions before final development. Postlicensing trials are often performed to determine efficacy even further in different populations and to gather information to optimize production. The recruitment of volunteers on an ethical basis for testing candidate vaccines has become an important consideration. The first vaccines were tested on institutionalized children or prisoners. Properly designed randomized, double-blind controlled field studies with natural challenge are now required prior to licensure. Vaccines are not used if they are expensive and not cost effective.

Prior to clinical trials, vaccines should be evaluated in animals. Clinical trials should be performed with the same batches of vaccine used in preclinical studies. The purity, consistency, and antigenic load should be standardized between batches. Manufacturing techniques to address these issues should be well established before starting clinical trials. The initial clinical evaluation of a new vaccine is designed to test safety, immunogenicity, and efficacy. In the United States, Phase I and Phase II trials are subject to federally mandated guidelines to provide intense laboratory evaluation of the vaccines under investigation before they are tested on a wider basis in field trials. In Phase I trials, dosage, vaccine interval, and immunogenicity, based on both humoral and cell-

TABLE 1 Examples of Vaccines

Antigen	Target	Source of Antigen	Delivery	Ref.
Live virus	Influenza virus	Temperature-sensitive mutant	Intranasal	17
Live bacterium	*Salmonella typhimurium*	Auxotrophic mutant	Oral	18
Surface antigen	Hepatitis B virus	Recombinant product	Liposomes, injection	27
Surface antigen	*Shistosoma mansoni*	Recombinant product	Injection	71–73
Urease B subunit	*Helicobacter pylori*	Purified protein	Oral	75
Surface antigen	Sperm (fertility)	Purified protein	Injection	78
Nucleoprotein	Influenza virus	Nucleoprotein DNA	Injection (gun into skin)	45
Circumsporozoite surface antigen	*Plasmodium falciparum*	Recombinant gene	Oral in avirulent *Salmonella typhi*	67, 119
Cholera toxin B subunit	*Vibrio cholerae*	Recombinant gene	Transgenic plants	126, 127

mediated responses, are evaluated in a small number (less than 50) of well-informed consenting volunteers. Subjects for both Phase I and Phase II trials must be in good health, be interested in the study, have reasonable motivation for participation, and be dependable and cooperative in returning for postvaccination examinations. In Phase IIa, more extensive safety and immunogenicity studies are performed. In Phase IIb, the preliminary efficacy is determined with challenge performed where possible under well-controlled conditions. During Phase II, inoculation schedule, dosage, and the best route of administration are determined. Studies are performed in outpatient clinics with good care, or if necessary, in hospitals under closer observation. The clinical protocol must be carefully designed, including the parameters to be used for evaluation. Study design with issues concerning informed consent, data collection, and justification of the risks involved in the study should be addressed to meet federal investigational new drug regulations and to withstand review by institutional ethical review boards.

During Phases III and IV, field trials vaccines are rigorously tested for safety, efficacy, and effectiveness. Field trials can assess postinoculation immune responses, or determine whether a recently licensed vaccine is safe and protective. The most important clinical field trial involves a carefully designed experiment in a population that is normally at risk of developing the disease for which the vaccine is targeted. These studies must be randomized, unbiased, and controlled. Lack of bias should include the selection of study groups, double-blind administration of test vaccine(s) or placebo, and interpretation of data.

In these studies, two different approaches are used to evaluate vaccines. Efficacy trials are designed to maximize the detection of protective immunity induced by a vaccine in a population at risk likely to respond to the vaccine allowing the detection of immune response. Effectiveness trials are designed to predict how well a vaccine will perform in actual practice in a population at risk and who would be targeted for vaccination after licensure. The efficacy trial is performed under optimal conditions to demonstrate a favorable immune response to a vaccine, whereas an effectiveness trial compares a test vaccine to a standard vaccine if possible under conditions as close as possible to real condition. Informed consent of participants is very important. For in depth guidelines, readers are referred to other sources [143,144].

Veterinary vaccine production in the United States is regulated by the US. Department of Agriculture (USDA), specifically the Veterinary Biologics Division of the Animal and Plant Health Inspection Service (APHIS). The guidelines for vaccine development are outlined in Title 9, *Code of Federal Regulations*. Licensure of a veterinary vaccine requires efficacy testing similar to that for human vaccines. The efficacy of a vaccine depends on statistically valid challenge studies performed on the host animal. These studies must be performed on the youngest animals to be vaccinated, with the lowest level of antigen and highest passage level of the master seed of the organism used to make the vaccine. Field efficacy trials are only performed when challenge studies are not possible. Field safety tests are required, intended to detect unexpected reactions that were not observed during development studies. The tests are performed on the host animal, using large numbers of susceptible animals of all ages under different husbandry practices [145]. More detailed information about regulations concerning the production of veterinary vaccines is given in Title 9, *Code of Federal Regulations*.

Production

The production of vaccines involves the use of microorganisms for the production of inactivated or attenuated vaccines, of subunit vaccines, and recombinant material. For each situation, strict control of conditions for the growth of these microbes is necessary to assure the purity of the final product without contaminating substances or organisms, and maintain consistency in the final product. Highly pure water, nutrients, and a sterile system for culturing the product material are required. The number of infectious agents per milliliter or total immunogen content must be standardized for every batch of product. The phase and conditions (nutrients, gas mixture, stirring rate, etc.) of growth of these organisms at harvest must be standardized to maximize the expression of the desired immunogenic factors with minimal toxic components [146].

Vaccine production has been boosted tremendously by the use of biotechnology to generate safer, highly selective, immunogenic, more economical products. Recombinant vaccines such as for hepatitis B with a predicted market of $100 million have been released and promise to revolutionize the vaccine industry. Other factors are contributing to an increase in vaccine production. For many years, the profit margin for vaccine production was very low and therefore did not provide for the necessary research and development to generate improved vaccines. High litigation costs also impeded development and production of vaccines. Litigation for adverse reactions to pertussis vaccines alone discouraged further vaccine development and for a period of time threatened the availability of these vaccines as companies spent as much or more money on litigation fees as they made in sales. Changes in liability laws limiting the amount of awards for adverse vaccine reactions has lessened the impact of litigation. The medical community and health insurance industry have recognized the cost benefit of preventative medicines which has shown that with very expensive vaccines the return on such preventative measures saves money in treatment costs. The World Health Organization efforts to increase vaccine availability, especially to children, has further increased awareness of the need to reduce the incidence of preventable infectious disease. It is likely that increased commercial success will encourage the development of better and safer vaccines, depending on production and development costs to bring a product to market. Biotechnology will increase the cost of manufacturing initially until the industry is equipped to produce vaccines in this manner. Then the actual cost of production should decrease. However, newer adjuvants may offset these savings inasmuch as they are much more costly, contributing 10-50% of the cost of a vaccine instead of 0.01% for the standard alum adjuvants. Patent and licensing rights may be another source of costs as certain patents, such as for recombinant hepatis B, require licensing agreements from one company at present. It is hoped that new delivery systems permitting intranasal or oral administration will reduce cost by eliminating the need for sterile needles and syringes which have to be disposed. Overall, the present climate for vaccine production looks favorable with many new companies entering the market. Demand for vaccines for diseases such as hepatitis B, HIV, and herpes virus alone, with estimated markets in excess of $225 million, will certainly encourage development [147].

Acknowledgments

This study was supported in part by a grant from the Pacific Corporation.

References

1. Fynan, E.F., Webster, R.G., Fuller, D.H., Haynes, J.R., Santoro, J.C., and Robinson,

H.L., DNA vaccines: protective immunizations by parenteral, mucosal, and gene-gun inoculations, *Proc. Nat. Acad. Sci.-USA*, 90:11478-11482 (1993).
2. Webster, R.G., Fynan, E.F., Santoro, J.C., and Robinson, H., Protection of ferrets against influenza challenge with a DNA vaccine to the haemagglutinin, *Vaccine*, 12:1495-1498 (1994).
3. Lowrie, D.B., Tascon, R.E., Colston, M.J., and Silva, C.L., Towards a DNA vaccine against tuberculosis, *Vaccine*, 12:1537-1540 (1994).
4. Bisno, A.L., Group A streptococcal infections and acute rheumatic fever, *N. Engl. J. Med.*, 325:783-788 (1991).
5. Benjamin, J.B., Berzofsky, J., and East, I., The anitgenic structure of proteins: a reappraisal, *Ann. Rev. Immunol.*, 2:67-78 (1984).
6. Hopp, T.P., and Woods, K.R., Prediction of the protein antigenic determinants from amino acid sequences, *Proc. Nat. Acad. Sci. USA*, 78:3824-3828 (1978).
7. Chou, P.Y., and Fasman, G.D., Prediction of the Secondary Structure of Proteins from their Amino Acid Sequences. In: *Advances in Enzymology*, Wiley, New York, 1978, pp. 45-148.
8. Kyte, J., and Doolittle, R.F., A simple method for displaying the hydropathic character of a protein, *J. Mol. Biol.*, 157:105-132 (1982).
9. Garnier, J., Osguthorpe, D.J., and Robson, B., Analysis of the accuracy and implications of simple methods for predicting the secondary structure of globular proteins, *J. Mol. Biol.*, 120:97-120 (1978).
10. Tanier, J.A., Getzoff, E., and Paterson, Y., The atomic mobility component of protein antigenicity, *Ann. Rev. Immunol.*, 3:501-510 (1985).
11. Laver, W.G., Air, G.M., Webster, R.G., and Smith-Gill, S.J., Epitopes on protein antigens: misconceptions and realities, *Cell*, 61:553-559 (1990).
12. Buus, S., Sette, A., and Grey, J.M., The interaction between protein-derived immunogenic peptides and IA, *Immunol. Rev.*, 98:115-125 (1987).
13. Parkman, P.D., Meyer, H.M. Jr., Kirschstein, R.L., and Hopps, H.E., Attenuated rubella virus. I. Development and laboratory characterization, *N. Engl. J. Med.*, 275:569-574 (1966).
14. Bunyak, E.B., Hilleman, M.R., Weiber, R.E., and Stokes, J., Jr., Live attenuated rubella virus vaccines prepared in duck embryo cell culture. I. Development and clinical testing. *JAMA.*, 204:195-200 (1968).
15. Plotkin, S.A., Farquhar, J., Katz, M., and Ingalls, T.H., A new attenuated rubella virus grown in human fibroblasts: evidence for reduced nasopharyngeal excretion, *Am. J. Epidemiol.*, 86:468-477 (1967).
16. Sabin, A.B., and Boulger, L., History of Sabin attenuated poliovirus oral live vaccine strains, *J. Biol. Stand.*, 1:115-118 (1973).
17. Richman, D.D., Murphy, B.R., Spring, S.B., Coleman, M.T., and Chanock, R.M., Temperature sensitive mutants of influenza virus: IX. Genetic and biological characterization of TS-1 [E] lesions when transferred to a 1972 (H3N2) influenza A virus, *Virology*, 66:551-562 (1975).
18. Chatfield, S.N., Roberts, M., Dougan, G., Hormaeche, C., and Khan, C.M.A., The development of oral vaccines against parasitic diseases utilizing live attenuated Salmonella, *Parasitology*, 110:S17-S24 (1995).
19. Mettenleiter, T.C., New developments in the construction of safer and more versatile Pseudorabies virus vaccines, *Dev. Biol. Stand.*, 84:83-87 (1995).
20. Kimman, T.G., Gielkens, A.L.J., Glazenburg, K., Jacobs, L., de Jong, M.C.M., Mulder, W.A.M., and Peeters, B.P.H., Characterization of live Pseudorabies virus vaccines, *Dev. Biol. Stand.*, 84:89-96 (1995).
21. Dorner, F., An overview of virus vectors, *Dev. Biol. Stand.*, 84:23-32 (1995).
22. Cirillo, J.D., Stover, C.K., Bloom, B.R., Jacobs, W.R., Jr., and Barletta, R.G., Bacterial vaccine vectors and Bacillus Calmette-Guerin, *Clin. Inf. Dis.*, 20:1001-1009 (1995).

23. Berzofsky, J.A., Cease, K., and Cornette, J., Protein antigenic structures recognized by T cells: potential applications to vaccine design, *Immunol. Rev.*, 98:9-19 (1987).
24. Randall, R.E., Solid matrix-antibody-antigen (SMAA) complexes for constructing multivalent subunit vaccines, *Immunol. Today.*, 10:336-341 (1989).
25. Mowat, A.McI., Donachie, A.M., Reid, G., and Jarrett, O., Immune-stimulating complexes containing Quil A and protein antigen prime class I MHC-restricted T lymphocytes in vivo and are immunogenic by the oral route, *Immunology*, 72:317-322 (1991).
26. Maloy, K.J., Donachie, A.M., O'Hagan, D.T., and Mowat, A.McI.: Induction of mucosal and systemic immune responses by immunization with ovalbumin entrapped in poly(lactide-*co*-glycolide) microparticles, *Immunology*, 81:661-667 (1994).
27. Manesis, E.K., Cameron, C., and Gregoriadis, G., Hepatitis B surface antigen-containing liposomes enhance humoral and cell-mediated immunity to the antigen, *FEBS Lett.*, 102:107-111 (1979).
28. Connors, M., Collins, P.L., Firestone, C., and Murphy, B.R., Respiratory syncytial virus (RSV) F, G, M2 (22K), and N proteins each induce resistance to RSV challenge, but resistance induced by M2 and N proteins is relatively short-lived, *J. Virol.*, 65:1634-1637 (1991).
29. Murphy, B.R., Hall, S.L., Kulkarni, A.B., Crowe, J.E., Jr., Collins, P.L., Connors, M., Karron, R.A., and Chanock, R.M., An update on the approaches to the development of respiratory syncytial virus and parainfluenza virus type 3 vaccines, *Virus Res.*, 32:13-36 (1994).
30. Sato, Y., Kimura, M., and Fukumi, J., Development of a pertussis component vaccine in Japan, *Lancet*, 1:122-129 (1984).
31. Noble, G.R., Bernier, R.H., and Escher, C.E., Acellular and whole-cell pertussis vaccines in Japan: report of a visit by US scientists, *JAMA*, 257:1351-1357 (1987).
32. Fox, J.L., Several acellular pertussis vaccines appear safe, effective, *ASM News*, 61:506-508 (1995).
33. Brown, F., Dougan, F., Hoey, E.M., Martin, S.J., Rima, B.K., and Trudgett, A., *Vaccine Design*, Wiley, New York, 1993, pp. 107-118.
34. Diakun, K.R., and Matta, K.L., Synthetic antigens as immunogens: III. Specificity analysis of an anti-anti-idiotypic antibody to a carbohydrate tumor-associated antigen, *J. Immunol.*, 142:2037-2040 (1989).
35. Grzych, J.M., Capron, M., Lambert, P.H., Dissous, C., Torres, S., and Capron, S., An anti-idiotypic vaccine against experimental schistosomiasis, *Nature (London)*, 316:74-76 (1985).
36. Zanetti, M., Secarz, E., and Salk, J., The immunology of new generation vaccines, *Immunol. Today*, 8:18-22 (1987).
37. Wiley, D.C., Wilson, I.A., and Skehel, J.J., Structural identification of the antibody-binding sites of Hong Kong influenza haemagglutinin and their involvement in antigenic variation, *Nature (London)*, 289:373-378 (1981).
38. Zweerink, H.J., Askonas, B.A., Millican, D., Courtneidge, S.A., and Skehel, J.J., Cytotoxic T cells to type A influenza virus; viral haemagglutinin induces A-strain specificity while infected cells confer cross-reactive cytotoxicity, *Eur. J. Immunol.*, 7:630-635 (1977).
39. Mbawuike, I.N., and Wyde, P.R., Induction of CD8+ cytotoxic T cells by immunization with killed influenza virus and effect of cholera toxin B subunit, *Vaccine*, 11:1205-1213 (1993).
40. Yap, K.L., Ada, G.L., and McKenzie, I.S.C., Transfer of specific cytotoxic T cells protects mice inoculated with influenza viruses, *Nature (London)*, 273:238-239 (1978).
41. Eichelberger, M., Allan, W., Zijlstra, M., Jaenisch, R., and Doherty, P.C., Clearance of influenza virus respiratory infection in mice lacking class I major histocompatibility complex-restricted CD8+ T cells, *J. Exp. Med.*, 174:875-880 (1991).

42. Oehen, S., Waldner, H., Kundig, T.M., Hengartner, H., and Zinkernagel, R.M., Antivirally protective cytotoxic T cell memory to lymphocytic choriomeningitis virus is governed by persisting antigen, *J. Exp. Med.*, 176:1273-1281 (1992).
43. Hou, S., Hyland, L., Ryan, K.W., Portner, A., and Doherty, P.C., Virus specific CD8+ T cell memory determined by clonal burst size, *Nature (London)*, 369:652-654 (1994).
44. Rimmelzwaan, G.F., and Osterhaus, A.D.M.E., Cytotoxic T lymphocyte memory: role in cross-protective immunity against influenza, *Vaccine*, 13:703-705 (1995).
45. Ulmer, J.B., Donelly, J.J., Parker, S.E., Rhodes, G.H., Felgner, P.L., Dwarki, V.J., Gromkowski, S.H., Deck, R.R., DeWitt, C.M., Friedman, A., Hawe, L.A., Leander, K.R., Martinez, D., Perry, H.C., Shiver, J.W., Montgomery, D.L., and Liu, M.A., Heterologous protection against influenza by injection of DNA encoding a viral protein, *Science*, 259:1745-1749 (1993).
46. Pela, P., and Askonas, B.A.: Low responder MHC alleles for Tc recognition of influenza nucleoprotein, *Immunogenetics*, 23:379-387 (1986).
47. Nowak, M.A., Anderson, R.M., McLean, A.R., Wolfs, T.F.W., Goudsmit, J., and May, R.M., Antigenic diversity thresholds and the development of AIDS, *Science*, 254:963-969 (1991).
48. Gooding, L.R., Virus proteins that counteract host immune defenses, *Cell*, 71:5–14 (1992).
49. Greve, J.M., Davis, G., and Meyer, A.M., The major human rhinovirus receptor is ICAM-1, *Cell*, 56:839-846 (1989).
50. Doherty, P.C., Allan, W., Eichelberger, M., and Carding, S.R., Roles of $\alpha\beta$ and $\gamma\delta$ T cell subsets in viral immunity, *Ann. Rev. Immunol.*, 10:123-134 (1992).
51. Gonzalez, R.N., Cullor, J.S., Jasper, D.E., Farver, T.B., Bushnell, R.B., and Oliver, M.N., Prevention of clinical coliform mastitis in dairy cows by a mutant *Escherichia coli* vaccine, *Can. J. Vet. Res.*, 53:301-305 (1989).
52. Baumgartner, J.D., O'Brien, T.X., Kirkland, T.N., Glauser, M.P., and Ziegler, E.J., Demonstration of cross-reactive antibodies to smooth gram-negative bacteria in antiserum to *Escherichia coli* J5, *J. Infect. Dis.*, 156:136-143 (1987).
53. Giannini, G., Rappuoli, R., and Ratti, G., The amino acid sequence of two nontoxic mutants of diphtheria toxin: CRM45 and CRM197, *Nucleic Acids Res.*, 12:4063-4069 (1984).
54. Vella, P.P., and Ellis, R.W., *Haemophilus* B Conjugate Vaccines. In: *Vaccines: New Approaches to Immunological Problems*, Marcel Dekker, Inc., New York, 1992, pp. 1-22.
55. Schneerson, R., Robbins, J.R., Parke, J.C., Bell, C., Schlesselman, J.J., Sutton, A., Wang, Z., Schiffman, G., Karpas, A., and Shiloach, J., Quantitative and qualitative analyses elicited in adults by *Haemophilus influenzae* type B and *Pneumococcus* type 6A capsular polysaccharide–tetanus toxoid conjugates, *Infect. Immun.*, 52:519-528 (1986).
56. Black, R.E., Levine, M.M., Clements, M.L., Young, C.R., Svennerholm, A.M., and Holmgren, J., Protective efficacy in humans of killed whole-vibrio oral cholera vaccine with and without the B subunit of cholera toxin, *Infect. Immun.*, 55:1116-1120 (1987).
57. Maskell, D., Frankel, G., and Dougan, G., Phase and antigenic vaiation-the impact on strategies for bacterial vaccine design, *Trends Biotech.*, 11:506-510 (1993).
58. McQueen, C.E., Boedeker, E.C., Reid, R., Jarboe, D., Wolf, M., Le, M., and Brown, W.R., Pili in microspheres protect rabbits from diarrhea induced by *E. coli* strain RDEC-1, *Vaccine*, 11:201-206 (1993).
59. Edelman, R., Russell, R.G., Losonsky, G., Tall, B.D., Tacket, C.O., Levine, M.M., and Lewis, D.H., Immunization of rabbits with enterotoxigenic *E. coli* colonization factor antigen (CFA/I) encapsulated in biodegradable microspheres of poly(lactide-*co*-glycolide), *Vaccine*, 11:155-158 (1993).
60. Reid, R.H., Boedeker, E.C., McQueen, C.E., Davis, D., Tseng, L.Y., Kodak, J., Sau, K., Wilhelmsen, C.L., Nellore, R., Dahal, P., et al., Preclinical evaluation of microen-

capsulated CFA/II oral vaccine against enterotoxigenic *E. coli*, *Vaccine*, 11:159-167 (1993).

61. Tacket, C.O., Reid, R.H., Boedeker, E.C., Losonsky, G., Naataro, J.P., Bhagat, H., and Edelman, R., Enteral immunization and challenge of volunteers given enterotoxigenic *E. coli* CFA/II encapsulated in biodegradable microspheres, *Vaccine*, 12:1270-1275 (1994).

62. Morton, R.J., Panciera, R.J., Fulton, R.W., Frank, G.H., Ewing, S.A., Homer, J.T., and Confer, A.W., Vaccination of cattle with outer membrane protein-enriched fractions of *Pasteurella haemolytica* and resistance against experimental challenge exposure, *Am. J. Vet. Res.*, 56:880-884 (1995).

63. Good, M.F., Berzofsky, J.A., and Miller, L.H., The T cell response to the malaria circumsporozoite protein: an immunological approach to vaccine design, *Ann. Rev. Immunol.*, 6:663-669 (1988).

64. Good, M.F., A malaria vaccine strategy based on the induction of cellular immunity, *Immunol. Today.*, 13:125-130 (1992).

65. Nardin, E.H., and Nussenzweig, R.S., T cell response to pre-erythrocyte stages of malaria: role in protection and vaccine development against pre-erytrocyte stages, *Ann. Rev. Immunol.*, 11:687-727 (1993).

66. Weiss, W.R., Sedegah, M., Beaudoin, R.L., and Miller, L.H., CD8+ T cells (cytotoxic/suppressors) are required for protection in mice immunized with malaria sporozoites, *Proc. Nat. Acad. Sci. USA*, 85:573-576 (1988).

67. Gonzalez, D., Hone, D., Noriega, F.R., Tacket, C.O., Davis, J.R., Losonsky, G., Nataro, J.P., Hoffman, S., Malik, A., Nardin, E., Sztein, M.B., Heppner, G., Fouts, T.R., Isibasi, A., and Levine, M.M., *Salmonella typhi* vaccine strain CVD908 expressing the circumsporozoite protein of *Plamsodium falciparum*: strain construction and safety and immunogenicity in humans, *J. Infect. Dis.*, 169:927-931 (1994).

68. Good, M.F., Malon, W.L., Lunde, M.N., Margalit, H., Cornette, J.L., Smith, F.L., Moss, B., Miller, L.H., and Berzofsky, J.A., Construction of synthetic immunogen: use of new T-helper epitope on malaria circumsporozoite protein, *Science,* 235:1059-1062 (1987).

69. Donelson, J., *The Biology of Parasitism: A Molecular and Immunological Approach,* Alan Liss, New York, 1988.

70. Sher, A., and Coffman, R.L., Regulation of immunity to parasites by T cells and T cell-derived cytokines, *Ann. Rev. Immunol.*, 10:385-390 (1992).

71. Balloul, J.M., Grysch, J.M., Pierce, R.J., and Capron, A.: A purified 28,000 Dalton protein from *Schistosoma mansomi* adult worms protects rats and mica against experimental schistosomiasis, *J. Immunol.*, 138:3448-3453 (1987).

72. Wolowczuk, I., Auriault, C., Bosus, M., Boulanger, D., Gras-Masse, H., Mazingue, C., Pierce, R.J., Grezel, D., Reid, F.D., Tartar, A., and Capron, M., Antigenicity and immunogenicity of a multiple peptide construction of the *Shistosoma mansomi* SM28 GST antigen in rat, mouse and monkey. 1. Partial protection of Fischer rats after active immunization, *J. Immunol.,* 146:1987-1995 (1991).

73. Khan, C.M., Vellarreal-Ramos, R.J., Pierce, R.J., Demarco de Hormeache, R., McNeill, H., Ali, T., Chatfield, S., Capron, A., Dougan, G., and Hormaeche, C.E., Antigenicity and immunogenicity of multiple peptide constructions of the *Schistosoma mansoni* SM28 GST antigen in rat, mouse, and monkey. 1. Partial protection of Fischer rats after active immunization, *J. Immunol.*, 146:1985-1987 (1994).

74. Willadsen, P., Eisemann, C.H., and Tellam, R.L., 'Concealed' antigens: expanding the range of immunolical targets, *Parasitol. Today*, 9:132-135 (1993).

75. Corthesy-Theulaz, I., Porta, N., Glauser, M., Saraga, E., Vaney, A.C., Haas, R., Kraehenbuhl, J.P., Blum, A.L., and Michetti, P., Oral immunization with *Helicobacter pylori* urease B subunit as a treatment against Helicobacter infection in mice, *Gastroenterology,* 109:115-121 (1995).

76. Lee, A., Fox, J.G., Otto, G., and Murphy, J., A small animal model of human *Helicobacter pylori* active chronic gastritis, *Gastroenterology*, 99:1315-1323 (1990).
77. Krieg, A.M., Yi, A-K., Matson, S., Waldschmidt, T.J., Bishop, G.A., Teasdale, R., Koretzky, G.A., and Linman, D.M., CpG motifs in bacterial DNA trigger direct B-cell activation, *Science*, 374:546-549 (1995).
78. Primakoff, P., Lathrop, W., Woolman, L., Cowan, A., and Myles, D., Fully effective contraception in male and female guinea pigs immunized with the sperm protein PH20, *Nature (London)*, 335: 543-546 (1988).
79. Muir, W., Husband, A.J., Gipps, E.M., and Bradley, M.P., Induction of specific IgA responses in rats after oral vaccination with biodegradable microspheres containing a recombinant protein, *Immunol. Lett.*, 42:203-207 (1994).
80. Nash, H., Talwar, G.P., Segal, S.J., Luukkainen, T., Johansson, E.D.B., Vasquez, J., Coutinho, E., and Sundaram, K., Observation on the antigenicity and clinical effects of a candidate anti-pregnancy vaccine: beta subunit of human chorionic gonadotropin linked to tetanus toxoid, *Fertil. Steril.*, 34:328-335 (1980).
81. Carelli, C., Audibert, F., Giallard, J., and Chedid, L., Immunological castration of male mice by a totally synthetic vaccine administered in saline, *Proc. Nat. Acad. Sci. USA*, 79:5392-5395 (1982).
82. Miller, S.E., Chamow, S.M., Baur, A.W., Oliver, C., Robey, F., and Dean, J., Vaccination with a synthetic zona pellucida peptide produces long-term contraception in female mice, *Science*, 246:935-938 (1989).
83. Fitchen, J., Beachy, R.M., and Hein, M.B., Plant virus expressing hybrid coat protein with added murine epitope elicits autoantibody respnse, *Vaccine*, 13:1051-1057 (1995).
84. Dong. P., Brunn, C., and Ho, R.J.Y., Cytokines as Vaccine Adjuvants: Current Status and Potential Applications. In: *Vaccine Design: The Subunit and Adjuvant Approach*, Plenum Press, New York, 1995, pp. 625-643.
85. Brokstad, K.A., Cox, R.J., Olofsson, J., Jonsson, R., and Haaheim, L.R., Parenteral influenza vaccination induces a rapid systemic and local immune response, *J. Infect. Dis.*, 171:198-203 (1995).
86. Fontanilla, B.C., Silvano, F., and Cumming, R.: Oral vaccination against Newcastle disease of village chickens in the Philippines, *Prevent. Vet. Med.*, 19:39-44 (1994).
87. Lawrence, D.N., Goldenthal, K.L., Boslego, J.W., Chandler, D.K.F., and La Montagne, J.R., Public Health Implications of Emerging Vaccine Technologies. In: *Vaccine Design: The Subunit and Adjuvant Approach*, Plenum Press, New York, 1995, pp. 43-60.
88. Service, R.F., Triggering the first line of defense, *Science*, 265:1552-1554 (1994).
89. Hornquist, E., Lycke, N., Czerkinsky, C., and Holmgren, J., Cholera Toxin and Cholera B Subunit as Oral-Mucosal Adjuvant and Antigen Carrier Systems. In: *Novel Delivery Systems for Oral Vaccines*, CRC Press, Inc., Ann Arbor, MI, 1994, pp. 157-173.
90. Roberts, M., Chatfield, S.N., and Dougan G., Salmonella as Carriers of Heterologous Antigens. In: *Novel Delivery Systems for Oral Vaccines*, CRC Press, Inc., Ann Arbor, MI, 1994, pp. 27-58.
91. McGhee, J.R., Mestecky, J., Dertzbaugh, M.T., Eldridge, J.H., Hirasawa, M., and Kiyono, H., The mucosal immune system: from fundamental concepts to vaccine development, *Vaccine*, 10:75-93 (1992).
92. Dale, J.W., Dellagostin, O.A., Norman, E., Barrett, A.D.T., and McFadden, J., Multivalent BCG Vaccines. In: *Novel Delivery Systems for Oral Vaccines*, CRC Press, Inc., Ann Arbor, MI, 1994, pp. 87-109.
93. Weng, C.N., Tzan, Y.L., Liu, S.D., Lin, S.Y., and Lee, C.J., Protective effects of an oral microencapsulated *Mycoplasma hypopneumoniae* vaccine against experimental infection in pigs, *Res. Vet. Sci.*, 53:42-46 (1992).
94. Mirchamsy, H., Hamedi, M., Fateh, G., and Sassani, A., Oral immunization against diphtheria and tetanus infections by fluid diphtheria and tetanus toxoids, *Vaccine*, 12:1167-1172 (1994).

95. Husby, S., Jensenius, J.C., and Svehag, S.-E., Passage of undegraded dietary antigen into the blood of healthy adults. Further characterization of the kinetics of the uptake and the size distribution of the antigen, *Scand. J. Immunol.*, 24:447-455 (1986).
96. Eaton, K.A., and Krakowka, S., Chronic active gastritis due to *Helicobacter pylori* in immunized gnotobiotic piglets, *Gastroenterology*, 103:1580-1586 (1992).
97. Baintner, K., *Intestinal Absorption of Macromolecules and Immune Transmission from Mothers to Young*, CRC Press, Inc., Boca Raton, FL., 1986.
98. Clemens, J.D., Sack, D.A., Harris, J.A., Khan, M.R., Chakraborty, J., Chowdhury, S., Rao, M.R., Van Loon, F.P.L., Stanton, B.F., Yunus, M.C., Ali, M.D., Ansaruzzaman, M., Svennerholm, A.-M., and Holmgren, J., Breast feeding and the risk of severe cholera in rural Bangladeshi children, *Am. J. Epidemiol.*, 131:400-411 (1990).
99. Smith, N.C., Wallach, M., Miller, C.M.D., Morgenstern, R., Braun, R., and Eckert, J., Maternal transmission of immunity to *Eimeria maxima*: Enzyme-linked immunosorbent assay analysis of protective antibodies induced by infection, *Infect. Immunol.*, 62:1348-1357 (1994).
100. Newman, M.J., and Powell, M.F., Immunological and Formulation Design Considerations for Subunit Vaccines. In: *Vaccine Design: The Subunit and Adjuvant Approach*, Plenum Press, New York, 1995, pp. 1-42.
101. Gupta, R.K., Relyveld, E.H., Linblad, E.B., Bizzini, B., Ben-Efraim, S., and Gupta, C.K., Adjuvants—a balance between toxicity and adjuvanticity, *Vaccine*, 11:293-306 (1993).
102. Ott, G., Barchfeld, G.L., Chernoff, D., Radhakrishnan, R., van Hoogevest, P., and Van Nest, G., Design and Evaluation of a Safe and Potent Adjuvant for Human Vaccines. In: *Vaccine Design: The Subunit and Adjuvant Approach*, Plenum Press, New York, 1995, pp. 277-296.
103. Audibert, F.M., and Lise, L.D., Adjuvants: Current status, clinical perspectives and future prospects, *Immunol. Today*, 14:281-284 (1993).
104. Eldridge, J.H., Staas, J.K., Meulbroek, J.A., McGhee, J.R., Rice, T.R., and Gilley, R.M., Biodegradable microspheres as a vaccine delivery system, *Mol. Immunol.*, 28:287-294 (1991).
105. Rhodes, J., Chen, J., Hall, S.R., Beesley, J.E., Jenkins, D.C., Collins, P., and Zheng, B., Therapeutic potentiation of the immune system by costimulatory Schiff-base-forming drugs, *Nature (London)*, 377:71-74 (1995).
106. Gupta, R.K., Rost, B.E., Relyveld, E., and Siber, G.R., Adjuvant Properties of Aluminum and Calcium Compounds. In: *Vaccine Design: The Subunit and Adjuvant Approach*, Plenum Press, New York, 1995, pp. 229-248.
107. Cleland, J.L., Powell, M.F., Lim, A., Barr-n, L., Berman, P.W., Eastman, D.J., Nunberg, J.H., Wrin, T., and Vennari, J.C., Development of a single-shot subunit vaccine for HIV-1, *AIDS Res. Hum. Retroviruses*, 10:521-526 (1994).
108. Bienenstock, J., The Nature of Immunity at Mucosal Surfaces—A Brief Review. In: *Bacterial Infections of Respiratory and Gastrointestinal Mucosae*, IRL Press, Oxford, 1988, pp. 9-34.
109. Quiding, M., Nordstrom, I., Kilander, A., Andersson, G., Hanson, L.A., Holmgren, J., and Czerkinsky, C., Intestinal immune responses in humans. Oral cholera vaccination induces strong intestinal antibody responses, gamma-interferon production, and evokes local immunological memory, *J. Clin. Invest.*, 88:143-151 (1991).
110. Hadden, J.W., T-Cell Adjuvants, *Int. J. Immunopharmac.*, 16:703-710 (1994).
111. Jones, T., Stern, A., and Lin, R., Potential role of granulocyte-macrophage colony-stimulating factor as vaccine adjuvant, *Eur. J. Clin. Microbiol. Infect. Dis.*, Suppl. 2:47-53 (1994).
112. Bussiere, J.L., McCormick, G.C., and Green, J.D., Preclinical Safety Assessment Considerations in Vaccine Development. In: *Vaccine Design: The Subunit and Adjuvant Approach*, Plenum Press, New York, 1995, pp. 61-79.

113. Gregoriadis, G., Immunological adjuvants: A role for liposomes, *Immunol. Today*, 11:89-97 (1990).
114. Buiting, A.M.J., van Rooijen, N., and Classen, E., Liposomes as antigen carriers and adjuvants in vivo, *Res. Immunol.*, 143:541-548 (1992).
115. Childers, N.K., and Michalek, S.M., Liposomes. In: *Novel Delivery Systems for Oral Vaccines*, CRC Press, Inc., Ann Arbor, MI, 1994, pp. 241-254.
116. Gluck, R., Liposomal Presentation of Antigens for Human Vaccines. In: *Vaccine Design: The Subunit and Adjuvant Approach*, Plenum Press, New York, 1995, pp. 325-345.
117. Tomizawa, H., Aramaki, Y., Fujii, Y., Hara, T., Suzuki, N., Yachi, K., Kikuchi, H., and Tsuchiya, S., Uptake of phosphatydylserine liposomes by rat Peyer's patches following intraluminal administration, *Pharm. Res.*, 10:549-557 (1993).
118. Gluck, R., Mischler, R., Brantschen, S., Just, M., Althaus, B., and Cryz, S.J., Immunopotentiating reconstituted influenza virosome (IRIV) vaccine delivery system for immunization against hepatitis A, *J. Clin. Invest.*, 90:2491-2495 (1992).
119. Forrest, B.D., Clinical Evaluation of Attenuated *Salmonella typhi* Vaccines in Human Subjects. In: *Novel Delivery Systems for Oral Vaccines*, CRC Press, Inc., Ann Arbor, MI, 1994, pp. 59-85.
120. Ellis, R.W., New Technologies for Making Vaccines. In: *Vaccines*, 2nd ed. (S.A. Plotkin and E.A. Mortimer, Jr., eds.), W.B. Saunders Co., Philadelphia, 1994, pp. 867-888,
121. Oggioni, M.R., Manganelli, R., Contorni, M., Tommasino, M., and Pozzi, G., Immunization of mice by oral colonizaion with live recombinant commensal streptococci, *Vaccine*, 13:775-779 (1995).
122. Nguyen, T.N., Hansson, M., Stahl, S., Bachi, T., Robert, A., and Domaig, W., Cell-surface display of heterologous epitopes on *Staphylococcus xylosus* as a potential delivery system for oral vaccination, *Gene*, 128:89-94 (1993).
123. Wells, J.M., Wilson, P.W., Norton, P.M., Gasson, J.J., and LePage, R.W.F., *Lactobacilus lactis*: high-level expression of tetanus toxin fragment C and protection against lethal challenge, *Molec. Microbiol.*, 8:1155-1162 (1993).
124. Zaronzinski, C.C., Fynan, E.F., Slein, L.K., Robinson, H.L., and Welsh, R.M., Protective CTL-dependent immunity and enhanced immunopathology in mice immunized by particle bombardment with DNA encoding an internal virion protein, *J. Immunol.*, 154:4010-4017 (1995).
125. Sizemore, D.R., Branstrom, A.A, and Sadoff, J.C., Attenuated *Shigella* as a DNA delivery vehicle for DNA-mediated immunization, *Science*, 27:299-303 (1995).
126. Arntzen, C.J., Mason, H.S., Shi, J., Haq, T.A., Estee, M.K., and Clements, J.D., Production of Candidate Oral Vaccines in Edible Tissues of Transgenic Plants. In: *Vaccines 94: Modern Approaches to New Vaccines Including Prevention of AIDS*, Cold Spring Harbor Press, 1994, pp. 339-345.
127. Haq, T.A., Mason, H.S., Clements, J.D., and Arntzen, C.J., Oral immunization with a recombinant bacterial antigen produced in transgenic plants, *Science*, 268:714-716 (1995).
128. Mason, H.S., Lam, D.M.K., and Arntzen, C.J., Expression of hepatitis B surface antigen in transgenic plants, *Proc. Nat. Acad. Sci. USA*, 89:11745-11751 (1992).
129. Langer, R., New methods of drug delivery, *Science*, 249:1527-1533 (1990).
130. Wilding, I.R., Davis, S.S., and O'Hagan, D.T., Optimizing gastrointestinal delivery of drugs, *Bailliere's Clin. Gastroenterol.*, 8:255-270 (1994).
131. Morris, W., Steinhoff, M.C., and Russell, P.K., Potential of polymer microencapsulation technology for vaccine innovation, *Vaccine*, 12:5-11 (1994).
132. O'Hagan, D.T., Microparticles as Oral Vaccines. In: *Novel Delivery Systems for Oral Vaccines*, CRC Press, Inc., Ann Arbor, MI, 1994, pp. 175-205.
133. Hanes, J., Chiba, M., and Langer, R., Polymer Microspheres for Vaccine Delivery. In: *Vaccine Design: The Subunit and Adjuvant Approach*, Plenum Press, New York, 1995, pp. 389-412.

134. Kossovsky, N., Gelman, A., Hnatzszyn, H.J., Rajguru, S., Garrell, R.L., Torbati, S., Freitas, S.S.F., and Chow, G-M., Surface modified diamond nanoparticles as antigen delivery vehicles, *Bioconj. Chem.*, 6:507-511 (1995).
135. Moldoveanu, Z., Novak, M., and Huang, W-Q., Oral immunization will influence virus in biodegradable microspheres, *J. Infect. Dis.*, 167:84-90 (1993).
136. Le Fevre, M.E., and Joel, D.D., Peyer's Patch Epithelium, an Imperfect Barrier. In: *Intestinal Toxicology*, Raven Press, New York, 1984, pp. 45-58.
137. Eldridge, J.H., Hammond, C.J., Meulbroeck, J.A., Staas, J.K., Gilley, R.M., and Tice, T.R., Controlled vaccine release in the gut-associated lymphoid tissues, I. Orally administered biodegradable microspheres target the Peyer's patches, *J. Control. Rel.*, 11:205-214 (1990).
138. Ebel, J.P., A method for quantifying particle absorption from the small intestine of the mouse, *Pharm. Res.*, 7:848-856 (1990).
139. O'Hagan, D.T., Intestinal tranlocation of particulates—implication for drug and antigen delivery, *Adv. Drug Deliv. Rev.*, 5:265-277 (1990).
140. Parkman, P.D., and Hardegree, M.C., Regulation and Testing of Vaccines. In: *Vaccines* (S.A. Plotkin and E.A. Mortimer, eds.), 2nd ed., W.B. Saunders, Philadelphia, 1994, pp. 889-901.
141. Gug, M., Veterinary vaccines in an economic and sociopolitical context. The viewpoint of the veterinary pharmaceutical industry, *Dev. Biol. Stand.*, 79:31-36 (1992).
142. Sauer, F., Regulatory framework of immunologicals in the European union, *Biologicals*, 22:307-311 (1994).
143. Hopps, H.E., Meyer, B.C., and Parkman, P.D., Regulation and Testing of Vaccines. In: *Vaccines*, 1st ed. (S.A. Plotkin and E.A. Mortimer, eds.), Philadelphia, W.B. Saunders, 1988, pp. 576-797.
144. *Code of Federal Regulations*, Title 21, parts 600-680, Subchapter F—biologics, Government Printing Office, Washington, 1993.
145. Espeseth, D.A., and Greenberg, J.B., Licensing and Regulation in the U.S.A. In: *Vaccines for Veterinary Applications*, Butterworth-Heinemann Ltd., Oxford, 1993, pp. 321-434.
146. Cryz, S.J., Jr., and Gluck, R., Large-Scale Production of Attenuated Bacterial and Viral Vaccines. In: *New Generation Vaccines* (G.C. Woodrow, and M.M. Levine, eds.), Marcel Dekker, Inc., New York, 1990, pp. 921-932.
147. Clarke, J.R., and Samways, G.R., Commercial Aspects of the Vaccine Industry. In: *New Generation Vaccines* (G.C. Woodrow, and M.M. Levine, eds.), Marcel Dekker, Inc., New York, 1990, pp. 933-950.

TERRY L. BOWERSOCK
KINAM PARK

Vaginal Delivery and Absorption of Drugs

Introduction

A small survey conducted to evaluate the preferences of females with regard to the use of intravaginal medications showed a positive market outlook for this mode of delivery [1]. Pharmaceutical dosage forms available on the prescription and over-the-counter (OTC) markets for intravaginal delivery consist primarily of those used to treat specific gynecological conditions. Products available include antifungals, antimicrobials, cleansers, vaginal contraceptives, deodorants, and lubricants. These products are formulated as capsules, creams, films, foams, gels, ointments, solutions, suppositories, or tablets. Currently, there are numerous prescription and OTC medications that are intended only for local activity in the vagina. However, the absorption capabilities of the vagina provide a potential route for systemic drug delivery with direct entry into the bloodstream (Fig. 1). There are already a few pharmacologically active molecules, such as progesterone and estradiol, that are delivered intravaginally for systemic activity. The use of the vaginal route for noninvasive drug delivery has received increased attention recently, particularly with the new focus on therapeutic agents that are subject to extensive hepatic "first-pass" elimination such as proteins and peptides. This article describes the physiology of the human vagina and its characteristics of absorption and permeability. The reader will also be familiarized with current research trends in vaginal delivery and absorption of drugs.

The Human Vagina
General Anatomy

The vagina is a canal extending from the vulva to the cervix (Fig. 1). Extensive investigations on its morphology and anatomy have been compiled [2]. Physiologically, the vagina serves a number of functions, acting primarily as a conduit for the passage of seminal fluid, an excretory duct for menstrual discharge, and as the lower part of the birth canal [3]. The anterior portion of the vagina in an adult averages 6 to 7 cm in length, the posterior wall is approximately 7.5 to 8.5 cm.

The vagina is characterized by an exceptional elasticity, and has its greatest resiliency at parturition. A layer of relatively thick connective tissue is located between the anterior vaginal wall and the urinary canal as well as between the posterior vaginal wall and the intestinal tract. The vaginal wall itself consists of three layers: the epithelial layer, the tunica adventitia, and the muscular coat. The epithelial layer is made up of an epithelial lamina and a lamina propria. It consists of noncornified, stratified squamous epithelial cells that are subject to changes with age. The epithelium atrophies from birth to puberty when hormonal activity increases the thickness and resistance of this layer. In the subepithelial layer rests a network of elastic fibers around the lamina propria and collagenous fibers around the tunica adventitia, creating a connection to the mus-

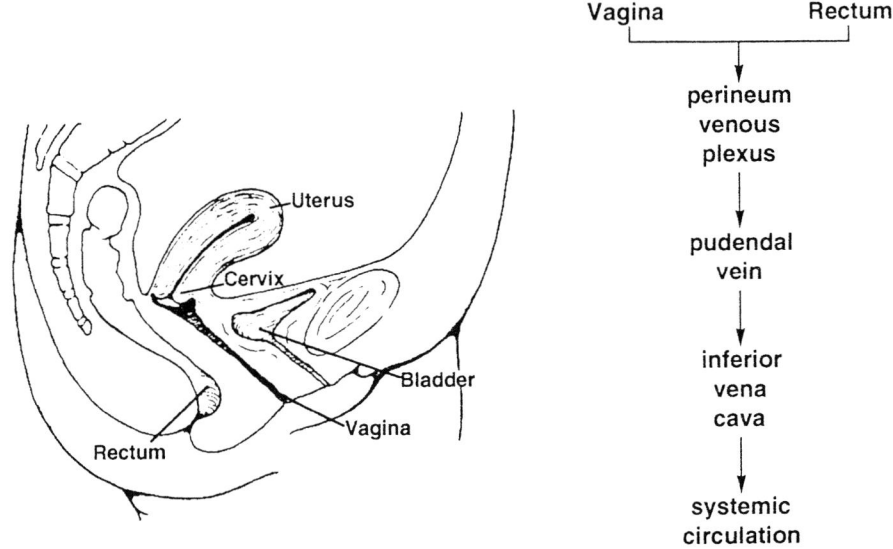

FIG. 1. Lateral view of the female pelvis showing the absorption route to the systemic circulation.

cular coat. Changes in the cytology of the vaginal epithelium occur with the cyclical stages in women. The epithelium is thickest in the proliferative stage, peaking at ovulation and diminishing with the secretory phase. The muscular coat of the vagina is composed of smooth muscle and elastic fibers. A spiral arrangement of these fibers provides support to withstand stretching without rupturing the vagina. The tunica adventitia is formed of loose connective tissue that is attached to the muscular coat. Fluctuations in the volume of the vaginal lumen occur due to alterations in the tension of this layer. The vagina is encompassed by a vascular supply of arteries, veins, and lymph capillaries, as well as sensory and autonomous nerves.

Cellular Structure

Histological studies of vaginal biopsies from healthy volunteers (premenopausal, postmenopausal, and following ovariectomy) have been conducted to characterize the ultrastructure of the vaginal mucosa by electron microscope [4]. The epithelium of the vaginal mucosa is found to have five layers of different cells: the basal, parabasal, intermediate, transitional, and superficial layers (Fig. 2). The cellular types that make up these different layers renew continuously as they are stimulated by hormonal action and intracellular communication. The basal cells are typically columnar or squamous in shape with microvilli present on the surface of the cell membrane. Parabasal cells are similar to the basal cells in size and structure, but have a greater formation of surface microvilli and interdigitations. Their polygonal shapes are formed by adapting to spaces left free from neighboring cells. The cells of the intermediate layer are of the largest cell type and also exhibit microvilli. The transitional cells that follow show noticeable signs of involution and surface characteristics of diminishing and thinning microvilli and intercellular junctions (desmosomes). Superficial cells, as indicated by

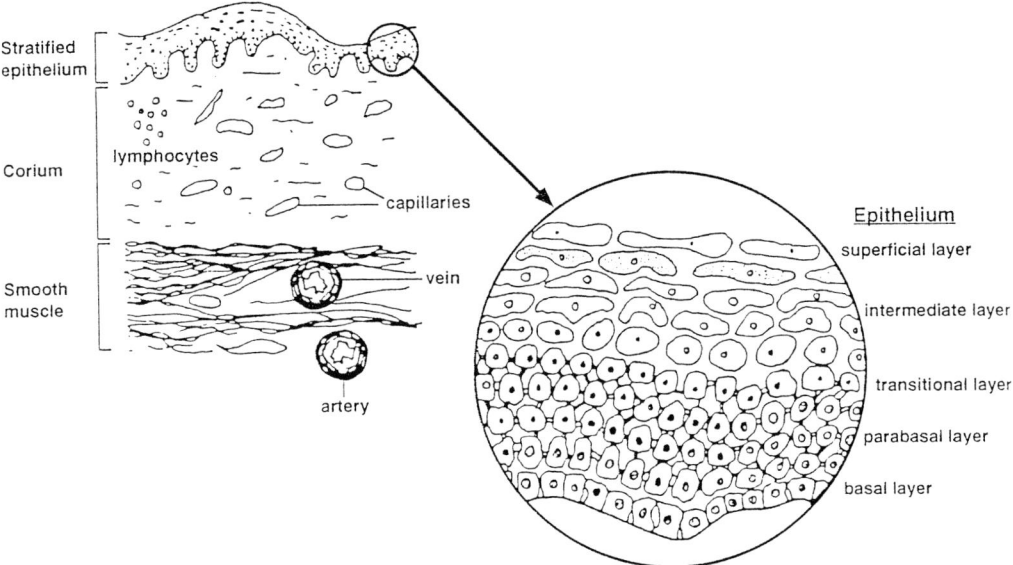

FIG. 2. Cross-sectional view of the vaginal wall with magnification of the stratified epithelial layers. Based on Ref. 6.

their nomenclature, are the cells of the outermost layer during the follicular phase of the cycle.

The vaginal epithelium contains a network of intercellular channels that continuously undergo development, reaching a maximum during the ovulatory and luteal phases. The channels present in the transitional and superficial layers do not change with the cycle as do those in the basal, parabasal, and intermediate layers. These channels provide a supply of nutrients and transport metabolites from one epithelial layer to another. Since secretory glands are absent from the vagina, lubrication is provided via these channels. Intercellular junctions, including desomosomes and tight junctions, have also been identified. Desmosomes are most prominent in the intermediate layer and progressively become less toward the superficial layer, which may play a role in the desquamation of vaginal cells.

Because the vaginal epithelium is affected by ovarian hormones, a cyclical variation occurs (Fig. 3). Although less intense than the uterine modifications, changes include proliferation, differentiation, and desquamation. During the follicular phase, the time period from the end of menstruation to the day of ovulation, mitosis increasingly occurs in the cells of the basal and parabasal layers, creating an increase in the number of layers and the thickness of the epithelium. The desquamating layers grow until ovulation, after which the layers diminish and are sloughed away through the vaginal lumen. During the luteal phase, the period following ovulation, the transitional cells become superficial due to the absence of the normal superficial layer.

It has been found that the basal cells replicate continuously to provide a self-cleaning mechanism to the epithelial layer. Autoradiographic studies [5] of cell proliferation on normal human cervix and vagina indicate that the basal layer is relatively inactive with a cell population turnover rate of 33 days, whereas the parabasal layers have an

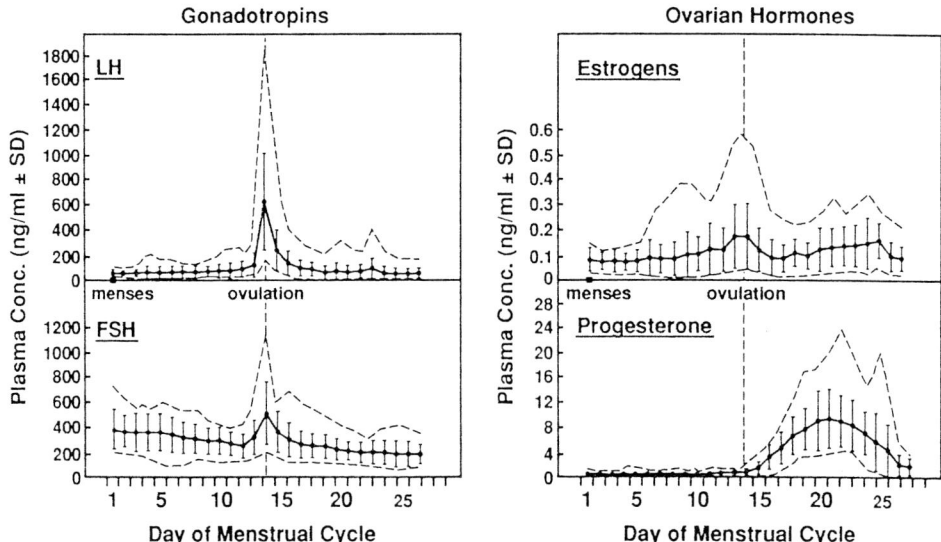

FIG. 3. Profile of the gonadotorpin and ovarian hormones during a normal menstrual cycle. The number of cell layers in the vaginal epithelium rises from 22 layers at approximately day 10 of the cycle to 45 layers at ovulation, and drops to 33 layers around day 20. Based on Refs. 87 and 164.

active proliferation with a turnover rate of three days. The intermediate and superficial layers were found to have inactive differentiation.

Fluids and Enzymes

Despite the paucity of glands, the vaginal epithelium is usually maintained moist by a surface film. This film, known as vaginal fluid, consists of cervical mucus and exfoliated cells from the vagina itself. Transudation from the blood vessels, through the intercellular channels to the lumen, can also contribute to the chemical composition [4]. The fluid may contain carbohydrates, amino acids, aliphatic acids, protein, and immunoglobulins [6]. Nonserum-type proteins in human vaginal secretions have recently been identified [7,8]. Typically, the vaginal fluid in healthy, mature women has a pH in the range of 4 to 5 [9]. This acidic environment is produced by the presence of microflora such as lactobacilli which convert carbohydrates to lactic acid. The cervical mucus, a principal component of the vaginal fluid, is produced by glandular units within the cervical canal and has a pH in the range of 6.5 to 9. The cervical mucus changes in composition and physical characteristics with the menstrual cycle, facilitating sperm migration during ovulation. At the time of ovulation, an augmented amount of cervical secretions results in an increase in the volume of vaginal fluid. The mucus produced at ovulation has increased spinnbarkeit (fibrosity), ferning (crystallization of the mucus dried on a slide), pH, and mucin content [10]. Additionally, there is a decrease in the viscosity, cellularity, and albumin concentration.

The existence of a variety of enzymes in the vagina is an important concern in the development of vaginal delivery systems, particularly with proteases and their effect on protein and peptide candidates [11]. The outer cell layers of the vagina contain varying amounts of β-glucuronidase, acid phosphatase, α-naphthylesterase, diphosphopyridine nucleotide-diaphorase (DPND), phosphoamidase and succinic dehydrogenase [9]. Enzymatic activity has also been shown in the basal cell layers with the presence of β-glucuronidase, succinic dehydrogenase, DPND, acid phosphatase, and α-naphthylesterase.

The vaginal lumen is a nonsterile environment inhabited by a variety of microorganisms, mainly the species of *Lactobacillus, Bacteroides,* and *Staphylococcus epidermidis*, as well as potentially pathogenic aerobes [12]. In addition to enzymes, the existence of these microbes and their metabolites may also have a detrimental effect on the intravaginal stability of a vaginal drug delivery device.

Physiology and Dynamics

The unstimulated vagina anatomically consists of a luminal space that exists potentially rather than actually. However, in response to sexual excitement some tension-induced anatomic variations occur which may have effects on vaginal delivery systems and their long-term intravaginal drug delivery. These variations are reflected in the four phases in a sexual response cycle as outlined by Masters and Johnson [13].

The first sign of physiological response to stimulation is the production of a vaginal lubricating fluid, which appears on the vaginal mucosa surface within 10-30 s after an effective stimulation (excitement phase). As sexual tension progresses, individual droplets of transudation-like mucoid material appear scattered throughout the rugal folds of the vaginal lumen, coalescing to form a smooth coating over the entire vaginal mucosa surface. This transudative mucoid material results from the activation of a massive localized vasocongestive reaction and marked dilation of the venous plexus that encircles the entire vaginal lumen. This sweating phenomenon provides complete lubrication of the vagina. There is lengthening and distention of the inner two-thirds of the vaginal lumen. As sexual tension mounts toward the plateau phase, the vaginal wall in this area expands involuntarily and then partially relaxes in an irregular, tensionless manner. The demand to expand gradually overcomes the tendency to relax. In addition to the expansive effect in the vaginal fornices, the cervix and corpus pull slowly backward and upward into the false pelvis position. This cervical elevation creates a "tenting effect" at the transcervical depth in the midvaginal plane. This phenomenon always occurs in a normal anteriorly positioned uterus (Fig. 4). The vagina of either nulliparous or multiparous women, regardless of prior degree of vaginal expansion or lengthening, increases substantially in length and transcervical width with sexual stimulation.

With attainment of the plateau phase level of sexual tension, a marked localized vasocongestive reaction develops in the outer one-third of the vaginal lumen. The entire area becomes grossly distended with venous blood, and its central lumen is reduced by at least a third compared to the distention previously established in the excitement phase. The increase in the width and depth of the vaginal lumen is minimal. The production rate of vaginal lubricating fluid gradually slows down at this point, particularly if this level of sexual tension has been experienced for an extended period of time.

During the orgasmic phase, the basic response of the inner vaginal lumen is essentially expansive rather than constrictive in character. Conversely, the bulbar vasoconstriction at the orgasmic platform in the outer one-third of the vaginal lumen contracts strongly in a regularly recurring pattern. The intercontractile intervals lengthen in duration, and the intensity of the contractions progressively diminishes.

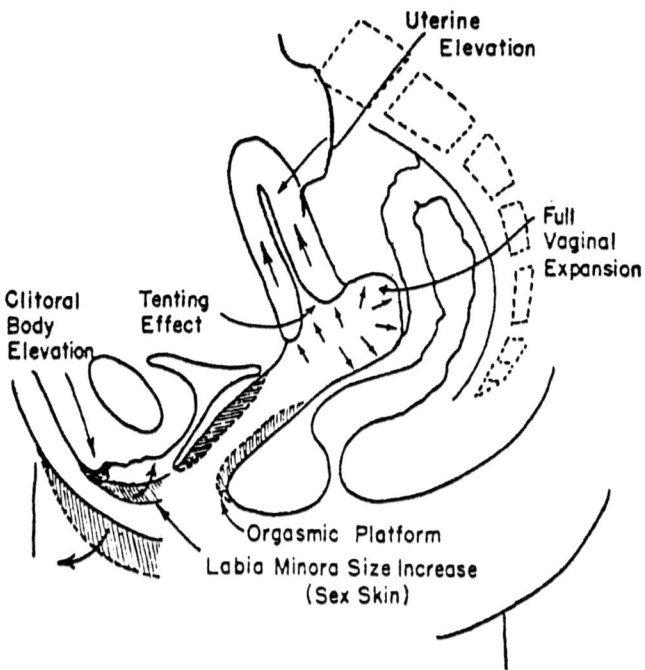

FIG. 4. Lateral view of the female pelvis showing the stimulated vagina. Based on Ref. 13.

Along with the onset of the resolution phase, retrogressive changes develop first in the outer one-third of the vaginal lumen. The localized vasocongestion is dispersed rapidly, leading to an increase in the diameter of the central lumen of the outer one-third of the vagina. The previously expanded inner two-thirds of the vaginal lumen also gradually shrinks back to the original collapsed, unstimulated state. This shrinking process is an irregular, zonal-type relaxation of the lateral and posterior walls. The anterior wall and the cervix of the anteriorly positioned uterus descend rapidly toward the vaginal floor, leading to a quick resolution of the tenting effect created earlier during the excitement phase.

Menopause

The natural aging process results in significant changes in the vagina, which include a reduction in vaginal size, loss of elasticity, decrease in vascularity, and a thinning of the mucosa [14]. The cytology of the vagina is variable, and many aspects are addressed by Steger and Havez [14]. The epithelium becomes markedly thinner and is often invaded by leukocytes. Areas can be completely denuded of epithelial covering, exposing the subepithelial connective tissue. On the surface of the vagina, the number of exfoliating cells and microridges are greatly reduced. Collagen replaces many of the elastic fibers in the lamina propria, causing the loss of elasticity. Glycogen is very low or completely absent, contributing to the change in vaginal microbiology and pH. Vaginal secretions become scant and watery and the pH increases from 4.5–5.5 to 7.0–7.4. Resistance to bacterial and fungal infections is diminished due to the lower population of acidophilic organisms [15]. The enzymes present in the vagina also increase with the onset of menopause, particularly β-glucuronidase, acid phosphatase, and nonspecific esterases [14].

Unlike other tissues, the vagina is greatly affected by hormone-replacement therapy. Estrogen replacement is often used to treat vaginal manifestations of menopause. The reduction in thickness and the increase in permeability of the vaginal epithelium after menopause should be taken into consideration with vaginal drug delivery. The absence of epithelial changes results in less fluctuation in absorption, affecting both systemic and local drug delivery.

Vaginal Absorption

Much has been written in the literature discussing vaginal absorption. The first experimental studies using animals date back to 1918. At that time, the histological characteristic of the vaginal wall was known to exist in only three simple layers: the connective tissue, the muscularis, and the mucosa, collectively resembling the skin without the stratum corneum. Originally, the vagina was regarded as an organ impermeable to exogenous agents. Reports began to surface, however, which indicated vaginal absorption of foreign materials as the cause of toxicity and even death in several cases. Studies in dogs and cats, using a wide variety of compounds including alkaloids, inorganic salts, esters, and antiseptics, demonstrated the occurrence of vaginal absorption [16]. Later work showed the vaginal absorption of compounds such as hydrocyanic acid, pilocarpine, atropine, and insulin [17]. Using rabbits, cats, and dogs, the vaginal absorption of quinine bisulfate and oxyquinoline sulfate was investigated in the interest of emphasizing vaginal applications of medicine [18]. A unidirectional transmission of agents was proposed to occur from the vagina to the blood, with no transmission in the reverse direction [19,20].

An extensive review of the literature has been made recently which documents the absorption of carbohydrates, fats and proteins [21,22]. Glucose has been shown to be absorbed and rapidly oxidized. Peanut protein was one of the first proteins that was demonstrated to be absorbed vaginally [23]. The vaginal permeation of spermatozoal and bacterial antigens has also been shown [22]. Bacterial antigens play an important role in triggering the local immunological mechanism involved in protecting the area against infection. Other classes of compounds reported to be absorbed intravaginally include steroids (e.g., estrogens, progesterone, and testosterone), prostaglandins, antimicrobials, nonoxynol-9, and methadone. The vaginal delivery of estrogens and progesterone have been well documented over the years and used clinically in dosage forms such as vaginal creams and suppositories.

Vaginal absorption of drugs is dependent upon such physicochemical properties as lipophilicity, ionization, molecular weight, molecular size, chemical structure, and interaction with vaginal secretions and tissues. Absorption is also modified by the thickness of the vaginal wall as affected by the ovarian cycle or by pregnancy [21]. Other factors include changes in the vaginal epithelium and pH with menopause. Prior to absorption, drugs must be in solution. The vaginal fluid can help to dissolve drugs, but when the cervical mucus secretion is present in abundance, it may instead create a barrier and remove a drug from the site [11]. Dosage forms have varied absorption profiles due to the differing dissolution patterns in vaginal fluid. For example, products such as creams, inserts, and tablets remain for different periods of time in the vagina. A comparison of vaginal inserts versus creams showed the cream to have a longer contact time [24].

Permeability

The three primary mechanisms of transport across the vaginal membrane are passive diffusion through the cells (the transcellular route), diffusion through the tight junctions between cells (the intercellular route), and vesicular or receptor-mediated transport [11,25]. Vaginal permeation studies have been conducted using the rabbit as an animal model [26,27]. The female rabbit does not exhibit an estrus cycle, and its vaginal tissues show a constancy in their histological, biochemical, and physiological properties not ordinarily seen among mammals [28]. The lack of a sexual cycle is therefore expected to produce a minimal variability in the permeability of the vaginal mucosa, making the measurements of vaginal drug permeation more controllable and accessible [26,27,29].

The vaginal mucosa permeability of the doe rabbit has been studied by continuous perfusion of straight-chain alkanols and alkanoic acids [26,27]. Similar to the vaginal absorption of ethynodiol diacetate (Fig. 5), the vaginal uptake of both alkanols and alkanoic acids was observed to follow a first-order kinetics process. The results are consistent with a physical model having a hydrodynamic diffusion layer in series with the mucosal membrane, which itself consists of two parallel pathways, a lipoidal pathway and an aqueous "pore" pathway (Fig. 6). Immediately behind the mucosa (serosal side), a perfect sink is maintained by hemoperfusion.

The apparent permeability coefficient P_{app} for vaginal membrane permeation is defined by Eqs. (1) to (2),

$$P_{app} = \frac{1}{\frac{1}{P_{aq}} + \frac{1}{P_v}} \tag{1}$$

or

$$P_{app} = \frac{1}{\frac{1}{P_{aq}} + \frac{1}{P_p + P_l}} \tag{1a}$$

since

$$P_v = P_p + P_l \tag{2}$$

where P_{aq}, P_v, P_p, and P_l are the permeability coefficients of the aqueous diffusion layer, the vaginal membrane, the aqueous pore pathway, and the lipoidal pathway, respectively.

The vaginal permeation kinetics of a series of straight-chain alkanols was investigated [26]. Using methanol as a reference permeant, a normalized permeability coefficient P_{app} (alkanol/MeOH) was determined for each of the alkanols. The normalized

Vaginal Delivery and Absorption of Drugs

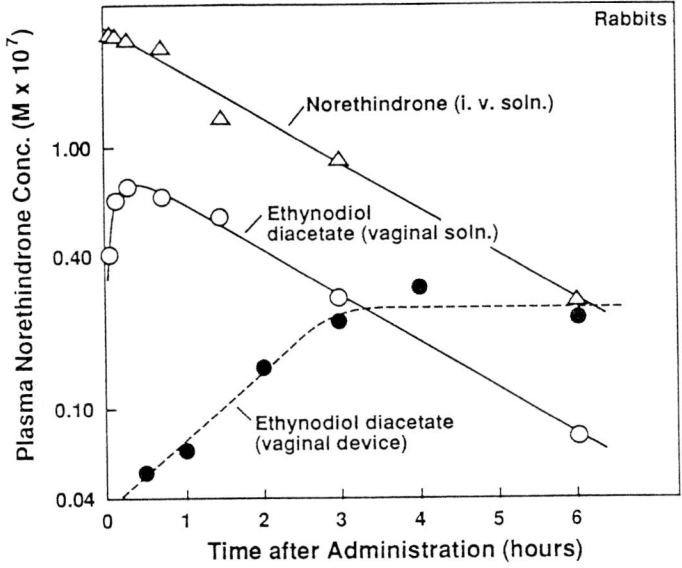

FIG. 5. Rabbit plasma concentration profiles of norethindrone following the intravenous administration of a single dose (solution) of norethindrone. Also shown is the intravaginal absorption of ethynodiol diacetate from a solution dose and from a vaginal delivery device. Based on Ref. 37.

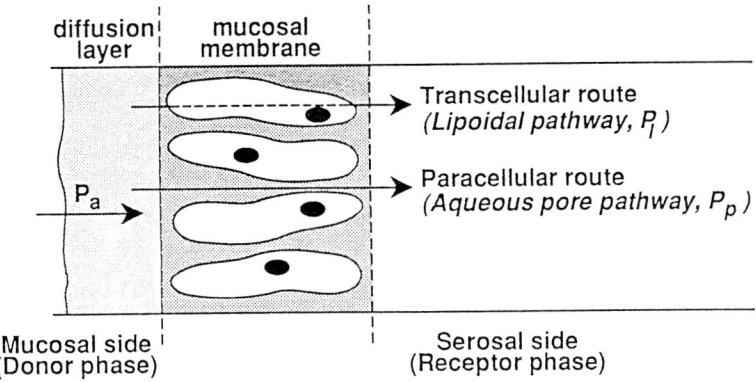

FIG. 6. Schematic of the vaginal membrane as a transport barrier. Based on Ref. 25.

permeability coefficient was observed to increase in value as the alkyl chain length of the alkanols increased (Table 1). This increased permeability can be attributed to the increase in the permeability coefficient for the lipoidal pathway P_1 [Eq. (2)]. It is estimated that with the addition of each methylene (CH_2) group, the P_1 value increases by 2.5 for straight-chain aliphatic alcohols and by 3.5 for the series of straight-chain alkanoic acids [26,27].

For the vaginal absorption of ionizable compounds, such as the homologous series of n-alkanoic acids, the apparent permeability coefficient P_{app} becomes pH dependent and is defined by Eq. (3),

$$P_{app}(n, \mathrm{pH}) = \cfrac{1}{P_{aq}(n) + \cfrac{1}{\cfrac{[H]}{Ka + [H]} P_1^0 10^n \pi + P_p}} \quad (3)$$

where n is the number of methylene (CH_2) groups in the alkyl chain; [H] is the concentration of protons; Ka is the dissociation constant of the acid; P_1^0 is the permeability coefficient of the lipoidal pathway for the hypothetical acid with zero carbon atoms ($n = 0$); and π is the methylene group incremental constant, that is, 3.5 for straight-chain alkanoic acids.

As illustrated earlier for the homologous series of n-alkanols, the normalized permeability coefficient of n-alkanoic acids shows a dependence on alkyl chain length (Table 2). In addition, the straight-chain alkanoic acids demonstrate a pH dependence in their normalized permeability coefficients [27]. It should be noted that the rabbit's vaginal secretion has an effective pKa value of 6.3 ± 0.1. However, the rate of vaginal secretion is relatively small, which leads to a surface pH of approximately 2.0 [30]. This acidic surface pH affects the extent of dissociation of n-alkanoic acids and thus the magnitudes of P_1 and P_{app} [Eq. (3)].

The vaginal uptake of steroids has also been studied and found to follow a first-order kinetics process [31]. The normalized permeability coefficient of steroids appears to be dependent upon steroidal structure (Table 3). The permeability coefficient across the vaginal mucosa (P_v) shows the same trend of structure dependence; the lipophilic steroids (progesterone and estrone) were better absorbed than the more polar steroids (hydrocortisone and testosterone). However, the P_{aq} value, the permeability coefficient

TABLE 1 Effect of Alkyl Chain Length on the Normalized Permeability Coefficients of Straight-Chain Alkanols[a]

Alkanol	$CH_3(CH_2)_n OH$	P_{app} (Alkanol/MeOH)[b]
Methanol	n = 0	1.00
Propanol	n = 2	1.11
Butanol	n = 3	1.13
Pentanol	n = 4	1.20
Hexanol	n = 5	1.48
Heptanol	n = 6	1.91
Octanol	n = 7	2.15

[a]Based on data from Ref. 26.
[b]Normalized permeability coefficient = P_{app}(alcohol)/P_{app}(methanol). Mean value from three rabbits at pH 6.0 and 37°C.

TABLE 2 Effect of Alkyl Chain Length and pH on the Normalized Permeability Coefficients of Straight-Chain Alkanoic Acids[a]

Acids	P_{app} (Acid/MeOH)[b]		
	pH 3	pH 6	pH 8
Acetic	1.22	0.73	0.25
Butyric	1.62	1.94	0.34
Hexanoic	1.89	2.06	0.81
Octanoic	1.74	2.49	1.24
Decanoic	—	—	1.26

[a]Based on data from Ref. 30.
[b]Normalized permeability coefficient = P_{app}(acid)/P_{app}(methanol). Mean value from three experiments involving different rabbits at pH 3, 6, and 8.

across the hydrodynamic diffusion layer, is very much the same among the four steroids (Table 3). For drugs with high P_v values such as progesterone and estrone (6.1–7.6 × 10^{-4} cm/s), vaginal absorption is mainly controlled by their permeability across the hydrodynamic diffusion layer on the surface of the vaginal mucosa ($P_v > P_{aq}$). Conversely, for drugs with low P_v values, such as testosterone and hydrocortisone (5.8–7.5 × 10^{-5} cm/s), vaginal uptake is determined predominantly by their molecular permeation through the vaginal mucosa ($P_v \ll P_{aq}$) [32]. A linear relationship between vaginal permeability and lipophilicity has been shown for a series of progestins in vitro using rabbit epithelium [33].

The apparent permeability coefficient P_{app}, related to the first-order rate constant for the disappearance of drug from vaginal lumen (k_v), is given by Eq. (4),

$$P_{app} = k_v \frac{V_v}{S_v} \qquad (4)$$

where V_v is the volume of vaginal fluid and S_v the geometric surface area of the vaginal lumen.

Additional permeability studies have been performed with rabbits by measuring electrical conductance and permeation flux of 6-carboxyfluorescein, a hydrophilic fluo-

TABLE 3 Vaginal Permeation Parameters of Representative Steroids[a]

Steroids	P_{app}[b]	$P_v \times 10^4$ (cm/s)	$P_{aq} \times 10^4$ (cm/s)
Estrone	1.00	7.60	2.81
Progesterone	0.93	6.10	2.80
Testosterone	0.29	0.75	2.76
Hydrocortisone	0.23	0.58	2.79

[a]Based on data from Ref. 31.
[b]Normalized permeability coefficient = P_{app} (steroid)/P_{app} (methanol).

rescent probe [34]. Membrane permselectivity was evaluated by KCl diffusion potential or charge-discriminating ability. The fluorescein probe is known to permeate via the paracellular route. The permeation of 6-carboxyfluorescein through several biological membranes was investigated and found to follow the order: intestine ≈ nasal ≥ bronchial ≥ tracheal > vaginal ≥ rectal > corneal > buccal > skin. The permselectivity was negative, that is, the K^+ ion was more permeable than the Cl^- ion. There was no difference in permselectivity for all the biological membranes listed above. Using low molecular weight polyvinyl alcohol, the molecular weight cut-off for the rat's vaginal epithelium was shown to be higher than for other mucosae, such as for the gastrointestinal epithelium [35]. Permeability trends have also been evaluated using the spermicide nonoxynol-9 [36]. A linear correlation was observed between permeability and partitioning of nonoxynol-9 oligomers using lamb vaginal mucosa, suggesting the importance of the lipoidal pathway for this particular agent.

Pharmacokinetics

Assuming that the absorption, distribution, and elimination of a drug molecule after its release from a vaginal drug delivery device can be described by the following pharmacokinetic sequences,

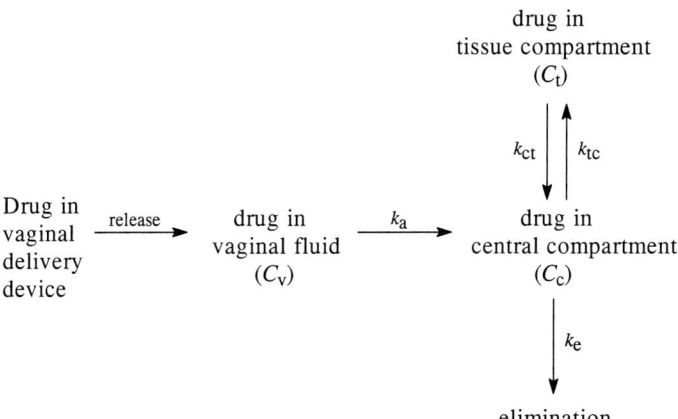

the instantaneous rate of change in drug concentration in the central compartment can be expressed by Eq. (5),

$$\frac{d(C_c)}{dt} = k_{tc}C_v + K_{tc}C_t - (k_{ct} + k_e)C_c \qquad (5)$$

where k_a, k_e, k_{ct}, and k_{tc} are the rate constants for absorption, elimination, and central compartment/tissue compartment exchange, respectively, and C_v, C_c, and C_t are the drug concentrations in the tissue fluid surrounding the vaginal device, in the central compartment, and in the tissue compartment, respectively.

The vaginal absorption of drug following its release from a vaginal drug delivery device may alternatively be described by a simplified one-compartment open model with

Vaginal Delivery and Absorption of Drugs

first-order drug absorption (Fig. 5) [37]. Using this simplified model, Eq. (5) is reduced to Eq. (6),

$$\frac{d(C_c)}{dt} = k_a C_v - k_e C_B \qquad (6)$$

where C_v and C_B are, respectively, the drug concentrations in the vagina and in the body (including blood, tissues, and related compartments with fast drug-exchange rates).

At steady state (Fig. 7), the change in the body concentration of the drug is relatively small ($d(C_B)dt \cong 0$). For example, the body concentration of norethhindrone (C_B), the major metabolite of ethynodiol diacetate, is related to the amount of ethynodiol diacetate (Q) released at time t as shown by Eq. (7),

$$C_B = \frac{k_a \Sigma R_v}{2k_e} \left(\frac{Q}{t}\right)_v \qquad (7)$$

where ΣR_v is the total diffusional resistance across the vaginal wall. Equation (7) suggests that the norethindrone concentration (C_B) in the body of each test animal should be directly proportional to the amount of ethynodiol diacetate released from the vaginal device, $(Q/t)_v$, for a given duration of intravaginal residence. The magnitude of ΣR_v can be estimated from the slope of the C_B vs. $(Q/t)_v$ plot and the values of k_a and k_e obtained from vaginal absorption studies of the same drug in solution.

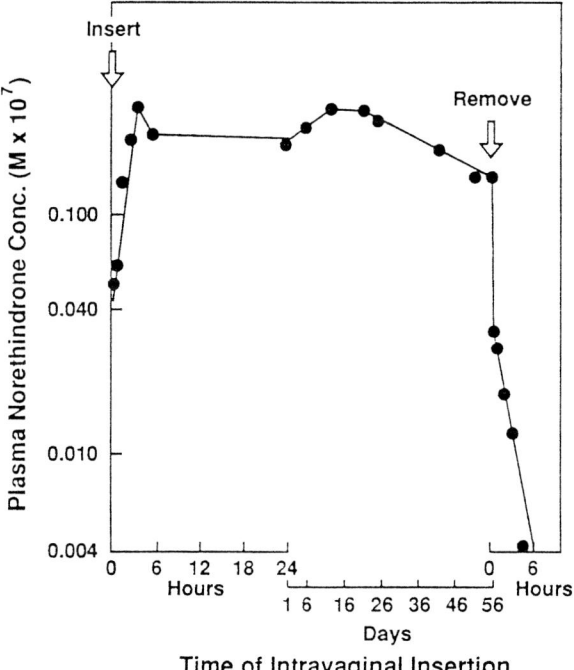

FIG. 7. Plasma profile of norethinedrone following the intravaginal insertion of ethynodiol diacetate-releasing vaginal devices in rabbits for 56 days and after device removal. Based on Ref. 37.

Cyclic Variability

As mentioned previously, the rabbit appears to be an ideal animal model for studying vaginal mucosa permeation due to the absence of an estrus cycle. However, the absence of a rhythmic pattern of hormones makes the doe rabbit an unsuitable animal model for investigating long-term vaginal absorption since it lacks the typical cyclic variations observed in the human vaginal tract. In the human female, the cyclic secretion of estrogenic hormones in the ovarian cycle induces some variations in the histology, biochemistry, and physiology of vaginal tissues. It is therefore reasonable to expect that the vaginal mucosa undergoes a corresponding cyclic variation in its membrane permeability.

The macaque rhesus monkey has an ovarian cycle of approximately 28 days, as do humans, and exhibits an estrus pattern very similar to that of the human female. It is widely believed by researchers in the fertility field that rhesus monkeys and humans have comparable anatomy and physiology, as well as similar reproductive functions [38]. The female rhesus monkey is therefore a superior animal model for studying the vaginal absorption of various drugs from a drug delivery system designed for use in human females.

The effect of the estrus cycle on the permeability of vaginal mucosa has been demonstrated in the vaginal absorption of a small molecule, like methanol, which has a vaginal membrane-controlled permeation, and a larger molecule, such as n-octanol, in which vaginal permeation is controlled by the hydrodynamic diffusion layer (Fig. 8). Further studies using intact and ovariectomized monkeys could not establish any systematic relationship between vaginal membrane permeability and the menstrual cycle [39]. Conflicting observations were also reported in the vaginal absorption of penicillin in humans [40,41] as well as in rats [42,43].

The vaginal permeability of a cycling monkey during the period immediately following menstruation is lower than that of a noncyclic rabbit (Fig. 9). This difference is greater for hydrophilic molecules, such as the short-chain alkanols (e.g., methanol), whose permeability is controlled by vaginal membrane permeation. The difference lessens as the alkyl chain length of alkanols increases, since molecular lipophilicity increases as the expense of hydrophilicity. At ovulation, the monkey's vaginal permeability is several-fold lower than that of the noncyclic rabbit [31].

The rhesus monkey's variation in vaginal permeability with the rhythmic pattern of their sexual cycle suggests that the absorption data they generate are highly reflective of human variations. The rhesus monkey is therefore a good animal model for the research and development of intravaginal delivery devices.

Types of Vaginal Drug Delivery Systems

Human Applications

Recent publications on vaginal drug delivery examine extensively the many types of vaginal delivery systems under development or commercially available [44,45]. In the development of vaginal dosage forms, several considerations should be addressed [44]:

- Maintenance of an optimal pH for vaginal epithelium,
- Ease of application,

Vaginal Delivery and Absorption of Drugs

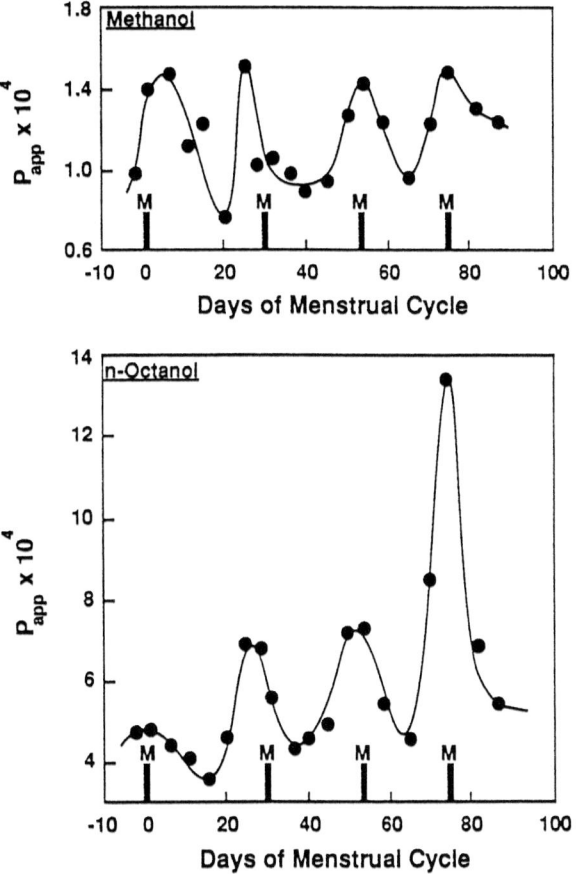

FIG. 8. Cyclic variation in the apparent permeability coefficient, P_{app}, of methanol and n-octanol in the female rhesus monkey in response to its estrus cycle. The bars indicate the time of observed menstruation. Based on Ref. 31.

- Even distribution of the drug,
- Retention time in the vagina, and
- Compatibility with coadministered medicines.

There should also be no offensive odor, staining, tissue irritation, or pain during sexual intercourse. With regard to systemic delivery, one key advantage of intravaginal administration is avoidance of the presystemic elimination associated with oral dosage forms. The perineum venous plexus, which drains the vaginal tissue and rectum, flows into the pudendal vein and ultimately into the vena cava, which circumnavigates the liver on its first pass. This is in marked contrast to gastrointestinal blood circulation which drains into the portal vein and passes directly through the liver before entering the systemic circulation. The vaginal route is preferable for drug entities associated with gastrointestinal irritation and for the localized treatment of vaginal disorders requiring minimal systemic absorption.

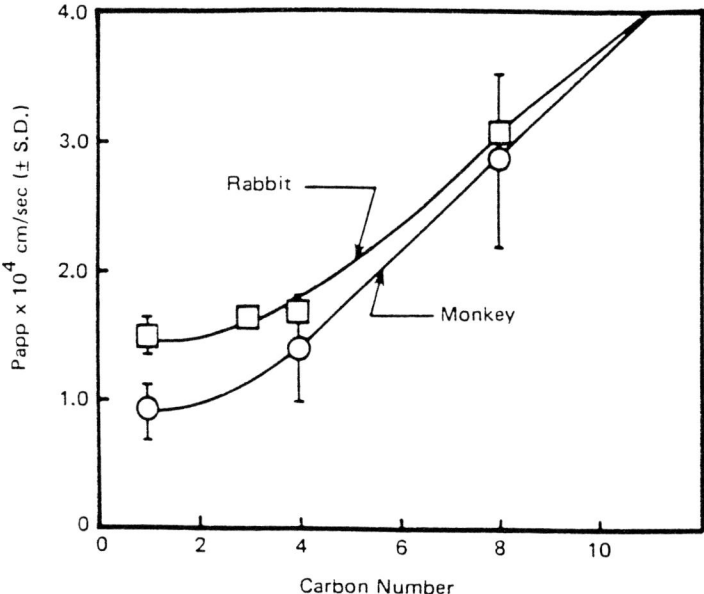

FIG. 9. Comparison of apparent permeability coefficients, P_{app}, for the vaginal absorption of straight-chain alkanols in noncyclic rabbits and cyclic rhesus monkeys. Based on Refs. 16 and 165.

Creams, Foams, Jellies

These types of vaginal products are likely to be the most familiar to consumers. Many OTC preparations are available in these forms. Common products are contraceptive creams, foams, gels, suppositories, sponges, and films, each of which contains a spermicidal agent such as nonoxynol-9 or octoxynol. A more recent addition to the OTC market came about with the FDA approval of vaginal preparations for treating yeast infections. Women with recurring conditions can now obtain their usual creams or suppositories, without a prescription, from their local grocery store or pharmacy. This ease of availability has encountered opposition among some medical professionals who feel that self-treatment may compound problems such as benign physiological lukorrhea, yeast vulvovaginitis, cervicitis, sexually transmitted diseases, and pelvic inflammatory disease [46]. For treatment of menopausal symptoms, estrogen products are available as vaginal creams. A relatively new product for postmenopausal women, Replens, is also available as a vaginal bioadhesive moisturizer. It has been shown to be as safe and effective as estrogen vaginal creams in increasing moisture, fluid volume, and elasticity, and in returning the vaginal pH to its premenopausal state [47]. Available by prescription, low-pH lactate gels have been dispensed for cases of bacterial vaginosis. Application of these gels leads to a disappearance of abnormal discharge and malodor, restores normal acidity, and facilitates recolonization of lactobacilli. Localized treatment of vaginosis by intravaginal delivery of antimicrobials may be preferable to an oral regimen, particularly during pregnancy [48].

Vaginal Rings

Vaginal rings, under development since 1970, provide a means of delivering a pharmacologically active agent to the systemic circulation at a controlled release rate. An

Vaginal Delivery and Absorption of Drugs

advantage of this method over conventional oral administration is best illustrated by the example shown in Fig. 10. After oral ingestion, medroxyprogesterone acetate (MPA) reaches a peak plasma concentration within 2 h and then declines over the next 22 h. Intermittent use of this dosage form would produce alternately surging and ebbing plasma levels. Conversely, intravaginal controlled delivery of MPA from a vaginal ring attains a steady plasma plateau, also within 2 h, which is maintained throughout the course of treatment until removal of the ring. This continuous "infusion" of drugs through the vaginal mucosa bypasses the hepatogastrointestinal "first-pass" metabolism and thus

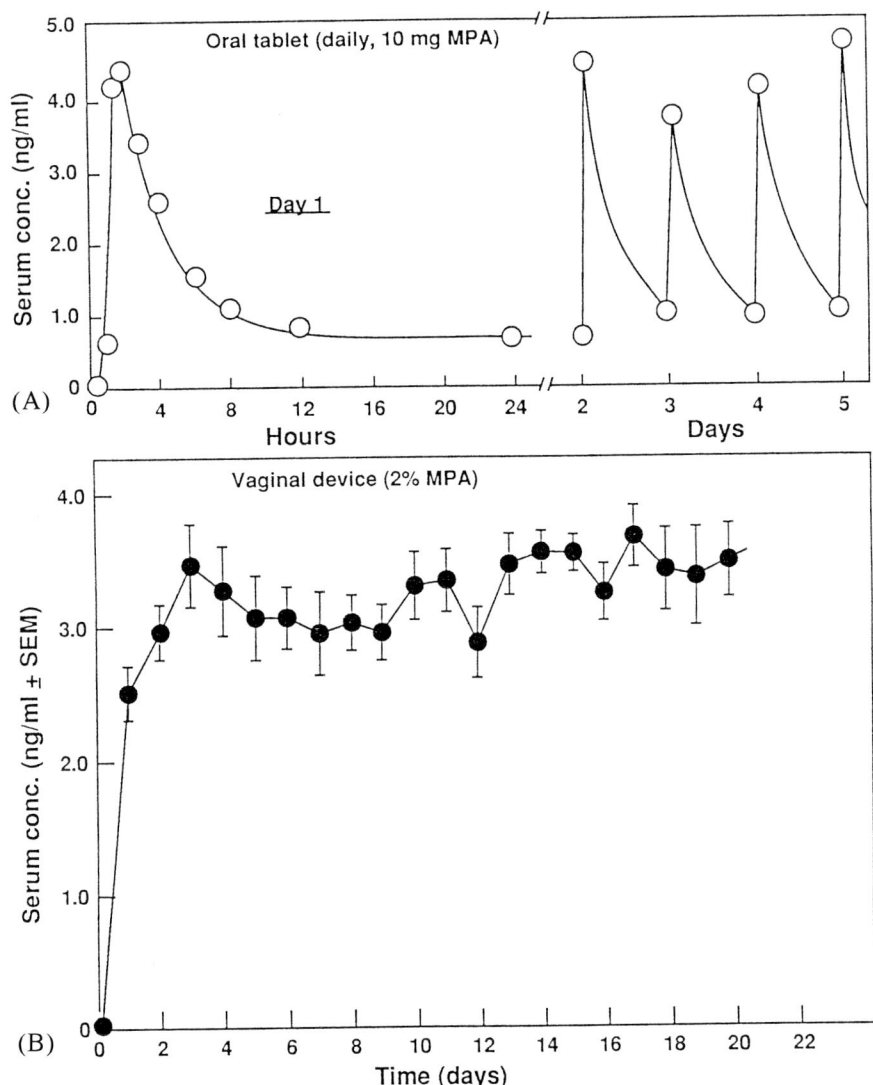

FIG. 10. (A.) Serum concentrations of medroxyprogesterone acetate after a daily oral administration of a medroxyprogesterone acetate tablet (10 mg) taken by a healthy woman before breakfast for five consecutive days. (B.) Daily serum concentrations of medroxyprogesterone acetate in women wearing medicated silicone vaginal rings (2% medroxyprogesterone acetate) for 20 days. Based on Ref. 53.

avoids the relatively inefficient therapeutic activity resulting from variable plasma levels [31]. The vaginal rings developed to date are primarily for contraception and have been reviewed in the literature [45,49]. Therapeutic agents delivered in this form include medroxyprogesterone acetate [50–56], estradiol [57], norgestrel [58,59], levonorgestrel [60–64], and combinations of progestins and estrogens [65–70]. Another area of interest is in the application of prostaglandin-containing vaginal rings for cervical ripening and induction of labor or pregnancy termination [71]. Most of the prostaglandin delivery systems previously developed have been in the form of suppositories or pessaries [72–82]. More research in this area has been performed recently due to the recognition of prostaglandins as an alternative to surgical abortion. This will be discussed later.

Vaginal rings have traditionally been made of silicone elastomer, which consists of an inert ring-shaped core coated by a layer of medicated (drug-containing) elastomer. Vaginal rings are inserted and positioned around the cervix. Those designed for contraception are kept intravaginally for 21 days and then removed for 7 days to allow for menstruation. The frequent occurrence of bleeding irregularities with early ring designs prompted the development of a new generation of sandwich-type vaginal rings in which the drug-dispersed silicone polymer matrix was coated by a nonmedicated silicone polymeric membrane. The design was intended to reduce the initial spike of drug concentration frequently observed at the beginning of a treatment cycle following insertion of the contraceptive ring. The effect of the overcoat on the release rate profile of d-norgestrel is demonstrated in Fig. 11. It shows that the addition of an overcoat minimizes or eliminates the burst release of d-norgestrel and shifts the non-zero-order drug-release profile to a constant zero-order release rate profile. The concept of intravaginal dual-controlled delivery of progestin and estrogen in combination was recently extended to the development of a combined contraceptive vaginal ring. This new design, shown in Fig. 12, is constructed with two drug-reservoir compartments. The larger compartment consists of a core loaded with 3-keto-desogestrel, a potent progestin, whereas the smaller compartment contains a combination of 3-keto-desogestrel and ethinylestradiol, a synthetic estrogen. These compartments are partitioned by two steroid-impermeable glass closures and covered by a rate-controlling silicone membrane through which the steroids are released at a fixed ratio [67]. Serum profiles of 3-keto-desogestrel and ethyinylestradiol from two prototype vaginal rings are shown in Fig. 13.

Veterinary Applications

Pessaries

Intravaginal drug delivery has been a useful tool in animal husbandry to control the estrus cycle of sheep and cattle. Synchronization of a herd's estrus cycle facilitates the management of these domestic animals. Fluorogestone acetate, an effective ovulation-inhibitory progestin in the ewe, has been formulated into a vaginal pessary. The pessary is placed intravaginally for a predetermined period of time; removal enables the sheep to regain its estrus and ovulate within 2 to 4 days. If all treated ewes are inseminated upon ovulation, this procedure results in a high rate of pregnancy among the herd. Commercially available delivery systems include Syncro-Mate vaginal pessary (S.D. Searle & Co.) and Chronogest vaginal pessary (Intervet S.A.), both containing

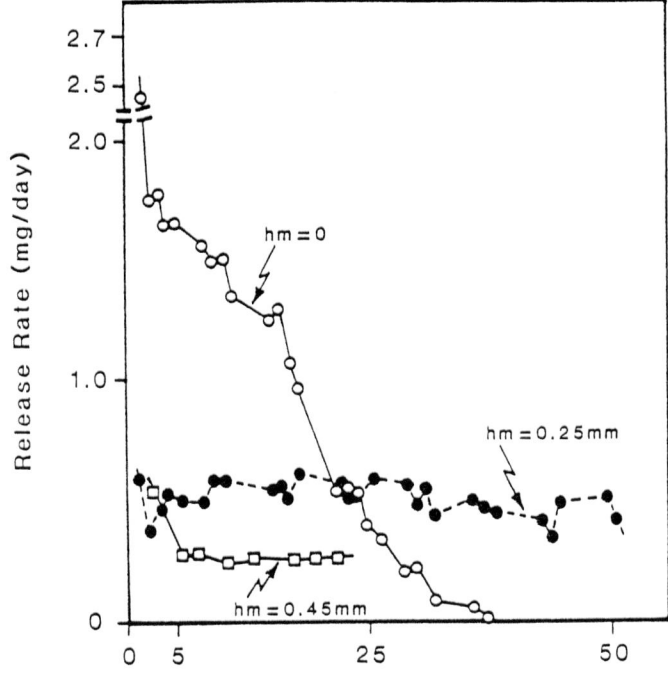

FIG. 11. Comparative in vitro release rate profile of levonorgestrel from a vaginal ring containing a homogeneous dispersion of drug in a silicone-based polymer matrix (open circles) and from one containing an inert overcoat covering the drug reservoir layer (closed circles and squares). The effect of overcoat thickness h_m on the release rate of levonorgestrel is also shown. Based on Ref. 25.

fluorogestone acetate, and PRID vaginal insert for dairy cattle (Sanofi Animal Health Ltd.), which contains a combination of progesterone and estradiol benzoate. A medroxyprogesterone acetate sponge has been used in research to evaluate the preovulatory gonadotropin surge in ewes [83].

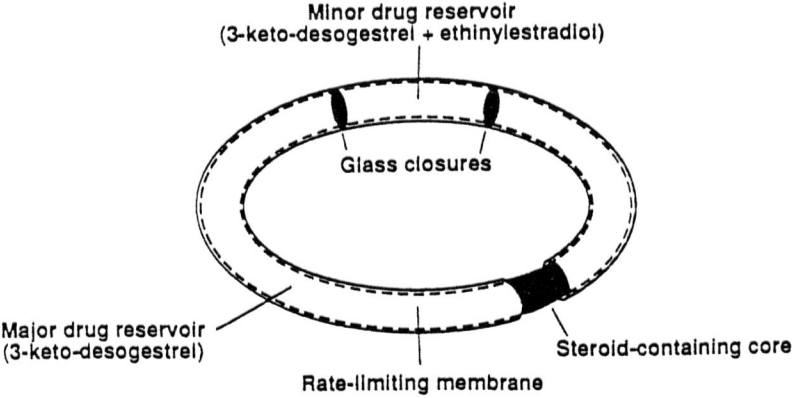

FIG. 12. Structural components of a contraceptive vaginal ring containing the combination of 3-keto-desogestrel and ethinylestradiol. Based on Ref. 67.

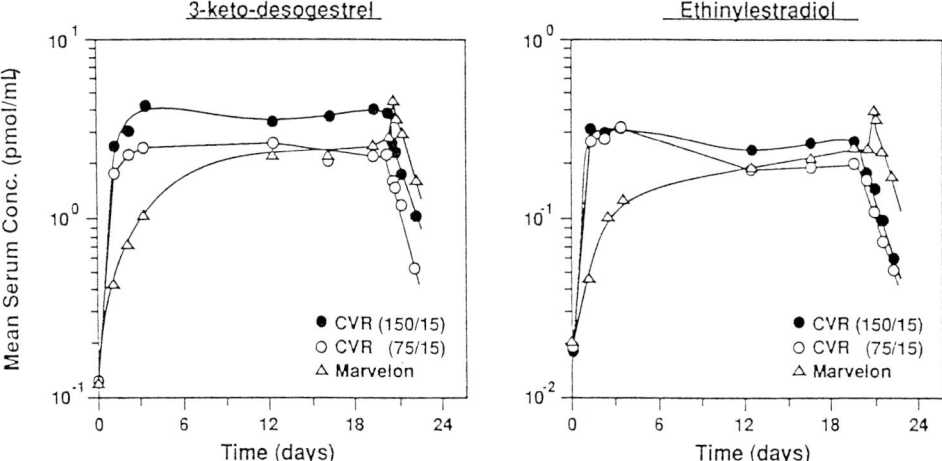

FIG. 13. Mean serum profiles of 3 keto-desogestrel and ethinylestradiol after a 21-day continuous intravaginal administration of two prototype combination contraceptive vaginal rings (CVR). The profiles from an oral combination tablet (Marvelon) is plotted for comparison. Based on Ref. 67.

Modified Vaginal Pessaries

The Syncro-Mate vaginal pessary is fabricated by dispersing a progestin, such as fluorogestone acetate, uniformly throughout a porous polyurethane sponge. This traditional design has been reworked with the aim of overcoming non-constant matrix-type release and absorption profiles, minimizing loading dose, and improving systemic bioavailability. Researchers began by studying the in vitro and in vivo release rates of a cylindrical drug-free polyurethane vaginal sponge coated with a laminate of fluorogestone-containing silicone matrix and partially covered by a drug-free silicone membrane [84–86]. As less membrane was used and more of the drug-releasing silicone laminate was exposed to direct contact with the vaginal wall, the dose delivered increased. This effort has resulted in two new pessary designs (Fig. 14). Both types have made use of the polyurethane sponge as the mechanical support for vaginal insertion and retention, but the drug reservoir has been relocated from the porous sponge matrix to a sheet-type rate-controlled silicone laminate that covers the circumferential surface of the sponge. The type-I rate-controlled silicone device consists of a homogeneous dispersion of drug in a silicone polymer matrix. The type-II drug-dispersing polymer matrix is sandwiched between two sheets of silicone membrane to form a three-layer laminate.

Potential Developments, Bioadhesives

Novel intravaginal delivery systems include those that employ bioadhesive materials. The mucoadhesive properties of polymers such as hydrogels provide a delivery system with a prolonged residence and intimate contact with the vaginal epithelium. Many hydrophilic polymers have been used in vaginal products, including starch, collagen, proteins, gelatin, and cellulose derivatives (hydroxypropyl methylcellulose, hydroxypropyl cellulose and sodium carboxymethylcellulose) [48]. Two synthetic hydrogels that have been evaluated for potential vaginal drug delivery are polyethylene oxide and

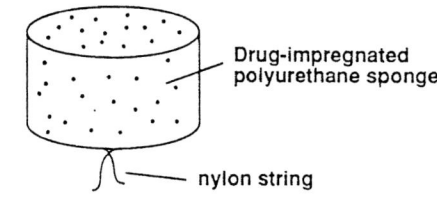

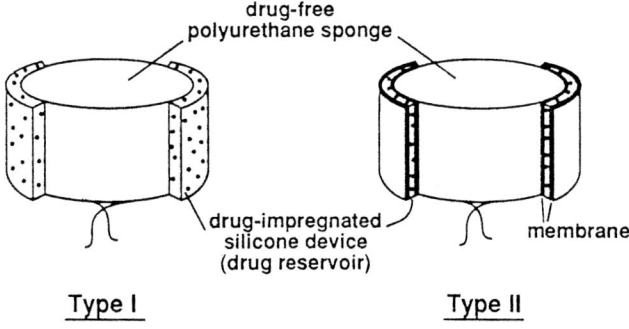

FIG. 14. Comparison of newer progestin-releasing vaginal pessaries (Type I and II) with an older (Syncro-Mate) pessary design. Based on Ref. 25.

polyacrylic acid. Mucoadhesion is thought to involve an interaction of the hydrophilic polymer with the mucosal surface in which an initial attraction between surface polarities leads to interpenetration of the mucosal surface by the polymer chains of the hydrogen [87].

According to recent reviews of vaginal bioadhesive formulations, bioadhesive tablets have been used for localized treatment of diseased vaginal tissue [48,87]. Bleomycin, an antitumor agent, was incorporated into a flat-faced, disk-shaped vaginal tablet fabricated from hydroxypropyl cellulose and polyacrylic acid (Carbopol 934) [88]. The tablet was designed to release bleomycin at a slow rate to minimize inflammation of healthy mucosa. Another vaginal tablet has been formulated by the combination of polyacrylic acid with hydroxypropyl methylcellulose and ethylcellulose [89]. Other polymer combinations evaluated for potential bioadhesive vaginal delivery include polyacrylic acid and sodium carboxymethylcellulose with Avicel PH102 (methylcellulose) added as the diluent [90]. A cross-linked polyacrylic acid gel was found to adhere onto the vaginal surface of alloxan-induced diabetic rats and rabbits and was used for intravaginal delivery of insulin [91]. Emulsion-based formulations with bioadhesive properties have been designed to deliver antifungal agents intravaginally, although little has been reported in the literature [48]. Bioadhesive microparticles, currently used in nasal and oral drug delivery, also have the potential for further development into an intravaginal delivery system [48]. The mucoadhesive benzyl ester of hyaluronic acid has been used to construct microspheres for the intravaginal delivery of salmon calcitonin to rats [92]. As mentioned previously, Replens, which consists of a cross-linked polycarbophil system, is marketed as a bioadhesive moisturizer which remains in the vagina for 2 to 3 days [93].

Drug Candidates for Vaginal Administration
Antimicrobials

Antimicrobials, along with antifungals, have been important drug candidates for the treatment of gynecological conditions. Investigations have been made in this area on the use of such drugs as metronidazole [94–96], clindamycin [97,98], feticonazole [99], and clotrimazole [99,100]. Metronidazole has been prescribed for the treatment of amoebiasis, trichomoniasis, lambliasis, and anaerobic infection [96]. It is administered vaginally as a gel, normally twice a day (every 12 hours) for 7 days, for the treatment of bacterial vaginosis. The gel yields low serum concentrations with negligible adverse systemic effects [94]. The low lipid solubility of metronidazole probably contributes to its poor vaginal absorption [95]. A comparison of vaginal and oral delivery of metronidazole from film-coated tablets showed that the maximum serum concentrations attained by vaginal delivery are sufficient only to kill the most susceptible anaerobic germs systematically [96]. Earlier research has used antimicrobials such as penicillin and sulfanilamide [22].

Clindamycin has also been indicated for the treatment of bacterial vaginosis. Its efficacy when delivered intravaginally from a 2% cream formulation has been found to be similar to that of oral metronidazole treatment [97]. Measurable amounts of clindamycin, corresponding to the frequency of intravaginal application, have been detected systematically at levels well below those of intravenous delivery [98]. Gentamicin, an aminoglycoside-type antibiotic, has been evaluated for vaginal administration in ovariectomized rats [101]. The results indicated the following order of absorption enhancers by effectiveness: palmitoylcarnitine (1%) > lysophosphatidylcholine (0.5%) > laureth-9 (1%) > citric acid (10%). Severity of desquamation of the vaginal epithelium was scored as lysophosphatidylcholine = laureth-9 > palmitoylcarnitine > citric acid.

The market for vaginal candidiasis treatments has been expanded in the last few years due to the availability of OTC products. Very recently the oral antifungal agent ketoconazole was approved for treatment of vaginal candidiasis. Earlier research comparing vaginal feticonazole to oral clotrimazole [99] and vaginal clotrimazole to oral fluconazole [100] concluded that in both cases the vaginal product was equally as effective and as well tolerated as the oral product. An important consideration in the choice of oral versus vaginal treatment is the contraindication of oral dosage forms during pregnancy. Vaginal treatment for recurrent vaginal conditions may be a good alternative in such a case [102].

Anticancer Agents

Intravaginal investigations into the local treatment of cervicovaginal cancers has made some progress over recent years. Treatment of cervical carcinoma by ^{3}H-fenticonazole has been evaluated in comparison with normal cervicovaginal mucosa and relapsing vulvovaginal candidiasis, with the results indicating that the treatment is devoid of risk to patients [103]. For patients with vaginal rhabdomyosarcoma and residual vaginal disease following surgery and chemotherapy, the effects of high-dose irradiation from vaginal molds loaded with iridium^{192} were examined [104]. Individualized molds were made with rapid-setting silastic foam and loaded with iridium wires. After the treatment, the patients were found to remain well and disease-free for at least 7 years. Vaginal delivery of another chemotherapeutic agent, ciclopirox olamine, has been evaluated in rabbits and in human patients. The results demonstrated that vaginal absorption was low with minimal penetration of drug into the deep tissue, which led to good local and systemic tolerability [105]. Cisplatin, a common anticancer agent, has been delivered as an intravaginal suppository prior to an operation [106]. The cisplatin penetration into the tumor surface needs further improvement in order to achieve effective local chemotherapeutic activity.

In the opposite vein, some cervicovaginal cancers have been linked to the use of vaginal pessaries [107]. A review of cancer cases reveals that many tumors were first detected at sites of ring insertion. Although chemical carcinogenesis cannot be ruled out, chronic local infection may be the main etiologic factor. The severity of cancer cases has declined in recent times due to the availability of more advanced surgery and radiation treatment with minimal complications.

Prostaglandins

Prostaglandins, primarily prostaglandin E_1 (PGE_1) and E_2 (PGE_2), have long been studied for cervical ripening and induction of labor, as well as for use as an abortifacient. The initial formulation of PGE_2 was a sustained-release pessary fabricated from a swellable, cross-linked polymer hydrogel [82]. Further work was conducted using a semicrystalline polyethylene oxide and polyurethane hydrogels impregnated with PGE_2 solution [108]. In this research, the cervical score measurement was linearly correlated with the controlled release of PGE_2, suggesting the applicability of controlled PGE_2 release for cervical ripening [109]. A number of investigations have been conducted using PGE_2 pessaries for cervical ripening and induction of labor. Pessaries were found to provide a higher degree of control in labor induction [110] and were preferable to intracervical gels [111]. Furthermore, the pessaries were associated with high efficacy and low incidence of side effects [112] and achieved a reduction in the incidence of Cesarean section from the high rate often seen with artifiical rupture caused by oxytocin infusion [113]. Although a PGE_2 pessary initiates active labor and reduces the need for oxytocin, it can also cause uterine hyperstimulation or fetal heart rate abnormalities which are reversed with removal of the pessary [114]. In addition, chemically stable and cost-effective tablet forms of PGE_2 have been developed [115,116]. The ease in the application of intravaginal PGE_2 delivery may allow for the shortening of post-date pregnancies in a safe and effective manner on an outpatient basis [117].

In addition, PGE_2 has been formulated as gels. A comparison of a triacetin-based gel with the tablet form showed a more favorable induction with the gel [118]. The use of PGE_2 gel in women with prelabor spontaneous membrane rupture significantly reduced the time of delivery without increasing the Cesarean-section rate or the maternal infective morbidity of the fetus [119]. The intravaginally administered gel was more efficacious than that given intracervically [120]. In comparing 6-h and 12-h dosage regimens, most of the 12-h subjects were able to achieve labor after a single dose. The interval of induction was similar in both groups, however [121].

Because of their labor-inducing characteristics, prostaglandins have been used as abortifacients. The combination of a PGE_1 vaginal pessary and an oral antiprogestin, mifepristone (RU486), has been used as a safe, efficient, low-cost outpatient method for pregnancy termination [122]. The PGE_1 product misoprostol was originally intended for the treatment of gastrointestinal ulcers caused by nonsteroidal anti-inflammatory agents. On its own, misoprostol can induce labor in females with late fetal death [123]. Although not yet approved as an abortifacient by the FDA, misoprostol has recently attracted the attention of medical professionals and the news media for being used in combination with methotrexate for early abortion. In this application, methotrexate, originally used as a chemotherapeutic agent in cancer and arthritis, is given intramuscularly followed by the intravaginal administration of misoprostol 3 days later. This is an effective abortion method for a gestation period of 56 days or less [124].

Spermicides

An intravaginal spermicide is intended for local rather than systemic activity. To achieve contraception, a common spermicide such as nonoxynol-9 acts by causing cessation of sperm motility which ultimately leads to sperm death. Initial absorption studies conducted with nonoxynol-9 in rabbit mucosa found the compound to be absorbed rapidly into the systemic circulation [125]. Later work pointed out that the previous research did not provide reliable quantitative data due to loss of nonoxynol-9 through the vaginal cavity by leakage and to ingestion by preening [126]. This reinvestigation found the absorption of nonoxynol-9 through the vaginal membrane to be very slow and suggested a dependence on the molecular weight of the component oligomers. Permeation studies have found the hydrophilic–lipophilic balance (HLB) of the oligomers also to play a role [36]. Spermicides have become more popular with the rise in social awareness and prevention of sexually transmitted diseases. The most widely available compounds in the United States are nonoxynol-9 and octoxynol, although many others are being evaluated for their spermicidal activity. Alkyloxynol-741 has been tested in dissolvable polyvinyl alcohol films for spermicidal activity in stump-tailed macaques and may be an inexpensive alternative in countries where nonoxynol-9 is not readily available [127]. A Canadian contraceptive sponge, Portectaid, is made with sodium cholate, nonoxynol-9, and benzalkonium chloride. Sodium cholate by itself has been shown to exhibit strong spermicidal and antiviral activity [28,128]. An acrosin-inhibiting serine protease from sperm, 4'-acetamidophenyl 4-guanidinobenzoate, has recently been found to be more potent and less irritating than nonoxynol-9 and to possess some activity against HIV [129].

Steroids

The steroids progesterone and estrogen have long been used for such purposes as hormone replacement and contraception. Vaginal estrogen cream has proved to be an effective alternative to oral estrogen replacement for the treatment of atrophic vaginitis, although the association with endometrial proliferation and hyperplasia suggests the coadministration of progestins [130,131]. Estrogen creams are not prescribed in situations where oral estrogen therapy is contraindicated. In addition, this mode of delivery is not yet recommended for the prevention of cardiovascular disease and osteoporosis. As mentioned previously, vaginal rings have been shown to be a safe and effective delivery mechanism for estrogen and more comfortable than a pessary [132].

Like estrogen, progesterone has been delivered intravaginally as creams, pessaries, and vaginal rings. Absorption and local redistribution of progesterone to the genital organs was observed in a study using young female pigs [133]. It was found that vaginal application provided enhanced delivery to the uterus compared to a standard intramuscular regimen [134]. Progesterone has also been delivered in a micronized form as a nonliquefying vaginal cream [135,136]. For systemic delivery of progesterone, doctors have prescribed a suppository compound of progesterone and cocoa butter. A new lactose-based progesterone tablet has been designed to deliver biologically effective amounts of progesterone for up to 48 h [48]. These tablets form a milky suspension which remains in the vagina for a relatively long period of time, making them ideal for the treatment of menstrual irregularities, functional uterine bleeding, luteal-phase defects, premenstrual tension, infertility, and osteoporosis.

Absorption and secretion characteristics of sodium prasterone sulfate have been evaluated in rats after vaginal administration. The absorption was found to be significantly affected by the estrus cycle and progression of pregnancy [137].

Protein and Peptides

Protein and peptides are primarily given parenterally because of their susceptibility to degradation by proteolytic enzymes in the gastrointestinal tract and by first-pass metabolism. The development of a novel delivery system for these molecules faces many challenges, such as hydrophilicity, poor epithelial permeability, large molecular size, short half-life, and low chemical and enzymatic stability [70]. Research into the intravaginal delivery of peptides and proteins has focused on insulin and leutinizing hormone-releasing hormone (LHRH) and their delivery into the systemic circulation. Insulin and thyroid-stimulating hormone have been shown to have some absorption from the vagina of rats and rabbits with a high dependency on the estrus cycle [91]. Hydrophilic compounds such as insulin and LHRH are absorbed predominantly through intercellular channels, so that absorption is higher with thinner epitheliums [48,138]. As commonly observed in other protein and peptide research, an enhancer is often needed to assist in this type of absorption. Because human testing of enhancers is extremely risky, most of the preliminary research is done on animal models such as the rat and the rabbit [48]. It has been found that hypoglycemia in rats is increased by vaginal administration of insulin using enhancers such as sodium taurodihydrofusidate, polyoxyethylene-9-lauryl ether, lysophosphatidylglycerol, lysophosphatidyl choline, and palmitoylcarnitine chloride [139]. Other therapeutic agents that have been investigated include leucine enkephalin [140], salmon calcitonin [93], and recombinant human relaxin [141,142]. Relaxin, structurally related to insulin, was formulated as a 3% methylcellulose gel for intravaginal delivery. In this form, it had limited permeability through nonpregnant rabbit and rhesus monkey vaginas.

Much work has been done using LHRH analogs, particularly leuprolide. Initial work with leuprolide indicated a higher potency in rats when using vaginal administration over rectal, nasal, or oral administration [143]. Enhancement of vaginal absorption by organic acids (citric, succinic, tartaric, and glycocholic) increased bioavailability by 20%. The acidifying and chelating abilities of these organic acids are the primary mechanisms of absorption enhancement [144]. Citric acid also loosens the blood–vaginal epithelium barrier. The reduction of pituitary activity by chronic intravaginal treatment of leuprolide causes regression of hormone-dependent mammary tumors in rats [145–147]. Vaginal administration of LHRH appears to be the preferred route according to a recent presystemic metabolism study of first-order LHRH degradation in rabbit homogenates [148]. The degradation half-life of vaginal homogenates was 9 to 12 times longer than that of rectal homogenates and three to four times longer than for nasal homogenates.

Vaccines and Antigens

Since the recognition of the Human Immunodeficiency Virus (HIV) as the cause of Acquired Immunodeficiency Syndrome (AIDS) in the early 1980s, it has commanded the attention of researchers and has challenged them to discover pharmacological agents for the prevention and treatment of the virus. Inasmuch as the infection can be sexually transmitted during vaginal intercourse, one area of research has been in the development of a vaccine for intravaginal immunization. If the vagina is capable of mounting an immune response, antibodies in genital secretions may be able to reduce the transmission of HIV [149]. Considerations in this approach include the number of administrations required for adequate protection and the practicality of the method of inducing immunity at the mucosal surface [150]. In one study, a human simian virus 1 (HSV) vaccine was formulated as an aqueous solution or a gel and administered to guinea pigs vaginally, intranasally, or subcutaneously [151]. The gel system was a controlled-release carbopol gel. The animals were challenged 3 to 5 weeks later with only the subcutaneous response producing IgG and IgA immunoglobulins. Anitbodies were elicited within those subjects administered by the nasal or vaginal routes, slightly reducing the severity of the disease, but showing no superiority to the subcutaneous route. In another study, rats immunized with a synthetic peptide from HIV envelope glycoprotein had a greater IgG and IgA response when using the enhancer lysophosphatidylglycerol [152]. The serum antibodies from subcutaneous and intravaginal delivery were able to recognize the glycoprotein (HIV 1 gp120), but no neutralizing activity against the virus was seen. An antigen delivery system consisting of lysophosphatidylcholine and degradable starch microspheres was evaluated in sheep and exhibited potential in intravaginal delivery [152]. Intravaginally administered tracers using fluorescein isothiocyanate (FITC)-bovine albumin, FITC-horseradish peroxidase, and FITC-horse ferritin have shown the vagina and cervix to be major sites of protein uptake [153].

Lactobacilli from the female genital tract have been developed as a vehicle to deliver continued doses of foreign antigen to the vaginal mucosa surface with the intention of stimulating a local immune response [154]. The lactobacillus fermentum was genetically altered and delivered intravaginally to guinea pigs. Although the altered lactobactillus persisted for only 5 days, the novel vaccination approach does present a potential method for triggering mucosal immunization. To study the effect of adjuvants on antibody titers, horse ferritin was evaluated in combination with aluminum hydroxide, muramyl dipeptide, monophosphoryl lipid A, dimethyldioctadecylammonium bromide, or cholera toxin [155]. The aluminum hydroxide combination was found to be the most effective. However, the doses of antigen used were larger than normal and consequently the drug combination may be inefficient at more realistic dosages. Additional work with horse ferritin has shown pelvic immunization at nonmucosal sites to be very effective in stimulating an IgA response in the mouse, more so than intravaginal delivery, possibly due to iliac lymph nodes not associated with the vagina [156].

As a potential means of treatment for gynecological conditions, candida albicans vaccine has shown an antibody response after intravaginal application [157]. Recurrent urinary tract infections have been evaluated for vaccine treatment. A vaccine containing heat-killed *E. coli* and non-*E. coli* uropathogens yielded serum antibody to some non-*E. Coli*, but no *E. coli* antibodies were found [158]. The vaccine was well tolerated and invites further development.

Inactivated polio vaccine has been investigated by intravaginal, intrauterine, mesopharyngeal, and intramuscular routes. The predominant secretory antibodies to polio viruses in the vagina were found to be IgA and IgG in the uterus. The genital tract is immunologically reactive and may play a role in protection against other infections such as gonococcus and genital herpes [159].

For veterinary use, dairy cattle research has looked at bovine herpes virus type 2 which causes ulcerative lesions in teats and udders. Vaccinations subcutaneously and intravaginally have proved beneficial in reducing the severity of the infection and show potential for the development of a vaccine for dairy cattle [160].

Other Candidates

Another chemical entity that has been researched for intravaginal delivery is tranexamic acid, an antifibrinolytic drug usually given by mouth for the treatment of menorrhagia associated with intrauterine devices. Further studies are needed, but the delivery was well tolerated and gastrointestinal side effects were avoided [161]. Bromocriptine is used for hyperprolactinemic women [162]. Tablet forms of the drug were administered intravaginally and were well absorbed, again avoiding side effects. Benzydamine, a nonsteroidal anti-inflammatory with local anesthetic and analgesic properties, is well absorbed orally. Therapeutic activity was evaluated at lower dose levels using mouthwash, dermal cream, and vaginal douche formulations [163].

Bibliography

Banja, A. K., *Therapeutic Peptides and Proteins: Formulations, Processing, and Delivery Systems*, Technomic Publishing Co., Lancaster, PA, 1995.

Chien, Y. W., *Novel Drug Delivery Systems*, Marcel Dekker, Inc., New York, 1992.

Hafez, E. S. E., and Evans, T. N., eds., *The Human Vagina*, North Holland Publishing Co., New York, 1978.

Lee, V. H. L., *Peptide and Protein Drug Delivery*, Marcel Dekker, Inc., New York, 1991.

References

1. Joglekar, A., Rhodes, C. R., and Danish, M., *Drug Dev. Ind. Pharm.*, 17:2103–2113 (1991).
2. Platzer, W., Poisel, W., and Hafez, E. S. E., Functional Anatomy of the Human Vagina.

In: *The Human Vagina* (E. S. E. Hafez and T. N. Evans, eds.), North Holland Publishing Co., New York, 1978, pp. 39-53.
3. Kistner, R. W., Physiology of the Vagina. In: *The Human Vagina* (E. S. E. Hafez and T. N. Evans, eds.), North Holland Publishing Co., New York, 1978, pp. 109-120.
4. Burgos, M. H., and Roig de Vargas-Linares, C. E., Ultrastructure of the Vaginal Mucosa. In: *The Human Vagina* (E. S. E. Hafez and T. N. Evans, eds.), North Holland Publishing Co., New York, 1978, pp. 63-93.
5. Averette, H. E., Weinstein, G. D., and Frost, P., *Am. J. Obstet. Gynecol.*, 108:8-17 (1970).
6. Wagner, G., and Levin, R. J., Vaginal Fluid. In: *The Human Vagina* (E. S. E. Hafez and T. N. Evans, eds.), North Holland Publishing Co., New York, 1978, pp. 121-137.
7. Itoh, Y., *Japan. J. Legal Med.*, 44:267-271 (1990).
8. Itoh, Y., Furuhata, A., and Sato, Y., *Japan. J. Legal Med.*, 45:26-29 (1991).
9. Schmidt, E. H., and Beller, F. K., Biochemistry of the Vagina. In: *The Human Vagina* (E. S. E. Hafez and T. N. Evans, eds.), North Holland Publishing Co., New York, 1978, pp. 139-149.
10. Moghissi, K. S., Composition and Function of Cervical Secretions. In: *Handbook of Physiology* (R. O. Greep and E. B. Astwood, eds.), Sect. 7, Vol. II, Part 2, American Physiological Society, Washington, 1978, pp. 25-48.
11. Richardson, J. L., and Illum, L., *Adv. Drug Del. Rev.*, 8:341-366 (1992).
12. Sparks, R. A., Purrier, B. G. A., Watt, P. J., and Elstein, M., *Br. J. Obstet. Gynecol.*, 84:701-704 (1977).
13. Masters, W. H., and Johnson, V. E., *Human Sexual Response*, Little, Brown and Co., Boston, 1966, pp. 68-100.
14. Steger, R. W., and Hafez, E. S. E., Age-associated Changes in the Vagina. In: *The Human Vagina* (E. S. E. Hafez and T. N. Evans, eds.), North Holland Publishing Co., New York, 1978, pp. 95-106.
15. Brown, W. J., Microbial Ecology of the Normal Vagina. In: *The Human Vagina* (E. S. E. Hafez and T. N. Evans, eds.), North Holland Publishing Co., New York, 1978, pp. 407-422.
16. Macht, D. D., *J. Pharmacol. Exp. Ther.*, 10:509-521 (1918).
17. Robinson, G. D., *J. Pharmacol. Exp. Ther.*, 32:81-88 (1927).
18. Macht, D. D., *J. Pharmacol. Exp. Ther.*, 34:137-145 (1928).
19. Millman, N., Hartman, C. G., Stavorski, J., and Botti, J., *Fed. Proc.*, 9:89 (1950).
20. Hartman, C. G., *Ann. N. Y. Acad. Sci.*, 83:313-327 (1959).
21. El-Sheikha, A. Z., and Hafez, E. S. E., Absorption of Drugs and Hormones in the Vagina. In: *The Human Vagina* (E. S. E. Hafez and T. N. Evans, eds.), North Holland Publishing Co., New York, 1978, pp. 179-191.
22. Benzinger, D. P., and Edelson, J., *Drug Metab. Rev.*, 14:137-168 (1983).
23. Rosenzweig, M., and Walzer, M., *Am. J. Obstet. Gynecol.*, 45:286-290 (1943).
24. Cunningham, F. E., Kraus, D. M., Brubaker, L., and Fischer, J. H., *J. Clin. Pharmacol.*, 34:1060-1065 (1994).
25. Chien, Y. W., Mucosal Drug Delivery. In: *Novel Drug Delivery Systems* (Y. W. Chien, ed.), Marcel Dekker, Inc., New York, 1992, pp. 197-228.
26. Hwang, S., Owada, E., Yotsuyanagi, T., Suhardja, L., Ho, H. F. H., Flynn, G. L., and Higuchi, W. I., *J. Pharm. Sci.*, 65:1574-1578 (1976).
27. Hwang, S., Owada, E., Suhardja, L., Ho, H. F. H., Flynn, G. L., and Higuchi, W. I., *J. Pharm. Sci.*, 66:781-784 (1977).
28. Bengtsson, L. P., *Acta Endocrinol.*, 13(Suppl.):5-75 (1953).
29. Yotsuyanagi, T., Molokhia, A., Hwang, S., Ho, N. F. H., Flynn, G. L., and Higuchi, W. I., *J. Pharm. Sci.*, 64:71-76 (1975).
30. Hwang, S., Owada, E., Suhardja, L., Ho, H. F. H., Flynn, G. L., and Higuchi, W. I., *J. Pharm. Sci.*, 66:778-780 (1977).

31. Flynn, G. L., Ho, N. F. H., Hwang, S., Owada, E., Molokhia, A., Behl, C. R., Higuchi, W. I., Yotsuyanagi, T., Shah, Y., and Park, J., Interfacing Matrix Release and Membrane Absorption Analysis of Steroid Absorption from a Vaginal Device in the Rabbit Doe. In: *Controlled Release of Polymeric Formulations* (D. R. Paul and F. W. Harris, eds.), American Chemical Society, Washington, 1976, pp. 87–122.
32. Ho, H. F. H., Suhardja, L., Hwang, S., Owada, E., Molokhia, A., Flynn, G. L., Higuchi, W. I., and Park, J., *J. Pharm. Sci.,* 65:1578–1585 (1976).
33. Corbo, D. C., Liu, J. C., and Chien, Y. W., *J. Pharm. Sci.,* 79:202–206 (1990).
34. Rojanasakul, Y., Wang, L. Y., Bhat, M., Glover, D. D. Malanga, C. J., and Ma, J. K., *Pharm. Res.,* 9:1029–1034 (1992).
35. Sanders, J. M., and Matthews, H. B., *Human Exp. Toxicol.,* 9:71–77 (1990).
36. Yu, K., and Chien, Y. W., *Int. J. Pharm.,* 125:81–90 (1995).
37. Chien, Y. W., Mares, S. E., Berg, J., Huber, S., Lambert, H. J., and King, K. F., *J. Pharm. Sci.,* 64:1776–1781 (1975).
38. Hartmann, C. G., *Endocrinology,* 25:670–682 (1939).
39. Behl, C. R., Ph.D. Dissertation, University of Michigan, Ann Arbor, 1979.
40. Rock, J., Barker, R. H., and Bacon, W. B., *Science,* 105:13 (1947).
41. Shudmak, M., and Hesseltine, H. C., *Am. J. Obstet. Gynecol.,* 62:669–671 (1951).
42. Baker, D. D., *Anat. Rec.,* 39:339 (1928).
43. Laug, E. P., and Kunze, F. M., *J. Pharm. Exp. Ther.,* 95:460–464 (1949).
44. Despande, A., and Rhodes, C. T., *Drug Dev. Ind. Pharm.,* 18:1225–1279 (1992).
45. Chien, Y. W., Vaginal Drug Delivery and Delivery Systems. In: *Novel Drug Delivery Systems* (Y. W. Chien, ed.), Marcel Dekker, Inc., New York, 1992, pp. 529–584.
46. Kabongo, M. L., *Am. Family Phys.,* 48:579 (1993).
47. Nachtigall, L. E., *Fertil. Steril.,* 61:178–180 (1994).
48. Holst, E., and Brandberg, A., *Scand. J. Inf. Dis.,* 22:625–626 (1990).
49. Brannan-Peppas, L., *Adv. Drug Delivery Rev.,* 11:169–177 (1993).
50. Mishell Jr., D. R., Talas, M., Parlow, A. F., and Moyer, D. L., *Am. J. Obstet. Gynecol.,* 107:100–107 (1970).
51. Mishell Jr., D. R., Lumkin, M., and Stone, S., *Am. J. Obstet. Gynecol.,* 113:927–932 (1972).
52. Cornette, J. C., Kirton, K. T., and Duncan, G. W., *J. Clin. Endocrinol. Metab.,* 33:459–466 (1971).
53. Hiroi, M., Stanczyk, F. Z., Goebelsmann, U., Brenner, P. F., Lumkin, M. E., and Mishell Jr., D. R., *Steroids,* 26:373–386 (1975).
54. Thiery, M., Vandekerckhove, D., Dhondt, M., Vermeulen, A., and Decoster, J. M., *Contraception,* 13:605–617 (1976).
55. Vermeulen, A., Dhondt, M., Thiery, M., and Vandekerckhove, D., *Fertil. Steril.,* 27:773–779 (1976).
56. Landgren, B. M., Aedo, A. R., Johannisson, E., and Cekan, S. Z., *Contraception,* 49:139–150 (1994).
57. Schmidt, G., Andersson, S. B., Nordle, O., Johansson, C. J., and Gunnarsson, P. O., *Gynecol. Obstet. Inv.,* 38:253–260 (1994).
58. Victor, A., Edquist, L. E., Lindberg, P., Elamsson, K., and Johansson, E. D. B., *Contraception,* 12:261–278 (1975).
59. Stanczyk, F. A., Hiroi, M., Goebelsmann, U., Brenner, P. F., Lumkin, M. E., and Mishell, Jr., D. R., *Contraception,* 13:279–298 (1975).
60. Koetsawang, S., Ji, G., Krishna, U., Cuadros, A., Dhall, G. I., Wyss, R., Rodriquez la Puenta, J., Andrade, A. T., Khan, T., Kononora, E. S., et al., *Contraception,* 41:105–124 (1990).
61. Burton, F. G., Skiens, W. E., Gordon, N. R., Veal, J. T., Kalkwarf, D. R., and Duncan, G. W., *Contraception,* 17:221–230 (1978).

62. Landgren, B. M., Johannisson, E., Masironi, B., and Diczfalusy, E., *Contraception*, 26:567–585 (1982).
63. Landgren, B. M., Johannisson, E., Xing, S., Aedo, A. R., and Diczfalusy, E., *Contraception*, 26:581–601 (1985).
64. Landgren, B. M., Aedo, A. R., Cekan, S. K., and Diczfalusy, E., *Contraception*, 26:473–497 (1986).
65. Mishell, Jr., D. R., Moore, D. E., Roy, S., Brenner, P. F., and Page, M. A., *Am. J. Obstet. Gynecol.*, 130:55–62 (1978).
66. Nash, H. A., Controlled Release Systems for Contraception. In: *Medical Applications of Controlled Release* (R. S. Langer and D. L. Wise, eds.), CRC Press, Boca Raton, FL, 1984, pp. 35–64.
67. Sam, A. P., In: *Minutes of 5th International Pharmaceutical Technology Symposium on New Approaches to Controlled Drug Delivery* (A. A. Hincal, et al., eds.), Editions de Santè, Paris, 1991, pp. 271–284.
68. Timmer, C. J., Apter, D., and Voortman, *Contraception*, 42:629–642 (1990).
69. Chien, Y. W., *Methods Enzymol.*, 112:461–470 (1985).
70. Hermans, W. A., *Pharm. Weekblad*, 14:253–257 (1992).
71. Witter, F. R., Rocco, L. E., and Johnson, T. R., *Am. J. Obstet. Gynecol.*, 166:830–834 (1992).
72. Lauersen, N. H., and Wilson, K. H., *Prostaglandins*, 12(Suppl.):63–79 (1976).
73. Lauersen, N. H., and Wilson, K. H., *Contraception*, 13:697–705 (1976).
74. Roseman, J. J., and Spilman, C. H. In: *Controlled Release Systems* (S. K. Chandrasekaran, ed.), AICHE Symp. Series 206, Vol. 77, American Institute of Chemical Engineers, New York, 1981.
75. Cohen, L. J., and Lordi, N. G., *J. Pharm. Sci.*, 69:955 (1980).
76. Spilman, C. H., Roseman, T. J., Baker, R. W., Tuttle, M. E., and Lonsdale, H. K., A Polymeric Controlled Release Delivery System for Prostaglandins. In: *Controlled Release Delivery Systems* (T. J. Roseman and S. A. Mansdorf, eds.), Marcel Dekker, Inc., New York, 1983, pp. 133–140.
77. Duenhoelter, J. H., Ramos, R. S., Milewich, L., and MacDonald, P. C., *Contraception*, 17:51–59 (1978).
78. Karim, S. M. M., and Ratnam, S. S., *Br. J. Obstet. Gynecol.*, 84:135–137 (1977).
79. Karim, S. M. M., Ratnam, S. S., Prasad, R. N. V., and Wong, Y. M., *Br. J. Obstet. Gynecol.*, 84:269–271 (1977).
80. Spilman, C. H., and Roseman, T. J., *Contraception*, 11:409–418 (1975).
81. Spilman, C. H., Beuving, D. C., Forbes, A. D., Roseman, T. J., and Larion, L. J., *Prostaglandins*, 12(Suppl.):1–16 (1976).
82. McNeill, M. E., and Graham, N. B., *J. Control. Rel.*, 1:99–117 (1984).
83. Currie, W. D., Joseph, I. B., and Rawlings, N. C., *J. Reprod. Fertil.*, 92:407–414 (1991).
84. Kabadi, M. B., and Chien, Y. W., *J. Pharm. Sci.*, 73:1464–1468 (1984).
85. Kabadi, M. B., and Chien, Y. W., *Drug Dev. Ind. Pharm.*, 11:1271–1312 (1985).
86. Kabadi, M. B., and Chien, Y. W., *Drug Dev. Ind. Pharm.*, 11:1313–1316 (1985).
87. Knuth, K., Amiji, M., and Robinson, J. R., *Adv. Drug Delivery Rev.*, 11: 137–167 (1993).
88. Machida, Y., Masuda, H., Fujiyama, N., Ito, S., Iwata, M., and Nagai, T., *Chem. Pharm. Bull.*, 27:93–100 (1979).
89. Gürsoy, A., and Bayhan, A., *Drug Dev. Ind. Pharm.*, 18:203–221 (1992).
90. Gürsoy, A., Sohtorik, I., Uyanik, N., and Peppas, N. A., *STP Pharma*, 5:886–892 (1989).
91. Morimoto, K., Takeeda, T., Nakamoto, Y., and Morisaka, K., *Int. J. Pharm.*, 12:107–111 (1982).
92. Bonucci, E., Ballanti, P., Ramires, R. A., Richardson, J. L., and Benedetti, L. M., *Calcif. Tissue Int.*, 56:274–279 (1995).
93. Leung, S. H. S., and Robinson, J. R., *Polymer News*, 15:333–342 (1990).

94. Cunningham, F. E., Kraus, D. M., Brubaker, L., and Fischer, J. H., *J. Clin. Pharmacol.,* 34:1060–1065 (1994).
95. Salas-Herrera, I. G., Lawson, M., Johnston, A., Turner, P., Gott, D. M., and Dennis, M. J., *Br. J. Clin. Pharmacol.,* 32:621–623 (1991).
96. Hoffmann, C., Focke, N., Franke, G., Zschiesche, M., and Siegmund, W., *Int. J. Clin. Pharm. Ther.,* 33:232–239 (1995).
97. Fischbach, F., Petersen, E. E., Weissenbacher, E. R., Martius, J., Hosmann, J., and Mayer, H., *Obstet. Gynecol.,* 82:405–410 (1993).
98. Borin, M. T., *J. Clin. Pharmacol.,* 30:33–38 (1990).
99. Lawrence, A. G., Houang, E. T., Hiscock, E., Wells, M. B., Colli, E., and Scatigna, M., *Curr. Med. Res. Opinion,* 12:114–120 (1990).
100. Boag, F. C., Houang, E. T., Westrom, R., McCormack, S. M., and Lawrence, A. G., *Genitourinary Med.,* 67:232–234 (1991).
101. Richardson, J. L., Minhas, P. S., Thomas, N. W., and Illum, L., *Int. J. Pharm.,* 56:29–36 (1989).
102. Merkus, J. M., *J. Am. Acad. Dermatol.,* 23:568–572 (1990).
103. Novelli, A. Periti, E., Massi, G. B., Masi, R., Mazzei, T., and Periti, P., *J. Chemother.,* 3:23–27 (1993).
104. O'Connell, M. E., Hoskin, P. J., Mayles, W. P,., McElwain, T. J., and Barrett, A., *Clin. Oncology,* 3:236–239 (1991).
105. Coppi, G., Silingardi, S., Girardello, R., De Aloysio, D., and Manzardo, S., *J. Chemother.,* 5:302–306 (1993).
106. Fujii, T., Naito, H., Kioka, H., Tanioka, Y., Murakami, J., Sanada, M., Tanimoto, H., Nakagawa, H., Tanaka, T., Furui, J., et al., *Japan. J. Cancer Chemo.,* 22:99–103 (1995).
107. Schraub, S., Sun, X. S., Maingon, P., Horiot, J. C., Daly, N., Keiling, R., Pigneux, J., Pourquier, H., Rozan, R., and Vrousos, C., *Cancer,* 69:2505–2509 (1992).
108. Embrey, M. P., Graham, N. B., and McNeill, M. E., *Br. Med. J.,* 281:901–902 (1980).
109. Taylor, A. V., Boland, J., and MacKenzie, I. Z., *Prostaglandins,* 40:89–98 (1990).
110. Taylor, A. V., Boland, J., Bernal, A. L., and MacKenzie, I. Z., *Prostaglandins,* 41:585–594 (1991).
111. Lyndrup, J., Nickelsen, C., Guldbaek, E., and Weber, T., *Eur. J. Obstet. Gynecol. Repr. Bio.,* 42:101–109 (1992).
112. Bennett, M. J., Horrowitz, S. D., and Wass, D. M., *Austr. New Zealand J. Obstet. Gynecol.,* 31:44–47 (1991).
113. Kurup, A., Chua, S., Arulkumaran, S., Tham, K. F., Tay, D., and Ratnam, S. S., *Austr. New Zealand J. Obstet. Gynecol.,* 31:223–226 (1991).
114. Rayburn, W. F., Wapner, R. J., Barss, V. A., Spitzberg, E., Molina, R. D., Mandsager, N., and Yonekura, M. L., *Obstet. Gynecol.,* 79:374–379 (1992).
115. Stampe Sorensen, S., Palmgren Colov, N., Andreasson, B., Bock, J. E., Berget, A., and Schmidt, T., *Acta Obstet. Gynecol. Scand.,* 71:201–206 (1992).
116. Bugalho, A., Bique, C., Machungo, F., and Bergstrom, S., *Gynecol. Obstet. Invest.,* 39:252–256 (1995).
117. Sawai, S. K., O'Brien, W. F., Mastrogiannis, D. S., Krammer, J., Mastry, M. G., and Porter, G. W., *Obstet. Gynecol.,* 84: 807–810 (1994).
118. Greer, I. A., McLaren, M., and Calder, A. A., *Acta Obstet. Gynecol. Scand.,* 69:621–625.
119. Mahmood, T. A., and Dick, M. J., *Obstet. Gynecol.,* 85:71–74 (1995).
120. Seeras, R. C., *Int. J. Gynecol. Obstet.,* 48:163–167 (1995).
121. Seeras, R. C., Olatunbosun, O. A., Pierson, R. A., and Turnell, R. W., *Clin. Exp. Obstet. Gynecol.,* 22:105–110 (1995).
122. Hill, N. C., Ferguson, J., and MacKenzie, I. Z., *Am. J. Obstet. Gynecol.,* 162:414–417 (1990).

123. Bugalho, A., Bique, C. Machungo, F., and Bergstrom, S., *Acta Obstet. Gynecol. Scand.,* 74:194–198 (1995).
124. Creinin, M. D., and Vittinghoff, E., *JAMA,* 272:1190–1195 (1994).
125. Chapvil, M., Eskelson, C. D., Stiffel, V., Owen, J., and Droegemuller, W., *Contraception,* 22:325–339 (1980).
126. Walter, B. A., Agha, B. J., and Digenis, G. A., *Toxicol. Appl. Pharmac.,* 96:258–268 (1988).
127. Diao, X. H., Zou, S., Quigg, J., Kaminski, J., and Zaneveld, L. J., *Contraception,* 42:677–682 (1990).
128. Psychoyos, A., Creatsas, G., Hassan, E., Georgoulias, V., and Gravanis, A., *Human Reprod.,* 8:866–869 (1993).
129. Bourinbaiar, A. S., and Lee-Huang, S., *Contraception,* 51:319–322 (1995).
130. Baker, V. L., *Obstet. Gynecol. Clin. N. Amer.,* 21:271–297 (1994).
131. Handa, V. L., Bachus, K. E., Johnston, W. W., Robboy, S. J., and Hammond, C. B., *Obstet. Gynecol.,* 84:215–218 (1994).
132. Henriksson, L., Stjernquist, M., Boquist, L., Alander, U., and Selinus, I., *Am. J. Obstet. Gynecol.,* 171:624–632 (1994).
133. Einer-Jensen, N., Kotwica, J., Krzymowski, T., Stefanczyk-Krzymowska, S., and Kaminski, T., *Acta Vet. Scand.,* 34:1–7 (1993).
134. Miles, R. A., Paulson, R. J., Lobo, R. A., Press, M. F., Dahmoush, L., and Sauer, M. V., *Fertil. Steril.,* 62:485–490 (1994).
135. Kimzey, L. M., Gumowski, J., Merriam, G. R., Grimes, Jr., G. J., and Nelson, L. M., *Fertil. Steril.,* 56:995–996 (1991).
136. Norman, T. R., Morse, C. A., and Dennerstein, L., *Fertil. Steril.,* 56:1034–1039 (1991).
137. Sakaguchi, M., Sakai, T., Adachi, Y., Kawashima, T., and Awata, N., *J. Pharmaco. Dyn.,* 15:67–73 (1992).
138. Okada, H., Yashiki, T., and Mima H., *J. Pharm. Sci.,* 72:173–176 (1983).
139. Richardson, J. L., Illum, L., and Thomas, N. W., *Pharm. Res.,* 9:878–883 (1992).
140. Sayani, A. P., Chun, I. K., and Chien, Y. W., *J. Pharm. Sci.,* 82:1179–1185 (1993).
141. Chen, S. A., Reed, B., Nguyen, T., Gaylord, N., Fuller, G. B., and Mordenti, J., *Pharm. Res.,* 10:223–227 (1993).
142. Chen, S. A., Perlman, A. J., Spanski, N., Peterson, C. M., Sanders, S. W., Jaffe, R., Martin, M., Yalcinkaya, T., Cefalo, R. C., Chescheir, N. C., et al., *Pharm. Res.,* 10:834–838 (1993).
143. Okada, H., Yamazaki, I., Ogawa, Y., Hirai, S., Yashiki, T., and Mima H., *J. Pharm. Sci.,* 71:1367–1371 (1982).
144. Okada, H., Yamazaki, I., Yashiki, T., and Mima H., *J. Pharm. Sci.,* 72:75–78 (1983).
145. Okada, H., Sakura, R., Kawaji, H., Yashiki, T., and Mima H., *Cancer Res.,* 43:1869–1874 (1983).
146. Okada, H., Yamazaki, I., Sakura, Y., Yashiki, T., Shimamoto, T., and Mima, H., *J. Pharm. Dyn.,* 6:512–522 (1983).
147. Okada, H., Yamazaki, I., Yashiki, T., Shinamoto, T., and Mima, H., *J. Pharm. Sci.,* 73:298–302 (1984).
148. Han, K., Park, J. S., Chung, Y. B., Lee, M. J., Moon, D. C., and Robinson, J. R., *Pharm. Res.,* 12:1539–1544 (1995).
149. O'Hagan, D. T., Rafferty, D., Wharton, S., and Illum, L., *Vaccine,* 11:660–664 (1993).
150. Eldridge, J. H., Staas, J. K., Chen, D., Marx, P. A., Tice, T. R., and Gilley, R. M., *Sem. Hematol.,* 30(Suppl.):16–24 (1993).
151. Bowen, J. C., Alpar, H. O., Phillpotts, R., and Brown, M. R., *Research Virol.,* 143:269–278 (1992).
152. O'Hagan, D. T., Rafferty, D., McKeating, J. A., and Illum, L., *J. Gen. Virol.,* 73:2141–2145 (1992).

153. Parr, M. B., and Parr, E. L., *J. Reprod. Immunol.*, 17:101–114 (1990).
154. Rush, C. M., Hafner, L. M., and Timms, P., *J. Med. Microbiol.*, 41:272–278 (1994).
155. Thapar, M. A., Parr, E. L., and Parr, M. B., *J. Reprod. Immunol.*, 17:207–216 (1990).
156. Thapar, M. A., Parr, E. L., and Parr, M. B., *Immunology*, 70:121–125 (1990).
157. Waldman, R. H., Cruz, J. M., and Rowe, D. S., *J. Immunology,* 109:662–664 (1972).
158. Uehling, D. T., Hopkins, W. J., Dahmer, L. A., and Balish, E., *J. Urology*, 152:2308–2311 (1994).
159. Ogra, P. L., and Ogra, S. S., *J. Immunology*, 110:1307–1311 (1973).
160. Smee, D. F., and Leonhardt, J. A., *Intervirology,* 37:20–24 (1994).
161. Moodley, J., Cohen, M., Devraj, K., and Dutton, M., *S. African Med. J.,* 81:150–152 (1992).
162. Ginsburg, J., Hardiman, P., and Thomas, M., *Lancet*, 338:1205–1206 (1991).
163. Baldock, G. A., Brodie, R. R., Chasseaud, L. F., Taylor, T., Walmsley, L. M., and Catanese, B., *Biopharm. Drug. Disp.*, 12:481–492 (1991).
164. Vande Wiele, R. L., and Dyrenfurth, I., *Pharmacol. Rev.*, 25:189–207 (1973).
165. Owada, E., Behl, C. R., Hwang, S. S., Suhardja, L., and Flynn, G. L., *J. Pharm. Sci.,* 66:216–219 (1977).

KAREN YU
YIE W. CHIEN

Validation of Pharmaceutical Processes

Process validation is a requirement of current Good Manufacturing Practices (cGMPs) for finished pharmaceuticals (21 CFR 211) and of the GMP regulations for medical devices (21 CFR 820) and therefore applies to the manufacture of both drug products and medical devices.

According to the FDA *Guidelines on General Principles of Process Validation* [1], process validation is defined, ". . . as establishing documented evidence, which provides a high degree of assurance, that a specific process will consistently produce a product meeting its predetermined specifications and quality characteristics." The process for making a drug product consists of a series (flow diagram in logically defined steps) of unit operations (modules) that result in the manufacture of the finished pharmaceutical.

There is much confusion regarding the definition of process validation and what constitutes process validation documentation. The term validation is used here generically to cover the entire spectrum of cGMP concerns, most of which are essentially facility, equipment, component, method, and process qualification. Based upon the FDA process validation guidelines [1], the specific term should be reserved for the final stage(s) of the product and process development sequence. The essential or key steps or stages of a successfully completed development program are shown in Table 1.

The end of the development sequence, which should be assigned to formal (three-batch) process validation, derives from the fact that the specific exercise of process validation should never be designed to fail. Failure in carrying out the formal process validation assignment is often the result of incomplete or faulty understanding of the process capability, in other words, what the process can and cannot accomplish under a given set of operational requirements.

In a well-designed validation program, most of the effort should be spent on facilities, equipment, components, methods, and process qualification. In such a program, the formalized, final three-batch validation sequence provides only the necessary process validation documentation required by the FDA to show product reproducibility and a manufacturing process in a state of control. Such a strategy is consistent with the FDA preapproval inspection program directive [2].

Process Validation Options

The guidelines on general principles of process validation [1] mention three options: prospective process validation (also called premarket validation), retrospective process validation, and revalidation. Actually there are four, if concurrent process validation is included.

Prospective validation is carried out prior to the distribution of a new product or an existing product made under a revised manufacturing process where such revisions may affect product specifications or quality characteristics. The prospective approach

TABLE 1 Process Validation is the Last Step in Development

Developmental Stage	Batch Size
Product design Product characterization Product selection Process design	1 X
Product optimization Process characterization Process optimization Process qualification	10 X
Process qualification Process validation Process certification	100 X
Process revalidation	100 X to 1000 X

features critical step analysis in which the unit operations are challenged during the process qualification stage to determine those critical process variables that may affect overall process performance, using either worst-case analysis or a fractional factorial design. During formal, three-batch, prospective validation, critical process variables should be set within their operating ranges and should not exceed their upper and lower control limits during process operation. Output responses should be well within finished-product specifications.

Retrospective validation is recognized in both cGMPs (21 CFR 211.110(b)) and the process validation guidelines [1]. It involves accumulated in-process production and final product testing and control (numerical) data to establish that the product and its manufacturing process are in a state of control. Valid in-process results should be consistent with the final specifications of the drug product and shall be derived from previous acceptable process average and process variability estimates where possible and determined by the application of suitable statistical procedures (quality control charting) where appropriate.

The retrospective validation option is chosen for established products whose manufacturing processes are considered to be stable and when, on the basis of economic considerations and resource limitations, prospective qualification and validation experimentation cannot be justified. Prior to undertaking either prospective or retrospective validation, the facilities, equipment, and subsystems used in connection with the manufacturing process must be qualified in conformance with cGMP requirements.

Concurrent validation studies are carried out under a protocol during the course of normal production. The first three production-scale batches must be monitored as comprehensively as possible. The evaluation of the results is used in establishing the acceptance criteria and specifications of subsequent in-process control and final product testing. Some form of concurrent validation, using statistical process control techniques (quality control charting) may be employed throughout the product manufacturing life cycle.

Validation of Pharmaceutical Processes

Revalidation is required to ensure that changes in the process and/or in the process environment, whether introduced intentionally or unintentionally, do not adversely affect product specifications and quality characteristics [2]. There should be a quality assurance system (change control) in place which requires revalidation whenever there are significant changes in formulation, equipment, process, and packaging that may impact on product and manufacturing process performance [3]. Furthermore, when a change is made in a raw material supplier, the drug manufacturer should be made aware of subtle, potentially adverse differences in raw material characteristics that may adversely affect product and manufacturing process performance.

It is recommended that every requested change be reviewed by the validation committee, group, or team. Such a committee should judge if a change is significant for revalidation and decide upon a course of action to be taken. The following conditions require revalidation study and documentation:

1. Change in a critical component (usually refers to active drug substance, key excipients, or primary packaging);
2. Change or replacement in a critical piece of modular (capital) equipment;
3. Significant change in processing conditions that may affect subsequent unit operations and product quality;
4. Change in a facility and/or plant (usually location, site, or support systems);
5. Significant increase or decrease in batch size that affects the operation of modular equipment; and
6. Sequential batches that fail to meet product and process specifications.

In some situations process performance requalification studies may be required prior to undertaking specific revalidation assignments. With the exception of sterile products manufacture, periodic revalidation is not required at the present time. The performance and state of control of the product and its manufacturing process can be adequately covered during the annual product and process review. The FDA has issued an interim guidance document that addresses what constitutes major and minor formulation and manufacturing changes for immediate-release solid dosage forms [4]. Such documentation and others to follow should simplify manufacturing decisions about the need to revalidate.

The Validation Committee

In most companies, the validation committee, group, or team is charged with the responsibility of establishing and operating the complete validation program. In some companies the program is led by a validation manager whereas in others, quality assurance personnel have taken on expanded responsibilities in this regard.

Specific process validation assignments are carried out by those with the necessary training and experience. The specifics of how the committee, group, or team is organized to conduct process validation assignments is beyond the scope of this article. The responsibilities that must be carried out and the traditional organizational structures best equipped to handle each of these assignments are outlined in Table 2.

TABLE 2 Composition of the Process Validation Committee

Representative of	Function
Engineering	Qualifies for plant, facilities, equipment, and support systems
Development	Qualifies for product and manufacturing process
Manufacturing	Operates plant, facilities, equipment, support systems and manufacturing process
Quality assurance	Audits plant, facilities, equipment, support systems, manufacturing process, and product

Validation Master Plan

The creation of a master plan permits the development of a logical overview of the validation effort. It lays out in a logical sequence the activities and/or key elements to be performed in accordance with the approximate time schedule in a Gantt or PERT chart format. The master plan establishes the critical path through the chart against which progress can be monitored.

The validation program starts with the design and development of raw materials and components, followed by the IQ/OQ of facilities, equipment, and systems through performance and process qualification stages, and terminates in the protocol-driven, three-batch, formal process validation program. Most of these activities move forward in series. However, by combining activities and elements and moving in parallel, where possible, on independent tracks with respect to bulk pharmaceutical chemicals (BPC)s, analytical methods development, facilities, equipment, support systems, and the drug product design and manufacturing process development, a great deal of time can be saved before the individual elements or grouping of activities are combined prior to the formal process validation program. A Gantt chart is shown in Fig. 1.

Installation Qualification (IQ)

This includes procedures and documentation to show that all important aspects of the installation of the facility, support system, or piece of modular equipment, having been properly calibrated, meet its design specifications and that the vendor's recommendations had been suitably considered.

Operational Qualification (OQ)

Following IQ, procedures and documentation show that the facility, support system, or piece of modular equipment perform as intended throughout all anticipated operating ranges under a suitable load.

Performance Qualification (PQ)

Following IQ and OQ, actual demonstrations during the course of the validation program show that the facility, support system, or piece of modular equipment perform according to a predefined protocol and achieve process reproducibility and product acceptability.

Validation of Pharmaceutical Processes

		Qualification stage			Validation stage	
Key elements	Design stage	Installation	Operational		Prospective	Concurrent
Facilities and equipment	Engineering phase →	(Validation protocols)	→	Manufacturing start-up →	(Batch records and validation documentation)	
Process and product Including BPC and analytical methods	Developmental phase (formula definition and stability testing)	↗	Scale-up phase (process optimization and pilot production) →	↑		QA and manufacturing pahse (full production)
			Time line for new product introduction			

FIG. 1. Validation progress Gantt chart.

Validation Protocol and Report

The following validation protocol and format for the completed validation report have been suggested in the WHO *Guidelines on Validation of Manufacturing Processes* (TRS 823) [5].

1. Purpose (for the whole validation) and prerequisites
2. Presentation of the whole process and subprocesses including flow diagram and critical step analysis
3. Validation protocol approvals
4. Installation and operational qualifications, including blueprints or drawings
5. Qualification report(s)
   a. Subprocess 1
   b. Purpose
   c. Methods and procedures
   d. Sampling and testing procedures, release criteria
   e. Reporting function
   f. Calibration of test equipment
   g. Test data
   h. Summary of results
   i. Approval and requalification procedure

   a. Subprocess 2 (repeat)
6. Product qualification, test data from prevalidation batches
7. Product validation, test data from three formal validation batches
8. Evaluation and recommendations (include revalidation and requalification requirements)
9. Certification (approval)
10. Summary report with conclusions

The validation protocol and report may also include copies of the product stability report or its summary as well as validation documentation on cleaning and analytical methods.

Pre-Approval Inspection

The FDA Pre-approval Inspection Program [2] is designed to provide a basis for determining the adequacy and accuracy of reported and factual information in New Drug Application (NDA) and Abbreviated New Drug Application (ANDA) submissions with respect to the suitability of cGMP product development, analytical laboratory, and manufacturing facilities.

A preapproval inspection checklist should include the following documentation which may be required prior to the formal inspection:

1. Active drug substance development and validation report(s) including impurity profile and polymorphic forms;

Validation of Pharmaceutical Processes

2. Pharmaceutical (dosage form) development report;
3. Stability and clinical batch records and history, including phase-III program;
4. Data for active drug substance and key excipients used in the manufacture of clinical and biobatches;
5. Bioequivalency report;
6. Technical transfer report (development to manufacturing/QA/QC);
7. Copy of the CMC section of the NDA including information on suppliers and vendors;
8. Copy of proposed production monograph and master batch record;
9. Equipment validation report establishing IQ and OQ;
10. Cleaning validation report;
11. Analytical methods validation and computer systems validation reports;
12. Stability report establishing expiry dating; and
13. Process validation protocol for formal three-batch validation of production-size batches.

During preapproval inspection, the FDA accepts a process-validation protocol based upon the company's commitment to complete successfully three production-size validation batches prior to product launch. In some situations a prevalidation (process qualification) production-size batch is completed or the entire formal three-batch program is carried out.

Pilot Scale-Up and Technical Transfer

The pilot-production program may be carried out as a shared responsibility between the development laboratories and their appropriate manufacturing counterpart or as a process demonstration by a separate, designated pilot-plant or process development department. Supporting technical transfer documentation applies to both the specific process and system being qualified and validated and the related testing standards and testing methods. The formal technical transfer is normally made from the development laboratories or the process development pilot-plant to pharmaceutical production function.

In actuality, a number of technical transfer points and documents are generated as prospective validation proceeds through the various stages of product development. These stages of technical transfer in terms of scale-up are illustrated in Fig. 2.

Solid pharmaceutical dosage forms (tablets and capsules) are used to illustrate the various stages of product and process development. These principles and practices also apply in a general way to the development of liquid and semisolid pharmaceutical dosage forms (not discussed here).

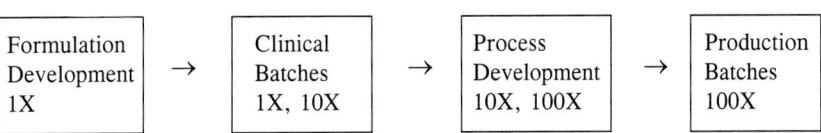

FIG. 2. Technical transfer stages.

Stages of Validation

Elements of the validation concept should be incorporated during each of the various stages of the product and process development continuum. These stages can be summarized as follows:

Preformulation Studies: BPCs
    Stage I   Product design and development
    Stage II   Preparation of clinical and biobatches
    Stage III Process scale-up and evaluation
    Stage IV Formal process validation

Preformulation Studies: Bulk Pharmaceutical Chemicals

Preformulation testing of the specific active drug substance of interest and key excipients to be used in the product design stage, alone and in combinations with the active drug substance, should be included as a preliminary first step in the product and process development sequence. A simple check list of items worth consideration in preformulation studies with bulk pharmaceutical chemicals (both active drug substances and important or critical excipients) is provided below.

- Active drug substance
- Key excipients
    Fillers and diluents
    Binders
    Disintegrants
    Glidants and lubricants
- Chemical and physical compatibility
- Minimum lot-to-lot variability in properties
- Worldwide availability from comparable suppliers
- Properties for possible evaluation
    Color, odor, taste, solubility;
    Particle morphology (DSC, TGA, x-ray diffraction);
    Particle size distribution and surface area;
    Crystal and bulk density, and compaction index;
    Angle of repose and flowability index;
    Spectrophotometry (UV, FTIR, NMR, OR);
    Water content, LOD, moisture uptake;
    Microbial limits and heavy metals;
    HPLC assay and impurity profile.

Before preformulation studies are undertaken, two-way technical communication between the manufacturers of the active drug substance (laboratory and plant) and the pharmaceutical product development laboratories must be established. It should start early and be maintained through-out the product and process development program.

In addition to potency, purity, and stability considerations of the active drug substance, the product development department is especially interested in the chemical and

Validation of Pharmaceutical Processes

physical form (free acid or base, salts, esters, amides, polymorphs, solvates, particle size and shape) of the active drug substance. Time spent early in the cycle in establishing these particular factors often aids and/or simplifies the subsequent product and process development program.

Not every subject shown above must be tested or addressed. However, aspect, particle morphology and size, compaction and flowability, water content, spectrophotometric and chromatographic data should be studied and monitored throughout the product and process development program [6,7].

Since key excipients are well established in most new product and process development programs, the same degree of preformulation scrutiny is often not required. Compatibility studies with the active drug substance, however, should be performed to study possible untoward interactions between the active ingredients and the excipients. It should be kept in mind that small or minor changes in physical and possibly chemical properties upon intimate contact in binary studies with key excipients should not automatically exclude a favored excipient without further critical testing.

Stage-I Product Design and Development

Following successful preformulation studies, the active drug substance is transferred to the formulations laboratory for preliminary product design and development studies. In most cases, the drug is mixed with an appropriate diluent or filler and glidant combination and filled into two-piece opaque hard-shell capsules for preliminary stability and subsequent phase I clinical studies vs. matching placebo capsules [8]. At or about the same time, initial studies of a prototype tablet formulation should be started. The key steps in the product design and development sequence are given below.

- Stage-I Product Design: 1X Laboratory Scale (1–10 Kg)
  Hard-shell capsule (phase I clinical trials) followed by prototype tablet dosage form
  Direct compression vs. wet granulation
  Maximum chemical and physical stability
  Minimum product and process costs
  Product characterization
  Product selection
  Process design
- Excipients are selected from the following:
  Binder, diluents, and disintegrants including alginates, calcium phosphate, cellulose dextrates, gelatin, povidones, starch and derivatives, sorbitol, sucrose, and derivatives. Glidants and lubricants including colloidal silicon dioxide, hydrogenated vegetable oil, mineral oil, PEG, silica gel, sodium lauryl sulfate, stearates, talc.

Although the work is conducted in the research or formulations laboratory using small-scale processing equipment, it is important to gain early experience with colorant systems that have been selected for the finished tablet product; color aids in blend-uniformity evaluation.

In addition to excipient screening and selection, it is important to gauge processing prarameters that are more fully explored during the scale-up phases. These processing factors include flowability, compaction and compressibility of powders and granules, content uniformity of powder and granule blends and finished tablets, moisture uptake, in vitro dissolution release profiles, and subsequent full-scale stability testing.

Products used in human clinical trials must, of course, conform to good laboratory, good clinical, and good manufacturing practice requirements [1,9].

Stage-II Process Development: Pilot Laboratory (Clinical)

After the (1X) "go" laboratory batch has been determined to be both physically and chemical stable, based upon accelerated, elevated temperature testing (1 month at 45°C or 3 month at 40 or 40°C and 80% relative humidity) the next step (stage II) is to scale the product and its process to (10X) pilot-laboratory size batch(es). This batch represents the first replicated scale-up of the designated formula. Its size usually ranges between 10 and 100 kg, 10 and 100 L, or 10,000 to 100,000 units. Often these pilot-laboratory batches are used in clinical trials and bioequivalency studies. According to the FDA, the minimum requirement for a biobatch is 100,000 units [10].

Pilot-laboratory batches are usually prepared in small pilot equipment within a designated cGMP approved facility. The number and size of these pilot-laboratory batches may vary, depending on one or more of the following factors:

- Equipment availability
- Active drug substance availability
- Cost of raw materials
- Inventory requirements for both clinical and nonclinical studies

Process development (process qualification) or process capability studies are normally started in this important stage II of the scale-up sequence. The scope of stage-II process development consists essentially of product optimization and process characterization studies.

- Product Optimization:
  Establish formula rationale and boundary conditions for active substance and excipients
- Process Characterization:
  Define unit operations, process variables, and response parameters.
  Define critical process variables and response parameters using simple experimental designs.
  Establish provisional control limits for critical process variables and their response parameters based upon process replication.
- Maintain product stability.
- Unit operations for solid dosage-form development:
  Granulation
  Drying
  Sizing
  Blending and mixing
  Encapsulation and tablet compression
  Coating

Validation of Pharmaceutical Processes

Unit operations are selected for the development of a tablet (coated or not coated) or capsule (hard shell or soft-gel) process [11]. Unit operations that are considered to be critical are determined through an analysis of the process variables and their respective measured responses in each unit operation (Table 3) [12–14].

In order to apply the critical control parameters and their unit operation, constraint analysis techniques [15] followed by fractional factorial designs (Table 4) are used to challenge the tentative control limits (so-called worst-case analysis) established for the process at this intermediate stage. Time and effort spent to qualify the process at the 10X stage often simplifies the work that follows during stages III and IV.

Von Doehren, et al. [13] and Chowhan [16] have described the various stages of solid dosage form process development as it relates to technology transfer and process validation. Their respective approaches to the topic have been integrated in this article.

TABLE 3 Control Parameters for Solid-Dosage-Form Development

Unit Operation	Process Variables (X)[a]	Measured Responses (Y)[b]
Granulation (Power type)	Load Speed (main chopper) Liquid addition rate Granulation time	Power consumption
Drying	Load Inlet temperature Air-flow rate Drying time	Moisture content Bulk density
Sizing (Screening)	Load Screen size Speed Feed rate	Particle size distr. Bulk density
Blending (Mixing)	Load Speed Mixing time	Blend uniformity
Encapsulation	Fill volume Tamper setting Speed Glidant (type, amount)	Capsule weight Moisture content Dissolution Content uniformity Potency
Tablet compression	Press speed Feed rate Precompression force Compression force	Tablet weight Moisture content Hardness/friability Thickness Dissolution/disintegration Content uniformity Potency
Coating (Film type)	Load Pan speed Spray rate Air flow	Weight gain

[a]7-23 possible variables.
[b]11-16 possible responses.

TABLE 4 Fractional Factorial Design for Process Development[a]

Trials	Key Variables[b]							Sums
	X_1	X_2	X_3	X_4	X_5	X_6	X_7	
1	−	−	−	−	−	−	−	0/7
2	−	−	−	+	−	−	−	1/6
3	−	−	+	−	−	+	−	2/5
4	+	+	−	−	+	−	−	3/4
5	+	+	−	−	−	+	+	4/3
6	+	−	+	+	+	−	+	5/2
7	−	+	+	+	+	+	+	6/1
8	+	+	+	+	+	+	+	7/0
Sums	4/4	4/4	4/4	4/4	4/4	4/4	4/4	28/28

[a]Adapted from Hendrix, C. D., What every technologist should know about experimental design, *CHEMTECH* (March 1979).
[b]Key variables are randomly assigned an "X" value.

Fahrner [17] raises the following issues regarding the new role for pilot plants in product development.

- Too much time is devoted to preliminary or applied research and not enough to the proper development of the process.
- Often a suitable manufacturing strategy is lacking during the early phases of the program, which results in poorly planned technology transfer and an inappropriate division of responsibility with respect to the overall program.
- Most laboratory processes are rarely scalable, since piloting is a scaled-down version of manufacturing not a scaled-up version of the laboratory batch.

Fahrner makes the case for a separate pilot facility (process development function) to bridge the communication gap between R & D and production.

Stage-III Pilot Production

The technical transfer of the product and process from the traditional product development function to a separate process development (pilot plant) function or production itself is normally carried out at the (100X) pilot-production batch stage (100–1000 kg):

- Full-scale production batch
- For possible future commercial clinical use
- Evaluate critical process parameters; product and process are scaled to another order of magnitude (100X)
- Process optimization
  Mixing and blending times
  Drying times
  Milling operations
  Press speed, compression force

Validation of Pharmaceutical Processes

Encapsulation speed, tamping settings
Speed, air flow, spray settings, temperature
- Process qualification (prevalidation batches); determine process capability, challenge in-process control limits
- Maintain product stability

The creation of a separate pilot plant or process development unit has been favored in recent years because it is ideally suited to carry out key process qualification and/or process validation studies in a timely manner [18,19].

The objective of the pilot-production batch is to scale the product and its process by another order of magnitude (100X). For most solid dosage forms it represents a full production scale batch in standard equipment. The technical transfer documents should include the technical package normally required for preapproval inspection:

1. Preformulation information
2. Product development report
3. Product stability report
4. Analytical methods report
5. Proposed manufacturing formula, manufacturing instruction, in-process and final product specifications at the 100X-batch size

The objectives of prevalidation trials at stage III (100X pilot production) is to qualify and optimize the process in full-scale production equipment and facilities.

Rushing through the first (100X) pilot-production batch in order to proceed with formal validation should be discouraged. Small problems that often arise during (100X) scale-up should be addressed immediately and not ignored. Such problems are often best addressed by returning to the laboratories (10X) for supplemental process characterization and qualification studies.

Many companies, however, proceed directly to three-batch formal validation without stage III prevalidation work and often complete formal trials prior to preapproval inspection. The downside of this alternative strategy is that finished production batches often remain in the warehouse beyond their approved expiry dating period.

When faced with a choice of strategies, there is no one ideal way of completing the pilot scale-up and validation sequence other than depending upon prior experience with related products and processes.

Stage-IV Formal Process Validation

In the normal course of events and following a successfully completed preapproval inspection, formal, three-batch process validation is carried out in accordance with the protocol approved during the preapproval inspection. The primary objective of the formal process validation exercise is to establish process reproducibility and consistency. The program is not designed to challenge upper and lower control limits (so-called worst-case analysis) of critical process variables. Such upper and lower control limit challenging is normally conducted during the stage II (10X size) process characterization, optimization, and qualification program, using suitable and reasonable experimental designs (Table 4).

The documentation to be established before, during, and after formal process validation is shown below. The protocols and the subsequent formal validation studies are designed to establish uniformity among the three batches with respect to granulation, blend, finished tablet, and finished capsule stages [1,2,10].

100X Production Batches

- Complete product development program and report
- Prepare protocol for prospective process validation
- Complete preapproval inspection requirements; conduct three-batch formal process validation, establish reproducibility for mixing, blending, and compression or encapsulation operations
- Establish process documentation
  Preformulation report
  Analytical methods validation report
  IQ/OQ and cleaning validation reports
  Formula development report
  Process feasibility report
  Manufacturing bioequivalency report
  Product development report
  Process validation protocol
  Process validation report
  Product stability report

In that respect, the following test data and results are used to show process reproducibility and consistency among validation batches: particle or granule size distribution, bulk density, moisture content, hardness, thickness, friability, weight uniformity, potency uniformity, disintegration–dissolution profile, and product stability. Not every one of these categories have to be addressed nor followed both during in-process and final product testing. Nevertheless, testing must be sufficient to establish process reproducibility and demonstrate, with a high degree of certainly, that the product and process are under control.

Whenever possible, formal validation studies should continue through packaging and labeling operations (whole or in-part), so that machinability and stability of the finished product can be established and documented in the primary container–closure system.

Change Control

Procedures with respect to establishing change control should be in place before, during, and after the completion of the formal validation program. A change control system maintains a sense of functionality as the process evolves and provides the necessary documentation trail that ensures that the process continues in a validated, operational state, even when small noncritical adjustments and changes have been made. Such minor, noncritical changes in materials, methods, and machines should be reviewed by the validation team (development, engineering, production, and QA/QC) to ensure all that process integrity and process comparability has been maintained and documented before the specific change that has been requested can be approved by the head of the quality control unit.

The change control system, based upon an approved standard operating procedure(s) (SOPs), takes on added importance as the vehicle or instrument through which innovation and process improvements can be made more easily and more flexibly without prior formal review on the part of the NDA and ANDA reviewing function of the FDA. If more of the supplemental procedures with respect to the chemistry and manufacturing control sections of NDAs and ANDAs could be covered through annual review documentation procedures, with appropriate safeguards, process validation will become more innovative. [20–22].

Out-of-Specifications

Probably the single most important technical issue facing the pharmaceutical industry at the present time is the question: what constitutes process or batch failure in terms of an out-of-specification (OOS) assay value? The concept of product and/or process failure appears twice in the cGMPs [3].

According to 21 CFR Sect. 211.165(f), "Drug products failing to meet established standards or specifications and other relevant quality control criteria shall be rejected." In CFR Sect. 211.192 it is stated:

> Any unexplained discrepancy (including a percentage of theoretical yield exceeding the maximum or minimum percentages established in master production and control records) or the failure of a batch or any of its components to meet any of its specifications shall be thoroughly investigated [regardless] whether the batch has already been distributed. The investigation shall extend to other batches of the same drug product and other drug products that may have been associated with the specific failure or discrepancy. A written record of the investigation shall be made and shall include the conclusions and follow-up.

The key to establishing product and/or process failure is to verify the accuracy, relevance, and reproducibility of deviant assay value(s), test result(s), and recorded number(s) that are reported [23]. All companies should have SOPs in place that cover first the verification of deviant numbers in the quality control laboratories and, following that investigation and a report showing the test result to be deviant, a second set of SOPs covering follow-up actions taken such as the following steps:

1. A written procedure for full investigation when not a verified laboratory error,
2. Scientific criteria for retesting and resampling during the formal investigation,
3. Description and results of the formal investigation into possible causes of the OOS result(s),
4. Results of all testing involved during the investigation,
5. A scientific basis and justification for discarding any OOS test result and accepting the batch in question,
6. Final determination of conformity to appropriate specifications and justification of the actions taken, and
7. Signature of individual(s) responsible for final decision(s) and the action(s) taken.

Even though the responsibility for batch acceptance or rejection lies with the head of the quality control unit, the help of the validation team should prove useful in reviewing the process of OOS investigation and arriving at a recommendation for action taken.

Cleaning Validation

According to 21 CFR Sect. 211.67, Equipment Cleaning and Maintenance of cGMP regulations [3], equipment and utensils should be cleaned, maintained, and sanitized at appropriate intervals to prevent malfunction or contamination that would alter the safety, identity, strength, quality, or purity of the drug product. Written procedures shall be established and followed for cleaning and maintenance of equipment. These procedures shall include, but are not limited to the assignment of responsibility for cleaning and maintaining equipment; maintenance, cleaning, and sanitizing schedules where appropriate; description in sufficient detail of methods, equipment, and materials used in cleaning and maintenance operations, and the methods of disassembling and reassembling equipment as necessary to assure proper cleaning and maintenance; removal or obliteration of previous batch identification, protection of clean equipment from contamination prior to use; and inspection of equipment for cleanliness immediately before use. Records shall be kept of maintenance, cleaning, sanitizing, and inspection.

The objective of cleaning validation of equipment and utensils is to reduce the residues of one product below established limits so that the residue of the previous product does not affect the quality and safety of the subsequent product manufactured in the same equipment.

According to 21 CFR Sect. 211.63, Equipment Design, Size, and Location, of cGMP regulations [3], equipment used in the manufacture, processing, packing, or holding of a drug product shall be of appropriate design, adequate size, and suitably located to facilitate operations for its intended use and for its cleaning and maintenance. Some of the equipment design considerations include type of surface to be cleaned (stainless steel, glass, plastic), use of disposables or dedicated equipment and utensils (bags, filters, etc.), of stationary equipment (tanks, mixers, centrifuges, presses, etc.), of special features (clean-in-place systems, steam-in-place systems), and identifying the difficult-to-clean locations on the equipment (so-called hot spots or critical sites).

The specific cleaning procedure should define the amounts and the specific type of cleaning agents and/or solvents used. The cleaning procedure should give full details as to what is to be cleaned and how it is to be cleaned. The cleaning method should focus on worst-case conditions, such as highest-strength, least-soluble, most difficult to clean formulations. Cleaning procedures should identify the time between processing and cleaning, cleaning sequence, equipment dismantling procedure, need for visual inspection, and provisions for documentation.

The choice of a particular analytical method (HPLC, TLC, spectrophotometric, total organic carbon, pH, conductivity, gravimetric, etc.) and sampling technique chosen (direct surface by swabs and gauze or by rinsing) depends on the residue limit to be established, based upon the sampling site, type of residue sought, and equipment configuration (critical sites vs. large surface area) considerations. The analytical and sampling methods should be challenged in terms of specificity, sensitivity, and recovery.

Validation of Pharmaceutical Processes

The established residue limits must be practical, achievable, verifiable, and assure safety. The potency of selected drug and presence of degradation products, cleaning agents, and microorganisms should be taken into consideration.

The following residue limits have been suggested: not more-than (NMT) 10 ppm or NMT 0.001% of the dose of any product appears in the maximum daily dose of another product and no residue visible on the equipment after cleaning procedures have been performed.

Bulk Pharmaceutical Chemicals

Bulk pharmaceutical chemicals (BPCs) are components of finished drug products and are therefore active drug substances or key or critical excipients (inert ingredients). Key or critical excipients are BPCs that affect the final specifications and/or quality attributes of the finished drug product and are recognized by the USP/NF. A list of key excipients for solid dosage forms is given below.

- Diluents, Fillers, and Binders
  Calcium phosphate, dibasic
  Dextrates
  Dextrin
  Lactose (anhydrous, fast flow)
  Mannitol
  Starch (corn)
  Sugar, compressible
- Tablet Disintegrants
  Cellulose, microcrystalline
  Croscarmellose sodium
  Crospovidone
  Sodium starch glycolate
  Starch, pregelatinized
- Tablet and Capsule Lubricants
  Magnesium stearate
  Mineral oil, light
  Polyethylene glycol
  Sodium stearyl fumarate
  Stearic acid, purified
  Talc
  Vegetable oil, hydrogenated
- Other Excipients
  Carboxymethylcellulose sodium
  Cellulose acetate phthalate
  Ethylcellulose
  Hydroxypropyl cellulose
  Hydroxypropyl methylcellulose
  Hydroxypropyl methylcellulose phthalate
  Methacrylic acid copolymer

Polysorbates
Polyvinyl acetate phthalate
Povidone
Sodium lauryl sulfate

A chemical is considered to be a BPC if it is intended for medicinal purposes. Regulatory agencies however, place greater emphasis and priority on the manufacture and validation of active drug substances.

According to Sect. 501 (a)(2)(b) of the Food, Drug and Cosmetic (FD&C) Act, all drugs must be manufactured, processed, packed, and held in accordance with cGMPs. No distinction is made between BPCs and finished drug products.

Elements common to both BPCs and finished drug products include facilities and equipment qualification (IQ/OQ, and PQ), cleaning validation, validation of water supplies, microbial limits for nonsterile material, manufacture of sterile and pyrogen-free material, in-process blending and mixing, analytical methods validation, laboratory controls and in-process testing, change control procedures and revalidation, reprocessing, packaging and labeling, and stability testing.

Process

There are four primary processes used in the manufacture of BPCs. They are chemical synthesis, fermentation, extraction, and purification. A flow diagram (Fig. 3.) and a description of the chemistry involved are helpful in defining the process. The process description should include appropriate parameters, such as charging quantities or volumes of reactants or solvents, reaction times, temperatures, pressures, etc. Critical processing steps and critical operating parameters should be maintained to ensure batch-to-batch consistency, product yield, and quality.

Where in the chain of unit operations (chemical process) does BPC validation start? As long as key intermediates are made in the plant, they and their reaction and processing steps should be subjected to an appropriate cGMP and process qualification-validation program. A key intermediate is defined as an intermediate in which an essential molecular characteristic, usually related to stereochemical configuration, is introduced into the final BPC structure (moeity).

Physical Characteristics

Besides purity (chemical potency), the physical characteristics and properties of the BPC are extremely important to the end user (drug product manufacturer). Characteristics such as crystal morphology, particle size and shape, bulk density, melting point, optical rotation, etc., have a profound effect upon the drug product and its performance and stability. In addition to the reaction or extraction step, crystallization, milling, and blending unit operations must be subject to qualification and validation.

Impurity Profile

The USP permits up to 2% of ordinary nontoxic impurities. However, impurities above 0.1% should be fully characterized and quantified. Impurities may include starting materials, by-products, intermediates, degradation products, reagents, catalysts, heavy

Validation of Pharmaceutical Processes

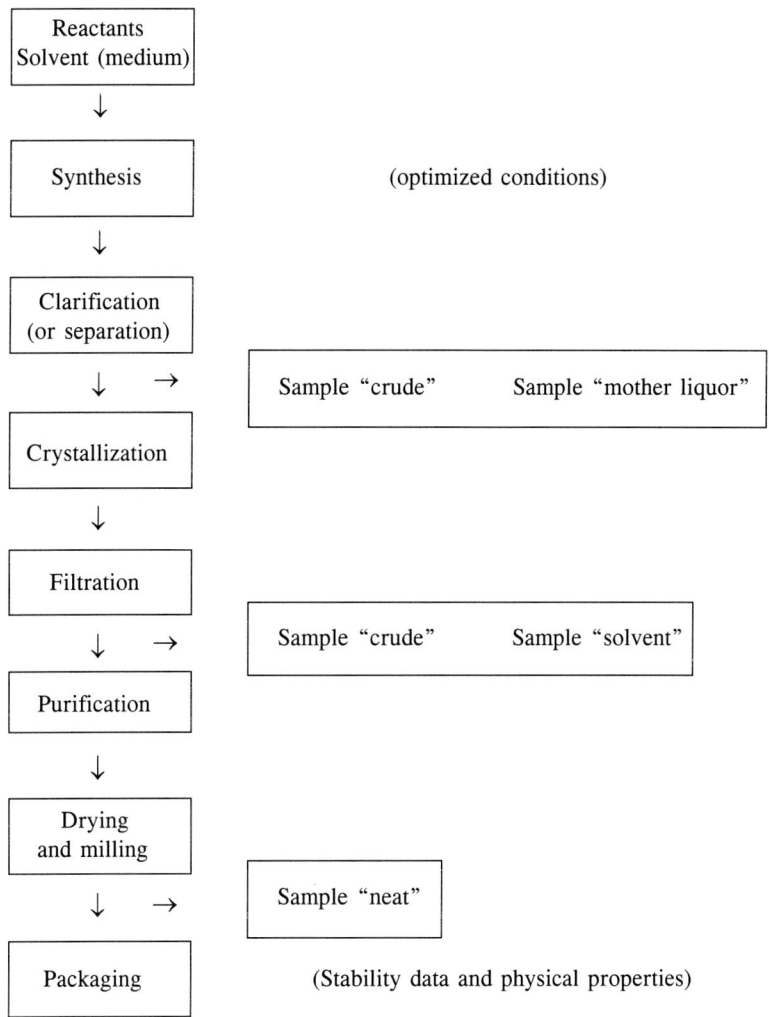

FIG. 3. Manufacture of bulk pharmaceutical chemicals.

metals, electrolytes, filter aids, and residual solvents. Known toxic impurities must be held to a tighter standard, i.e., below 0.1%.

The ISO Quality Standards Series

The ISO 9000 Series was developed in 1987 by the International Organization for Standardization (ISO) in Geneva, Switzerland. It is a comprehensive set of management standards governing the operation of quality assurance to help develop and document a quality system that is useful for individual companies.

The ISO 9000 Quality Management and Quality Assurance Standards, Guidelines for Selection and Use, provide basic definitions and concepts and explain how to use the rest of the series (9001, 9002, 9003, and 9004).

TABLE 5 Meeting Quality Standards

	ISO 9000 Series	cGMPs
1.	Management responsibility	Organization, personnel
2.	Quality system	Organization, personnel
		Laboratory Controls
		Records, reports
3.	Contract review	Holding, distribution
4.	Design control	Production and process controls
5.	Document control	Records, reports
6.	Purchase products	Control of components, drug product containers, closures
7.	Supplied product	Holding, distribution
8.	Product identification, traceability	Packaging and labeling control
9.	Process control	Production and process control
10.	Procedures for inspection, testing	Laboratory controls
11.	Inspection, measuring, testing equipment	Laboratory controls
		Production, and process controls
12.	Inspection, testing status	Laboratory controls
13.	Control of nonconforming products	Returned and salvaged drug products
14.	Corrective action	Records, reports
15.	Handling, storage, packaging, delivery	Packaging and labeling control
		Holding, distribution
16.	Quality records	Records, reports
17.	Internal quality audits	Laboratory controls
18.	Training needs	Organization, personnel
19.	Servicing procedures	Equipment
20.	Statistical techniques	Building, facilities
		Production and process controls

The ISO 9001 Quality System—Model for Quality Assurance in Design and Development provides for quality assurance in the areas of design, installation, servicing, development, and production. It is useful primarily for companies that design and develop their own products.

The ISO 9002 Quality System—Model for Quality Assurance in Production, Installation and Service applies to manufacturers, distributors, and service vendors whose products have been designed and serviced by a subcontractor. Such companies are exempt from design control requirements. Both ISO 9001 and ISO 9002 are directly applicable to cGMPs. The connection between the two independent systems is shown in Table 5. Except for language, shades of meaning, and stresses the documents are similar.

The ISO 9003 Quality Systems—Model for Quality Assurance in Inspection and Testing, designed for testing laboratories and equipment distributors only requires conformance to final inspection and testing procedures.

The ISO 9004 Quality Management and Quality Systems Elements—Guidelines provide standards and guidelines for quality management planning and implementation.

Appendix
Glossary of Terms Used in Process Validation

Acceptance activities
Acceptance criteria
Analytical methods validation
Audit of suppliers

Bulk pharmaceutical chemicals (BPCs)

Calibration
Certification
Challenge testing
Chemistry and manufacturing control (CMC)
Cleaning validation
Component
Computer qualification
Concurrent validation
Critical processing variables

Design change
Design of experiments
Design history
Design input
Design output
Design review
Design transfer
Design validation
Design verification
Development report

Equipment suitability

Good manufacturing practices

In-process control
Installation qualification (IQ)
ISO 9000 series

Manufacturing process
Master plan
Master record
Methods validation
Module

Operating range
Operational qualification (OQ)
Out-of-specifications

Packaging validation
Policy
Performance qualification (PQ)
Preapproval inspection
Prequalification
Prevalidation

Process
Process capability
Process characterization
Process optimization
Process flow diagram
Process optimization
Process parameters
Process performance
Process qualification
Process suitability
Process validation
Proven acceptable range
Product attribute
Product optimization
Product performance
Product qualification

Protocol

Qualification
Qualified person
Quality
Quality assurance
Quality audit
Quality control
Quality policy
Quality system

Representative sample

Reprocessing

Requalification
Retrospective validation
Revalidation

Technical transfer
Time limitation
Total quality managment
Traceability
Unit operation

Worst case
Validation
Validation change control
Validation committee, group, team
Validation manager
Validation master plan
Validation protocol
Validation report
Verification

Bibliography

Carleton, F. J., and Agalloco, J. P., eds., *Validation of Aseptic Pharmaceutical Processes*, Marcel Dekker, Inc., New York, 1986.

Chow, S-C., and Liu, J-P., eds., *Validation, Process Controls and Stability, Statistical Design and Analysis in Pharmaceutical Science,* Marcel Dekker, Inc., New York, 1995.

Loftus, B. T., and Nash, R. A., eds., *Pharmaceutical Process Validation,* Marcel Dekker, Inc., New York, 1984.

Sucker, H., ed., *Validation in Practice*, Wissenchaftliche Verlagsgesellschaft GmbH, Stuttgart, 1983.

Validation of Manufacturing Processes , Fourth European Seminar on Quality Control, Geneva, Sept. 25, 1980.

References

1. FDA, *Guideline on General Principles of Process Validation*, FDA, Rockville, MD, May 11, 1987.
2. FDA, *Pre-approval Inspection/Investigations Guidance Manual*, 7346.832, Rockville, MD, Oct. 1, 1990.
3. *Fed. Reg.* 43(190), Human and veterinary drugs, current Good Manufacturing Practice in manufacturing, processing, packing or holding, Sept. 29, 1978, pp. 45,014–45,089.
4. Lucisano, L. J., and Franz, R. M., FDA Proposed guidance for CM and C changes: A review and industrial Perspective, *Pharm. Technol.,* 19(5): 30–40 (1995).
5. WHO, *Good Manufacturing Practices for Pharmaceutical Products—Guidelines on the Validation of Manufacturing Processes*, WHO, Geneva, 1993.
6. Skelly, J. P., et al., Scale-up of immediate-release oral solid dosage forms, *Pharm. Res.,* 10: 313–316 (1993).
7. Skelly, J. P., et al., "Scale-up of oral extended-release dosage forms, *Pharm. Res.,* 10: 1800–1804 (1993).
8. Bolton, S., Process validation for hard gelatin capsules, *Drug Cosm. Ind.,* 134(3): 42–48, 85–87 (1984).
9. Avallone, H. L., Development and scale-up of pharmaceuticals, *Pharm. Eng.,* 10(4): 38–41 (1990).
10. FDA, *Guide to Inspections of Oral Solid Dosage Forms Pre/Post Approval Issues for Development and Validation*, FDA, Rockville, MD, January 1994.
11. Berry, I. R., Process validation for soft gelatin capsules, *Drug Cosm. Ind.,* 134(4): 26–35 (1984).
12. Nash, R. A., Process validation for solid dosage forms, *Pharm. Technol.,* 3(6): 105–107 (1979).
13. von Doehren, P. J., St. John Forbes, F., and Shively, C. D., An approach to the characterization and technology transfer of solid dosage form processes, *Pharm. Technol.,* 6(9): 139–156 (1982).
14. Sucker, H., ed., *Validation in Practice*, Wissenschaftliche Verlagsgesellschaft GmbH, Stuttgart, 1983.
15. Berry, I. R., and Nash, R. A., eds., *Pharmaceutical Process Validation*, 2nd ed., revised and expanded, Marcel Dekker, Inc., New York, 1993.
16. Chowhan, Z. T., Development of a new drug substance into a compact tablet, *Pharm. Technol.,* 16(9): 58–67 (1992).

17. Fahrner, R., New role for pilot plants in product development, *Biopharm.*, 6(3): 34–37 (1993).
18. Avallone, H. L., and D'Eramo, P., Scale-up and validation of ANDA/NDA products, *Pharm. Eng.*, 12(6): 36–39 (1992).
19. Bala, G., An integrated approach to process validation, *Pharm. Eng.*, 14(3): 57–64 (1994).
20. Chapman, K. G., A history of validation in the United States, Part I, *Pharm. Technol.*, 15(10): 82–96 (1991).
21. Akers, J., Simplifying and improving process validation, *J. Parent. Sci. Technol.*, 47: 281–284 (1993).
22. Tomamichel, K., et al., Pharmaceutical quality assurance: basics of validation," *Swiss Pharma*, 16(3): 13–23 (1994).
23. Bolton, S., When is it appropriate to average and its relationship to the Barr decision, *Clin. Res. Reg. Affairs*, 11: 171–179 (1994).

ROBERT A. NASH

Validation of Pharmaceutical Water System

Introduction

The validation of water systems for pharmaceutical applications encompasses system-design qualifications, and attention to the regulatory requirements and the necessary documentation thereof. Among the system-design considerations are the decision points for choosing among alternative purification units and their proper operations. This includes materials of construction, system sanitizations, clearing of foulants, etc. The engineering requirements of water volume and flow balancing include definitions of pumps and pipe sizes. Other considerations involve documentary, microbiological, regulatory, and unit process operational issues relating to the validation issues.

This article is limited to the nonengineering aspects of water-system validation. It describes the validation exercise in terms of what is required to demonstrate by documented experimental effort the confirmation of the purported actions of the individual water purification units comprising pharmaceutical water systems. In keeping with the concept of process validation, the validation of each unit operation of a water system will, in sum, establish the validation of the total system. The validation exercise, however, is infinitely more than the demonstration that each individual purification unit performs as designed and intended. The intention of the validation effort is to establish that the system as a whole functions consistently, when operated in accordance with the standard operating procedures (SOPs) defined for that purpose, to produce water of the quality required for the given pharmaceutical application. The adequacy of the relevant SOPs is supported by documented data that the system does consistently produce water of the specified quality. Consistency becomes validated over a span of time long enough to encompass seasonal feedwater changes, and to define the renewals, refurbishings, and replacements necessary to ensure prolonged system operations.

Validation

There are many different definitions of validation. The 1987 FDA definition [1] states:

> Validation is the attaining and documenting of sufficient evidence to give reasonable assurance, given the current state of science, that the process under consideration does, and/or will do, what it purports to do.

A less eloquent but serviceable definition [2] is given in the FDA *Guidelines on Sterile Drug Products by Aseptic Processing*:

> Establishing documented evidence which provides a high degree of assurance that a specific process will consistently produce a product meeting its predetermined specifications and quality attributes.

In essence, validation seeks answers to two questions. Does the process or device accomplish what it is intended to do? If so, for how long? With regard to water systems, Artiss [3] defined validation as ensuring that the particular system consistently produces water of predictable quality when operated in the prescribed manner.

The FDA requires that each of the manufacturing processes whereby drugs or drug components are prepared be validated. Each step or piece of equipment utilized in the process must be demonstrated and documented to be performing the function that it is purported to do. As a consequence of such demonstrated suitability, the entire process (the total assemblage of each proven component and operation) will, by inexorable logic, have ensured its ability to fulfill its intended function. In the case of a water system, frequent testing before and after each purification stage, particularly when translated into trend lines, attests to its purported operation. The test frequency is such as to span time durations wherein expected variations can occur. Thus, it is revealed whether each purification unit operates properly, unaffected by the variations that may occur over time. Such intense and frequent testing serves to validate each unit and ultimately the entire process as operating dependably and consistently.

Process Validation

The FDA places dependency upon process validation, an exercise wherein the proper performance of each stage in a chain of manipulations and/or devices serves to ensure the logical and desired outcome of the entire operation. Analyses serve only, though importantly, to confirm the continuing appropriateness of the validation. Process validation is therefore said to be "building quality in," as distinct from a sole reliance on end-product testing analysis. The latter could be made to serve as a separation of the acceptable from the unacceptable as produced by the same process. What is desired is an assurance that the process produces only the "good."

The FDA is correct in its insistence upon process validation. It requires, as pointed out previously, that the process consistently and reliably produces only acceptable product. This is in contrast to a reliance upon analysis to differentiate between "good" and "bad." Since analyses are relied upon in either instances, in both the validation and in assessing the product, it may be asked why analysis can be depended upon in one case but not in the other. The subtlety involved here arises from the nature of the hypothetical proposition in scientific logic: If A, then B. Confirming the antecedent A, confirms the consequence B. However, confirming the consequence B does not confirm the antecedent A. If the process A, is valid, the product water, B, is suitable. But finding through analysis that B, the product, is acceptable, does not establish that the process is validly dependable. In this instance B may be confirmed for some reason other than A. Therefore, analysis of the product water alone cannot be used to establish the validity of the process in producing only acceptable product. Process validation itself is required.

The FDA requires that each of the manufacturing processes whereby drugs or drug components are prepared be validated. Each step or piece of equipment utilized in the process must be demonstrated and documented to be performing the function that it is supposed to perform.

Documentation and Information

As part of the validation requirements, a documentation and information master file has to be established. It must include a full description of the system, specifying its accept-

Validation of Pharmaceutical Water System

able ranges and limits. It also contains schematics of the electrical, mechanical, and water flow details. This enables subsequent verification of the proper installation of the several purification units, the control devices, the safety and alarm systems, and the provisions for instrument calibrations.

The documentation lists the activities necessary to the consistent production of the stipulated grade of pharmaceutical water. Perhaps the most important of these are the SOPs, the standard operating procedures, that set forth in detail the measures required for the dependable production of waters of requisite quality. A subset of the SOPs developed later is the standard maintenance procedures, SMPs, for the given water purification system. They detail the replacements, regenerations, renewals, sanitizations, and maintenance operations necessary to extend the system's reliability. Another subset of the SOPs will set forth the procedures relative to sampling, testing, and equipment calibration. Documentation of all that is entailed is an important part of the validation exercise. The FDA inspectors investigate the adherence to the pharmaceutical company's policy regarding validation, as set forth in the SOPs and allied protocols and as revealed by the documented data and the conclusions drawn.

The documentation gathered during the validation process can be substantial. Its management and control require considerable effort at organization; lists of equipment, instruments, materials, computer hardware, etc., are included. The subjects covered range from critical instrument check lists to specifications involving flow rates and pipe diameters. Each of the qualification steps, soon to be discussed, include equipment receipt verifications, installation verifications, calibration and instrument checks, change-control related documents, etc. The documentation includes articles associated with vendor audits.

Architectural and engineering firms and other consultant services are available which, on the basis of long experience, are competent to deal with the designing of plants and systems and with the assembling and organizing the documentation in the form of validation control files. They and the equipment manufacturers can be counted upon to be helpful in collecting the information that should constitute the necessary document for the validation plan. Inevitably, however, that file bears the imprint of the individual water processor and must reflect the operational knowledge gained from that company's particular proceeding.

Documentation is a Good Manufacturing Practice (GMP) requirement. Extensive records are to be kept as a check on procedures, constituting a paper trail of information demonstrating process control. This permits auditing of a company's practices.

The documentation aspect of the validation process is extremely important. A high proportion of the FDA investigation is involved with it. Documentation of the operations and of the results obtained are the only evidence that these activities have been performed. They are, therefore, the focus of FDA auditors during an inspection. The documentation enables an after-the-fact review of the validation process. Such retrospective examinations of the data permit an FDA auditor to judge the appropriateness of the procedures and of the conclusions reached. To make this possible, the raw recorded data, and the written conclusions drawn by the system operators must be available in clear documented form for the FDA to examine.

Keer [4] summarizes the documentation needs as follows:

> Documentation of a water system is a continuous exercise that starts at the very beginning of the project and ends when the facility is closed. A systematic approach to the task will yield the proper documentation to give the owner and regulatory authorities the confidence

in the system's control. The owner's objective is to meet all regulatory requirements in a cost-effective manner. The regulatory agencies want to ensure that there is no compromise or adulteration of products. Full and organized documentation satisfy the inspector's concern with minimal interruption to a facility's operation and at a small relative cost.

Validation Steps

A sequence of steps is involved in the validation of a pharmaceutical water system. The definition and design of the total system, and hence of its constituting purification units or modules comes first. The design qualifications of each separate unit are ascertained, to be succeeded by the installation qualification wherein the correct linking of the several purification units is made. Each of the linked modules is tested and challenged in an operational qualification that demonstrates its and the system's operating capability. The long-term suitability of the system's functioning and the establishing of its dependable reproducibility is attested to in the performance or process qualification step that follows. Traditionally, these steps are identified as design qualification (DQ), installation qualification (IQ), operational qualification (OQ), and process qualification (PQ). Some groups add a performance qualification prior to the process qualification; others call the process qualification the validation.

However performed, a logical progression of one qualification to another is required. For example, it is inappropriate to pursue a process qualification before completion of an installation or operational qualification. If the system has not been properly installed and verified to operate over the required range of conditions, water testing of the system PQ is not warranted. The final validated condition is a sum total of the preceding qualifications.

Control of the system's reliable operation is again required to be demonstrated following the implementation of alterations and changes that may be instituted from time to time. The question to be answered is whether the changes involved are substantive enough to significantly affect the quality of the product water. If so, revalidation is required.

Validation Sequence*

Design Qualification

The design of the equipment constituting the water purification system obviously comes first. It derives from the requirements of the water purification process. With a pharmaceutical water system, the quality of the water minimally meets either USP Purified Water or Water for Injection specifications, depending on its usage. The design documents set the standards and goals of the hardware.

Next, the process capacities should be defined such as the total volume needed per hour or day, the average consumption, the peak demand requirements, the reserve capacity, the minimum circulation needs, and whether elevated temperature storage is necessary, etc. In other words, early on in the project the functional definition of the project

---

*This section is based upon information and text supplied by Dan Meshnick, Validation Project Manager, Foster Wheeler USA, Perryville Corporate Park, Clinton, NJ.

Validation of Pharmaceutical Water System

or process should be formulated in order to provide a clear understanding of how the system must perform. After this document has been approved by the responsible groups, it becomes the basis of the system design.

The succeeding procedures and reports document how the manufacturing system was designed to address these requirements. This link between the intended purpose and the final design of the system is important. Too often, the qualification process begins with the system after it has been purchased, and there is no clear statement of user requirements. The end user is ultimately required to provide the criteria to judge the system, and not the system manufacturer or fabricator. What is important is not that a system meets an equipment manufacturer's specifications, but that what the vendor has provided meets the process requirements of the water preparer.

This functional definition is a valuable document for describing the system during an inspection, upgrading or repairing the system, and especially for controlling the validated condition of the water system as part of a change-control procedure.

The functional design basis is easily included for new construction, but it is not so simple to obtain or develop with existing water systems. Still, some description of the construction and design of the system must be provided for an existing water system. This is important for future reference, especially to individuals who may not have been involved with the validation, but who may have to redesign and revalidate at a later date. It is especially useful to someone who may have to explain the design and validation during an inspection five years later. It is difficult to defend a report or procedure without a clear statement of the design basis and functional goals.

Unfortunately, there are no meaningful design or construction standards currently in use for water production in the drug industry. All too often, the information and recommendations forthcoming from equipment suppliers must be relied upon. These are necessarily limited to their own expertise and are not always objective. The critical considerations of operational suitability, microbial control, and adherence to regulatory needs should first be set forth. The engineering design should then be formulated to meet these needs. Therefore the design qualification should, from the onset, include the participation of all appropriate groups, such as engineering design, production operations, quality assurance, analytical services, etc. The need for a team approach is necessitated by the complexity of the undertaking. Materials selection, equipment suitability, operational controls, construction techniques, cleaning and sanitization procedures, component compatibility, preventive maintenance, sterilization programs, sampling and regulatory requirements are all involved. It is essential that an adequate address to all these considerations be designed into the system. Where an insufficiency of guidance from other disciplines is involved, additions and amendments result in an effort to correct an inadequate system design.

The appropriate group to consider the design qualifications can be expanded to include the eventual users, representatives of technology development services and informational systems facilities, and system analysts, as well as consultants and vendors. Inclusion of the last facilitates the vendor–user relationship, enabling vendors to better serve the user needs.

Even before the validation exercise begins, a description and print of the entire system, from start to finish, must be available. The location of the sampling ports should be clearly marked. This will set forth the process and equipment design whose purpose is the achievement of consistent product water specifications.

The design qualification lists the activities necessary for the consistent production of the stipulated grade of water. It contains a full description of the system, specifying its acceptable operating ranges and limits. It supplies full schematics of the electrical, mechanical, and water flows for subsequent verification of their proper installation. It identifies the specific purification units, the various control devices, and the safety and alarm systems. It also provides for the calibration of critical instruments. The design qualification sets the microbial action and alert limits, specifies sampling plans and ports for chemical and microbial testing, stipulates sanitizing methods, and defines procedures for the analysis and plotting of data.

According to the PDA workshop [5], the basic design package should include the following:

1. Flow schematics for the proposed water system showing all of the instrumentation, controls, and valves necessary to operate, monitor, and sterilized the system. All major valves and components should be numbered for reference.
2. A complete description of the features and function of the system. This is of critical importance to enable production and quality assurance personnel, who may be unfamiliar with engineering terminology, to fully understand the manner in which the system is to be designed, built, operated, monitored, and sterilized.
3. Detailed specifications for the equipment to be used for water treatment and pretreatment.
4. Detailed specifications for all other system components such as storage tanks, heat exchangers, pumps, valves, and piping components.
5. Detailed specifications for sanitary system controls and a description of their operation.
6. Specifications for construction techniques to be employed where quality is of critical importance. These techniques should be suitable for exacting sanitary applications.
7. Procedures for cleaning the system, both after construction and on a routine basis.
8. Preliminary SOPs for operating, sampling, and sterilization. These procedures will be cross-referenced to the valve and component numbers on the system schematics.
9. Preliminary SOPs for filter replacement, integrity testing, and maintenance.
10. Preliminary sampling procedures to monitor both water quality and the operation of the equipment.
11. Preliminary system certification procedures.
12. Preliminary preventive maintenance procedures.

The design package should be as complete as possible to enable all disciplines involved to understand what the final system will entail.

Validation Plan or Master File

As stated above, the functional definition is often included as part of a validation plan. This document is not an FDA requirement, but it has become almost an industry standard. The FDA performs an in-depth evaluation of the validation data because without a validation plan a firm is more likely to overlook some required activity. It is advisable to include such a document as part of the validation, as it sets the overall goals and limits that will be followed during the validation, and can be referred to throughout the project, but especially later, well after the study has been completed. As a reference document, the plan permits a reviewer immediately to understand the scope of the validation, and to ensure that all parts of the system are validated.

The validation plan promulgates the facility organization responsible for the activity. It defines the responsibilities, gives the available resources and scheduling, and specifies the tools, techniques, and methodologies to be employed in the task.

The validation plan should contain all the information relevant to the water system. It is a repository for the basic design information, drawings, specifications, procedures, and protocols. It states the reasons for equipment selection, cleaning and sanitization frequencies, and component replacements and renewals. It contains the records for equipment modification and procedural alterations, the equipment and filter logs, and any recertification data. In short, it constitutes the major reference file for the entire water production system. As such, it serves internal investigatory purposes, and forms the basis for outside regulatory reviews. It is, therefore, critical that the validation plan be carefully controlled as part of a change-control or overall-quality system.

The validation plan may have its counterpart as a validation file or master file. (The term master file should not be confused with the various master files used by the FDA.) Meshnick [6] differentiates between a master file and the validation plan. The former is readily accessible, under liberal control, permitting easy modification of the change-control system. It is available to maintenance personnel, engineering staff, etc. without the strict control accorded the validation plan. Consequently the master file may often be in an incomplete status, drawings may be on an engineer's desk, manuals may be lost. The master file is a useful concept, but can often be out of control. By contrast, the validation plan or the master file for the validated system must be under strict control by the manager of the change-control activity or by someone with QC or GMP responsibility.

The validation plan is used to set the limits of the validation, to define the scope of the project, the systems included and not included in the qualifications, and to define what the project attempts to prove. For example, if the project includes the use of deionized water to feed a clean-steam generator, the validation plan would define which components would be involved in the preparation of such a water; what general quality attributes each purification unit would be expected to achieve; the length of time the system will undergo sampling and at what frequency, etc. Issues involving choices should be addressed in the validation plan, including the reasons for the choices. It must be made apparent why the selected decisions are appropriate. The validation plan must be consistent with the company QC policies and previous projects. It will be much appreciated in a later review, as in response to an out-of-tolerance condition, in a quality audit, or in a revalidation.

Installation Qualification

The installation qualification (IQ) is usually the first validation document prepared. It consists of a system description followed by a procedures section. Before the operational characteristics of the system can be investigated, the proper installation and assembly of the various articles of equipment require verification. This follows a careful check that each piece of equipment ordered and received is identical to that stipulated in the system design. All the critical features of the articles and their installation must conform to the written and approved specifications. As advised by Artiss [5]:

> Consideration should be given to conducting an inspection of the equipment before it is shipped from the supplier. Features of operational function and compliance with specifications can be verified and any deviations can be corrected without incurring the cost and time delay of reshipment.

The installation qualification ascertains that all of the unit components are installed as per specifications and according to the design drawings. It provides a construction verification in that the established specifications have been complied with. This also involves instrument connections. Included in this operation is a review of process and instrumentation drawings (P&ID) and isometric representations, verification of materials of construction, examination and documentation of welds, inspections for dead legs (in pipes) and correct pipe slopes, verification of stainless steel passivation, etc. The installation qualification confirms the "as built" drawings, and ensures the suitability of the completed system. The absence of leaks, which may provide pathways for invading organisms, can be ensured by vacuum testing, or by the use of pressurized air or water.

As stated in the FDA Guidelines [2]:

> This phase of validation includes examination of equipment design; determination of calibrations, maintenance, and adjustment requirements; and identifying critical equipment features that could affect the process and product. Information obtained from these studies should be used to establish written procedures covering equipment calibration, maintenance, monitoring, and control.

The first step in the installation qualification should be a detailed description of the water-purification system; this constitutes the system description. It is to be followed by a procedure section, setting forth a plan on how to proceed in performing the specific requirements. The protocol should define the procedures to be performed, the documents to be assembled, and the articles to be checked and verified. The plan thus set forth is to be approved before the qualification work begins. Subsequent changes may become indicated. These require being quantified, recorded, and approved in the final report.

The installation qualification procedures are generally in the form of check sheets that verify components or details critical to the validated condition of the equipment. Confirmation of details such as materials of construction, surface finishes, weld mapping and inspection documents, major equipment inventories (pumps, filters, UV lights, control valves, etc.), process instrument lists, utility connections (including drains), etc., define the system as installed.

In developing these IQ check sheets, individual components must first be identified, as in the system description or in a comprehensive equipment listing. Vital characteristics, necessary to the proper operation of the components, are included, along with the specific criteria that must be met. Spaces must be provided for the verification of each item with the date and the initials of the individual checking.

Specific acceptance criteria are required, set prior to beginning the qualification. The raw data gathered as part of the verification must be included as part of the final re-

Validation of Pharmaceutical Water System

port, along with a description of the procedures used during the check. Space should be provided for any actions or correspondence taken to address "out-of-specification" results. These check sheets should be prepared with the intent of being taken into the field and completing them as the work is performed. Raw data recorded on separate sheets must be included with the completed check lists.

Process and instrumentation drawings (P&IDs) are ideal documents for providing a clear description of where critical instrumentation and major system components are located. "As-built" construction drawings, showing actual measured piping layouts, filter locations, sampling stations, an absence of dead legs, pipe pitches, etc., are necessary as verification of how these critical articles are installed. A component is commonly verified by initialing the drawings along with the date. Any notes or comments regarding the verification should be recorded on the drawing or attached and referenced.

Areas that are often overlooked during installation qualification are those usually contracted to service groups. Cleaning and passivation documents, especially procedures, types and concentrations of acids and neutralizers, and the pH results of the various rinses are often neglected. These data should be requested beforehand and signed and dated by the technicians performing the work. This is especially important for documents such as weld certifications, where quality procedures are sometimes lax. The welders must document the welds as they are made, not at the end of the day or at the end of project. The purpose of the inspections and verification is to ensure careful, precise welds. The actual construction techniques used for system installation should be carefully monitored to ensure compliance with the written specifications.

The installation qualification should be well documented with regard to its flow of logic. This can prove critical to change control, serving as a basis upon which subsequent changes to the water purification system can be explained and justified.

Instruments and Controls

Instrumentation and control systems fall between the installation qualification and the operational qualification. These systems contain issues that could be included in either or both.

The first step in qualifying instruments and controls is to make a list of all system instruments. This must be available for inclusion in the installation qualification. Such a comprehensive list should be available as part of the P&ID. At this point, determinations must be made, classifying each instrument as critical or noncritical to the process.

Critical instrumentation (needed for direct process control and monitoring and recording) requires periodic calibration under 21CFR, sections 211.68 and 211.160 of the GMPs. These calibrations must be traceable to a recognized standards organization, such as the National Institute for Standards and Technology (NIST). Critical instruments include remote temperature detectors, tank level sensors, chart recorders that provide documents for monitoring records, resistivity meters and controls, and flow meters used to control resin-bed regeneration. Procedures must be available for the calibration of these instruments, which include the method of calibration, the range and accuracy of the instruments, and an appropriate schedule for performing these calibrations. Records of the results of these calibrations must be kept in order to comply with the GMPs. Instrument ID number and a sticker indicating the dates of the last and the next calibration must be clearly visible on all critical instruments.

Noncritical instruments, such as air regulator gauges or redundant pressure or temperature instruments, do not need rigorous calibration schedules. However, noncritical instruments must still be identified and logged into a calibration program. There must be a clear statement on such an instrument that it is not used for process control.

Calibration of instrumentation can be performed at the end of the installation qualification and recorded as part of the IQ, or at the beginning of the operational qualification. Either way, before operational testing is begun, all system instruments must be verified as calibrated.

The complete information is included not only as part of the qualification package, but also as the company's metrology, or instrumentation program which ensures that the controls and recordings from the system are consistently accurate and reliable. It contains documented calibration procedures, schedules, calibration results, and response to out-of-specification calibrations.

Operational Qualification

After the installation of the equipment assemblage has been verified as being correct, the operational qualification of the system can proceed. The system should be carefully cleaned and all construction debris removed to minimize contamination of corrosion. Cleaning is followed by passivation and verification. Cleaning and passivation should be the last steps of IO or the first steps of the operational qualification. Once cleaning and passivation have been completed, the equipment should be started up and carefully checked for proper operation in order to demonstrate that each component functions throughout all the anticipated operating ranges. The operational or equipment qualification of the water-purification system assumes defined acceptable product specifications.

As stated, operational qualification verifies the capability of the processing equipment to perform satisfactorily within operational limits. Considerations of feedwater quality, system capacity, temperature controls and flow rates are involved in this step, where the equipment design is examined to identify features critical to the process and product. The goal of the operational qualification is to evaluate the limits of control within which the validated system is expected to perform and obtain information to evaluate changes to the operation. The focus is on defining the critical areas and practices. Alarm conditions for utilities such as low steam pressure or instrument air; diverter conditions resulting from low condensate resistivity; differential pressure limits, high or low, are a few examples of events that should be confirmed as functioning correctly.

The protocol should begin with an introduction, and a description section, describing the operations of the system; some details may have been described before.

Subsequent to writing the operational qualification requirements and procedures, the specific acceptance criteria are to be promulgated by which the system's results will be judged. Specification of the acceptance criteria is the key to the protocol development effort. It defines the bounds within which the system is to be controlled. Acceptance criteria are required which, while they challenge the system, are appropriate to the system's operation; exaggerated standards are unnecessary. However, the criteria that are set must adequately assure the proper product-water quality. The system's specifications should be precisely defined and adequate for its operation.

Performance Qualification

The purpose of the performance qualification is to provide rigorous testing to demonstrate the effectiveness and reproducibility of the total integrated process. This results in a documentation of the system's consistent performance as designed and operated. The set points, control sequences, and operating parameters are probed. All the acceptance criteria are to be met under the worst-case process conditions. Failures should be identified and corrected, and tests should be rerun to confirm the elimination of their causes. Consistency of acceptable product water quality is sought, and documentation of every operation involved in attaining this aim is required.

The performance verification ensures the suitability of the system's function. The proper operation of equipment and controls should result in consistent system and product characteristics. This is established by repeated start-ups and shut-downs, simulating manual, automated, and emergency conditions. This process confirms operational SOPs and protocols for operations are finalized. The goal is to achieve the production of a dependable product in a continuous mode. A procedural verification of the written SOPs is sought. The limits of the product quality are explored by sampling and analytical testing, chiefly of electrical resistivity, total organic content (TOC) content, and bacterial and endotoxin levels. Long-term trends and evaluation are explored. The general strategy of how the process is challenged should be a part of the validation plan, and the PQ protocol should elaborate on its specifics.

As will be seen, the customary plan of the PQ includes intensive sampling for a relatively short time, one or two months, while the system is operated under normal conditions. As much information as possible concerning operating conditions should be gathered during this phase. Some firms attempt to challenge the system to the limits of the operating ranges during this testing, while others run the system as close to the center of the operating ranges as possible. Both have their merits; however, challenging the limits may have detrimental effects on the study, such as random failures, and certainly presents difficulties in determining which combination of variables would represent the most appropriate challenges. Thus, it is easier to operate under normal conditions. The water produced may be used, provided this intensive period of investigation so indicates.

After the intensive monitoring phase has been successfully completed, the system should undergo a long-term evaluation, for perhaps a year or more. It is considered qualified or validated, based upon the data from the first monitoring phase, but due to time-dependent effects, including the variability of feedwater supply, the effects of wear or deterioration of components such as UV lights, and the ability of organisms to adapt to harsh conditions, longer-term evaluation is appropriate before a system is considered validated.

The developed program should be described in the validation plan, and detailed in the process qualification protocol. If the two-phase (or longer) program is implemented, the data review and summary reports must be approved as each phase is completed. The validated condition of the system should be determined before the end of an extended monitoring program, especially if the water is being used.

A smoothly operating water system may undergo departures for reasons other than alterations in its water supply. Time-dependent changes may be involved, which have to be elucidated, defined, and documented. Purification units, such as ion-exchange beds, may become exhausted, reverse-osmosis (RO) membranes require cleaning, tanks and pipes may need sanitizations, etc. In general, the devices and accoutrements constituting the system periodically require maintenance-related activities, such as replenishment, refurbishing, cleaning, sanitization, replacements, and renewals of different kinds. Furthermore, various areas require attention on different time schedules. The necessary documentation therefore will include a body of information relating to the proper maintenance of each piece of equipment. Much of this is supplied by the equipment suppliers, and may, indeed, constitute stipulations connected with their guarantees of equipment performance. The relevant documentation composes the standard maintenance procedures necessary to the correct handling.

On a time-limit basis, the installation qualification and operational qualification are performed at the time of the installation of the purification and ancillary equipment and the preparation of the water (Fig. 1). This leads to the commissioning of the system and the qualification of its performance. The validation exercise can be divided into three phases. On the time-line basis, start-up overlaps both the operational qualification and the prospective phase of the validation. The performance parallels the concurrent and retrospective phases. Another view of the overall purification process is shown in Fig. 2. The entire operation should be reviewed at least annually to ensure the ongoing appropriateness of the product water and operational specifications. The system must be revalidated after any significant change in design, both mechanical or operational.

Qualification and Validation Final Reports

Once the validation has been planned, the design documented, the procedures written and executed, and the data collected, the last and the most important step of the process is the evaluation and reporting of the study.

Meshnick [6] advises as follows:

> "The final report is your opportunity to focus the study. It is where you describe what the data means. Take this opportunity. Results are not self-explanatory. The report should include a section which summarizes the raw data in tables, figures and drawings, graphs or other means. Review, explain and finally, conclude what the data support, based upon the acceptance criteria in the protocol. The review section should specifically review each point

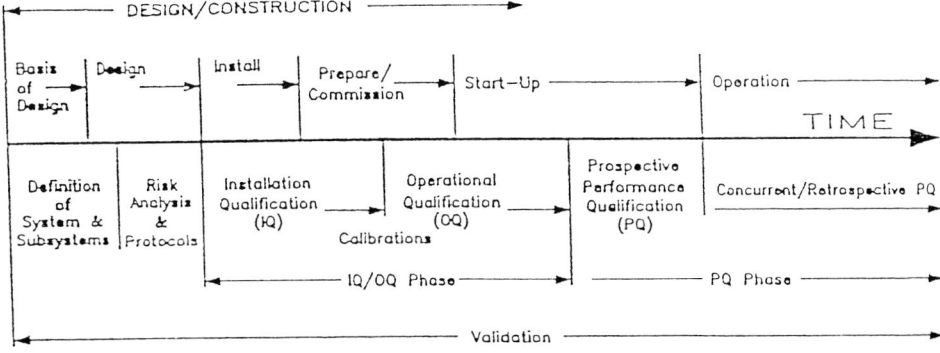

FIG. 1. The validation time line. From Ref. 11; permission granted, The United States Pharmacopeial Convention, Rockville, MD.

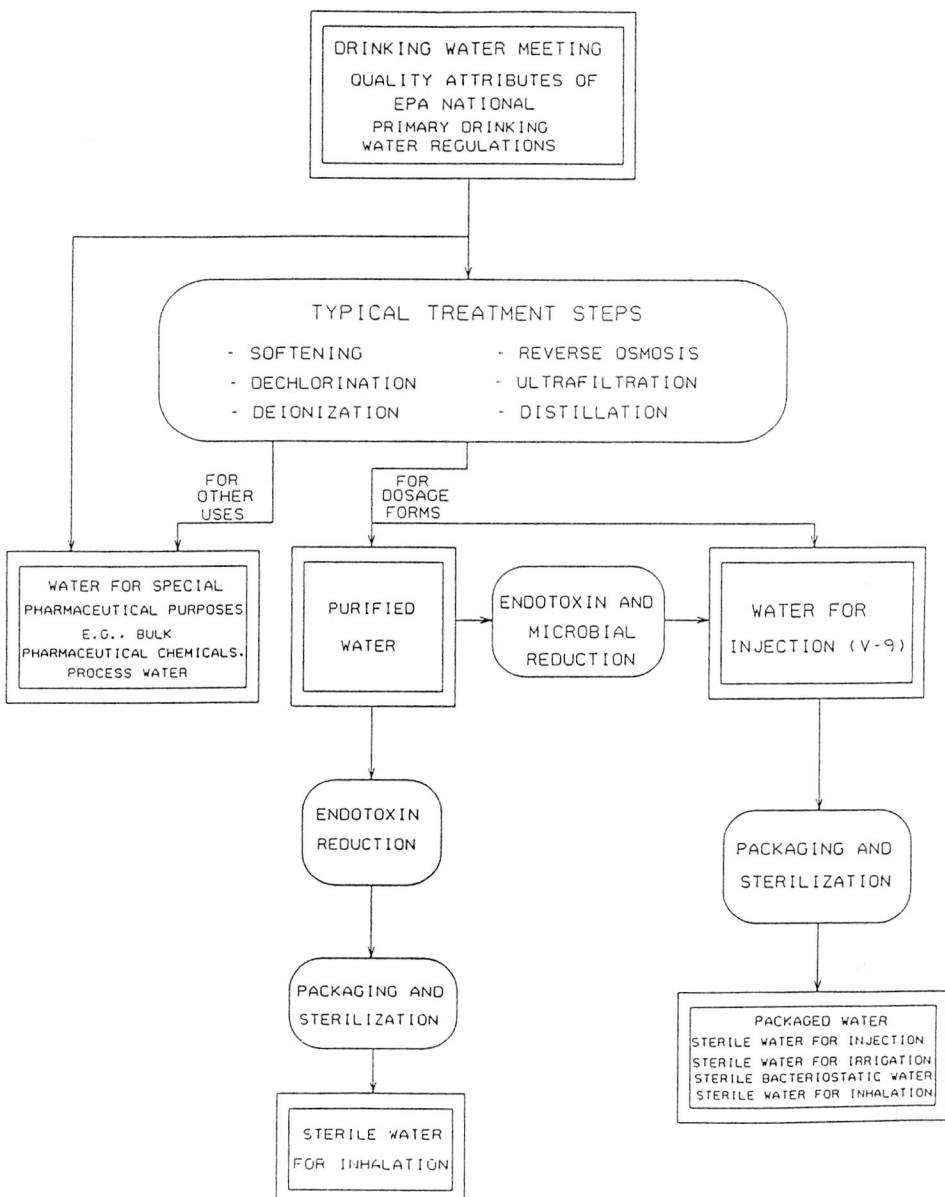

FIG. 2. Water for pharmaceutical purposes. From Ref. 12, p. 7543; permission granted, The United States Pharmacopeial Convention, Rockville, MD.

in the protocol acceptance criteria, and state whether the criteria were met. Then, based upon this review, the conclusion section should state whether the system is considered qualified or validated. In any event, do not just present the raw data in the report, or fail to make a conclusion. Do not allow the reviewer to judge the data alone, since he may not come to the same conclusions as you did. In a properly formatted and concluded report, there may still be disagreements, but at least there is a clear stand as to what the data mean. Without this, there is an open invitation to a differing view.

The final report must be written as an adjunct to the individual protocols, relating the observations recorded during the study, to the procedures and acceptance criteria in the protocol. Most often, the procedure employed during an audit review is to begin with the protocol and perform a step-by-step comparison with the report. It is critical that the protocol be followed, and that deviations be documented and justified. Often, when the procedure is being implemented, it becomes obvious that it cannot be performed as planned, or a better procedure becomes apparent. At this point some groups feel a protocol rewrite is needed, with the resulting effort for circulating the documents for review and approvals.

Deviations from an approved protocol require being dealt with carefully. They must be the exception, and not the rule. Consider what effect deviations have on the protocol and the validation plan. If the protocol is substantially changed by the deviations, then a rewrite is in order. Even major excursions from the protocol can be addressed in a deviations section of the report, provided they are justified and approved by authorized individuals. But consider the consequences. Lost or destroyed information, failures to follow SOPs, and other faux pas may indicate to investigators an insufficiency in the required technique." [It will also indicate that the personnel developing the protocols are inadequately trained in this area.]

The Validation Exercise

Several organizations in the United States are involved in defining the activities appropriate to pharmaceutical water-system validations: the Pharmaceutical Research and Manufacturing Association (PhRMA), whose Water Quality Committee is advising the United States Pharmacopeial Convention on the subject, the USP itself, free to accept or reject the proffered advice, and the FDA. The views of these three organizations are largely congruent, but not identical, on all validation matters. None has dealt deeply with the specifics of particular unit purification process validation requirements. All regard water-system validation as consisting of a series of consecutive stages:

- A prospective phase
- A concurrent validation phase
- A retrospective phase

According to an FDA spokesperson, in the prospective phase of the validation, daily samples are to be assayed for a minimum one-month period, for chemical and microbiological quality at each unit of the water purification system and at each point of use. The data obtained during this first period are used to develop the SOPs and confirm that they, the operational SOPs, are adequate. During the second period of a month or so, the concurrent validation phase, the same frequency of testing is to be observed. The resulting data serve to establish the short-term consistency of the water system operated according to the SOPs developed in the prospective phase. In essence, these four-week periods constitute the performance qualification. The long-term effects are yet to be explored. These will be investigated during the remainder of the year in phase three. During phase three, the retrospective validation step, microbiological testing of the Water For Injection (WFI) systems should be performed daily, with each point of use being tested at least weekly. For Purified Water systems, each point of use should also be tested weekly. It is to be emphasized that the analytical results are not to serve as pass/fail values but as alert and action levels. Their utility is to establish trend lines.

Validation of Pharmaceutical Water System

The USP monograph on the subject agrees that this one-year period should normally suffice for the validation exercise [7].

Underlying the setting of the time period for the initial phase of the validation is the assumption that the constancy of the feedwater composition is such that its management in the purification process can be defined and described in an SOP within a period of one month or so. However, a source water, particularly when processed by a municipality using mixes from different origins, may alter in character even on a daily basis. One American biotechnology company depends upon a municipal source that in answer to its own urgencies may, upon very short notice, mix well waters with river water containing large quantities of TOC of unknown compositions derived from industrial sources and farm runoffs. This particular source water changes often with dramatic frequency and suddenness. The system is made manageable only by the use of pretreatment purification units sufficiently exaggerated in size and scope so it can handle peak contamination loads. More than a few months were required to define an acceptable SOP for this water-purification system, and intensive ongoing daily monitoring is involved to ensure that the developed SOP suffices from day to day, the source water being of highly variable quality.

The three-phase validation scheme is proposed by the FDA for new systems. However, that agency is also prepared to accept other validation approaches. Some companies perform validations consisting only of the concurrent phase, a practice wherein the process is evaluated simultaneously with the manufacture of the product water. In this approach, individual batches may be utilized even before the entire validation has been completed. Concurrent validations entail much risk and may result in rejection of finished product.

Historical data may be relied upon solely to establish a retrospective validation in instances where the water has been produced for many years by the same process. This applies to validation of old systems. In such cases, documented evidence must firmly establish that there is a significant ongoing experience reflecting a constancy of practice. This signifies the existence of a rugged system giving consistent performance.

As stated in the FDA *Guidelines on General Principles of Process Validation* [1]:

> In some cases a product may have been on the market without sufficient premarket process validation. In these cases, it may be possible to validate, in some measure, the adequacy of the process by examination of accumulated test data on the product and records of the manufacturing procedures used.

The objective of retrospective validation is to demonstrate that the water-purification process has performed satisfactorily and consistently over time. Such documented evidence can serve to ensure that the specific process consistently produces water of the same quality in the future.

Microbiological Validation

It is the FDA whose views must be accorded with when performing the microbiological aspects of the validation process. It should be emphasized, however, that the pharmaceutical water processor is responsible for ascertaining that the validation exercise is sufficient and proper for his or her purposes. Complying with FDA regulations, advices, guidelines, etc. should lead to reassuring results. However, if despite FDA approval (or lack of disapproval) the "validated" system does not prove suitable for drug processing, the responsibility is that of the pharmaceutical manufacturer. The FDA imprimatur confers no immunity for the drug processor against untoward consequences.

Munson [8] divides the validation exercise into the three phases already discussed:

In phase 1, daily water samples are taken downstream from each unit in the treatment system and from each point-of-use in the holding/distribution system to assess the chemical and microbiological quality of the water. The data from the daily samples taken over a one-month period should be used to develop SOPs, appropriate maintenance and cleaning protocols, and analytical schedules for each unit in the system.

Daily sampling is continued in phase 2 for another month. During this phase the water system is operated according to the protocols and schedules developed during phase 1. The data from this phase are used to confirm that the operating and maintenance protocols and schedules are adequate and that the system can consistently produce water meeting its specifications. The data can also be used as the base-line data for trend analysis of the system. At the end of phase 2 the sampling schedule changes to that of routine monitoring. Chemical testing of pharmaceutical water systems should be performed at least weekly. Microbial testing of Water For Injection systems should be daily, with each point-of-use being sampled at least weekly. For Purified Water systems microbial testing should be performed on each point-of-use at least weekly.

Phase 3 of the validation program consists of reviewing the routine of monitoring data for at least 6 to 10 months. This time period will demonstrate that the operating protocols are adequate to handle variations in the quality, both chemically and microbially, of the incoming feedwater. At the end of phase 3, if all data indicate that the water system when operated according to its SOP consistently produces water that meets its specifications, the water system can be considered validated.

The validation program described is only a suggestion. It should not be interpreted as the only acceptable program that FDA will accept. Each water system, including the validation data and program, will be judged on its own merit.

The water generated during the validation phases 2 and 3 can be used to manufacture drug products."

Microbiological Levels

The bacterial endotoxin contents of Water For Injection is set up by USP 23 at the 0.25 EU/mL level (endotoxin units, EU). The microbiological content of Purified Water is not to exceed 100cfu/mL (colony-forming units), and that of Water For Injection is not to exceed 10cfu/100mL. These, however, are not rejection limits but are rather action levels [7,9]. The organism action level for Water For Injection permits little room for maneuver. The Purified Water action level can, however, be modified, depending upon the use to which it is put. The limit for Purified Water for antacid preparation may need to be reduced, depending upon the drug manufacturing process. For example, if heat is involved, the limit need not be so low. This is necessitated by the ease with which organisms grow at the alkaline pH of such preparations where preservatives are generally ineffective. A lower level would reduce the risk caused by the potential for organisms growth in the product. Oral medications might be permitted higher counts than otic, nasal, or topical wound preparations. Where one water system is dependent upon in the preparation of several products, the action level should be set in accordance with the needs of the product offering the highest risk for microbial growth. Room is, thus,

Validation of Pharmaceutical Water System

left for individual judgements with regard to the action levels for Purified Water, depending upon its ultimate use.

Munson, as spokesperson for the FDA [8], advises:

> Failure to meet these action limits does not mean automatic rejection of products. As the definition indicates, action limits are points which signal a drift from normal operating conditions and which require action on the part of the firm. When these limits are exceeded you should conduct an investigation designed to determine why the action limit is being exceeded. Then identify and implement the corrective action needed to restore the system to normal operation. You should also recheck products made prior to the corrective action to determine of the contamination has affected the quality of the product. You should increase your sampling rate for a period after the corrective action is implemented to insure that the system has returned to a state of control. This also does not mean that if you get a count of 110 cfu per mL for your Purified Water that you must shut down the system during the investigation.
>
> Because microbial tests results are already two to five days old you should not wait for two consecutive samples to exceed the action limit before you perform an investigation. This is when control charts or trend analysis can be a very useful tool. If the organism(s) isolated do not represent a potential problem and the historical profile of the system indicates that this single result is unusual and not part of an upward trend, then the follow-up action may simply consist of re-sampling or stepping up the rate of sampling for a short period so that a more accurate determination of whether the system is out of control or not can be made. The important thing is to document what follow-up action you took and that the problem was corrected. No documentation means no follow-up action and no correction.

Testing for Specific Organisms

The types of organisms present in Purified Water must be considered. Previously the FDA had excluded pseudomonads, which is, however, not the present FDA position [8]. *Pseudomonas species* do not have to be monitored for unless representing a potential hazard to the product. The burden for knowing whether that situation exists, as well as the consequences attendant upon it, rests on the drug manufacturers. It is their responsibility to learn and know the situation with regard to their products. It has been known that the presence of *P. aeruginosa* in topical can produce infections in persons with abraded skin or wounds. Therefore, these pseudomonads must be absent in waters used for topicals. In general, water systems are required to be free of particular organisms only if they represent pathogens or potential pathogens in the end products, that is, when their presence in the drug preparations poses a potential health hazard during use as directed. The relevant knowledge is the responsibility of the drug manufacturer.

As stated, the number of microbes restricted in the compendial waters by the alert and action limits is associated with a prohibition against objectionable organisms. The presence of opportunistic pathogens needs also to be considered, however. These may be pathogenic when applied to patients with compromised immunities, a situation not known in advance to the drug manufacturer, who is, nevertheless, liable for untoward consequences. It may be prudent, therefore, to maintain even Purified Water under self-sanitized storage at 80°C or in the presence of ozone. The use of a sterile Purified Water could eliminate the presence of undesirable organisms from the drug preparation. This would minimize dependency on preservatives whose action is sometimes uncertain.

Viable Nonculturable Bacteria

The possible presence of viable but nonculturable bacteria is being increasingly recognized. The question is whether their presence has disease-causing implications. The general belief is that they do not pose a significant threat to health. The practical consequences of their potential presence seems minimal.

Microbiological Assay Methods

There are different views concerning the performance of microbiological assays, whether by direct count, pour plate, etc., the nutrient media to be employed, the incubation times, and the incubation temperatures.

The recommendations of Water Quality Committee of the Pharmaceutical Research and Manufacturing Associations on this subject are as follows [10–12]:

Purified Water: Pour Plate Method
      Minimum sample, 1.0 mL
      Plate count agar
      Minimum 48 h incubation at 30–35°C
Water For Injection: Membrane Filtration Method
      Filtration on 0.45 μm porosity filter
      Minimum sample, 100mL
      Plate count agar
      Minimum 48 h incubation at 30–35°C

The responsibility for choosing or even for devising culturing techniques suitable for revealing organism types that may be present in a particular water is that of the pharmaceutical processor.

It should be noted that there is no one method that detects all possible organisms present in the water. The method chosen should adequately characterize the predominant organisms present. The most important aspect of monitoring is to look for changes in the numbers and types of microorganisms present.

Alert and Action Levels

Pharmaceutical water manufacturers set and utilize alert and action levels to guard their WFI and Purified Water from exceeding the specified microbial limits. The alert level indicates that a process may have drifted from its normal operating condition, and thus provides a warning. The action level signals such a departure from the normal range that investigation and corrective action are required.

It is helpful and prudent for the waters being prepared to attain normally an even greater purity than that stipulated. For example, the action level of a Purified Water is set at 100 cfu/mL, but it is normally purified to a higher degree, say, 50 cfu/mL. If a periodic analysis indicated a level of 70 cfu/mL, the water system operator would be alerted to check the accuracy of that finding by promptly repeating the analysis. Were the recount to affirm the higher level, action could be undertaken promptly to discover the cause of the deviation and implement remedial steps to bring the system back to normal.

The numerical values for alert and action levels are often set arbitrarily. It is desirable that they be set on a statistical basis. Trend analysis is used to interpret what the microbiological data signify by way of standard deviations. In some cases the limits are established as multiples of the standard deviation from the normal, namely, two times the standard deviation (or sigma) for the alert level, and three times the standard deviation for the action level. On this basis the alert level accounts for 95% of the data, and the action level covers 99%. A 1% outside the action level is considered normal. Exceeding this level is unusual and requires attention. There is also room for ambiguity in how the alert levels are responded to. The alert level may be addressed by the retesting of samples to confirm the higher values. The alert response may also include corrective actions in advance of those to be taken when the action limit is reached. Water processors are expected to set their own alert and action levels. The FDA inspectors insist, however, that the records show that these are respected and adhered to in practice, and that the USP action levels are GMP at this time. Action levels above those suggested by the USP have to be justified.

Conductivity Measurements and pH

The standards of chemical acceptability for Purified Water and Water For Injection are shown in Table 1, based on the relevant analytical procedures described in USP 23 [7,9]. A single conductivity measurement in conjunction with pH values is substituted for the total of the specific measurements for chloride, sulfate, ammonia, calcium, and carbon dioxide.

Testing the suitability of the product water is possible at each of three stages. At Stage 1, assays are performed by on-line conductivity tests, a situation presumably free of the influences of carbon dioxide and its ionic pH and conductivity consequences. The temperature of the water is read directly, not compensated for. Comparisons is then made of the conductivity/temperature values with those presented in an official table

TABLE 1 USP 23 Standards for Water Purity Numerical Interpretations[a]

Component	Purified Water	Water For Injection
pH	5.0–7.0	5.0–7.0
Chloride (mg/L)	0.2	0.2
Sulfate (mg/L)	1.0	1.0
Ammonia (mg/L)	0.1	0.1
Calcium (mg/L)	1.0	1.0
Carbon dioxide (mg/L)	5.0	5.0
Heavy metals (mg/L)	0.1 as Cu	0.1 as Cu
Oxidizable substances	Pass USP permanganate test	
Total solids (mg/L)	10.0	10.0
Pyrogens (Eu/mL by LAL[b])	—	0.25

[a]Numerical values are interpretations of procedures listed in the standards of the *United States Pharmacopeia* XXII.
[b]Limulus ambocyte lysate test.

of acceptable levels. The conductivity at the temperature value equal to or less than the measured temperature defines the acceptable limit: $\leq 1.3 \mu S/cm$ at $\geq 25°$ C.

If the conductivity is equal to or less than the tabulated value, the water quality is acceptable. If it is higher, a Stage 2 determination is made to determine whether the higher conductivity is due to the presence of carbon dioxide. In the Stage 2 assay, the water is stirred vigorously at $25 \pm 1°C$ to permit complete equilibration with the atmospheric carbon dioxide. Equilibration is measured by the levelling off of the periodically determined change in conductivity. When the net alteration falls below $0.1 \mu S/cm$ per 5 min, the sample conductivity is recorded. If it is no greater than $2.1 \mu S/cm$, the water is acceptable. If the conductivity value is higher, the possible influence of pH is ascertained in a Stage 3 assay as follows.

Saturated potassium chloride is added to the sample examined in the Stage 2 test, to allow measurement of its pH. Reference is made to a predetermined pH/conductivity requirements table to find the acceptable conductivity limit at the measured pH level. Unless the conductivity of the water is higher than the acceptable limit, or the pH is outside the 5.0 to 7.0 range, the water quality is judged to be proper (Table 2).

TABLE 2 Stage 3: pH and Conductivity Requirements[a,b]

pH	Conductivity Requirement ($\mu S/cm$)[c]
5.0	4.7
5.1	4.1
5.2	3.6
5.3	3.3
5.4	3.0
5.5	2.8
5.6	2.6
5.7	2.5
5.8	2.4
5.9	2.4
6.0	2.4
6.1	2.4
6.2	2.4
6.3	2.3
6.4	2.3
6.5	2.2
6.6	2.1
6.7	2.7
6.8	3.1
6.9	3.8
7.0	4.6

[a] For atmosphere and temperature equilibrated samples only.
[b] From *Pharmacopeial Forum*, 22(6) (1996). Courtesy The United States Pharmacopeial Convention, Rockville, MD.
[c] $\mu S/cm$ (microSiemen per centimeter) = $\mu mho/cm$ = reciprocal of M $\approx$-cm.

Validation of Pharmaceutical Water System

By the same token, if at either of the earlier stages of testing the conductivity is found to be acceptable, the pH, of necessity, must be within its proper range. Indeed, the original role of pH was to limit the concentration of ions not otherwise specifically identified. Therefore, the specific requirement to determine directly the pH of the water would seem to be redundant where the conductivity is suitable. Nevertheless, pH testing is required.

TOC Measurements

Measurements of TOC can be utilized as a substitute for the USP Potassium Permanganate Oxidizable Substances Test. The acceptability standard is set at 500 ppb.

The TOC measuring devices available in the market place differ significantly in their abilities to detect (by oxidation and its consequences) organic molecules of varying complexities. Any TOC monitor should be under consideration capable of measuring the presence of organic molecules likely to be found in pharmaceutical waters. The reference compound chosen for the instrument suitability test was 1,4-benzoquinone. It has the useful properties of being a powder at room temperature, readily available in pure form; it is relatively safe to handle and well defined chemically. In a multilaboratory testing exercise its average recovery was the lowest among the organic compounds examined. Its use as the standard for the TOC suitability test therefore suggests the greatest challenge to oxidation. This presents a prudent choice for TOC determinations. The 1,4-benzoquinone recovery is to be within the test limits of 80 to 115% for the TOC instruments to be acceptable. Sucrose serves as the TOC test standard.

Source-Water Testing

It is required that the pharmaceutical waters be prepared from sources of drinking-water quality as defined by the Environmental Protection Agency (EPA) or comparable by European Union or Japanese regulations [13]. For municipally treated feedwaters, quality certification can be obtained by the drug producer from the municipal authorities, perhaps on a quarterly basis. For unprocessed source waters, or when the pharmaceutical processor does the testing to establish in-house EPA certification, the fully panoply of EPA potable-water analyses, including testing for pesticides, should be carried out. An annual performance of such analyses should suffice. Yearly spot checks, including pesticide analyses, should also be made by users of municipal waters to see how well the levels found match those reported by the municipal suppliers.

Sampling Program

The defining of suitable protocols for sampling and testing, and a rigid adherence to the scheduling is part of the validation program. The positions of the sampling valves or sampling points should be evident on the drawings of the system layout. Sampling ports are best installed before and after each purification unit, and before and after storage tanks. All the sampling valves should be of the same kind. Each valve should be numbered or otherwise unambiguously identified. The valves should be of small inside dimensions. This permits their prompt, full opening and their flushing under high velocity to ensure the removal of organisms presumed to be contaminating the downstream side of the valve. In the distribution, samples should be taken at the points of use unless the water system is led through a hard pipe to a piece of equipment.

A description should indicate the actual manner in which the samples are taken, sample size, containers, method of identifying the sample with sampling location and time, equipment employed, points to be sampled, time frames for analysis to be initiated, and disposition and approval of results.

Inherent in sampling is the assumption that the sample is representative of the entire bulk of the water being characterized. Care should be taken not to invalidate that assumption. Artiss points out that point-of-use samples should be drawn using the hose or pipe employed in delivering the water for manufacturing or rinsing. In this way contamination problems possibly inherent in that pipe or hose will appear in the microbiological assay results [3].

Table 3 gives a sampling program, sampling sites, assays, and the frequency of testing. Such sampling schemes are required as part of the water-system validation.

Cleaning and Sanitizations

Periodic cleaning or sanitization and sterilization and flushing should be performed on the water lines, sampling points, unused legs, and hoses off water-transmission lines. Sanitization of the water system using hot water must be validated. A protocol, record of time and temperature, adequate raw data, formal review, and an evaluation of the final report should be prepared.

Sanitization using a chemical agent (e.g., peracetic acid, hydrogen peroxide, formalin, antimicrobial agent, etc.), or steam, should be followed by a routine analysis for chemical residues. These can be eliminated by flushing; residual analysis should be performed. Documentation consisting of formal logs should be kept of these activities. A record of sanitization, equipment replacement, and maintenance is required.

Pretreatments

Ion-exchange, reverse osmosis, and distillation are the principal methods of water purification in pharmaceutical system design. More recently, electrically driven purification units for continuous deionization have been introduced. At least in principle, to some extent any of these unit purification processes can furnish water of requisite pharmaceutical quality. (Source waters having high chloride ion contents may require two-pass, product-staged reverse-osmosis treatments.) The question is whether these processes provide realistic service lives to the purification units or whether the processes may be affected and be quickly overwhelmed by the quantity of impurities normally present in feedwaters. The purpose of pretreatment techniques is to prolong the useful service lives of the principal purification units. The appropriate pretreatment selectively removes or diminishes part of the impurity burden to the point where compromise of the principal purification unit is eliminated or becomes tolerable. For example, the presence of certain types of TOC in the feedwaters may serve to prematurely foul a reverse-osmosis (RO) purification unit. The use of an activated carbon bed in a pretreatment to remove all or some of the TOC by absorption can prolong the life of the RO to an extent that is operationally practical. The definition of what is "practical" in a water-purification context has an economic component. Water-purification exercises

Validation of Pharmaceutical Water System

are not simply technical practices; they are technico-economic undertakings. Since the pretreatment unit operations may greatly influence the principal purification results, they require being validated along with the principal units.

Impurities

The impurities that are the subject of the source water analysis are of concern for two reasons. First, their removal, at least to certain levels, is required according to the analytical specifications of Purified Water or Water For Injection as stipulated for these compendial waters in various national or regional pharmacopeias. Table 1 identifies the impurities listed in the *United States Pharmacopeia (USP)*, for example, calcium, sulfate, and chloride ions. Another group of impurities requires elimination because their presence would compromise the efficiency or service lives of the purification units, such as ion-exchange, reverse osmosis, or distillation, employed to prepare the compendial water. Silica is an example of such an impurity. Its presence, although not proscribed by the USP, can cause fouling of reverse-osmosis membranes, and vitrification of other surfaces.

There may be a third reason for analyzing for certain elements or compounds. In the United States, the USP specifies that pharmaceutical waters must be prepared from source waters of potable quality. This stipulation being made in the USP monograph section has the force of regulations, and is enforceable by the FDA. The specifications for potable water are the responsibility of the EPA. Their restrictions of heavy metals in potable waters are more stringent than those of the USP for Purified Water and Water For Injection. Therefore, analysis of the treated source water for heavy metals would seem to be unnecessary. Not all pharmaceutical source waters are of the potable quality which is usually a consequence of prior processing by a central water authority. Nonpotable source waters have, therefore, to be brought to potable water quality in the process of being purified to the suitable compendial standard. The original source water may contain, for example, heavy metals in unacceptable concentrations; the finished pharmaceutical water should not. It is not necessary to segregate the water during its purification into a potable water stage. It must, however, be ascertained that at some point in the purification process water of potable quality has been achieved.

In the case of *E. coli*, its absence must be ensured, as mandated by EPA potable water standards. This is usually achieved by the early chlorination of the source water. The absence of *E. coli* is thus provided and tested for, and subsequent testing in the prepared compendial waters need not be reaffirmed by analysis; the same applies to the testing for heavy metals.

Total Suspended Solids

It is necessary to reduce or remove suspended and colloidal matter from the feedwaters entering any of the principal purification units. Ion-exchange beds, in addition to their demineralizing functions, serve as deep-bed filters. They are composed of a packed volume and depth of resin beads, generally between 16 and 50 mesh size (0.3–1 mm), although the range of 20 to 40 mesh (0.425–0.850 mm) is often preferred. They accumulate particulate matter within their interstices precisely in the manner of deep-bed filters. The accumulated particulate material, the suspended matter present in the feedwater, causes elevated pressure differentials within the ion-exchange beds. This occur-

TABLE 3 Sampling Program[a]

Sampling Location and Assay	Frequency Validation	Frequency Operation	Comments
Raw water, potable			
Microbial	Daily	Daily	Review together to determine contact time
Residual Cl_2	Daily	Daily	Fast, low-cost test
Chemicals, TDS[b]	Daily	Weekly	Depend on source, season
Chemicals, complete	Weekly	Every 6 months	Depends on equipment
pH	Weekly	Every 6 months	
Sand filter			
Microbial	Daily	Daily	
Residual Cl_2	Daily	Daily	
Carbon filter[d]			
Microbial	Daily	Daily	
Residual Cl_2	Daily	Weekly	
Conductivity	Continuous	Continuous	
Total Solids, USP	Daily	Daily	Depends on Water use
pH	Daily	Daily	Depends on water use
DI equipment			Varies with service cycle
Microbial	Daily	Daily	
Pyrogen	Daily	Weekly	Depends on water use
Silica, colloidal and dissolved	Daily	Weekly	Depends on water use
Resin analysis	Initial	Every 6 months	Check individual modules
RO equipment			
Microbial	Daily	Daily	
pH	Continuous	Continuous	Critical on some equipment
Residual Cl_2	Continuous	Continuous	Critical on some equipment
Pyrogen	Daily	Daily	Depends on water use
Conductivity	Continuous	Continuous	
Chemicals USP	Daily	Daily	Depends on water use
Feedwater hardness	Daily	Daily	Critical on some equipment

Distillation equipment (USP VFI)			
Microbial	Frequently	Daily	Repeatability, stabilization
pH	Frequently	Daily	
Pyrogen	Frequently	Daily	
Conductivity	Continuous	Continuous	Inlet and outlet
Chemicals, USP	Frequently	Daily	
Blowdown chemicals, TDS[b]	Frequently	Weekly	
Particulates	Frequently	Weekly	
Storage			
Microbial	Frequently	Daily	
pH	Frequently	Daily	
Pyrogen	Frequently	Daily	If required for WFI
Chemicals, USP	Frequently	Daily	
Distribution use points			
Microbial	Daily	Weekly	On rotation
Pyrogen	Daily	[c]	
Chemicals, TDS[b]	Daily	Monthly	Fast low-cost test
Chemicals, USP	Weekly	[c]	
Particulates	Weekly	Monthly	
pH	Weekly	[c]	
Clean steam generator			
Blowdown chemicals, TDS	Daily	Weekly	To prevent scale build-up

[a]Adapted from Ref. 3.
[b]Total dissolved solids by conductivity.
[c]Sample only when indicated by failure to satisfy other tests.

rence slows the flow of water, may foul macroreticulated resin beads, and may otherwise offer spacial interferences that detract from the intended ion-exchange function.

In the case of reverse-osmosis operations, suspended matter blocks areas of the RO membrane, removing them from useful contributions. Unlike the ion-exchange beds, reverse-osmosis devices retain colloids, further interfering with the ion-removal function.

The accumulation of suspended matter in the still pot of distillers interferes with the designed heat-transfer effects and increases the likelihood of particle entrainment in the vapor. This is the object of the blowdowns, largely automatic, that are part of still operations.

To forestall the fouling occasioned by suspended matter such materials are removed by the use of sand filters and/or multimedia deep-bed filters in a pretreatment step. Colloids are removed by coagulation and flocculation, usually by the addition of alum or polyelectrolyte. This is the standard treatment in potable water preparations.

Scale-Forming Elements

Calcium, magnesium, alkalinity, sulfate, silica, pH, etc., in certain concentrations and combinations, produce precipitates and deposits that interfere with the principal purification-unit operations.

Of chief concern are the hardness elements. Calcium ions combine with sulfate ions to form insoluble calcium sulfate deposits. Such scale formation must be avoided in reverse-osmosis operations. Calcium carbonate can also be deposited as interfering scale; its formation from soluble calcium bicarbonate is a consequence of a shift in the pH of the water to the alkaline side. The Langelier solubility index provides a measure of the tendency of a water to form calcium carbonate scale and indicates the pH adjustment needed toward acidity to avoid such formation [14].

Scale and deposits of other compositions include calcium fluoride, voluminous magnesium hydroxide, and silica. Appropriate pH management, and the use of antiscalants (which require subsequent removal) can be effective in preventing scale; some of these may promote calcium sulfate supersaturation.

The most effective way of avoiding scale formation is a water-softening operation. Usually, ion-exchange resins in their sodium form are utilized to remove calcium, magnesium, barium, and strontium. The last two elements, if not removed in the water-softening pretreatment, can so irrevocably combine with cation-exchange resins that these cannot be regenerated. A deposit of insoluble barium sulfate scale, and, to a somewhat lesser extent, strontium sulfate on a reverse-osmosis membrane is almost impossible to remove. Therefore, barium and strontium should be analyzed for, and removed in the water-softening step.

Water softening also serves to remove soluble iron and manganese. These elements are commonly removed in a separate pretreatment step involving oxidation by chlorine or greensand zeolite, followed by the filtration of the insoluble oxidized product, usually by deep sand beds or by multimedia deep beds. Smaller quantities of iron and/or manganese are removed by way of cation-exchange resins.

The temporary water hardness due to bicarbonate ion is eliminated by the addition of acid to pH below 4.4. This converts the bicarbonate to water and carbon dioxide; the latter is removed from the system by a degasification or decarbonation unit.

Soluble silica can be removed by strong base ion-exchange or by rejection in the reverse-osmosis operation. Soluble silica should not be permitted to enter stills, although in certain water-purification operations it is actually present. Curiously, soluble silica is not removed in any pretreatment step, and none has been designed for that purpose, although strong base cation-exchange is a possibility.

Total Organic Carbon

The term total organic carbon (TOC) a misnomer. At most, it represents total oxidizable carbon as defined by an automated TOC analyzer. Several such TOC instruments are commercially available, each with different oxidizing capabilities. The definition of TOC may vary among them since each organic compound has its own susceptibility to oxidation, and very little is known about the TOC constituents of any water. The readings of the various TOC instruments are standardized by the use of reference compounds [11]. These developments are an improvement over the traditional USP Oxidizable Substances Test, an analysis noteworthy for its insensitivity.

There is no universal way of removing TOC from waters; it depends upon the specific nature of the organic compounds involved, and some cannot be removed efficiently. Usually the TOC is slowly absorbed on activated carbon granules, with low flow rates, about 1 gallon per minute per cubic foot of carbon. By contrast, chlorine is removed by activated carbon at double or triple these flow rates. Organic compounds, with some notable low molecular weight exceptions, such as phenols, acetic acid, and alcohols, are rejected by RO membranes. Ultrafiltration can also be used to retain organic compounds. Some still designs incorporate the means to oxidatively destroy organic materials in the still pots. Ion-exchange resins are also used to remove TOC. Organic molecules containing carboxylic acid moieties, usually the result of oxidation, can be removed by anion-exchange. Advantage can be taken of this fact to subject the TOC to oxidation by ozone, ultraviolet light, or hydrogen peroxide, or by various combinations of these agents. The oxidized TOC, bearing carboxylic acid groups that normally characterize one stage of the TOC oxidative degradation, can be removed by anion-exchange. The trihalomethanes (THM) that are end products of organic matter oxidized by chlorine, are exceedingly difficult to remove from water by any means, especially chloroform. Adsorption to activated carbon has only limited success. Some TOC can be removed by adsorption to ion-exchange resin beads because of the large surface areas these present. The danger is, however, that the beads may become excessively fouled, thereby compromising the function of ion-exchange. Resin beds are sometimes utilized, in a pretreatment mode, to remove TOC.

Microorganisms

Microorganisms are perhaps the most insidious of the impurities present in source waters. Other impurities once removed, remain removed, but organisms, even when removed to the state of sterility, can reinvade the water and multiply to significant populations. Organisms and their derivative pyrogenic lipopolysaccharides, the bacterial endotoxins, require strict concentration limitations in waters intended for parenteral pharmaceutical applications.

Once freed of microorganisms to the specified acceptable degree, the pharmaceutical water, both Purified Water or Water For Injection, needs to be so maintained to the same degree of microbiological and bacterial endotoxin purity during storage and transfer.

Ionic Constituents

The chemical impurities, whose presence and quantitation are the subjects of source water analyses, are almost all ionic in nature. Calcium, magnesium, barium, strontium, sodium, and potassium are all cations. The pH measurement gives the concentration of the hydrogen ion (more properly, hydronium ion), also cationic, or, at its higher values, of the hydroxyl anion. Sulfate, nitrate, and chloride are anions. Carbon dioxide, the anhydride of carbonic acid, is generated by bicarbonate or carbonate ions, which together with anionic hydroxyl ions constitute the water alkalinity. Ammonia is the anhydride of ammonium hydroxide. Added to water it yields hydroxyl ions through the feeble dissociation of ammonium hydroxide into ammonium cations and hydroxyl anions.

Ion-exchange practices and/or reverse-osmosis processes are the principal purification methods relied upon to remove these ionic impurities. Distillation is the other well-established purification method commonly utilized for this purpose. (Certain electrically powered techniques may also be utilized for deionizations or demineralizations. Their use, although small, is on the increase. Chief among these is an electrodeionization process called continuous deionization.) However, distillation does not suffice for the removal of carbon dioxide or other volatile impurities of significant water solubilities and which may remain to some degree in the condensed distillate.

System Design
The Purification Unit Processes

The concept of process validation can be expressed as follows: If each unit process of a water-purification system is demonstrated and documented to be operating as designed and expected, the sum of those units processes, the total system, must, of necessity, be dependable in its production of the water quality required for its intended purpose.

Since the design of water systems is site specific, it is difficult to generalize concerning the unit process components of a "typical" system. Broadly speaking, however, pharmaceutical water-purification arrangements consist of the following parts:

- A chlorination unit to supply the means of controlling the organism content of the feedwater
- A sand or multimedia bed to remove suspended solids down to 10 to 40 μm in size
- A water softener to remove scale-forming ions
- An activated carbon bed to remove chlorine and TOC

A decision to use RO involves the selection of the membrane type. Cellulose acetate RO, often chosen for pharmaceutical applications, entails acidification to about pH 5.5–6 and, where bicarbonate is present, carbon dioxide removal with the help of degasification equipment. Ozone, ultraviolet units, filters of various sorts and ratings, chemical antiscalants, and acids or alkalies for pH adjustments are also utilized.

Chlorination

Municipally treated waters generally arrive chlorinated, or containing a certain concentration of a biostat, usually chloramine. Otherwise, the source water is chlorinated as soon as it is acquired by the pharmaceutical plant. The chlorine content of the feedwater is adjusted to a residual of 0.5 to 2 ppm. On occasion, higher concentrations are used (2–6 ppm), if, for example, there is concern regarding *Legionella pneumophilia* [15].

Ozone

Ozone is a more efficient biocide than chlorine. It is more rapid in its killing action and more effective against a wider variety of microbes including viruses. Its action against *E. coli* is 3125 times as rapid as that of chlorine [16]. Indeed, no microorganisms seem to be immune to its lethal effects. Additionally, ozone offers the tremendous advantage of being removable in seconds by the destructive action of 254 nm UV radiation.

Ultraviolet Radiation

Ultraviolet wavelengths have germicidal effects producing photochemical reactions involving biomolecules in organisms. The resulting molecular alterations inhibit the growth of microorganisms, and in higher doses kill them. The germicidal effectiveness of UV radiation depends upon its wavelength, and different organisms show different sensitivities to various parts of the UV spectrum. Figure 3 illustrates the roughly Gaussian germicidal action curve whereby germicidal effectiveness is plotted against wavelength.

Multimedia Deep Beds

The use of deep-bed sand filters and multimedia deep-bed filters for the removal of suspended matter has been mentioned before. Silica sand is commonly used in sand-

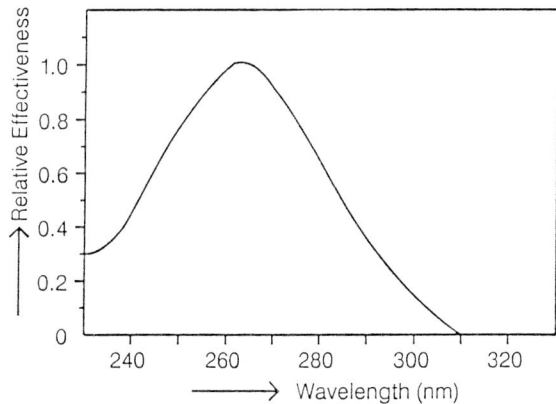

FIG. 3. Germicidal action curve in the ultraviolet region of the energy spectrum. From Meulemans, C. C. E., Basic Principles of UV Sterilization—Sterilization of Water. In: *Proceedings of the International Ozone Association* (W. G. Mashelem, ed.), European Community, Paris, 1986. Courtesy, International Ozone Association.

bed constructions [17]. Such beds have nominal porosities of 10 to 40 μm; newer beds have lower porosities. The size of the sand grains determines the packing densities. Retention of suspended matter takes place in the top 6 in. (15 cm) of the bed. The remaining depth serves to regulate the flow of water through the bed. At moderate flow rates (4–16 gal/min/ft^2 for rapid sand beds, 2–3 gal/min/ft^2 for slow sand beds), the flow volumes are defined by the extent of bed surface. Actual flow depends upon the silt density index of the feedwater. Pre-RO sand beds require flows as low as 1 gal/min/ft^2 to ensure complete removal of the suspended particles.

Carbon Bed Operation

An example of a successful carbon-bed operation may illustrate a diverse and sometimes contradictory experience. A pharmaceutical company has for some three decades utilized a carbon bed downstream from sand beds and separated by filters from downstream ion-exchange beds. The carbon tank or shell is 6 ft high (1.8 m) and 54 in. (137 cm) in diameter, and contains about 50% of freeboard. The normal effluent rate is about 120 gal/min. The beds are backwashed twice daily to cleanse them of iron deposits. The backwash is at the rate of 200 to 250 gal/min. Microbial assays are performed on alternating days, thrice weekly. Microbial alert limits are set at 600 to 700 cfu/mL. The action limit is 1000 cfu/mL for three consecutive days on the cold water system, ascertained as total heterotrophic plate counts. This action limit calls for hot (65°C) water sanitization. The heated water is flushed into the bed and trickled to a total volume of 500 to 1000 gal in an overnight operation during a weekend. Carbon fines are removed overnight from new beds by an upward flush (backwash), barely vigorous enough to overflow the fines to drain. The successful operation of the carbon bed is ascribed to its continuous recirculative flow from its inception. The flow, through a line (0.5–1 in.) capable of delivering about 30 gal/min ranges from 25 to 40 gal/min (approximately 10 to 20 gal/min/ft^2), regardless of whether water is being supplied to the downstream ion-exchange beds or not. The return loop to the carbon bed is by way of the preceding sand beds. In summary, the three elements of maintenance of this carbon bed are continuous recirculation, twice-daily automated backwashes, and weekly sanitizing with hot water (65°C).

The Water Softener

It is good practice to use two softeners that are by design out of phase, so that one is being regenerated while the other is operative. To avoid organism growth, softeners not in use should be kept in recharged condition with 26% brine, ready to be flushed free of the brine and thus make water operative on a moment's notice. The addition of calcium hypochlorite pellets to the salt supply helps to keep the latter sanitized. Wherever possible, hot water sanitization of the water softener should be performed at 65 to 90°C. The cation-exchange resin survives heating at 90°C.

Principal Unit Purification Processes

As stated, generalized pretreatment design would consist of chlorination of the source water; the removal of iron, manganese, and suspended matter by coagulation and flocculation and/or deep-bed filtration; water softening; and the removal of TOC followed

Validation of Pharmaceutical Water System

by elimination of the chlorine from the treated water. Each of these pretreatment steps requires documented experimental verification or validation to make certain it conforms to the operational SOPs and to ensure that its purported action is indeed attained. The pretreated water is ready for purification by any or all of the principal processing units.

Ion Exchange

Ion-exchange resins are polyelectrolytes immobilized by the cross-linking of large organic moieties. In cation-exchange resins the functional group is anchored to sulfonic acid substituents whose mobile hydrogen ions (actually hydronium H_3O^+) can exchange with other cations. The law of mass action, as modified by specific ion selectivities, governs these exchanges. The result is an uptake of cations by the spacially fixed resin and a release of hydrogen ions in exchange. The anion-exchange resins, of which like the cation-exchange resins there are several types, utilize spacially fixed quaternary amine groups associated with mobile hydroxyl ions. As anions are acquired by the anion exchangers, hydroxyl ions are liberated. The released hydrogen and hydroxyl ions interact to form water, largely undissociated into ions. The overall effect of cations and anions being removed from solution is one of demineralization or of deionization. This is the very purpose of the ion exchange purification unit.

Reverse Osmosis

The USP 23 approves the use of reverse osmosis along with distillation for the preparation of Water For Injection. It may, of course, also be utilized for the preparation of Purified Water. However, the FDA insists that reverse osmosis used for the preparation of WFI must be in the form of a two-pass, product–stage arrangement, where the product water effluent from the first reverse osmosis unit is used as feedwater for the second RO unit.

There are at least three different types of RO membranes available. The oldest type is composed of cellulose acetate. The more recent reverse osmosis units, based on polyamide membranes, have the advantage of better rejection qualities. However, the polyamide RO membrane is easily destroyed by chlorine. A third type is composed of polysulfonated polysulfone. It has the advantage that it is resistant to chlorine but it is little used.

Distillation

Stills vaporize water separating it from nonvolatile impurities. The water vapor is condensed, allowing its separation from volatile impurities. Unfortunately, stills furnishing large volumes of distillate require high heat inputs that provide opportunities for vapor entrainment of droplets, and consequently a carryover of impurities. This problem is addressed by still design and by the proper operation of the still. Proper operation is defined in the development of the SOP suitable to the distillation. The validation of the still operation must, therefore, involve documented experimental evidence that the SOP protocols appropriate for the still were adhered to. Still design is also concerned with minimizing the heating costs by optimization of the vaporizing and condensing functions.

Modified GMPs Related to Water Systems

The FDA has established a number of GMPs that pertain to the preparation of pharmaceutical waters. However, in practice, promulgation may have undergone modification, as a consequence of the FDA's ongoing and evolving understanding of pharmaceutical water systems.

21CFR §211.48 Plumbing

(a) Potable water shall be supplied under continuous positive pressure in plumbing systems free of defects that could contribute contamination to any drug product. Potable water shall meet the standards prescribed in the Public Health Service Drinking Water Standards set forth in Subpart J of 42 CFR Part 72. Water not meeting such standards shall not be permitted in the plumbing system.

The Fifth Supplement of USP 23 [13] in its Official Monograph section permits, as of November 1996, the use of waters comparable to European Union or Japanese regulations.

21CFR §212.49 Water and Other Liquid-Handling Systems

(a) Filters may not be used at any point in the water for manufacturing or final rinse piping systems.
(b) Backflow of liquids shall be prevented at points of interconnection of different systems.
(c) Pipelines for the transmissions of water for manufacturing or final rinse and other liquid components shall:
    (1) Be constructed of welded stainless steel (nonrusting grade) equipped for sterilization with steam, except that sanitary stainless steel lines with fittings capable of disassembly may be immediately adjacent to the equipment or valves that must be removed from the lines for servicing and replacement,
    (2) Be sloped to provide for complete drainage,
    (3) Not have an unused portion greater in length than six diameters of the unused pipe measured from the axis of the pipe in use.

Although objections still exist among FDA inspectors regarding the use of filters, the 1993 FDA *Guidelines to Inspection of High-Purity Water Systems* states:

If filters are used in a water system there should be a stated purpose for the filter (i.e., particle removal or microbial reduction), and an SOP (standard operating procedure) stating the frequency with which the filter is to be changed which is based on data generated during the validation of the system.

Piping need not be of stainless steel construction. Indeed, the manufacture of certain proteins, particularly susceptible to denaturation by transistion elements, excludes iron, nickel, chrominum, etc., ions, but polymer piping may be used. Extractables and mechanical properties, particularly at elevated temperatures, are of concern. These are, however, satisfied by several polymeric compositions.

Validation of Pharmaceutical Water System

Dead legs are conventionally, if unofficially, defined by length-to-diameter ratios as low as 3:1.

21CFR §211.225 Water For Manufacturing or Final Rinsing

Water used as component or as a final rinse for equipment or product contact surfaces shall:
(c) Be stored in a suitable vessel or system including a piping network for distribution to points of use:
  (1) At a temperature of at least 80°C under continuous circulation, or
  (2) At ambient or lower temperatures for not longer than 24 hours, after which time such water shall be discarded to drain.

Pharmaceutical waters are still largely stored as described above. However, they may be stored under any conditions validated to preserve their required qualities. Storage under ozone is widely practiced. Storage at ambient temperatures in conjunction with periodic heating to and at 80°C is not uncommon. A prudent practice involves the stored water being maintained at 80°C at least for 4 h weekly. This is meant to address biofilm sanitization concerns as wells as kill of planktonic organism.

Among the GMPs not modified into less rigorous practices is the strong imperative for careful, complete, and conscientious record keeping and documentation.

Specific Unit Process Validations

The operation of each individual purification unit, part of the operational validation, requires its own focus and assessment. After the system has been correctly designed and installed, how is it to be validated? A number of questions must be answered in the validation exercise:

What component or unit of the system is being addressed?
What is its function?
What is the measure of its performance?
What are its normal maintenance requirements?
What additional maintenance may occasionally need to be performed?
When are sanitizations to be carried out?
What sanitization method is to be utilized?

An example is the carbon-bed purification unit. Its chief purpose is dechlorination, although it may also be relied upon to reduce the TOC load. Its performance is assessed by measuring the chlorine content of both the incoming and effluent waters, or the TOC, using an on-line TOC monitor. What would be the measure of the carbon bed's performance? In the case of dechlorination, complete chlorine removal would be expected. Therefore, the effluent water should contain zero chlorine. The performance standard for the TOC could be set variously. It could, for instance, be judged against a goal of less than 1 ppm, or the target could be a reduction of 50% of the original TOC burden, etc., whatever seems appropriate. Next would be to list and carry out the normal maintenance needs, for instance, backwashing, bumping (to eliminate channeling), and rinsing. Shall these operations be performed, as in a multimedia bed on the basis of pressure drop, or in response to a reduction in TOC uptake, in other words, in accordance with the achievement of a measured value? Alternatively, maintenance can be instituted on a time basis, say daily. The time basis can be set according to experience against an historically measured value, or in keeping with a prophylactic philosophy. Occasionally additional maintenance protocols must be observed, for example, replacement of the carbon bed.

When is the carbon bed to be sanitized? Shall it be in response to specific levels of organisms in the effluent water, or periodically on a time basis? How is the sanitization to be performed, by hot water or by steam?

Safety protocols must be observed. In the design of the water purification system, the installation of the necessary test ports, isolation valves, and protocols for microbiological and chemical assays are to be provided for. All performed operations and the data they generate will require analysis, documentation, and countersigning.

Municipally Treated Feedwater

It is generally considered advantageous to use municipally treated water, which is of potable quality, as is required for the starting waters of all pharmaceutical water manufacture. No doubt that is the case in most situations. However, in some instances problems occur in municipally treated waters. Such sources may contain quantities of aluminum ions, from excessive alum treatments, which, health implications aside, may contribute to the fouling of RO membranes. Iron fouling may occur where ferric chloride is used as the coagulating agent in place of alum. The use of chlorine, in conjunction with TOC, can create difficult-to-remove trihalomethanes, whereas efforts to avoid that situation by the neutralization of the chlorine with ammonia leads to the generation of chloramines which, although bacteriocidal, are objectionable. In such instances, the municipal water supply is not free of difficulties. Perhaps most important of all, as has already been alluded to, where the quality of municipal waters changes over relatively brief periods of time, validation can be a problem.

Batched Water Supplies

Batched water supplies offer advantages. The water isolated in storage can be characterized as fully as desired by pertinent analyses. The likelihood of chemical change is remote. Microbiological stability is less assured, depending upon the duration of storage, but is subject to control, particularly at high temperature conditions or containment under ozone. In essence, batched water can offer the security of a well-defined ingredient and the constancy of composition. The batching process, therefore, lends itself more easily to validations. By contrast, a system under continuous flow is not defined by its characterization at any given point. The changes it may undergo are less certain to be detected and plotted with confidence.

Batch-style operations are expensive in terms of capital outlay and are, therefore, justified only where the certainty of the batch water identity is required to ensure and protect a high product value. Batching operations demand careful design, in order to eliminate dead legs and guarantee batch integrity. Where large volumes of water are involved, as for both rinse and product water, batching may involve storage in several large tanks, which can be expensive. At this point, continuous-flow systems become advantageous. In continuous operations the necessary quantity of water is automatically maintained in the supply tank by the ongoing water production units. The piping requirements are simpler and are less likely to introduce dead legs [3]. Overall, continuous-flow requirements are less costly in terms of capital expenditures. With the need to keep constant the quality of an ever-flowing (and possible ever-changing) water product, a greater reliance must be placed on top sophisticated purification units. By the same token, the insurance of system predictability and of water quality constancy is more difficult to validate.

Another View of Validation

When a pharmaceutical company plans, constructs, equips, and operates a compendial water manufacturing facility, the responsible individuals and groups are expected by management periodically to report on the progress being made and on the status of the undertaking. The periodic reports would be illustrated and confirmed by relevant data obtained with reliable, and hence calibrated, instruments. The system design necessary to consistently produce water of the required quality in sufficient peak and total quantities would be decided upon. The correct constructions and dependable functioning of installed units would be checked and substantiated. Proof would be offered that the system designs, their constructions, and safe operations are on target. Pertinent documents relating to safety, drawings and descriptions of equipment, operational protocols, sampling, and testing procedures would be collected and retained. The reports and documented presentations would be intended to demonstrate to management that the assignment was being carried out correctly. Ultimately, the successful completion of the task would be attested to in a final report. The claims of an operationally functional water-purification system, dependable over long durations and safe in its operation, would be supported by an adequacy of appropriate data and documentation. Consistency in the stipulated quality of the product water over prolonged periods of time would be the proof of the attained goal.

It can be useful to regard such a company report as the essential system validation required by the FDA. Its purpose would be the twofold one of ensuring that the purification system is indeed capable of consistently producing compendial quality water in a dependable fashion. Since this twofold goal is the very aim of the FDA validation requirements, to address the FDA regulatory strictures becomes an important but secondary exercise.

The need to validate the pharmaceutical water system to ensure its dependable performance carries a regulatory burden. The postulation of validation originated from the FDA. It is, therefore, not unusual to hear the question, "What does the FDA require of the validation activity?" To repeat, the FDA validation exercise is meant to answer two questions: Does the system work? Does it do so consistently? Supportive experimentally secured documented data in substantiation of positive responses constitute the validation of the pharmaceutical water system.

Post-Validation Activities

The validation in its several phases having been completed, the water system requires periodic examination and testing as long as it remains in use. Change control is a serious issue. Have alterations, additions, or deletions, been made to the system? Have operational changes been made? What are the risk implications of such alterations? Are the drawings of the system kept up to date? Periodic follow-up checks should be made. If changes are made to the system by the substitution, for instance, of a pump, was the same or a different type of pump used? Was an RO unit added? Were substantial physical changes instituted? If so, these should be added to the P&ID list, and the system drawings should be updated. In particular, changes to the SOPs should be documented.

Routine data analysis should be performed on an ongoing basis by the QC laboratory to determine that the system continues to function satisfactorily. How are out-of-specification results explained; was the sampling or the system at fault? What was the cause of the deviation? What action was taken to correct it? Deviations from the SOPs must be explained, and deviation reports are required. For example, if the SOP states that sanitizations are needed every three days, and such an action was taken only after five days, the reason for the deviation must be stated. Were ultraviolet lamps cleaned or replaced in accordance with the standard maintenance schedule? Routine audits should, therefore, be made of the maintenance records, for instance, of the sanitization practices. The FDA inspector will certainly examine maintenance logs.

The data, particularly the microbiological, should be plotted, at least monthly. Identification should be made of organisms that are present. In particular, changes in the types and numbers of organisms should be looked for. The risk assessment of such changes should be made.

These routine and periodic examinations constitute an internal audit of the water system. In addition, the FDA inspectors in their audits will look at the validation data compiled by the drug manufacturer and by vendors. The pharmaceutical processor should also audit the vendors' data.

Periodic checks should be made of the validation data, protocols, and procedures, to ensure that the operational instructions are being followed. The FDA investigators will, for their part, do so during their inspections.

The Water System Audit*

The water system audit, whether performed by the FDA or by the drug manufacturer, is essentially an inquiry into the postvalidation actions. The documentation contains the

---

*Use has been made of the teaching of John Y. Lee, Executive Director, PCA Pharmaceutical Compliance, North Massapequa, NY.

activities pertinent to the proper operation of the water system, and establishes what was in fact performed in the actual exercise. The recorded test and operational data will be examined in the compliance audit for their adequacy to support the conclusions. The regulatory investigators require explanation of the discrepancies between promise and performance. For example, the responses to bacterial excursions will be examined. What corrective action was taken?

The audit covers system design, calibration, and maintenance, the monitoring program, remedial actions to alert and action limits, and the qualifications of the water system in general. The system design is examined, including the sampling ports before and after each of the purification units, such as carbon beds, softeners, deionization (DI) beds, RO, UV lights, filters stills, and the product-water holding tanks. The feedwater quality is examined by analytical data. The system design considerations with regard to recirculation, constructions of stainless steel or polymeric materials, and the possibilities for heat sanitization and hot storage is checked.

In particular, inspection is made of sanitary fittings, pitched piping, the absence of threaded joints, pressure-relief rupture disks, diaphragm valves, and the avoidance of dead legs. The absence of in-line filters is preferred. Heat-exchangers are inspected for their double-tube sheet constructions, or for the ongoing monitoring of constant positive pressure to their thermal-fluid transference side.

With regard to the RO units, the auditors ascertain that the pretreatment of the feedwater is performed as specified, and that the RO unit is not followed by DI beds with their inevitable tendency to organism growths. As in the case of the heat exchangers, the inspectors will make reference to the FDA *Inspection Technical Guide*.

The utilization of ion-exchange resins is audited. Where in-situ regeneration is performed, purity specifications for the regenerant chemicals, and a testing protocol for their eventual removal are implemented. With regard to DI resin for portable units, dedicated resins and containers are preferred where individual or bulk regeneration is involved. The maintenance program for nondedicated resins should include vendor certification of the industries serviced to ensure the absence of resins used in electroplating shops with their concomitant heavy metal impurities. Vendor assurances of such restricted uses, the vendor's particulars and records on resin regeneration, storage, and delivery should be supplied. Stand-by resin beds are to have time limits for the stand-by intervals, and suitable storage and maintenance controls over organism growth, such as recirculation and refrigeration, should be inspected.

In addition, auditing the maintenance programs involves examining records for the backflushing, sanitizing, and periodic replacement of the activated carbon beds, as also the sanitization, whether by chemicals, hot water, or steam of the water distribution and storage facilities. With regard to filters for venting or water flow, the frequency of sanitizations and change, as prescribed in the maintenance procedures, is examined. Regulatory investigators inspect whether proper maintenance is being performed on UV lamp installations. Periodic checks and recordings of lamp intensities are compared with their operating requirements. Conformity with lamp cleaning and replacement schedules is ensured. Records are examined for the correct flow rates through the UV units. It could be helpful to check microbiologically for the recovery of atypical organism morphologies following UV irradiation.

The microbiological assays and procedures are closely examined. Time limits and storage requirements indicated for microbiological samples should be obeyed. The frequency of testing at appropriate locations is checked. It will be ascertained whether aseptic techniques and sterile utensils were utilized in the performance of the microbiological assays, along with the proper nutrient media, and incubation times and temperatures stipulated in the SOP. The appropriateness of the supporting data to the claim of microbiological validation is closely examined.

Documentation is inspected to ensure the adequacy of record keeping. The various qualification steps, installation, qualification, purification-unit qualification, performance qualification, etc., are inspected. Data supporting claims of validation are examined for the correctness of the conclusions being drawn.

The questions asked by FDA investigators do not necessarily reflect established regulations and practices, nor do they imply that satisfactory techniques or approaches are necessarily available to the industry. The obligation of the investigator is to establish an overall balanced judgment in complicated situations where contradictory factors may be at work. An extensive and even overreaching probing may be a useful device in such circumstances. Opportunities abound for investigators, at times, to arrive at apparently contradictory conclusions. The different inspectors may each have his particular expertise and technique. Not every inspection is meant to cover the entire system. A given inspector may be intended for a particular investigative purpose. Therefore, an absence of adverse observations on the inspector's 483 form does not constitute an endorsement of any unmentioned operation, nor does it exempt the pharmaceutical processor from untoward consequences. The general intent, however, is clear: to safeguard the public safety while separating acceptable practices from those that require improvement and optimization.

The pharmaceutical water producer should be prepared, and should not hesitate, on the basis of documented experimental data, to dispute the FDA investigator's adverse judgements and observations where these seem to be erroneously derived. In the resolution of such contradictory points of view lies the potential for the ongoing developmental progress of pharmaceutical water systems.

The audit examines the documented evidence upon which are based the multifaceted design and operation of the water system in all its complexity to learn whether the claims made for the system's adequacy and validation are justified. The operational data are then evaluated for the support they provide to the assertion that the operation of the water system is in keeping with the validation scheme, that it performs satisfactorily, and is so maintained as to generate water of acceptable quality in a consistent manner. In the reconciliation of the differences, if any, between what the system purports to do and what it actually does, lies the attainment of the requisite first rate pharmaceutical water system.

Acknowledgment

This article is based on Meltzer, T. H., *Pharmaceutical Water Systems: Their Design and Validation*, Tall Oaks Publishing Co., Littleton, CO, ISBN-0-927-188-6-6, 1997.

Bibliography

Code of Federal Regulations, 1976. Human and Veterinary Drugs, 21CFR, Parts 201, 207, 210, 211, 229; *Fed. Register* 41(31): 6878-6894; Human Drugs—CGMPs for LVPs and SVPs, 21CFR, Part 212, *Fed, Register*, 41(106): 22202-22219; "Tree Nuts and Peanuts," 21CFR, Part 128f; *Fed. Register*, 41(127): 27000-27002; Nonclinical Laboratories Studies, 21CFR, Parts 3e, 8, 121, 312, 314, 430, 431, 514; *Fed. Register*, 41(225): 51206-51230.

Code of Federal Regulations, 1978. For Parenteral Injection; Related to Asbestos-Containing or other Fiber Releasing Filters, 21CFR, E211, 40, p. 63.

References

1. FDA, *Guidelines to General Principles of Process Validation*, Food and Drug Administration, Rockville, MD, 1978.
2. FDA, *Guideline on Sterile Drug Products Produced by Aseptic Processing*, Center for Drugs and Biologics and Office of Regulatory Affairs, Washington, June 1987.
3. Artiss, D. H., Water System Validation. In: *Validation of Aseptic Pharmaceutical Processes* (F. J. Carleton and J. P. Agalloco, eds.), 1st ed., Marcel Dekker, Inc., New York, 1986, Chap. 9.
4. Keer, D., *Gathering Validation Documentation for Pharmaceutical Water Systems*, Rust, Bensalem, PA, 1995.
5. Artiss, D. H., *PDA Workshop on Validation of Pharmaceutical Water Systems*, Parenteral Drug Association, Bethesda, MD, 1978.
6. Meshnick, D., *The Role of Documentation in the Validation Process*, Foster Wheeler USA, Clinton, N.J., (in press).
7. *United States Pharmacopeia*, 23rd ed., The United States Pharmacopeial Convention, Rockville, MD., Water For Pharmaceutical Purposes, p. 1984; Official Monograph, Water, 1995, pp. 1636-1637.
8. Munson, T. E., *FDA Views on Pharmaceutical Water*, Food and Drug Administration, Rockville, MD, 1993.
9. FDA, *Guide to Inspections of High Purity Water Systems*, Division of Field Investigation, Office of Regulatory Affairs, Washington, July 1993, p. 4.
10. Water Quality Committee, Pharmaceutical Manufacturers Association, Updating requirements for pharmaceutical grades of water: microbial considerations, *Pharmacop. Forum*, 18(6): 4397-4399 (1992).
11. Water Quality Committee, Pharmaceutical Manufactures Association, Updating requirements for pharmaceutical grades of water: validation and technology selection, *Pharmacop. Forum*, 19(6): 6633-6645 (1993).
12. Water Quality Committee, Pharmaceutical Manufacturers Association, Updating requirements for pharmaceutical grades of water: proposed revisions, *Pharmacop. Forum,* 20(3): 7526-7544 (1994).
13. *United States Pharmacopeia*, Fifth Supplement to USP 23rd ed., The United States Pharmacopeial Convention, Rockville, MD, 1996.
14. Kemmer, J., ed., *The Nalco Water Handbook*, McGraw Hill Book Co., New York, 1988.
15. Muraca, T. W., and Goetza, Yu V. L., Disinfection of water distribution systems for *Legionella*—Review of applications, processes, and methods, *Infect. Contr. Hosp. Epidemiol.*, 11(7): 79-88 (1990).

16. Meltzer, T. H., and Rice, R. G., Ultraviolet and Ozone Systems. In: *Biological Fouling of Industrial Water Systems: A Problem Solving Approach* (M. W. Mittelman and G. G. Geesey, eds.), Water Micro Associates, San Diego, CA, 1987.
17. Ogedengbe, O., Characterization and specification of local sands for filters, *Filtr. Sep.*, 21(4): 331–334 (1984).

THEODORE H. MELTZER

Veterinary Uses of Drugs

History of Veterinary Pharmacy

Historically, pharmacists have had little to do with the care of animals. Veterinarians have been, for the most part, solely responsible for the diagnosis, treatment, and dispensing of medications for companion animals for many years. The same has been true for large animals (including pleasure animals, such as horses, and feed animals, such as sheep, cattle, and pigs) with the exception of feed stores and catalogs for the distribution of some medications. The role of the pharmacist has been only to fill an occasional prescription for "Rover Jones," for a human medication which is not readily available to the veterinarian. This historical practice has given the veterinarian full control of the dispensing aspect of his practice. However, it also ties up the veterinarian time wise and often results in the veterinarian seeing fewer patients in a day's time.

In recent years, there has been small growth in a group of practicing veterinary pharmacists. These professionals are very helpful in veterinary hospitals. They have been useful to the veterinarians in determining compatibility of medications, instructing in sterile solutions, and problem solving in areas such as providing large volume intravenous solutions to a horse without restraining it. In community practice, these specialized pharmacists can help prevent accidental poisoning of pets by advising customers on the use of over-the-counter (OTC) medications for pets [1].

These professionals have also been helpful to veterinary schools by becoming involved in teaching students the necessity of providing sterile conditions in the operating room, sterile technique in making intravenous solutions, and drug interactions. This information can save the lives of some animals and reduce unnecessary medical bills for other animals [2].

The Future of Veterinary Pharmacy

The best possible scenario for potential veterinary pharmacists is to develop a rapport with the local veterinarians. Pharmacists in the retail setting have a good opportunity to be available to the local veterinarians as consultants and drug experts. Once the veterinarians are able to appreciate the importance of pharmacists as a source of valuable information, the relationship can begin. This relationship must be nurtured and carefully developed, as most veterinarians prefer to be self-sufficient and will look down upon anyone who, they feel, is attempting to step on their "turf." After the relationship is fully developed, the veterinarian begins to give up certain aspects of dispensing to the pharmacist, realizing that he or she can see more patients if not burdened with the dispensing of medications. He or she will then send the caretaker of the animal to the pharmacy which specializes in veterinary medications or devices. The veterinary pharmacist can serve as a source of information to the consumers on the use of OTC medications for their pets, since some animals do not tolerate various medications and others require a drastic dosage adjustment [3]. These pharmacies display a "Veterinary Center" for OTC treatments and devices, and also have a veterinary section in the prescription area. Needless to say, the same pharmacy serves human patients as well.

Veterinary pharmacy in the hospital setting is most likely restricted to animal hospitals, especially those associated with a veterinary school. The need for a veterinary pharmacist in a human hospital is unlikely. There could conceivably be a need for a veterinary pharmacist in a large independent veterinary practice, especially if it is dealing with both companion and domestic animals.

Many of the companies within the pharmaceutical industry have a veterinary branch and provide various medicinals to veterinarians. These companies could benefit from the expertise of a veterinary pharmacist as a consultant to provide them with expert information dealing with the veterinary aspect of pharmacy.

Drugs for Companion Animals

Dogs

Dogs have always been popular companion animals, with both children and elderly in need of companionship. Today, more and more hospitals and nursing homes are allowing patients to be visited by dogs. Some hospitals allow such visits even to critically ill patients in the intensive care areas. Research has shown that a positive mental outlook is helpful in the recuperation process. In addition, companion animals, especially dogs, are often times responsible for improving mental outlook, therefore reducing the recovery time from accidents or illnesses.

Common Ailments

Anal sac disease often occurs in dogs due to the failure of soft feces to properly express the anal glands. These glands empty into the rectum during bowel movements or at times of fright. Sometimes the rectal opening becomes blocked with fecal matter and does not allow for the glands to empty. The gland then becomes filled and possibly infected. Dogs with this problem drag their rear end on the ground in an attempt to squeeze out the accumulation. They may bite at the anal area and show pain or discomfort on defecation. It was often believed that this activity indicated the presence of worms. This is not necessarily true, as the anal glands can be the problem as well. It is important to obtain the proper diagnosis before any treatment is administered as treatment with a dewormer in a constipated dog can lead to toxic effects. The glands should be checked first, and if they are full, the fluid can be easily expressed by squeezing. The veterinarian can show the dog owner where the glands are located and how to empty them. They should be checked routinely every six months to prevent blockage. In addition, dry dog food and dog biscuits are helpful, as they produce a firm stool, which promotes expression of fluid from the glands, therefore preventing blockage. Infected sacs require local and/or systemic antibiotic therapy. Exercise is also helpful in preventing anal sac disease. In extreme cases of blocked anal glands that are not treated, other problems such as lameness (due to pressure on the spine), itching, and tonsillitis (due to licking the anal area) may occur [4,5].

Veterinary Uses of Drugs

Arthritis occurs in older dogs, especially those that are obese. Minimizing the weight gain as the dog grows older can reduce this problem. This condition can become crippling. Various treatments are available, including steroids (in severe or advanced cases), buffered aspirin, or phenylbutazone. The dog should be kept in warm and dry quarters to minimize discomfort [6].

Cardiac conditions can develop in elderly canines, especially those who are overweight. Usually the first signs of a heart condition are coughing and enlargement of the abdomen due to ascites. Poor circulation often arises, leading to edema, and congestive heart failure. Diuretics such as furosemide are useful in this situation. Dogs with congestive heart failure are often prescribed digoxin and have their diets adjusted. In serious situations, many of the human cardiotonics are useful in dogs as well, such as dobutamine, amrinone, milrinone, and sodium nitroprusside [7].

Diabetes is another common disease, often occurring in the overweight animal. It is usually seen over the age of four. Symptoms are similar to those of human diabetes mellitus, frequent urination and increased thirst. This is followed by weight loss, increased appetite, and possibly emaciation. In severe cases, uncontrolled vomiting may occur. If diagnosis is made early, the disease may be controlled by diet alone. The diet that is recommended is a low carbohydrate, high protein diet. Cases which cannot be controlled by diet alone, may need the help of either Neutral Protamine Hagedorn (NPH) or Protamine Zinc insulin injections. This method is usually successful [8,9].

Epilepsy is a fairly common ailment in dogs, especially cocker spaniels and poodles as well as other breeds of small dogs. There are a wide variety of types and frequency of seizures in dogs, similar to the variation in human seizures from petite mal to grand mal. The frequency may be as infrequent as once a year or as frequent as several times a day. Usually the seizures do not last long. Quite often excitement triggers a seizure in a dog. Commonly, seizures can be controlled by agents such as primidone, phenytoin, or potassium bromide. Once it has been established that the prescribed drug can control the seizures, the dose is often adjusted to a maintenance level [10,11].

Urinary incontinence is extremely common in aging female dogs, especially those that are spayed. It is believed to be a hormone problem and is often treated, at least initially with diethylstilbestrol administered orally. This is given daily until the urination becomes controlled again, and then can be decreased to several times a week as a maintenance dose. Some male dogs with incontinence problems respond to doses of testosterone. An alternative therapy for urinary incontinence is the use of phenylpropanolamine at a dose of 2–4 mg/kg per day in divided doses. The mechanism of action is not completely understood.

Common Infectious Diseases

Prophylaxis against canine infectious diseases is given in Table 1. Canine distemper is caused by a virus related to the human measles virus known as a paramyxovirus. This virus infects the central nervous system, and in addition to upper respiratory tract and intestinal tract symptoms, causes chorea (twitching of muscles) which may affect the legs, one side of the body, or the tail. Secondary bacterial infections are common. This should not be confused with rabies, another infection of the central nervous system. Distemper cannot be spread through the bite of an infected animal, rather it is spread through the air or on clothing inasmuch as it is highly contagious. Treatment is frustrating, as there are no antiviral agents. Treatment may include antibiotics in the case

TABLE 1 Canine Prophylaxis[a]

Organism	Disease	Vaccine Type	Schedule	Comments	Classification
Borrelia bronchiseptica	Kennel cough	Modified live or bacterin	Multiple initial doses beginning at 6 weeks of age, annual revaccination	Use if there is a problem with this organism in the area	Optional
Borrelia burgdorferi	Lyme disease	Bacterin	Initial 2-dose series beginning at 12 weeks of age, annual revaccination	Use in dogs who spend a great deal of time out doors	Optional
Coronavirus	Coronavirus infection	Killed	Initial 2-dose series beginning at 3 months of age, annual revaccination	Use for dogs who spend time in kennels or at shows	Optional
Canine distemper virus	Distemper and kennel cough	Modified live	Multiple initial doses beginning at 6 weeks of age, annual revaccination	Part of the recommended "puppy shots"	Recommended
Canine adenovirus Type 1 (CAV-1)	Hepatitis	Modified live	Multiple initial doses beginning at 6 weeks of age, annual revaccination	Part of the recommended "puppy shots"	Recommended
Canine adenovirus Type 2 (CAV-2)	Kennel cough	Killed	Multiple initial doses beginning at 6 weeks of age, annual revaccination	Gives cross protection with CAV-1, may be used as part of the "puppy shots"	Recommended

Leptospira sp.	Leptospirosis	Bacterin	Multiple initial doses beginning at 6 weeks of age, annual revaccination	Part of the recommended "puppy shots"	Recommended
Parvovirus	Parvoviral infection	Modified live or killed	Multiple initial doses beginning at 6 weeks of age, annual revaccination	Part of the recommended "puppy shots"	Recommended
Canine parainfluenza virus	Kennel cough	Modified live	Multiple initial doses beginning at 6 weeks of age, annual revaccination	Part of the recommended "puppy shots"	Recommended
Rabies virus	Rabies	1-year or 3-year killed	2-Dose initial series with revaccination annual or every 3 years	Must be certified by a veterinarian	Required
Dirofilaria immitis	Heartworm	Ivermectin	Doses given monthly after negative blood test	Oral prophylaxis	Recommended

[a]From Refs. 138–141.

of secondary bacterial infections, and good nursing is essential. Some dogs may require anticonvulsants as well. Many sick animals stop eating. This has to be counteracted by coaxing the animal to eat, or even tube feeding. An antiserum is available, which is extremely helpful in the early stages. A vaccine is also available for this infection. It should be administered to puppies at eight weeks of age with a booster several weeks later, followed by annual revaccination. Puppies that were bottle fed for one reason or another should be vaccinated with the human measles vaccine as early as three weeks of age, since they do not get antibodies from the mother's milk [12,13]

Canine parvoviral infection is characterized by enteritis with an acute onset which results in severe diarrhea and loss of fluids and electrolytes. The virus is shed in the feces and spread usually via ingestion of contaminated feces by uninfected animals. Mortality is most common in puppies, and death is usually a result of electrolyte imbalance and dehydration. Some animals display myocarditis which can also be fatal. Diagnosis can be made by isolating the organism from the stool. Treatment is purely symptomatic, since there are no antiviral agents against this organism. Fluid and electrolyte replacement are essential to survival. Both a live, attenuated vaccine, and an inactivated vaccine are available for this infection. Weaned puppies should be vaccinated every two to three weeks until they reach an age of 16 to 18 weeks, and then receive an annual revaccination. A similar infection, corona virus infection, is caused by a virus which is difficult to distinguish from the parvovirus [14].

Hepatitis is another viral infection, caused by the canine adenovirus, type I (CAV-1). This virus is usually spread via the urine of infected dogs. The initial symptoms of this infection are fever, conjunctivitis, and intestinal symptoms such as vomiting and diarrhea. The dog's eyes develop corneal opacity which gives the eyes a blue or white coloration, resulting in temporarily blindness. Eventually the liver becomes infected, and chronic hepatitis can develop. Treatment includes blood transfusions and intravenous fluids; antibiotics may be used against secondary bacterial infections. A live, attenuated vaccine is available and is usually administered along with the distemper vaccine on the same schedule. CAV-2 (see kennel cough below) protects also against CAV-1 but does not produce the side effect of corneal opacity [15,16].

Rabies is a disease which can affect all mammals, including wild, domestic, and companion animals as well as humans. The virus is spread primarily through saliva, although exposure to infected brain tissue can also spread the disease. Rabies infects the central nervous system, causing paralysis of various muscles throughout the body, beginning in the throat and progressing to the hind limbs. The infection of the central nervous system often leads to a drastic personality change in the animal. Shy animals become extremely aggressive, whereas aggressive animals become docile. The rabid animal may exhibit one of two basic personality types: those with "dumb rabies," who sit with their mouths hanging open, and those with "furious rabies," who attack someone or something which they would never have attacked previously. Sometimes animals with "dumb rabies" are thought to have something stuck in their mouth. A person may stick their hand in the mouth to help, and suddenly become bitten. Never stick your hand in any animal's mouth. Some, but not all, rabid animals drool, that is they produce frothy saliva which drips out of their mouths. This is a helpful diagnostic tool, but not all animals show this symptom. There are a variety of vaccines available, and in many states vaccination of companion animals is required by law and its administration must be certified [17,18].

Kennel cough, or infectious tracheobronchitis, is a highly contagious infection which may be caused by a virus, such as canine adenovirus, type 2 (CAV-2), canine distem-

Veterinary Uses of Drugs

per virus, or parainfluenza virus (CPI). Bacteria such as *Bordetella bronchiseptica* are often secondary invaders. This infection is generally a mild, self-limiting infection involving the bronchi and trachea. Often stress and environmental factors such as cold, drafts, high humidity, and so on increase the dog's susceptibility. The designation "kennel cough" came about since many dogs developed the infection when they were boarded in kennels. This is a stressful situation in itself, and a change in the animal's environment. Therefore, kennel cough was common in boarded animals. Now, reputable kennels require proof of vaccination against this infection in order for an animal to be boarded. The infection's major symptom is a hacking cough which lasts several weeks. The cough is often followed by retching or gagging and is easily produced by gentle palpation of the larynx. Secondary bacterial pneumonia is a common problem with this infection. Treatment includes antitussives such as codeine and butorphanol as well as antihistamines. Antibiotics should be used in secondary bacterial infections. In severe cases, steroids can be used to reduce inflammation. Vaccines are available for the four pathogens listed above. Immunization to the viruses are part of the routine beginning at puppyhood. Vaccination against *Bordetella bronchiseptica* is reserved for geographical areas which experience difficulties with bacterial kennel cough due to adverse local and systemic reactions [19].

Leptospirosis is a bacterial infection caused by a *Leptospira* species. This infection, which is transmissible to humans, can cause kidney and liver damage. It is carried by rats, and is often spread in rat-infested areas by urine. The mucous membranes of the mouth become inflamed and the skin sloughs off. Treatment is difficult; sometimes a combination of tetracycline and streptomycin is successful. Uremic animals can be saved by peritoneal dialysis, although the inconvenience and cost must be taken into consideration by the animal owner. The vaccine for this disease is part of the routine puppy immunization program [20,21].

Lyme disease affects the veterinary world in the same way as it affects humans. This is a tick-borne infection caused by the spirochete *Borrelia burgdorferi*. Although deer ticks are the major vector, other ticks such as the dog tick and wood tick as well as biting flies and other biting insects are also implicated. Symptoms in dogs are similar to those in humans, except that the red rash is often missing or at least not noticed due to the thick coat which many dogs have. The predominant canine symptoms are fever and arthritis, which mainly affects the larger joints. This infection may be recurrent or develop into a chronic arthritis. Various antibiotics are useful, including ampicillin and tetracycline. A vaccine is available which is administered at 12 weeks of age with a booster three weeks later. Annual revaccination is recommended [22].

Heartworm, a parasitic infestation caused by *Dirofilaria immitis*, is a major concern for dog owners today. The parasite is spread to dogs via the mosquito, usually during the warmer months of the year. The parasite makes its home in the heart where it multiplies. Infestation leads to shortness of breath (especially during and following exercise), cough, and lack of stamina. Ultimately, death can occur. Treatment of this condition is difficult. The parasite is a roundworm which reaches lengths of 27 cm (10 in.). When the dog is treated with anthelmintics such as arsinamine or dithiazanine iodide, the worms often move through the body, and may become lodged in vital veins, arteries, and ducts. This may be the cause of the animal's death. Treatment success often depends on the number of adult worms present in the heart. A better way of dealing with this infestation is to prevent it by yearly blood work to determine whether the dog is infested or not. If the test is negative, a preventative regimen can begin. The two major preventatives on the market are diethylcarbamazine or ivermectin. The latter can be administered every 30 days during the mosquito season. Veterinarians in some areas are now recommending that the preventative be administered year round. Ivermectin is also available in combination with pyrantel pamoate [23,24].

Cats

Cats are very different pets from dogs. They are much more independent and difficult to restrain. It seems that most people either love or hate cats. There does not appear to be much middle ground.

Common Ailments

Digestive disorders in cats are relatively common. These disorders may appear as constipation or diarrhea due to an improper diet, or hairballs. Constipation is often caused by insufficient water in the diet or small bones. A diet of strictly dry food with little water consumption can lead to constipation. A teaspoonful of vegetable oil on the food or the addition of milk to the diet helps to prevent constipation. Diarrhea is often seen in the pampered cat who receives treats such as hot dogs, bologna, or spicy foods on a regular basis. When the diarrhea is noticed, food should be withheld except for water to prevent dehydration. Kaopectate (one teaspoon) can be administered every 3 h as needed for loose bowel movements. Since diarrhea can be a symptom of an infectious disease, cases that do not respond after 12 h of treatment should be reported to a veterinarian. Hairballs occur when the cat cleans itself; they are a particularly difficult problem in cats with long hair. The hair mats in the stomach and forms a wad which may be 6-8 in. (15-20 cm) long and 2-3 in. (5-7.6 cm) in diameter. Cats often regurgitate hair balls, but if not, severe problems can arise. These large wads can cause constipation or intestinal obstruction. There are products on the market specifically flavored for cats. Most of these products contain mineral oil, milk of magnesia, or castor oil. These products can be administered alone, but the flavoring is helpful in getting the cat to accept the medication [25].

Poisoning of cats is not infrequent. Sometimes the poisoning is intentional, caused by cat haters or mischievous children. However, some poisoning is unintentional. Both phenol and warfarin poisoning can be prevented. Cats are extremely sensitive to phenols and can be poisoned by the ingestion of water from the toilet which has been cleaned with Lysol products, or from licking their paws after walking across a floor which has been recently cleaned with Lysol or a similar product. A cat can be prevented from drinking from the toilet by keeping the lid closed or from walking across a recently washed floor which should be thoroughly rinsed. Treatment includes the induction of vomiting, intravenous fluids, soothing preparations to the gastrointestinal tract, and good nursing. Warfarin is found in mouse and rat poisons. It causes death by internal bleeding. Rat poisons must be kept out of the cat's reach and should be well hidden. Dead rodents should be removed as the cat can be poisoned by ingesting the dead rodent. Poisoning due to warfarin can be treated with vitamin K which is an antagonist to warfarin. Blood transfusions and intravenous fluids may also be necessary. It is important to get the cat quickly to the veterinarian as time is of the essence [26,27].

Urinary calculi are often seen in male cats, many of which have been castrated. There is some controversy as to whether castration itself can predispose the cat to this condition. More important to this condition is urinary pH. If the pH of the urine re-

Veterinary Uses of Drugs

mains acidic, the likelihood of the cat developing urinary calculi declines. Some authorities believe that the ash and mineral content of the cat food may contribute to this condition. However, the predominant opinion is that the pH of the urine is the major factor, and there are foods on the market which reduce the urine pH to help prevent this condition. Maintaining a urinary pH of 6.0–6.4 minimizes urinary problems. Treatment of urinary calculi is not easy. As long as the calculi are being passed, treatment should be targeted at decreasing the urine pH. If one of the calculi becomes lodged in the urethra, the situation is more serious. The bladder becomes distended and hard, urine backs up in the kidneys, and eventually uremia, which can be fatal, develops. This requires catheterization, or some other method to dislodge the calculi and prevent toxemia. Antibiotics may be administered following the traumatic treatment to prevent infections [28].

Common Infectious Diseases

Feline distemper or panleukopenia is a highly contagious infection caused by a parvovirus. This infection strikes very quickly and may even cause death before any sign of illness. Sometimes this infection is confused with poisoning. As the name suggests, there is marked leukopenia in this disease, as well as fever, vomiting, diarrhea, weakness, and depression. Fluids and blood transfusions are useful in preventing death in some cats. Antidiarrheals and other symptomatic treatment are helpful. The best way of dealing with possible infection is prevention with a vaccine; both live and inactivated vaccines are available. The recommendations for disease prophylaxis in cats are given in Table 2. An antiserum gives temporary protection following exposure to the virus [29,30].

Feline infectious peritonitis (FIP) is caused by a coronavirus. The major symptoms involve the central nervous system where granulomatous lesions are formed. Neurological effects begin with paraparesis and progress to tetraparesis. The mortality rate approaches 100%. In the acute phases, the infection mimics an upper respiratory infection. In the chronic phase, lesions may form throughout the body. Likely sites are the kidneys, liver, lungs, eye, meninges, and brain. The immune response is not very good. In fact, it appears that FIP-positive cats are actually sensitized to subsequent exposure to other FIP strains which results in an acute, fulminating fatal disease. Treatment is ineffective, although a vaccine is available which is administered by the intranasal route. It is recommended that FIP-negative cats be kept away from FIP-positive cats, if at all possible [31].

Feline lymphosarcoma and leukemia are two very common forms of cancer in cats which have been linked to the feline leukemia virus. The disease is spread from cat to cat via the saliva. There is no evidence that the virus is spread to humans. Some cats experience a subclinical infection and develop immunity. Other cats become persistently infected. Still others develop one of the malignancies. The greatest incidence of malignancy is in homes where other cats have the disease. The symptoms of malignancy are similar to malignancies in humans, such as chronic wasting, pain, development of tumors (in the case of lymphosarcoma), anorexia, and lethargy. Other symptoms depend on the location of tumors. The feline leukemia virus is also capable of causing a nonmalignant infection which appears as a nonregenerative anemia and immunosuppression. A closely related virus is capable of causing feline acquired immune deficiency syndrome, very similar to HIV infection in humans. The malignancies are treated with

TABLE 2 Feline Prophylaxis[a]

Organism	Disease	Vaccine Type	Schedule	Comments	Classification
Feline calicivirus	Feline calicivirus infection	Modified live or killed	Multiple initial doses beginning at 6 weeks of age, annual revaccination	Part of the recommended "kitten shots"	Recommended
Chlamydia psittaci	Feline pneumonitis	Modified live or killed	Initial 2-dose series dose beginning at 9 weeks of age, annual revaccination	Part of the recommended "kitten shots"	Recommended
Coronavirus	Feline infectious peritonitis	Modified live (intranasal) or killed	Initial 2-dose series beginning at 16 weeks of age, annual revaccination		Optional
Feline leukemia virus	Feline leukemia	Modified live or killed	Multiple initial doses beginning at 10 weeks of age, annual revaccination	Follows a negative blood test	Optional
Parvovirus	Panleukopenia or feline distemper	Modified live or killed	Multiple initial doses beginning at 6 weeks of age, annual revaccination	Part of the recommended "kitten shots"	Recommended
Feline herpesvirus	Rhinotracheitis	Modified live or killed	Multiple initial doses beginning at 6 weeks of age, annual revaccination	Part of the recommended "kitten shots"	Recommended
Rabies virus	Rabies	1-year or 3-year killed	2-dose initial series with revaccination annual or every three years	Must be certified by a veterinarian	Required

[a]From Refs. 138–141.

Veterinary Uses of Drugs

conventional human antitumor agents and sometimes radiation therapy. Some cats respond quite well, developing long-lasting remissions. There is a vaccine for the feline leukemia virus, but some vaccinated cats develop an infection. The vaccine should be administered only after the cat has tested negative for the virus [32].

Like dogs, cats are susceptible to rabies. They are even more susceptible because of their inherent nature to roam and be territorial. They are more likely to challenge an invading animal, no matter who it is. The symptoms are similar to those for dogs. Treatment and prevention are also the same.

Feline respiratory disease complex is a group of infections with similar symptoms involving the upper respiratory tract. Feline rhinotracheitis (FVR) is caused by a herpesvirus. Cats that recover can become healthy carriers. The mortality is low, and the prognosis is good except for kittens and aged cats. Feline calicivirus infection (FCI) is also caused by a virus. This infection is characterized by mouth ulcerations in addition to upper respiratory symptoms, two strains of this virus have been known to cause the "limping syndrome." Feline pneumonitis (FPN) can be caused by a *Mycoplasma* species or *Chlamydia psittaci*. These bacterial infections often cause a conjunctivitis as well as upper respiratory symptoms, especially those caused by *Chlamydia*. Treatment of the viral infections is largely symptomatic with antihistamines such as chlorpheniramine maleate, cleansing of the eyes and nose, vasoconstrictor nose drops (epinephrine), and oxygen tents if breathing is a problem. Broad-spectrum antibiotics should be used for bacterial infections. There are two modified live vaccines available for FVR-FCI infections. One is a parenteral vaccine, the other an oronasal vaccine which is administered into the conjunctival sac and the nasal passages [33,34].

Abscesses are one of the more common infections in felines. Males are especially prone to this, as it is often a result of fights which result in puncture wound. Once the puncture wound heals, the abscess forms from within. It is best to have this lanced by a veterinarian, to clean out the wound, and allow it to heal. Broad-spectrum antibiotics should be administered as a wide variety of bacteria are often involved in these mixed infections [35].

Feline infectious anemia (FIA) is caused by the rickettsia *Haemobartonella felis*. This infection usually occurs in cats one to three years old, especially males. The mode of transmission is often a bite wound. The result is an autoimmune hemolytic anemia. Some of the symptoms include weakness, depression, emaciation, liver and spleen involvement, and dyspnea which can become severe in some chronic cases, requiring oxygen. Blood transfusions may be indicated, and treatment with one of the tetracyclines is usually effective [36].

Rabbits

Rabbits have been a fairly popular companion animal, especially for children. They are often allowed in apartments where dogs or a cats are excluded. They can be very tidy and do not bark.

Common Ailments

Dental malocclusion is a hereditary condition which affects the ability of the rabbit to eat. The rabbit's incisors, premolars, and molars grow throughout life. Normal tooth length is maintained by the constant grinding of opposing teeth. When the teeth are out of alignment, overgrowth of the teeth occurs. This not only makes eating difficult, but can also result in severe tongue or cheek lacerations. A temporary solution is to file or cut the teeth. Rabbits with this condition should not be bred [37,38].

Heat exhaustion is a relatively common occurrence in rabbits which are housed outdoors in areas where the summers are hot and humid. The best conditions for a rabbit are 60–70°F (15–21°C) and 40–60% humidity. If not treated, heat exhaustion can cause death. The rabbit will lie on its side and breathe rapidly. Treatment can include sprinkling with cool water, bathing in cool water, free access to cool or ice water, the use of a fan, or moving the rabbit to an air conditioned area [39].

Hutch burn occurs most frequently when the rabbit is housed in a wooden cage. The rabbit's urine soaks the wood and when the rabbit sits on it, the ammonia from the urine causes a chemical burn on the exposed area. The most common areas affected are the feet, the anal area, and the genitals. Proper cleaning and disinfection of the cages is a good preventative. Bland ointments can be applied to the affected area to hasten healing. Bacterial infections may follow and should be treated with topical and/or systemic antibiotics [40,41].

Moist dermatitis or wet dewlap occurs most frequently in does due to their large dewlap or flap of skin under the chin. When drinking from a bowl, water often drips on the dewlap. Eventually the dewlap becomes soggy and inflamed, and may become infected. If this occurs, topical or systemic antibiotics should be used. Moist dermatitis can be prevented by providing water in a bottle instead of a bowl. There is little dripping from the bottle, minimizing the moisture on the dewlap [39].

Common Infectious Diseases

Infectious myxomatosis is a viral disease that can affect domestic rabbits. It is caused by a poxvirus which is spread to the rabbits via mosquitos, biting flies, and direct contact. The first sign is conjunctivitis, which is quickly followed by a fever of 108°F (42°C) (normal body temperature for a rabbit is 102.5°F or 38.8°C), labored breathing, droopy ears, coma, and death as soon as in 48 h, but possibly up to two weeks later. There is no specific treatment but a vaccine is available [42].

Rabbits are also subject to rabies, although domesticated rabbits are less likely than cats and dogs to be exposed as they rarely run free out of doors.

There are three common infectious diseases in rabbits which affect the gastrointestinal tract. Enterotoxemia usually occurs in bunnies between the ages of four and eight weeks. It is characterized by an explosive diarrhea and death within 48 h. It is not uncommon for the bunny to die before the owner even realizes that it is sick. The causative agent is *Clostridium spiroforme*, which produces the exotoxin responsible for the symptoms. It is not completely understood how the rabbit becomes infected; diet seems to play an important role. Bunnies with a high fiber diet (consisting of hay or straw) rarely have a problem with this disease. Treatment is difficult due to the rapid death [40].

Mucoid enteropathy is a diarrheal disease which can occur at any age. Its etiology is unknown, but it seems to follow a period of constipation and is not an infectious disease per se. When the rabbit becomes constipated, its gastrointestinal tract responds by producing a gelatinous substance which helps to lubricate the feces for removal. Problems occur when there is an overproduction of this gelatinous substance and the result is a type of gelatinous diarrhea. This diarrhea becomes chronic and may persist for a week or two, but is generally followed by death. Treatment with rehydration and electrolyte replacement may be beneficial [40,43].

The third gastrointestinal infection is Tyzzer's disease, which is caused by the bacterium *Bacillus piliformis*. This too causes severe diarrhea and rapid death in young rabbits (usually six to twelve weeks of age), although it can affect rabbits of any age. The organism is introduced into the rabbit by ingestion, probably from poor sanitation in the cage. Death usually occurs in one to three days [44].

In addition to gastrointestinal problems, another common group of ailments in rabbits is known as pasteurellosis. It can occur in several areas of the rabbit's body from the skin, to the eye, to the genitals, and the lungs. The responsible organism is known as *Pasteurella multocida*. Abscesses can develop, usually in males, in an infected skin wound, caused by a fight or an injury within the cage. Treatment is often expensive, and the cost of treatment may be higher than replacement of the rabbit. Effective antibiotics include oxytetracycline and a combination of penicillin and streptomycin. In addition to abscesses, pasteurellosis can occur as conjunctivitis (due to dusty quarters or where sawdust is used for bedding), genital infections (especially in females, and due to poor sanitation in the cage), and an upper respiratory infection known as snuffles, which may be followed by pneumonia. Rabbits are exceptionally prone to the stresses of change in food, environment, and weather (outdoor rabbits). Infections often follow some form of stress in the rabbit's life. Snuffles is treatable, but pneumonia can cause death if not treated properly with is a solution of oxytetracycline in the drinking water for a week to ten days. Some rabbit owners use a preventative dose of oxytetracycline (half strength) following periods of stress or at the first sign of a sneeze. This is a good preventative method [45,46].

Coccidiosis is a parasitic infection which can cause diarrhea in young rabbits. Some do not show severe diarrhea, but fail to gain weight as they should, and some may even lose weight. This parasite can be transmitted via one of several intermediate hosts (birds, cats, sheep, as well as other animals). Without treatment, the animal often dies within 30 days. The best treatment is with sulfaquinoxaline in the food (0.025%) or the drinking water (0.04%) for 20 to 30 days [47,48].

There are no recommendations for disease prophylaxis in rabbits at the present time.

Birds

Birds are a unique group of pets in that they are capable of flying. No other group of pets (except for bats) have this capability. This may make their care difficult, if they take off when it is time to treat them. Birds require correct handling in order to prevent injury to both the bird and the owner.

Common Ailments

Feather loss is one of the most common reasons for veterinary visits for bird owners. It may be due to disease or to psychological factors. In the absence of infectious diseases, the bird may be picking the feathers out due to boredom. This can be resolved by providing toys and/or a mirror in the cage [49].

Gout is a painful condition in which uric acid is deposited in the joints and related membranes. Signs may include swelling of the joints and/or difficulty urinating. It is believed that gout is a metabolic disease. Treatment may include hospitalization to increase fluid consumption and the use of antibiotics to prevent secondary bacterial infections. Allopurinol may be useful in some cases. Alkalinizing the drinking water with a small amount of bicarbonate of soda may be helpful [50].

Common Infectious Diseases

Budgie fledgling disease is a recently recognized infection of very young budgerigars caused by a papovavirus. Other psittacines may also become infected. There is a high mortality rate in very young birds. Symptoms include diarrhea, dehydration, swollen abdomen, and death within one or two days. There is also a lack of down on the back and abdomen. Tail feather and contour feather growth is delayed in birds that survive more than 15 days. French mould may actually be a mild form of this disease. There is no treatment, but a vaccine is showing great promise in this infection [51].

Pacheco's parrot disease is caused by a herpesvirus and primarily affects the psittacines. It is spread by direct contact or by fecal contamination of food and/or water. Birds that are most susceptible are the macaws, Amazon parrots, cockatoos, cockatiels, parakeets, and some conures. Symptoms include vomiting, bright yellow diarrhea, neurological symptoms in the terminal stages, and acute death in some cases. An inactivated vaccine is available [52].

Pox disease is caused by a family of poxviruses, depending on the strain of *Poxvirus avium* (canary, parrot, pigeon, fowl, and turkey). There are three clinical forms: cutaneous (series of crusty lesions occurs on unfeathered parts of the body, mortality is low), diphtheritic (extensive fibrinonecrotic lesions on the mucous membranes, mortality is high), and a combination of the two. Transmission is by direct contact with infected birds or via insect vectors. Parenteral vitamin A, vidarabine ointment, and antibiotics (to prevent secondary bacterial infections) are helpful. There are vaccines for specific species of birds, which protect only against that strain of the virus [53].

Viscerotropic velogenic Newcastle disease (VVND) is caused by a paramyxovirus and is a reportable disease. Common birds which are susceptible to this virus include cockatiels, cockatoos, Amazon parrots, and conures. Transmission is via respiratory aerosol, fecal contamination of food and/or water, and direct contact with infected birds. Symptoms include depression, anorexia, weight loss, upper respiratory tract symptoms, bright yellow-green diarrhea, and in prolonged cases neurological symptoms. Some birds die from this infection; only the symptoms can be treated. Vaccination is prohibited in imported birds due to the fact that it does not eliminate the carrier state and masks the virus during the quarantine stages [52].

Psittacosis (chlamydiosis or ornithosis) is a relatively common infection which affects nearly all imported and breeding collections of psittacines (parrots, budgerigars, and cockatiels). It is caused by *Chlamydia psittaci* and is transmissible to humans. The major symptoms of psittacosis include upper and lower respiratory symptoms, diarrhea, and rapid death. Secondary bacterial infections are common. Transmission is primarily due to inhalation of nasal exudates or fecal dust. The infection is treated by mixing chlortetracycline in the food for 30-45 days; vaccination is not effective [54].

Candidiasis or moniliasis is a very common fungal infection in birds. It is caused by *Candida albicans* and primarily affects young birds. However, birds of any age can be affected in some species, especially lovebirds. It can be caused by prolonged anti-

Veterinary Uses of Drugs

biotic therapy, vitamin A deficiency, and spoiled feed. Symptoms include unthriftiness, slow weight gain or weight loss, vomiting, and increased appetite. There are raised, white lesions on the mucous membrane of the mouth. Treatment includes antifungal agents such as nystatin, and ketoconazole; topical iodine and supplemental vitamin A may be helpful; there is no vaccine [55].

Recommended Disease Prophylaxis

Vaccines that are available for captive birds include an inactivated vaccine for Pacheco's disease and live, attenuated vaccines for pox disease in canaries. In addition, vaccines for pox disease in other species are being developed.

Reptiles
Common Ailments

Gout is seen in reptiles as in birds. Symptoms are similar to those seen in birds, but treatment is slightly different. A combination of allopurinol with colchicine is sometimes useful [56].

Common Infectious Diseases

Cutaneous ulcerative disease is an infection in turtles caused by *Citrobacter freundii*. *Serratia* sp. may become involved in the infection process and act synergistically with the *Citrobacter*. Symptoms include a purulent discharge, anorexia, lethargy, and petechial hemorrhages. Liver necrosis commonly accompanies these symptoms. Systemic antibiotics and good sanitation are essential to recovery and prevention of further episodes [57].

Infectious stomatitis is a common problem in snakes, lizards, and turtles. These animals can develop infection due to *Pseudomonas* sp. and *Aeromonas* sp. which begins as petechiae in the oral cavity. The infection can progress to the bony structures of the mouth. Respiratory and gastrointestinal infections may occur in poorly managed animals. Debridement, irrigation with antiseptics, and antibiotic therapy are necessary for recovery. In severe cases, surgery may be required. Vitamin A and vitamin C supplementation is recommended [58,59].

Ulcerative dermatitis or scale rot is a skin condition of snakes and lizards which can result in secondary bacterial infections due to the *Pseudomonas* sp. and the *Aeromonas hydrophilia*. Infection with these organisms can lead to septicemia and death. This condition is often a result of high humidity. Treatment with broad-spectrum antibiotics such as tetracycline administered topically and/or parenterally, as well as improved hygiene are essential to recovery; there is no vaccine [60].

Mycotic infections can occur in all species of reptiles. They are usually a result of high humidity and poor management. Fungi of the species *Aspergillus, Metarhizium, Mucor, Paeciolmyces*, and *Penicillium* are a few of the responsible organisms. Infections usually develop slowly and affect the respiratory tract. The gastrointestinal tract and skin, shell, or scales may also be involved [61].

There are no recommendations for disease prophylaxis in reptiles at this time.

Exotics

Exotics is a term used to describe any animal which is normally considered a wild rather than a domestic animal which is now being enjoyed as a companion animal. These types of animals are becoming more and more popular today. Ferrets are the most common exotic animals; they will be discussed further.

Common Ailments of Ferrets

Enteritis is one ailment relatively common to ferrets. The etiology of this disease is unknown. Symptoms include anorexia and bloody diarrhea. Death occurs in three to four days. In some cases, the condition becomes chronic, with intermittent diarrhea. Eventually the animal becomes emaciated and dies in three to five weeks. Treatment is symptomatic, including fluid and electrolyte replacement, and antibiotics for the prevention of secondary bacterial infections [67].

Common Infectious Diseases

Canine distemper is an infection to which ferrets are extremely susceptible. The symptoms are similar to those seen in dogs with death occurring in 12 to 14 days. In animals which initially survive, death may occur weeks to months later due to neurological disease. Vaccination with the modified live canine vaccine from chick embryo is recommended. Vaccination with the modified live canine vaccine of ferret origin has been known to transmit disease to these animals and is not recommended [63].

Human influenza can be easily spread to ferrets. The disease in the ferrets is usually mild and may require antihistamines. Some veterinarians have used the human influenza vaccine as a preventative for ferrets, but its use is not recommended [62].

All wild animals are susceptible to rabies. Animals that come from an area which has a high incidence of rabies in wildlife are at high risk of exposure. Vaccination is highly recommended in all exotics, but especially in those from high incidence areas [64].

Ferrets are susceptible to one or more types of botulism which is caused by *Clostridium botulinum*, types A, B, and C. Infection in ferrets usually occurs if the animal is fed noncommercial feeds. Ferrets can be protected by a trivalent botulism toxoid for active immunization [64].

Recommended Disease Prophylaxis

Canine distemper vaccine as well as rabies vaccine is recommended for disease prophylaxis in ferrets. Ferret owners should also investigate the need for heartworm and botulism preventatives.

General Care of Companion Animals

Internal Parasite Control

Internal parasites are a common problem in all companion animals. They are especially a problem in young animals (less than one year) and animals that roam outside rather than being indoor pets. It is not unusual to find a parasite infestation in a newborn animal, such as a puppy or kitten, even though the mother was wormed prior to conception. Internal parasites seen in companion animals include roundworms, tapeworms, whipworms, flukes, and protozoa. Over-the-counter "worm medications" often contain a mixture of anthelmintics and are not the best approach to the internal parasite problem. The better approach is to have stool samples checked on all adult animals every six to twelve months. If parasites are found, they should be treated with the most effective agent. For animals under one year of age as well as outdoor animals, stool samples should be examined every three to six months.

External Parasite Control

Companion animals can develop a variety of external parasite infestations, from mange and lice to ticks and fleas. Ticks and fleas cause by far the most problems and will be discussed here. As most people are aware, disease is spread by ticks, primarily Lyme disease. Therefore, it is important to daily check a pet for evidence of ticks by feeling the entire surface of the animal and checking for bumps, especially inside the ears, a good hiding place for ticks. The best way to remove a tick is by grabbing the arthropod firmly between thumb and forefinger, and pulling until it is released. The tick should be removed as smoothly as possible as it is not uncommon for its mouth parts to remain in the skin and later become infected. Other commonly used methods for tick removal include the use of a hot match, vaseline, organic solvents, and other means. These methods irritate the tick, who then injects enzymes into the skin, causing damage. It is best not to use these methods of tick removal unless absolutely necessary.

Fleas are another nuisance to companion animals. For animals who are allergic to flea bites the situation is difficult, in fact almost intolerable. For some animals, a single flea on the body can make them highly irritated with agitation from the itching which accompanies the flea bite. A severe flea infestation can be a real problem to the pet owner who sometimes is bothered by flea bites as well as the animal. The fleas are not only on the dog, cat, rabbit, or ferret, but in the animal's bedding, in the carpet, and throughout the house. Although flea removal from the animal is not easy, removal of fleas from the household is extremely difficult. Flea control has just become more manageable with the discovery of a new, orally administered insect-development inhibitor known as lufenuron or Program. This substance interferes with the production of chitin in fleas. Chitin is required for flea maturation. The end result is the inhibition of the growth of flea eggs and larvae. Lufenuron does not kill adult fleas, and therefore this treatment must be administered in combination with other types of flea control, such as sprays, dips, and powders. Adult fleas do, however, ingest the medication when feeding on the animal. The lufenuron then acts on subsequent offspring of the flea, which never reach maturity. It may take 30 to 90 days for this medication to work efficiently due to the fact that it effects only the offspring and not the adults. Program is administered orally according to the weight of the animal, and is given once a month. It is available for both dogs and cats. There are a variety of insecticidal agents used in flea control. In addition, insect growth regulators (IGR) are being used. The most commonly used insecticides fall into one of the following categories: pyrethrins, organophosphates, and carbamates. It is important when treating flea infestations, not to mix these different types of insecticides. Some combinations may be harmful to the pets. Of the three types, the pyrethrins are the most popular, probably because they have the best margin of safety. Another insecticidal agent, a cholinesterase inhibitor known as cythioate or Proban, is also available orally in tablet or liquid form. It is administered two times a week according to the animal's body weight, and is effective in killing adult fleas. Numerous topical agents (sprays, dips, powders, and collars) can be used alone or in conjunction with other products. In severe infestation, the pet's bedding, and the home and yard which the pet inhabits may need to be treated. Numerous OTC products (sprays, bombs, foggers, and powders) are available [65–70].

Domestic Animals

Sheep and Goats

Sheep and goats are becoming more and more popular as pets. In addition, they are useful for the production of wool, milk, and meat. Since the needs and problems of these two types of animals are similar, they are discussed here together. Sheep, in general, are less friendly than goats, and therefore are not as desirable as pets. However, if they are taken from the ewe at an early age and bottle fed, they can become friendly. Goats are more intelligent than sheep and escape easily. They can jump over fences and find various ways to escape other restraints. If either of these animals is allowed to roam freely on a small piece of property, caution is advised. They graze on whatever is available (especially goats), including azaleas, rhododendron, and other plants which may be poisonous. This can result in the loss of the animal.

Common Ailments

The most important condition occurring in sheep and goats is actually seen most often in sheep. Ketosis, also known as pregnancy disease, usually develops during the last weeks of pregnancy. This is a management problem which usually can be prevented by an astute sheep farmer. The initial symptoms are a "slow" ewe or doe, who seems to be disinterested in feed. As the disease progresses, the animal begins to stagger, go in circles, prop the body against a wall, and grind its teeth. As with ketosis in cattle, this disease is a carbohydrate disorder, characterized primarily by hypoglycemia. The best way of dealing with this disease is to keep a close eye on all pregnant ewes, segregate those ewes that appear "slow" at feeding time and feed them separately, concentrating on carbohydrates. They could be fed special treats at this time such as carrots, potatoes, stale bread, and extra grain with molasses. If this does not improve the behavior or if the disease has progressed too far, the ewe needs to be force fed with a good carbohydrate source such as propylene glycol. This is essential to keep the ewe alive until the young are born. Once the lambs are born, the health of the mother returns back to normal in a short time [71,72].

Common Infectious Diseases

Foot and mouth disease (FMD) or sore mouth is caused by a picornavirus. It is extremely contagious and can be transmitted to humans. It can be brought to a farm by a sheep shearer or new additions to the flock. The infection is manifested by a group of lesions in and around the mouth, also on the feet between the toes, and on the nose.

Veterinary Uses of Drugs

There is no cure, and treatment includes the feeding of soft, palatable foods, possibly even resorting to force-fed liquids (known as drenching). Antibiotics can be used in secondary bacterial infections. A live vaccine is available. The recommendation is that all new sheep be vaccinated and isolated for two to three weeks [73,74].

Pneumonia is often the cause of death in sheep, and survivors often show substantial weight loss. Once a ewe has had pneumonia, it is difficult for her to survive a pregnancy and nursing due to the strain on the body. Several bacteria and viruses can cause pneumonia. The infection often follows a stressful period. In addition to fever, the sheep show signs of difficulty breathing, puffing, and panting for air, and they go off feed. Since sheep easily loose their will to live, pneumonia must be treated early and aggressively. Infected sheep should be isolated and treated with antibiotics. Expectorants may be useful in breaking up the mucous in the lungs. Light exercise, sunshine, and steroids may be helpful. The appetite can be stimulated with treats such as apples, carrots, and oats with molasses [75,76].

Scours is a term for a fairly common diarrheal disease in sheep and goats. It can be caused by a number of bacteria and viruses, combined often with overeating. Lambs and kids should be observed for sticky tails indicating diarrhea. The area should be cleaned well, and the animal treated with appropriate antidiarrheals. Kaopectate works well as well as reducing the milk intake if possible. In older animals, scours is usually due to overeating grain or lush pastures. Other causes of diarrhea need to be taken into consideration. A good rule of thumb is to treat the animal, and then observe it for 24 h. If the diarrhea continues, a stool sample should be examined by a veterinarian [77,78].

Enterotoxemia or overeating disease is caused by the bacterium *Clostridium perfringens* type D. This disease is not easily treated, but can be prevented by active immunization with a toxoid. It is most often seen in feedlot situations, where the goal is rapid weight gain. It can, however, occur on small farms if the animals gain access to the feed bin, or if the ewes and does manage to invade the creep feeder. Symptoms include circling, pushing their heads against the wall, convulsions, unsteadiness, and rapid death. This disease can occur in lambs who drink too much milk. The toxoid is administered in two-dose series with annual boosters. Enterotoxemia due to *Clostridium perfringens* types B and C can also occur, but is less common [79,80].

All domestic animals are susceptible to tetanus. This infection is caused by a bacterium, one of several species of *Clostridium*; the same disease affects humans. Usually it follows some type of puncture wound; domestic animals are at risk in situations where their fields and pastures have nails, wires, poor fencing, and other miscellaneous items on which they can get hurt. First signs of this infection include stiffness in one or more of the limbs as well as refusal to eat. The tetanus antitoxin can be administered when an animal is injured, but it must be administered before symptoms occur. This disease is best prevented by administering the tetanus toxoid, initially in a two-does series, followed by annual booster doses [81,82].

Foot rot is a mixed infection, with *Candida albicans* being one of the common invaders. The first sign of this infection is lameness, followed by refusing food. The foot should be trimmed and cleaned out. The best treatment is copper sulfate and keeping the animal on a dry pasture or barn area [83].

Coccidiosis is a protozoal infection which usually causes stunted growth, diarrhea, and unthriftiness. The animals most likely to be seriously affected by coccidiosis are young lambs and kids. Older animals may be infested with this protozoa, but their body mass compensates for the infestation, and the animal is often asymptomatic. This infestation usually occurs in animals that are kept in a barn or stable. Animals kept on open pastures are rarely afflicted. The protozoa can be carried by other animals such as cats and birds. The infection can be treated by adding sulfas to the drinking water [84].

Recommended Prophylaxis

The recommendations for disease prophylaxis in sheep and goats depends on the infections which are prevalent in the area where the animals are being raised. Prophylaxis is available for a number of infections (Table 3).

Cattle

Most cattle are used for production of meat or milk and are extremely valuable to the farmer. The management of beef cattle and dairy cattle vary, mostly because of the regulations which the dairy farmer has to follow in order to sell the milk. Sanitation and cleanliness are extremely important to the dairy farmer, while the beef farmer is much less concerned with these issues. Treatment of diseases and infections is often determined by the use of the cow, bull, or steer.

Common Ailments

Bloat is often caused by overeating. Lush clover especially is the culprit. The result is an abnormal amount of gas formation, with relatively small bubbles which are difficult to expel via belching. The gas continues to collect. If the animal is untreated, it begins to stagger, show respiratory difficulties, pant, and collapse into a heap. Without treatment, death may occur. Treatment consists of the administration of defoaming agents, such as corn oil, peanut oil, safflower oil, or soybean oil. These oils allow the aggregation of the small gas bubbles into larger ones, which can be belched out. The oils are best administered before the animal is showing severe symptoms. If the animal is close to death, a trochar can be used. This is a sharp object similar to an awl, with a cannula which is inserted into the back of the animal, at the highest point of the bloat (usually on the left side, just in front of the hip). This allows the gas to escape from the animal through the opening in the trochar. When bloat is caused by overeating grain, the gas bubbles are usually large and can be removed by inserting a stomach tube and manipulating it to relieve each pocket of gas. This should be followed by administration of one of the bloat medications to combat further gas formation as the remainder of the grain is digested [85,86].

Ketosis, or acetonemia, is a result of poor management which occurs a few days to a few weeks after calving. This disease is similar to ketosis in sheep and goats, except that rather than occurring during pregnancy it follows. The disease is primarily a metabolic disorder associated with decreased carbohydrate metabolism. It is characterized by hypoglycemia with associated ketonemia, ketonuria, loss of appetite, weight loss, and decreased milk production. The incidence is highest in high-producing stall-fed cows. In cows the disease is self-limiting, since the reduction in food consumption leads to a reduction in milk production, which decreases the carbohydrate drain on the body. Susceptible cows should be maintained on a relatively high carbohydrate intake before calving. The level should be increased further after parturition. The feed of thin un-

TABLE 3 Caprine and Ovine Prophylaxis[a]

Organism	Disease	Vaccine Type	Schedule	Comments	Classification
Clostridium perfringens, Types C and D	Overeating disease	Toxoid	Two initial doses followed by annual revaccination	Antitoxin is available for passive protection	Recommended
Clostridium tetani	Tetanus	Toxoid	Two initial doses followed by annual revaccination	Antitoxin is available for passive protection	Recommended
Picornavirus	Foot and mouth disease or soremouth	Modified live	Two initial doses followed by annual revaccination		Optional
Rabies virus	Rabies	1-year killed	2-Dose initial series with revaccination annually	Must be certified by a veterinarian	Recommended

[a]From Refs. 139–141.

dernourished cows should be supplemented with carbohydrates such as propylene glycol [87,88].

Common Infectious Diseases

Bovine viral diarrhea (BVD) is caused by a togavirus. In severe cases, the main concern is severe diarrhea, accompanied by fever, hemorrhage in the alimentary tract, depression, and dehydration. Mild cases may not present with diarrhea. Embryonic death or abortion may occur in pregnant cows. In addition, BVD is an immunosuppressive infection and may therefore lead to concurrent infections. Transmission is due to direct contact with an infected animal or by indirect contact via contaminated food or water. Acute cases may lead to death in 48 h. The effect on the fetus depends on its age at infection and the strain of the virus. Diagnosis is difficult since many other infections mimic BVD. There is no specific treatment for this infection; supportive treatment is all that can be done. Both a modified live virus vaccine and an inactivated vaccine are available to provide protection [89,90].

Infectious bovine rhinotracheitis (IBR), infectious pustular vulvovaginitis (IPV), and associated syndromes are caused by bovine herpesvirus-1 (BHV-1). This organism is responsible for numerous manifestations such as respiratory infections, abortions, encephalitis, conjunctivitis, and genital infections. The manifestation depends on the route of infection, the age, and the immune status of the animal. In feedlot cattle, the respiratory infection is the most common, whereas in breeding animals, abortion causes most of the problems. As with most herpesviruses, after the initial infection, the virus remains dormant in the animal for an indefinite period of time. Stress can reactivate the infection like herpesviral infections in humans. In respiratory infections, secondary bacterial infections pose the largest threat to the animal. Abortions can occur whatever the disease manifestation is. The symptoms of these infections depend on the disease presentation. Although there is no specific treatment for these infections, modified live as well as inactivated vaccines are available, the former for intranasal or parenteral administration. Caution should be used, however, since the parenteral live vaccine can cause abortions in cows. Vaccination should be done at six to eight months of age and every one to two years thereafter [91]. Rabies in cattle should be treated in the same way as in other domestic animals.

Infectious keratitis or pinkeye, usually occurs in the summer months. The infection is caused by a number of organisms including *Moraxella bovis, Mycoplasma bovoculi*, and the infectious bovine rhinotracheitis virus. The organisms are primarily spread via flies which land on the animal around the eyes and then move on to the next animal. The eyes of infected animals usually begin to show lacrimation, the animal shows signs of photophobia, and the eyes look bloodshot. If left untreated, the affected eyes develop a cloudy film and eventually exhibit a bluish-white color. Blindness can occur. Upper respiratory symptoms may also occur if the causative agent is the infectious bovine rhinotracheitis virus. Ophthalmic solutions or ointments containing antibiotics with or without local anesthetics usually promote healing. If the eye becomes opaque, systemic steroids may be necessary to help clear up the infection. Vaccines are available for *Moraxella bovis* and the infectious bovine rhinotracheitis virus [92,93].

Pneumonia or bovine pneumonic pasteurellosis or shipping fever is a disease often brought on by stress. Change in weather or in feed, shipping, or confinement in damp quarters are several examples. Several bacteria are responsible for this infection, with

Pasteurella species the most common. Several viruses can also be involved. Initial symptoms include rapid, shallow breathing patterns, drop in milk production, and loss of appetite. Additionally, fever, nasal discharge, and a dry, nonproductive cough may develop. Eventually, the breathing becomes labored and the animal begins to grunt with every breath; death usually follows soon. Rapid treatment is essential to the well-being, and usefulness of the animal. Permanent damage in the lungs can occur if the disease is allowed to progress. Numerous antibiotics and antibiotic combinations are useful in treating this infection. A vaccine is available but not completely protective. It is best to administer the vaccine three weeks prior to shipment and again upon entry into the feedlot [94,95].

Blackleg is a bacterial infection caused by *Clostridium chauvoei* but also by *Clostridium septicum*. These organisms form spores which, like tetanus, live in the soil. The disease appears suddenly, and death occurs quickly. The animal may appear healthy in the evening and be dead in the morning. There may be a fever, but it is often missed. There is characteristic edema and crepitant swelling at various places over the body. Initially the swelling is hot and painful; as the infection progresses, the area enlarges and the skin becomes cold as the blood supply is reduced in the area. Some animals may exhibit prostration and tremors. Treatment is difficult due to the rapid progression of the disease. Penicillin is sometimes attempted, but rarely successful. A vaccine (bacterin) is available, and should be administered initially in a two-dose series. Booster doses can be given annually in high-risk areas or every five years in lower-risk areas. In the event of an outbreak, animals should be vaccinated and given penicillin prophylactically [96,97].

Bovine genital campylobacteriosis is a bacterial infection caused by *Campylobacter fetus*. This infection is transmitted either through sexual contact or through artificial insemination. Bulls become sometimes infected via contaminated bedding. The major symptoms are apparent infertility and early embryonic death. The major concern with this disease is the apparent infertility. Most likely, the cow becomes pregnant, and loses the fetus at a very early stage; this loss is not apparent. From the farmer's viewpoint, the cow never became pregnant, as the pregnancy never progressed to a point where it was evident. Some cows actually abort a larger fetus, which is evident. Some cows also show signs of cervicitis and/or vaginitis. The majority of cows recover with no treatment. Recovery may be boosted by administering intrauterine infusions of penicillin–streptomycin combinations. The bulls may also be treated by infusing penicillin–streptomycin into the prepuce on three consecutive days. The best method of bringing this infection under control is to use artificial insemination (with semen treated with a combination of penicillin and streptomycin) exclusively for approximately two years. At the end of this time, the herd can be considered disease free. If natural service is necessary, the best control is to vaccinate the herd bulls and replacement heifers. This requires two initial doses with annual booster doses. Cows should be vaccinated at least six weeks before breeding [98].

Brucellosis is another bacterial infection caused primarily by *Brucella abortus*. The disease is characterized by abortion and orchitis. Both sexes experience infertility. The disease is transmitted via ingestion of contaminated food or water, or by contact with infected uterine discharge, aborted fetuses, or placental material. The organism is also shed in the milk. Sexual transmission or transmission via artificial insemination is rare. Abortion is the obvious manifestation of this infection, but reduced milk production, an increase in retained placentas, and an increase in full-term dead calves also occur. Diagnosis can be made by either the brucellosis ring test (BRT), which screens the milk and is useful for dairy farmers, or by market cattle testing (MCT), which is a serum screen used on nondairy herds. Once a herd is disease free, it can be maintained that way by vaccination of all new animals which are brought into the herd. The vaccine requires two initial doses, with annual boosters [99].

Foot rot in cattle is primarily a bacterial disease, caused mainly by *Fusobacterium necrophorum*, although other organisms are implicated. Some species of fungi may also be involved. The first sign is sudden lameness in one foot, which may be swollen and pussy. If left untreated, dairy cattle will experience a decrease in milk production due to the resulting pain. The best treatment is iodine, which can be used prophylactically, in a foot bath throughout the year. This works well for dairy cattle which are moved into the milking parlor twice a day. Treatment may require broad-spectrum antibiotics [100,101].

Tetanus is a concern with cattle as with other animals. Treatment and prevention are the same [102].

Farmer's lung is a fungal infection caused primarily by *Micropolyspora faeni*. This infection is often acquired from moldy hay and can be spread to humans. The disease is characterized by a hypersensitivity pneumonitis, and is usually seen in animals stabled in the winter. Symptoms include respiratory distress, anorexia, coughing, weight loss, decrease in milk production, exercise intolerance, and congestive heart failure. Death is rare. Most cattle recover partially with corticosteroid therapy. A marked improvement is observed when they are turned outside in the spring. Prevention is difficult [103].

Bovine trichomoniasis is a protozoal disease caused by *Trichomonas foetis*. This protozoal disease is transmitted venereally or by artificial insemination, the major problems being infertility due to early embryonic death and abortions. Infected cows recover quickly, but the bulls remain permanently infected unless treated, acting as a permanent reservoir for infection. Semen can be treated with antibiotics to prevent transmission via artificial insemination. The best management of this disease is to use artificial insemination for two years, until the herd is disease free. Metronidazole, dimetridazole, or ipronidazole can be used to treat the bulls [104].

Recommended Disease Prophylaxis

The recommendations for disease prophylaxis in cattle depends on the infections which are prevalent in the area where the cattle are being raised. The infections for which prophylaxis is available are indicated in Table 4.

Horses

There are a variety of reasons for owning a horse, and at times, this reason may play a role in how diseases and infections are treated. Horses may be necessary for making a living (such as for the Amish farmer), they may provide a livelihood (such as for the competitive equestrian), or they may be used for pleasure (such as the backyard pony). The cost of the horse may also play a role in how aggressively the problem is treated.

Common Ailments

Colic, a general term for abdominal pain, is a common problem in horses, possibly due to the small size of the horse's stomach. Colic can be caused by overeating, eating grain followed by drinking excessively, drinking water when overheated, constipation, or bowel impaction. It is important to find the cause is before treating the horse. Colic is easily diagnosed by the horse's behavior. Often it paces about, trying to decide whether to lie down or stand up. It is often seen turning to look at its belly, and breathing hard and sweating. A colicky horse often rolls on the ground, due to pain. One of the biggest problems with his behavior is that rolling or thrashing can cause a torsion of the bowel, which can be fatal. In addition, rupture of the bowel or stomach can occur, as well as external injuries when the horse thrashes about. Because of these problems, it is essential to prevent the horse from lying down by walking it until the veterinarian arrives. A nasogastric tube should be inserted to relieve gas and fluid distention. Treatment depends on the cause of the pain. Laxatives, such as dioctyl sodium succinate (DSS) or mineral oil can be used to relieve mild impaction. Tranquilizers such as promazine and analgesics (meperidine, xylazine, pentazocine, and phenylbutazone) are sometimes helpful in keeping the horse comfortable until the situation is remedied. Corticosteroids may be needed to prevent or treat shock [105].

Common Infectious Diseases

Equine coital exanthema is most likely a mixed infection, although equine herpesvirus-3 is usually the primary invader. The infection occurs in both mares and stallions, and is primarily spread at coitus. It can also be spread via gynecological manipulation or artificial insemination. In mares, four to eight days after mating, multiple, circular red nodules, up to 2 mm in diameter develop in the vaginal area and the perineum. The vaginal mucosa is also inflamed. The lesions progress to vesicles and pustules that rupture and form shallow ulcers. Healing takes approximately three weeks, leaving unpigmented areas or scars. Accompanying systemic infection is usually absent. Similar lesions occur on the penis and prepuce of the stallions. The fertility of either sex is unaffected. Diagnosis is usually easy due to the characteristic lesions. Treatment of the lesions with topical antibiotics or antibiotic/steroid combinations promotes the healing process. The mating process may proceed after seven to ten days [106].

Equine encephalomyelitis is caused by a group of related arboviruses, although *Toxoplasma* species may also be involved. The most common causative agents are the Eastern equine encephalomyelitis virus (EEE), the Western equine encephalomyelitis virus (WEE), and the Venezuelan equine encephalomyelitis virus (VEE). A similar flavivirus, the Japanese encephalitis virus (JE) may also be involved. The disease is primarily spread via mosquitoes, although other insects may be carriers as well. Clinical symptoms begin within five days of infection. Death may occur in two to three days. Some typical symptoms include fever, impaired vision, irregular gait, wandering, reduced reflexes, circling, incoordination, drowsiness, head-pressing, paralysis, convulsions, and death. Mild cases recover slowly over a few weeks, but some have residual brain damage, leaving them as "dummies." The mortality rate ranges from 5 to 90%. Diagnosis can be made from the clinical signs or antibodies in the serum. There are no specific antivirals available for encephalitis. Treatment may include the use of anti-inflammatory agents or anticonvulsants as well as intensive nursing. Mosquito control may reduce the spread of this infection. Animals should be stabled during outbreaks. Inactivated vaccines of the various arboviruses are available either singly or in various combinations. These vaccines should be administered about one month prior to the mosquito season. The disease can be spread to humans [107,108].

TABLE 4 Bovine Prophylaxis[a]

Organism	Disease	Vaccine Type	Schedule	Comments	Classification
Togavirus	Bovine viral diarrhea	Modified live or killed	2-Dose initial series with revaccination annually		Optional
Clostridium perfringens, Types C and D	Overeating disease	Toxoid	2-Dose initial series with revaccination annually	Antitoxin available for passive protection	Recommended
Clostridium tetani	Tetanus	Toxoid	2-Dose initial series with revaccination annually	Antitoxin available for passive protection	Recommended
Camplyobacter fetus	Bovine genital campylobacteriosis	Bacterin	2-Dose initial series with revaccination annually		Optional
Bovine herpesvirus-1 (BHV-1)	Infectious bovine rhinotracheitis, infectious pustular vulvovaginitis, and infectious keratitis	Modified live or killed	2-Dose initial series with revaccination annually	Parenteral live vaccine can cause abortions	Optional

Veterinary Uses of Drugs

Moraxella bovis	Infectious keratitis	Killed or bacterin	2-Dose initial series with revaccination annually	Optional
Pasteurella haemolytica	Pasteurellosis or shipping fever	Bacterin	2-Dose initial series with revaccination annually	Antiserum available for passive protection	Optional
Pasteurella multocida	Pasteurellosis or shipping fever	Bacterin	2-Dose initial series with revaccination annually	Antiserum available for passive protection	Optional
Clostridium chauvoei	Blackleg	Bacterin	2-Dose initial series with revaccination annually or every 5 years, depending on risk		Optional
Rabies virus	Rabies	1-year killed	2-Dose initial series with revaccination annually	Must be certified by a veterinarian	Recommended

[a] From Refs. 138–141

Equine infectious anemia (or swamp fever) is a viral infection transmitted via blood. Blood-sucking flies are frequently to blame for its transmission. Once infected, the virus remains in the horses's white blood cells for life. The incubation period is variable, from one week to three months. Symptoms include intermittent fever, depression, progressive weakness, weight loss, and progressive anemia. In acute cases, the animal displays splenomegaly. Death does occur in some cases. Diagnosis is made with the aid of a Coggins test, an immunodiffusion test for the presence of antibodies. Foals nursing on infected dams give a positive Coggins test temporarily. Infected animals do not test positively for a week or more until the antibody level rises to detectable levels. There is no specific treatment or vaccine available for swamp fever. Supportive therapy is the only hope. Infected animals should be isolated and kept in an insect-proof barn. Animals can be stabled during the fly season to minimize the spread of this infection [109,110].

Equine influenza is very similar to human influenza. However, there are only two strains of the virus in equine influenza currently recognized, whereas there are many strains for human infection. This simplifies the vaccination issue for horses. Equine influenza is a highly contagious, febrile, upper-respiratory infection. The disease is only fatal in the very young and the very old animals. Symptoms include fever, symptoms of an upper respiratory infection, expiratory dyspnea, weakness, and stiffness. Mild cases recover spontaneously within two to three weeks. Severe cases may convalesce up to six months. Complications include secondary bacterial infections, chronic bronchitis, and chronic obstructive pulmonary disease. Restricting exercise, controlling dust, providing superior ventilation and good stable hygiene minimize these complications. Horses without complications need only rest and good nursing. Secondary bacterial infections require proper antibiotic therapy. Antipyretics are recommended for fevers over 105°F (40.5°C). Restricted exercise is mandatory. A bivalent inactivated vaccine is given as a two-dose series, followed by a booster six months later. A minimum of one booster every twelve months is recommended. Boosters can be given every three to six months [111].

Equine viral rhinopneumonitis is caused by equine herpesvirus-1. The primary infection is an upper respiratory infection, which is often seen to cycle annually. The outcome of exposure to this virus is dependent on the immune status, pregnancy status, and age of the horse. Mares may abort the fetus several weeks to several months after clinical disease or asymptomatic infection. Abortion is most common in months eight to eleven of the pregnancy, and usually occurs with no apparent warning. Future breeding performance is unimpaired. Transmission is from direct or indirect contact with virus-laden nasal discharge, aborted fetuses, or placentas. There are several strains of this virus which cause disease. After a short incubation period, the initial symptoms are those of an upper respiratory infection. It is not at all uncommon for a bacterial infection to follow this viral respiratory infection. Often a horse's bowels change to diarrhea or constipation. Mild to severe central nervous system symptoms may occur in some horses. Diagnosis is easy when examining the aborted foal and finding pulmonary edema and/or fetal hepatic necrosis. Diagnosis on the mare is difficult. Treatment is primarily symptomatic, and can include antipyretics for the fever. Secondary bacterial infections should be treated with appropriate antibiotics. There are several vaccines available, including a modified live vaccine and an inactivated vaccine. The inactivated form is recommended for breeding mares, and should be administered in the 5th, 7th, and 9th months of pregnancy. Young horses, geldings, and stallions can be vaccinated

Veterinary Uses of Drugs

with the live or inactivated vaccine, as an initial two-dose series with annual booster doses. The vaccines are not 100% protective, but there is evidence that the inactivated vaccine reduces the abortion rate in pregnant mares [112].

Like all mammals, horses are susceptible to rabies. Horse owners can choose to vaccinate their animals. However, the injection must be administered by a veterinarian and must be certified.

Potomac fever (or equine monocytic ehrlichiosis) is a bacterial infection caused by an *Ehrlichia* species. The infection is presumably spread by an arthropod since most cases occur near the Potomac and Susquehanna rivers, and its incidence corresponds to the presence of most arthropods. The initial signs are fever, depression, leukopenia, and loss of appetite. Within 48 h, most cases develop diarrhea which can be watery and projectile in some cases. The fatality rate approaches 30%, with death being primarily due to dehydration and hypovolemic shock. It is important to rule out salmonellosis in the diagnostic process. Treatment consists primarily of early fluid therapy; tetracyclines are helpful for recovery. An inactivated vaccine is available [113].

Strangles (otherwise known as distemper or shipping fever) is a bacterial infection characterized by upper respiratory symptoms as well as abscessation of the adjacent lymph nodes. This infection is caused by *Streptococcus equi*, a group C, β-hemolytic streptococcus. It is transmitted via the purulent discharge of infected animals, and the active disease may be stress induced. Symptoms include upper respiratory symptoms, loss of appetite, fever, and abscessation of the lymph nodes. The normal course of the infection is 10 to 14 days. Death may occur due to central nervous system involvement or asphyxiation of the larynx or pharynx due to compression. Diagnosis is relatively easy because of the high fever and abscess formation. However, it is useful to culture the organism. New horses added to a herd should be isolated for several weeks and observed for nasal discharge before joining the herd. Infected animals should be kept isolated until free of symptoms. Complete rest and good nursing are essential to the recovery of the infected horse. Hot packs over the abscesses speed up their maturation, they should then be incised and drained. Tracheostomy may be necessary in the event of pharyngeal or laryngeal compression. Antibiotics are not recommended for initial therapy as they retard abscess maturation and prevent immune response. They may, however, be used prophylactically in the case of exposed animals. A killed vaccine does not give very good protection. Other types of vaccines are being investigated [114,115].

Tetanus is a concern with horses as well as with other domestic animals. Prevention can be taken care of with the toxoid [116,117].

Thrush is an infection of the frog of the hoof and occurs due to improper management of the horse. With proper care and cleaning of the hooves, thrush is not a problem. Although it is usually a mixed infection, the dominant organism is the yeast *Candida albicans*. The foot usually displays a characteristic foul odor which makes diagnosis easy. Treatment includes the use of dry, clean bedding in the stall, keeping the horse out of wet pastures, cleaning the hooves regularly, and application of a copper sulfate solution. Surgery is required for extensive tissue damage to the hoof [118,119].

Recommended Disease Prophylaxis

The recommendations for disease prophylaxis in horses depends on the infections which are prevalent in the area where the horse is being raised. Prophylaxis is available for a number of infections (Table 5).

TABLE 5 Equine Prophylaxis[a]

Organism	Disease	Vaccine Type(s)	Schedule	Comments	Classification
Eastern equine encephalomyelitis virus	Encephalitis	Killed	2-Dose initial series with revaccination annually	Available as a monovalent, bivalent, or trivalent vaccine	Optional
Western equine encephalomyelitis virus	Encephalitis	Killed	2-Dose initial series with revaccination annually	Available as a monovalent, bivalent, or trivalent vaccine	Optional
Venezuelan equine encephalomyelitis virus	Encephalitis	Killed	2-Dose initial series with revaccination annually	Available as a monovalent, bivalent, or trivalent vaccine	Optional
Equine influenza A1 virus	Equine influenza	Killed	2-Dose initial series with revaccination every 6 to 12 months	Available as a bivalent vaccine	Optional
Equine influenza A2 virus	Equine influenza	Killed	2-Dose initial series with revaccination every 6 to 12 months	Available as a bivalent vaccine	Optional

Veterinary Uses of Drugs

Equine herpesvirus, Type 1 (EHV-1)	Equine viral rhinopneumonitis	Modified live or killed	2-Dose initial series with revaccination annually; killed form administered in the 5th, 7th, and 9th months of pregnancy	Killed vaccine administered during pregnancy reduces the number of abortions	Optional
Ehrlichia species	Equine monocytic ehrlichiosis or potomac fever	Bacterin or killed	2-Dose initial series with revaccination annually		Optional
Staphylococcus equi	Strangles	Bacterin	Multiple initial doses followed by annual revaccination	Optional	
Clostridium tetani	Tetanus	Toxoid	2-Dose initial series with revaccination annually	Antitoxin available for passive protection	Recommended
Rabies virus	Rabies	1-year killed	2-Dose initial series with revaccination annually	Must be certified by a veterinarian	Recommended

[a]From Refs. 138–141.

Swine

Pigs are highly intelligent, and are supposedly good watch animals. However, most pigs are raised as a food source rather than a pet or watch animal. They are very large and strong as adults, and this has to be taken into consideration when raising pigs.

Common Ailments

Anemia is a common problem in baby pigs which must be attended to by the farmer. Feeding iron supplements to the sow does not increase the iron content of her milk appreciably, and other measures must be applied. Anemia is a costly disease, because the piglets do not gain weight and never seem to catch up to other piglets of the same age who have adequate iron. This is costly to the farmer who makes his living by bringing those pigs to market. This condition can be treated by giving the baby pigs oral iron supplements, by swabbing the sow's udder daily with a mixture of iron, honey, and molasses, or by giving the piglets an iron injection. Once the piglets are eating solid foods, there is adequate iron in the mixture to prevent anemia [120].

Common Infectious Diseases

Hog cholera is a viral infection caused by a togavirus. This disease is highly contagious and fatal. Fortunately, strict control measures have reduced the problems due to this infection. Affected pigs have diarrhea, fever, and weakness in the hindquarters; red lesions and petechiae can develop. The mortality rate in young pigs approaches 100%. Treatment includes a hyperimmune serum which is effective only in the early stages of the disease. It is best prevented during the endemic infection by a vaccine. Once the disease is eradicated, the vaccine should be discontinued [121,122].

Transmissible gastroenteritis (TGE) is a viral infection caused by a coronavirus. This is a highly contagious disease which can affect pigs of all ages. The major symptoms are diarrhea, vomiting, and severe dehydration. The mortality rate is high in young pigs whose body mass cannot tolerate the severe dehydration. There is no specific treatment. However, a vaccine is available for protection. Some farmers intentionally infect pregnant sows approximately two to four weeks prior to farrowing to provide the piglets with adequate antibody protection via the sow's milk [123,124].

Pneumonia in swine is similar to pneumonia in sheep, goats, and cattle. It can be caused by a variety of bacteria and viruses. Pneumonia is a major cause of death in pigs. Treatment includes systemic antibiotics, isolation, and the use of expectorants if needed; there is no preventative available [125].

Atrophic rhinitis is a bacterial infection primarily caused by *Bordetella bronchiseptica* and/or *Pasteurella multocida*. The infection is an upper respiratory infection, characterized by a nasal discharge, sneezing, conjunctivitis, facial distortion, and nasal hemorrhage. Oral or injectable antibiotics are helpful in fighting this infection; a protective vaccine is available [126,127].

Brucellosis is a bacterial infection caused primarily by *Brucella suis* in pigs. This infection (caused by other species of *Brucella*) can also occur in humans and cattle. Some of the symptoms of brucellosis in pigs include abortion, and the production of small, weak piglets, lameness, and paralysis. New animals added to a farm should be tested. There is no good treatment for brucellosis. It is best to maintain a brucellosis-free herd. Vaccination is unreliable [128,129].

Veterinary Uses of Drugs

Erysipelas is a bacterial infection caused by *Erysipelothrix rhusiopathiae*. This infection can be a serious problem to the hog farmer, primarily to young pigs. Death can occur within four days. The primary symptoms include fever, pain, and characteristic purple diamond-shaped lesions on the sides, belly, and back. In animals that survive, the disease can become chronic accompanied by arthritis and endocarditis. Early treatment with penicillin is required. Additionally, an antiserum can be administered to exposed animals; this treatment can save lives. The condition is prevented by a live vaccine [130,131].

Necrotic enteritis or necro is associated with a dietary deficiency. Diets low in protein (such as all corn diets) seem to increase the likelihood of this infection. Affected pigs have a lack of appetite, low energy, fever, and diarrhea. Improvement of the diet often alleviates the condition which is sometimes accompanied by a bacterial infection treatable with antibiotics [132].

Necrotic rhinitis or bull-nose is caused by *Fusobacterium necrophorum*. This is primarily a disease of young pigs, characterized by suppuration and necrosis arising from wounds in the oral or nasal mucosa. This infection usually follows some type of injury either from a bite or a scrape. Symptoms include swelling and deformity of the face with occasional hemorrhaging. Other symptoms, similar to those of an upper respiratory infection, include snuffling, sneezing, a foul-smelling nasal discharge, conjunctivitis, and loss of appetite. Antibiotics are sometimes helpful in treating this infection. They should be administered as soon as possible. The condition can be prevented by avoiding injury and improving sanitation [127,133].

Coccidiosis in swine is similar to the same disease in sheep and goats. Symptoms and treatment are the same [134].

Recommended Disease Prophylaxis

The recommendations for disease prophylaxis in swine depends on the infections which are prevalent in the area where the pigs are being raised. Prophylaxis is available for a number of infections (Table 6).

General Care of Domestic Animals

Internal Parasite Control

Internal parasites are an ongoing problem in domestic animals. This is primarily due to their grazing behavior, as many parasites and their eggs can be found in grass and dirt. Animals that are close grazers, such as sheep, have an even greater problem. A large number of parasites should be of concern to animal owners. These include roundworms, tapeworms, hookworms, and flukes among others. Most farmers have a routine prevention program including the administration of deworming medications at various times throughout the year. There are many deworming medications available for the different species of domestic animals. Although most successful farmers rotate the deworming medications, some find success with one which they continue to use. Sometimes, however, the parasites do become resistant, or there may be one species that is not killed by the dewormer which can take hold and cause problems in the flock or herd. Other preventative measures include pasture rotation. It is recommended to keep one or more pastures fallow while other pastures are being grazed. This allows the grass to grow, and when pasture rotation occurs, the new pasture has long grass and the

TABLE 6 Porcine Prophylaxis[a]

Organism	Disease(s)	Vaccine Type(s)	Schedule	Comments	Classification
Coronavirus	Transmissible gastroenteritis (TGE)	Modified live or killed	2-Dose initial series with revaccination annually		Optional
Bordetella bronchiseptica	Atrophic rhinitis	Bacterin	2-Dose initial series with revaccination annually		Optional
Pasteurella multocida	Atrophic rhinitis	Bacterin	2-Dose initial series with revaccination annually		Optional
Erysipelothrix rhusiopathiae	Erysipelas	Bacterin	2-Dose initial series with revaccination annually	Antiserum available for animals exposed to this organism	Optional
Clostridium tetani	Tetanus	Toxoid	2-Dose initial series with revaccination annually	Antitoxin available for passive protection	Recommended
Rabies virus	Rabies	1-year killed	2-Dose initial series with revaccination annually	Must be certified by a veterinarian	Recommended

[a]From Refs. 138–141.

Veterinary Uses of Drugs

animals are not forced to graze close to the ground where most of the parasites and their eggs are. The pasture that was used previously can then begin to grow until it is needed again. In addition, a stool sample from each herd or flock should be examined once or twice a year for identification of parasites. This helps the farmer to determine the effectiveness of the deworming medication. Lastly, any animal with diarrhea should be treated for 24 h. If the diarrhea persists, a stool sample should be examined for parasites.

External Parasite Control

There are numerous external parasites which infest domestic animals, ranging from ticks, to fleas, mosquitoes, lice, and mange. Many of these parasites are irritating to the animal by causing itchiness. Some animals are so disturbed by these infestations that they stop eating, leading in dairy animals to a reduction in milk production. A variety of commercial products, such as insect repellents, can be used to discourage these parasites from settling on the animals. Other helpful remedies are bug "zappers" which kill insects in an electric field, fly paper, and spraying the barn with insect sprays. For disease prevention, it is sometimes necessary to keep animals in a closed barn with good screens. Biting flies are another nuisance, although they are not really parasites. The bite of these insects is painful and may cause an animal to charge or bolt. This can cause injury to other animals or to humans. Some insect sprays repel these flies, although they are quite persistent.

Zoo and Aquatic Animals

Zoo animals and animals kept in aquariums have special needs different from those of domestic and companion animals. Animals living in aquariums (both fish and marine mammals) are unique in that their environment is water. This is both an asset and a concern for the marine biologist who is charged with their care. If these animals get an infection, they can be treated orally, by injection, or by bathing in the medication. If a group of animals get a particular infection, they can be isolated into a separate tank, and the whole tank can be treated simultaneously. Oral medications can be administered in gelatin which contains the food ration. Sharks can receive their medication inside a fish which is fed to them. Surgery on marine animals is difficult, because of their need to breathe under water [135].

Zoo animals also provide a challenge for the veterinarian. Many of these animals are large, and some are aggressive. They all seem to show stress in difficult situations, which makes the job of the caretaker that much harder. Furthermore, many zoo animals are very intelligent, and refuse to take medication. This is especially true for the ape and monkey families [136].

Drugs Used for Tranquilization

It is not unusual for animals in a zoo to need tranquilization. Large animals that are sick and need to be isolated or placed in the hospital, or animals that escape from their cages are two examples of situations which might require tranquilization. Many of the medications which are used to tranquilize zoo animals are the same as those used in domestic and companion animals. In addition, some zoos are permitted to use a very powerful narcotic, known as etorphine, for the tranquilization of large animals. This helps the veterinarian, because the dose is much smaller than that required for conventional agents [136].

Common Ailments

Zoo animals get the same diseases as other animals and the treatment is the same. Many zoo animals are related to domestic and companion animals. For example, lions and tigers are related to the domestic cat, and often get the same diseases as cats do. What may differ, however, is the method of administration and the dose of a particular medication.

Recommended Disease Prophylaxis

Vaccination programs in zoos often follow those used for domestic and companion animals. As indicated above, many zoo animals have counterparts in domestic and companion animals. This is helpful in the area of disease prophylaxis. For example, the wolves in a zoo would be vaccinated for the same infections as domestic dogs. Zoo animals are often vaccinated for rabies.

Special Handling

Zoo animals require special handling compared to domestic and companion animals, because of their size, ferocity, and intelligence. Large animals such as elephants may require several people for routine procedures. Ferocious animals such as tigers are usually given injections by blow dart or dart gun. This is the simplest method of vaccinating or administering parenteral medications. Intelligent animals such as orangutans need keepers capable outsmarting them when medication is administered. If medicated darts are used, the keeper or veterinarian must be able to get out of the way quickly, because darts have been known to come flying back out of the cages of some orangutans. If the medication is to be administered orally, the keeper or veterinarian sometimes hides the medication in a "treat." However, all the animals in the cage would require an unmedicated "treat" since the animal which needs the medication may refuse the treat if the others are not given one [137].

Summary

Veterinary pharmacy is a growing area of specialty for the pharmacist to explore. It offers many opportunities in the various aspects of veterinary medicine. Pharmacists can work for an animals hospital, a zoo, an aquarium, or an retail pharmacy and be able to practice veterinary pharmacy. The future is full of opportunities for the pharmacist interested in animals.

References

1. Davidson, G., Intervening in animal health care, *Am. Pharm.*, NS34 (7): 58–59 (1994).
2. Decker, J., Veterinary pharmacy: I wouldn't trade it for anything, *Tomorrow's Pharmacist*, 17(1): 11–13 (1994).
3. Smoak, C.H., Veterinary pharmacy for the community pharmacist, *U.S. Pharmacist*, 21(1): 45–62 (1996).
4. *The Merck Veterinary Manual*, 6th ed., Merck and Company, Rahway, NJ, 1986, p. 133.
5. Spaulding, C. E., *A Veterinary Guide for Animal Owners,* Rodale Press, Inc., Emmaus, PA, 1976, p. 315.
6. *The Merck Veterinary Manual*, 6th ed., Merck and Company, Rahway, NJ, 1986, p. 419.
7. Ref. 6, pp. 49–53.
8. Ref. 6, pp. 266–267.
9. Spaulding, C.E., *A Veterinary Guide for Animal Owners,* Rodale Press, Inc., Emmaus, PA, 1976, pp. 300–301.
10. *The Merck Veterinary Manual*, 6th ed., Merck and Company, Rahway, NJ, 1986, p. 570.
11. Spaulding, C.E., *A Veterinary Guide for Animal Owners,* Rodale Press, Inc., Emmaus, PA, 1976, p. 304.
12. *The Merck Veterinary Manual*, 6th ed., Merck and Company, Rahway, NJ, 1986, pp. 326–328.
13. Spaulding, C.E., *A Veterinary Guide for Animal Owners,* Rodale Press, Inc., Emmaus, PA, 1976, pp. 301–302.
14. *The Merck Veterinary Manual*, 6th ed., Merck and Company, Rahway, NJ, 1986, pp. 329–330.
15. Ref. 14, pp. 337–339.
16. Spaulding, C.E., *A Veterinary Guide for Animal Owners,* Rodale Press, Inc., Emmaus, PA, 1976, p. 307.
17. *The Merck Veterinary Manual*, 6th ed., Merck and Company, Rahway, NJ, 1986, pp. 605–607.
18. Spaulding, C.E., *A Veterinary Guide for Animal Owners,* Rodale Press, Inc., Emmaus, PA, 1976, p. 313.
19. *The Merck Veterinary Manual*, 6th ed., Merck and Company, Rahway, NJ, 1986, pp. 731–732.
20. Ref., 19, pp. 379–380.
21. Spaulding, C.E., *A Veterinary Guide for Animal Owners,* Rodale Press, Inc., Emmaus, PA, 1976, p. 309.
22. *The Merck Veterinary Manual*, 6th ed., Merck and Company, Rahway, NJ, 1986, pp. 461–462.
23. *Puppy Love; Easy Ways to Keep Your Dog Healthy and Happy,* Merck and Company, Inc., Rahway, NJ, Brochure, 1996.
24. Spaulding, C.E., *A Veterinary Guide for Animal Owners,* Rodale Press, Inc., Emmaus, PA, 1976, p. 316.
25. Ref. 24, pp. 337–339.
26. *The Merck Veterinary Manual*, 6th ed., Merck and Company, Rahway, NJ, 1986, p. 1399.
27. Spaulding, C.E., *A Veterinary Guide for Animal Owners,* Rodale Press, Inc., Emmaus, PA, 1976, pp. 345–346, 350.
28. Ref. 27, pp. 348–350.
29. *The Merck Veterinary Manual*, 6th ed., Merck and Company, Rahway, NJ, 1986, pp. 336–337.
30. Spaulding, C.E., *A Veterinary Guide for Animal Owners,* Rodale Press, Inc., Emmaus, PA, 1976, pp. 340–341.

31. *The Merck Veterinary Manual*, 6th ed., Merck and Company, Rahway, NJ, 1986, p. 335.
32. Ref. 31, pp. 42–43.
33. Ref. 31, pp. 729–731.
34. Spaulding, C. E., *A Veterinary Guide for Animal Owners,* Rodale Press, Inc., Emmaus, PA, 1976, pp. 347–348.
35. Ref. 34, pp. 332–333.
36. *The Merck Veterinary Manual*, 6th ed., Merck and Company, Rahway, NJ, 1986, pp. 29–30.
37. Messner, J., *Rabbit Diseases, Causes, Prevention, and Treatment*, American Rabbit Farms, Lancaster, pp. 31–32.
38. *The Merck Veterinary Manual*, 6th ed., Merck and Company, Rahway, NJ, 1986, p. 1000.
39. Ref. 38, p. 999.
40. Ref, 38, p. 995.
41. Spaulding, C.E., *A Veterinary Guide for Animal Owners,* Rodale Press, Inc., Emmaus, PA, 1976, p. 268.
42. *The Merck Veterinary Manual*, 6th ed., Merck and Company, Rahway, NJ, 1986, pp. 990–991.
43. Spaulding, C.E., *A Veterinary Guide for Animal Owners,* Rodale Press, Inc., Emmaus, PA, 1976, p. 270.
44. *The Merck Veterinary Manual*, 6th ed., Merck and Company, Rahway, NJ, 1986, pp. 995–996.
45. Ref. 44, p. 992.
46. Spaulding, C.E., *A Veterinary Guide for Animal Owners,* Rodale Press, Inc., Emmaus, PA, 1976, pp. 271–272.
47. *The Merck Veterinary Manual*, 6th ed., Merck and Company, Rahway, NJ, 1986, pp. 996–997.
48. Spaulding, C.E., *A Veterinary Guide for Animal Owners,* Rodale Press, Inc., Emmaus, PA, 1976, p. 266.
49. *The Merck Veterinary Manual*, 6th ed., Merck and Company, Rahway, NJ, 1986, pp. 967–968.
50. Ref. 49, p. 968.
51. Ref. 49, p. 960–961.
52. Ref. 49, p. 959.
53. Ref. 49, p. 959–960.
54. Ref. 49, p. 958.
55. Ref, 49, p. 961.
56. Ref. 49, p. 1014.
57. Ref. 49, p. 1011.
58. DeVosjoli, P., The general care and maintenance of red-eared sliders and other popular freshwater turtles, *Advanced Vivarian Systems*, Lakeside, CA, 1992, pp. 1–47.
59. *The Merck Veterinary Manual*, 6th ed., Merck and Company, Rahway, NJ, 1986, p. 1012.
60. Ref. 59, p. 1011.
61. Ref. 59, p. 1013.
62. Ref. 59, p. 946.
63. Ref. 59, pp. 945–946.
64. Ref. 59, p. 945.
65. Ackerman, L., Fleas and flea control, Part II, *Pet Focus*, 2 (3): 36–39 (1990).
66. Sinkora, S.B., Winning the battle, *Dog Fancy Magazine*, June: 54–59 (1995).
67. *Program*, Product Brochure, Ciba-Geigy Corporation, Greensboro, NC, 1994.
68. Gerhart, M.S., Flea and tick control, *Dog World*, July: 40 (1991).
69. Miles, Inc., Agricultural Division, Animal Health Prod. Technical Services Bulletin, Elkhart, IN, pp. 55–56.

Veterinary Uses of Drugs

70. Wilcox, B., Flea Control Requires A Two-Pronged Attack, *Dog Fancy Magazine,* January: 70–71 (1996).
71. *The Merck Veterinary Manual*, 6th ed., Merck and Company, Rahway, NJ, 1986, pp. 441–442.
72. Spaulding, C.E., *A Veterinary Guide for Animal Owners,* Rodale Press, Inc., Emmaus, PA, 1976, pp. 119–120, 154–155.
73. *The Merck Veterinary Manual*, 6th ed., Merck and Company, Rahway, NJ, 1986, pp. 375–378.
74. Spaulding, C.E., *A Veterinary Guide for Animal Owners,* Rodale Press, Inc., Emmaus, PA, 1976, p. 160.
75. *The Merck Veterinary Manual*, 6th ed., Merck and Company, Rahway, NJ, 1986, pp. 691–692.
76. Spaulding, C.E., *A Veterinary Guide for Animal Owners,* Rodale Press, Inc., Emmaus, PA, 1976, pp. 127–130, 156–158.
77. *The Merck Veterinary Manual*, 6th ed., Merck and Company, Rahway, NJ, 1986, pp. 177–180.
78. Spaulding, C.E., *A Veterinary Guide for Animal Owners,* Rodale Press, Inc., Emmaus, PA, 1976, p. 159.
79. *The Merck Veterinary Manual*, 6th ed., Merck and Company, Rahway, NJ, 1986, pp. 367–369.
80. Spaulding, C.E., *A Veterinary Guide for Animal Owners,* Rodale Press, Inc., Emmaus, PA, 1976, pp. 109–110, 151–152.
81. *The Merck Veterinary Manual*, 6th ed., Merck and Company, Rahway, NJ, 1986, pp. 369–370.
82. Spaulding, C.E., *A Veterinary Guide for Animal Owners,* Rodale Press, Inc., Emmaus, PA, 1976, pp. 132–133, 160.
83. Spaulding, C.E., *A Veterinary Guide for Animal Owners,* Rodale Press, Inc., Emmaus, PA, 1976, pp. 112–113, 153–154.
84. *The Merck Veterinary Manual*, 6th ed., Merck and Company, Rahway, NJ, 1986, p. 139.
85. Ref. 84, pp. 158–161.
86. Spaulding, C.E., *A Veterinary Guide for Animal Owners,* Rodale Press, Inc., Emmaus, PA, 1976, pp. 30–31.
87. *The Merck Veterinary Manual*, 6th ed., Merck and Company, Rahway, NJ, 1986, pp. 430–432.
88. Spaulding, C.E., *A Veterinary Guide for Animal Owners,* Rodale Press, Inc., Emmaus, PA, 1976, pp. 43–44.
89. *The Merck Veterinary Manual*, 6th ed., Merck and Company, Rahway, NJ, 1986, p. 162.
90. Spaulding, C. E., *A Veterinary Guide for Animal Owners,* Rodale Press, Inc., Emmaus, PA, 1976, p. 35.
91. *The Merck Veterinary Manual*, 6th ed., Merck and Company, Rahway, NJ, 1986, pp. 711–713.
92. Ref. 91, pp. 291–293.
93. Spaulding, C.E., *A Veterinary Guide for Animal Owners,* Rodale Press, Inc., Emmaus, PA, 1976, pp. 52–53.
94. *The Merck Veterinary Manual*, 6th ed., Merck and Company, Rahway, NJ, 1986, pp. 705–706.
95. Spaulding, C.E., *A Veterinary Guide for Animal Owners,* Rodale Press, Inc., Emmaus, PA, 1976, pp. 53–55, 64.
96. *The Merck Veterinary Manual*, 6th ed., Merck and Company, Rahway, NJ, 1986, pp. 364–365.
97. Spaulding, C.E., *A Veterinary Guide for Animal Owners,* Rodale Press, Inc., Emmaus, PA, 1976, pp. 29–30.

98. *The Merck Veterinary Manual*, 6th ed., Merck and Company, Rahway, NJ, 1986, p. 636.
99. Ref. 98, pp. 639–641.
100. Ref. 98, p. 488.
101. Spaulding, C.E., *A Veterinary Guide for Animal Owners,* Rodale Press, Inc., Emmaus, PA, 1976, pp. 39–41.
102. Ref. 101, pp. 67–68.
103. *The Merck Veterinary Manual*, 6th ed., Merck and Company, Rahway, NJ, 1986, pp. 710–711.
104. Ref. 103, pp. 637–639.
105. Spaulding, C.E., *A Veterinary Guide for Animal Owners,* Rodale Press, Inc., Emmaus, PA, 1976, pp. 189–190.
106. *The Merck Veterinary Manual*, 6th ed., Merck and Company, Rahway, NJ, 1986, p. 666.
107. Ref. 106, pp. 586–589.
108. Spaulding, C.E., *A Veterinary Guide for Animal Owners,* Rodale Press, Inc., Emmaus, PA, 1976, pp. 192–194.
109. *The Merck Veterinary Manual*, 6th ed., Merck and Company, Rahway, NJ, 1986, pp. 28–29.
110. Spaulding, C.E., *A Veterinary Guide for Animal Owners,* Rodale Press, Inc., Emmaus, PA, 1976, p. 208.
111. *The Merck Veterinary Manual*, 6th ed., Merck and Company, Rahway, NJ, 1986, pp. 716–717.
112. Ref. 111, pp. 717–719.
113. Ref. 111, p. 182.
114. Ref. 111, pp. 721–722.
115. Spaulding, C.E., *A Veterinary Guide for Animal Owners,* Rodale Press, Inc., Emmaus, PA, 1976, pp. 207–208.
116. *The Merck Veterinary Manual*, 6th ed., Merck and Company, Rahway, NJ, 1986, pp. 369–370.
117. Spaulding, C.E., *A Veterinary Guide for Animal Owners,* Rodale Press, Inc., Emmaus, PA, 1976, pp. 208–209.
118. *The Merck Veterinary Manual*, 6th ed., Merck and Company, Rahway, NJ, 1986, pp. 505–506.
119. Spaulding, C.E., *A Veterinary Guide for Animal Owners,* Rodale Press, Inc., Emmaus, PA, 1976, p. 201.
120. Ref. 119, pp. 225–226.
121. *The Merck Veterinary Manual*, 6th ed., Merck and Company, Rahway, NJ, 1986, pp. 342–344.
122. Spaulding, C.E., *A Veterinary Guide for Animal Owners,* Rodale Press, Inc., Emmaus, PA, 1976, pp. 228–229.
123. *The Merck Veterinary Manual*, 6th ed., Merck and Company, Rahway, NJ, 1986, pp. 191–192.
124. Spaulding, C.E., *A Veterinary Guide for Animal Owners,* Rodale Press, Inc., Emmaus, PA, 1976, p. 233.
125. Spaulding, C.E., *A Veterinary Guide for Animal Owners,* Rodale Press, Inc., Emmaus, PA, 1976, pp. 232–233.
126. *The Merck Veterinary Manual*, 6th ed., Merck and Company, Rahway, NJ, 1986, pp. 738–739.
127. Spaulding, C.E., *A Veterinary Guide for Animal Owners,* Rodale Press, Inc., Emmaus, PA, 1976, pp. 232.
128. *The Merck Veterinary Manual*, 6th ed., Merck and Company, Rahway, NJ, 1986, pp. 643–644.
129. Spaulding, C.E., *A Veterinary Guide for Animal Owners,* Rodale Press, Inc., Emmaus, PA, 1976, p. 226.

Veterinary Uses of Drugs

130. *The Merck Veterinary Manual*, 6th ed., Merck and Company, Rahway, NJ, 1986, pp. 373–374.
131. Spaulding, C.E., *A Veterinary Guide for Animal Owners*, Rodale Press, Inc., Emmaus, PA, 1976, p. 227.
132. Ref. 131, pp. 231–232.
133. *The Merck Veterinary Manual*, 6th ed., Merck and Company, Rahway, NJ, 1986, p. 741.
134. Spaulding, C.E., *A Veterinary Guide for Animal Owners*, Rodale Press, Inc., Emmaus, PA, 1976, pp. 226–227.
135. Frank Steslow, Marine Biologist, personal interview.
136. Keith Hinshaw, D.V.M., personal interview.
137. Donna Ialeggio, D.V.M., personal interview.
138. *Veterinary Pharmaceuticals and Biologicals*, 8th ed., Veterinary Medicine Publishing Company, Lenexa, KS, 1993–1994, pp. A-29 to A-61.
139. Grabenstein, J. D., Veterinary vaccinology, Part I. Introduction and companion animals, *Hosp. Pharm.*, 29(12): 1108–1119.
140. Grabenstein, J. D., Veterinary vaccinology: II. Horses, livestock, and other animals, *Hosp. Pharm.* 30(3): 222–228, 1994.
141. *Jeffers' Pet, Equine and General Catalog*, Fall, 1993. Product Information Catalog, Dothan, AL.

JOY B. REIGHARD

Water for Pharmaceutical Use

Introduction

The most widely used ingredient in pharmaceutical products is water. It is used in applications as an excipient, solvent, or vehicle. The process of manufacturing drugs uses water for drug synthesis, cleaning of equipment, heating and cooling, and in product testing.

Water is one of the pharmaceutical ingredients that is often overlooked because of its ubiquitous nature. The chemical and microbiological quality attributes of water are susceptible to contamination and degradation, resulting in adulteration of the pharmaceutical product and placing the patient at risk.

Pharmacopeial History

The first appearance of a modern quality standard for water to be used in pharmaceutical applications was in 1820 in the *United States Pharmacopeia* (USP I). Monographs for Aqua Fontana (Drinking Water) and Aqua Destillata (Distilled Water) were included, and a method of preparation was identified for distilled water. Over the years, the quality attributes for pharmaceutical water have evolved (Table 1) as new concerns with drug stability and patient safety were identified. Little information is available to support the development of the specific attributes. The general assumption is that they were identified to address specific concerns with regard to drugs or patients. Newer attributes are slowly being implemented to provide broad-spectrum tests for ionic and organic contaminants.

Water Monographs

All of the world pharmacopial compendia include monographs for water used in the preparation of pharmaceutical dosage forms (Table 2). The monographs generally include one section for Purified Water and another section for Water for Injection. The pharmacopoeia may additionally include monographs for water for specific applications, such as hemodialysis, inhalation, or irrigation. The types of water produced and the steps required are shown in Fig. 1.

Test methods were developed to permit the use of this water by the pharmacist for the verification of quality attributes. These were generally based on wet chemistry qualitative tests with no standard for comparison. The newer test methods are qualitative, instrumented methods that provide a consistent evaluation of the water quality.

TABLE 1 Introduction of Quality Attributes for Water in the USP

Attribute	Year of Introduction
Distilled water	1820
Sulfate	1840
Calcium	1840
Carbon dioxide	1850
Chloride	1890
Ammonia	1890
Oxidizable substances	1890
Heavy metals	1900
Total solids	1947
Coliforms	1947
pH	1970
Bacterial endotoxins	1983
Total organic carbon	1996
Conductivity	1996

Water Quality Attributes

The new quality attributes for Purified Water and Water for Injection, USP, are conductivity and total organic carbon. They provide a broad-spectrum analysis of the ionic and organic content of the water, and replace the specific ion attributes that have been in effect for over a century.

TABLE 2 Pharmacopeial Monograph Attributes for Water in the European (EP), Japanese (JP), and United States Pharmacopeia (USP)

Attributes	EP	JP	USP
Ammonia	0.2 ppm	0.05 mg/L	Deleted
Calcium	Pass/fail		Deleted
Conductivity			See description
Heavy metals	0.1 ppm Pb	Pass/fail	Deleted
Nitrates	0.2 ppm	Pass/fail	
Nitrite		Pass/fail	
Oxidizable substances	Pass/fail	Pass/fail	Pass/fail or TOC
pH	5–7	Acidity/alkalinity	5–7
Total organic carbon		0.50 mg/L	0.50 mg/L
Total solids	0.001%	0.001%	Deleted
Bacterial endotoxin (WFI)	0.25 IU/mL	0.25 EU/mL	0.25 EU/mL
Microbial attributes			
Purified water	10^2 org./mL		100 cfu/mL
WFI	10 org./100 mL		10 cfu/100 mL

Refer to the actual pharmacopeia for specific test attributes.

Water for Pharmaceutical Use

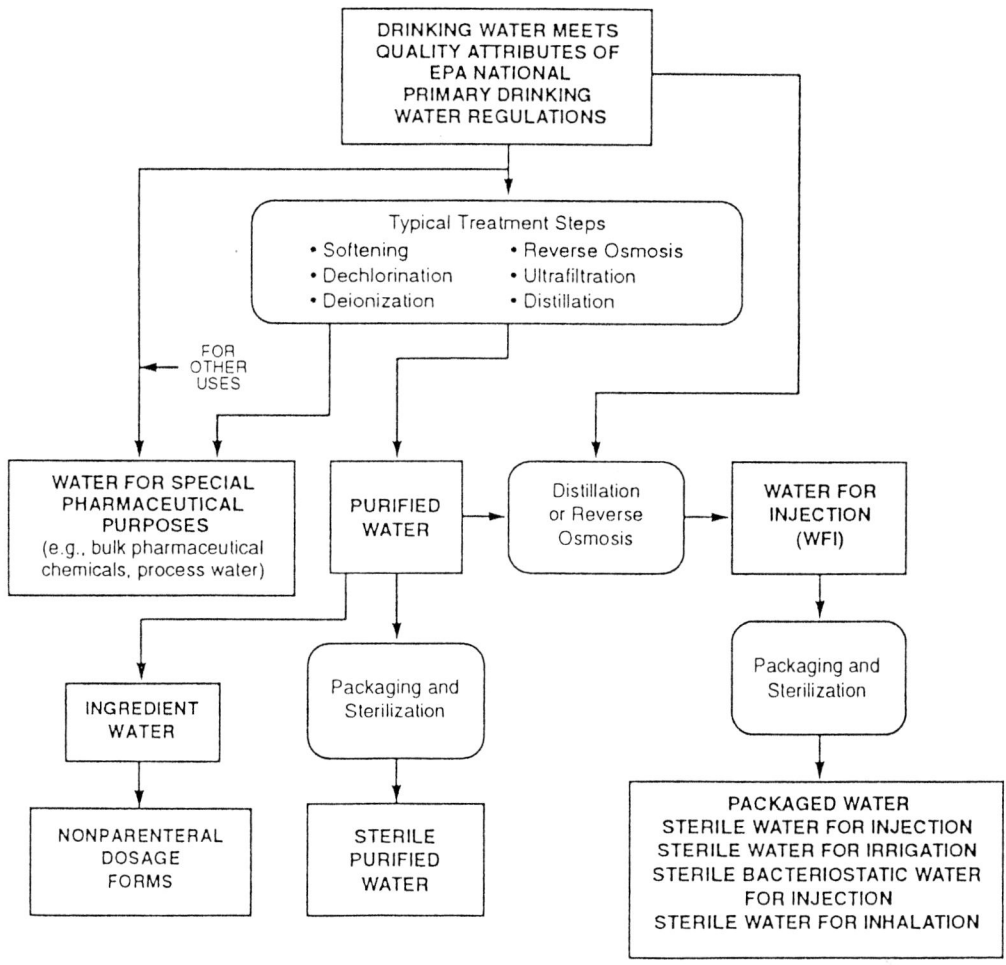

FIG. 1. Water for pharmaceutical purposes (USP/PF). (Courtesy of PhRMA Water Quality Committee.)

Conductivity

Electrical conductivity in water is produced by the presence of ionic chemicals. This attribute is made possible by a nonspecific determination of the concentration of the all the ions present. The source of the ions may be salts, gases, and some organic chemicals. Conductivity is at times measured as resistivity, the reciprocal of conductivity.

The unit of measure for conductivity is siemens per centimeter (S/cm) and was formerly referred to as mho per centimeter. The unit for resistivity is ohm-cm; S/cm = 1/(ohm − cm).

Conductivity is affected by the temperature of the solution being tested. This effect can be significant at values other than the standard temperature, generally 25°C. The conductivity value based on the temperature is at times compensated using correction algorithms. These equations are based on the conductivity deviation of known concentrations of ionic solutions, usually sodium chloride, potassium chloride, or carbon dioxide. The temperature-compensation algorithms are not valid for solutions of other ions. Because pharmaceutical water contains a mixture of ions, temperature compensation is not permitted in the pharmacopeial test method. Temperature-compensated conductivity values may be used for in-process evaluation of water quality.

Conductivity Instrumentation

Conductivity instruments are comprised of two sections, the conductivity cell and the meter that processes the information. The cell has two metal plates which are used to determine the conductivity of the water. Cells are available in various configurations. The most common are the dip-type cell which is placed directly into the test solution, and flow-through or in-line cells where the solution passes across the plates. Cells may also incorporate temperature-measurement sensors for temperature compensation.

The instrument must have the appropriate accuracy and be in a calibrated state before it can be used for compendial tests. The stated accuracy for the conductivity cell, expressed as a cell constant, must be $\pm 2\%$ for each scale reading. The meter must have a resolution of 0.1 µS/cm and have an accuracy of ± 0.1 µS/cm. Conductivity cell constants may be determined by using a solution of known conductivity, or by comparison with a reference cell. Cell constants are difficult to determine and it may be appropriate for the cell manufacturer to provide a calibration certificate for the probe. Meter accuracy is determined by using precision resistors with an accuracy of $\pm 0.1\%$ of the stated value or equivalent electrical circuitry such as a Wheatstone bridge.

Conductivity Test Method and Specifications

The Water Conductivity Test Method is described in USP 23, Supplement 5, pp. 3465–3467 including the attribute, instrumentation, test considerations, and test method. The variables affecting conductivity, pH, temperature, and atmospheric carbon dioxide are considered. The test method is specified in three stages, with each taking into account some of the variables and simplifying the test. Each stage is more laboratory intensive, but allows for a lower quality of water.

Stage 1 may be performed as an on-line test or in the laboratory. The instantaneous conductivity, not temperature compensated, and the temperature of the water are determined. The measured conductivity is compared to the conductivity corresponding to the next lower temperature value (Stage 1, Table 3). If the measured conductivity is lower than the table value, the requirements of the test are satisfied and no further testing is required. If the measured value is higher than the table value, Stage 2 is required.

Stage 2 is performed by equilibrating the temperature of the water to $25 \pm 1°C$, and equilibrating the carbon dioxide in solution with the atmospheric carbon dioxide. When the conductivity rate of change is less than 0.1 µS/cm per 5 min, the conductivity is noted. If the conductivity is not higher than 2.1 µS/cm, the requirements of the test are satisfied and no further testing is needed. If the measurement is above 2.1 µS/cm, Stage 3 is reached.

Stage 3 is to be performed within 5 min of completing Stage 2, while maintaining the sample at $25 \pm 1°C$. Saturated potassium chloride solution is added to attain a concentration of 0.3 mL per 100 mL of test specimen, and the pH is determined to the nearest 0.1 pH unit. The conductivity value from Stage 2 and the pH value from Stage

Water for Pharmaceutical Use

TABLE 3 Stage 1 Temperature–Conductivity Requirements[a]

Temperature (°C)	Conductivity Requirement (μS/cm)
0	0.6
5	0.8
10	0.9
15	1.0
20	1.1
25	1.3
30	1.4
35	1.5
40	1.7
45	1.8
50	1.9
55	2.1
60	2.2
65	2.4
70	2.5
75	2.7
80	2.7
85	2.7
90	2.7
95	2.9
100	3.1

[a]For non-temperature-compensated conductivity measurements only.

3 are then compared with the values in Table 4. If the measured values are not higher than those in the table, the water meets the requirements for conductivity. If the pH is outside the range of 5.0–7.0 or the conductivity is higher than the value in the table, the water does not meet the requirements.

Total Organic Carbon

The concentration of organic compounds dissolved in the water is determined by evaluating the total organic carbon (TOC) content. The organic compounds volatilizing when the solution is sparged with an inert gas are considered purgeable organic carbon (POC). Those remaining in solution are considered non-purgable organic carbon (NPOC). The total organic carbon is the sum of the two types. The level of POC in pharmaceutical water is relatively low compared to the limit value and can be considered negligible.

Many analytical methods are available to determine TOC levels. In all of them the organic compounds are oxidized with chemical oxidizing agents and/or ultraviolet to carbon dioxide. The instruments discriminate between inorganic carbon from carbon dioxide or bicarbonate and that produced from the oxidation reaction. The level of carbon dioxide is measured and expressed as carbon content.

TABLE 4 Stage 3 pH–Conductivity Requirements[a]

pH	Conductivity Requirement (μS/cm)[b]
5.0	4.7
5.1	4.1
5.2	3.6
5.3	3.3
5.4	3.0
5.5	2.8
5.6	2.6
5.7	2.5
5.8	2.4
5.9	2.4
6.0	2.4
6.1	2.4
6.2	2.5
6.3	2.4
6.4	2.3
6.5	2.2
6.6	2.1
6.7	2.6
6.8	3.1
6.9	3.8
7.0	4.6

[a]For atmosphere- and temperature-equilibrated samples only.
[b]μS/cm (microsiemen per centimeter) = μmho/cm = reciprocal of megohm-cm.

Instrumentation

The compendial test method does not identify any specific analytical method for TOC determination. Criteria are established for the instrumentation and for determination of its suitability. The instrument must have a manufacturer's specified limit of detection of 0.05 mg of carbon per liter (50 ppb) or lower, be in a calibrated state, and periodically demonstrate its suitability.

Test Method and Specifications

The TOC test may be performed on-line or in the laboratory. It determines the carbon that is contributed from all sources in addition to those in the water. Sampling equipment, techniques, and handling must be carefully evaluated to minimize the potential for extraneous contamination.

The TOC instrument must be in a calibrated state prior to use. It should be calibrated according to manufacturer's recommendations or other acceptable procedures. The system suitability test is performed to determine if the instrument will completely oxidize organic compounds of unknown structure.

Water for Pharmaceutical Use

The water used for the preparation of solutions (reagent water) must have a TOC level below 0.25 mg/L to minimize the bias that may be introduced during instrument evaluation. This TOC level will be used to correct for the background TOC levels. The system suitability test is performed by analyzing a solution of 1,4-benzoquinone of a concentration of 0.75 mg/L (0.50 mg of carbon per liter). The instrument response must by 85–155% of the theoretical concentration to be considered suitable. The system suitability test should be performed periodically to validate the instrument.

The standard solution is prepared from sucrose at a concentration of 1.19 mg/L (0.50 mg of carbon per liter). It is analyzed by the TOC instrument and corrected for the reagent water. The corrected response from the instrument is the TOC limit for pharmaceutical water analyzed by that instrument. This limit is theoretically 0.50 mg/L; other values may be due to the variables involved in performing the test.

Microbial Issues

Issues related to pharmaceutical water quality attributes are often due to microbiological concerns. The monographs establish attributes for bacterial endotoxins for WFI and additionally for sterility in the packaged forms of water. No attributes are included in the monographs for viable microorganism levels in Purified Water or WFI, although these often create serious problems. Microbiological attributes, other than sterility, are not include in the monographs because the test method for viable organisms has a broad range of reproducibility, and the results may vary. Microorganisms continue to grow after the test is performed.

The appropriate levels and corresponding test methods for microorganisms in pharmaceutical water are shown in Table 5. These action levels have withstood the test of time, but the specific levels for a particular use of water must be established as a function of the manufacturing process and the products in which it will be used.

Types of Water and Uses

Drinking (Potable) Water

Pharmaceutical water is prepared from water meeting the attributes of drinking water. These are established and regulated by government agencies, such as the United Stated Environmental Protection Agency (EPA). Individual pharmacopoeias have different

TABLE 5 Microbiological Action Levels and Test Methods

	Purified Water	Water for Injection
Action level	100 cfu/mL[a]	10 cfu/100 mL[a]
Method	Pour plate	Filtration
Minimum sample volume,	1 mL	100 mL
Media	Plate count agar	Plate count agar
Incubation time	48–72 h	48–72 h
Temperature	30–35°C	30–35°C

[a]Colony-forming units = cfu.

standards for drinking water. The USP permits water meeting the requirements of the United States, the European Community, or Japan to be used for preparing Purified Water or Water for Injection. The European Pharmacopeia requires that the potable water meet the requirements of the local authority.

The broad spectrum of quality attributes that are regulated by drinking water regulations ensure than a minimum level of contaminants is introduced into the water treatment system. Some attributes, such as lead and pesticides are regulated at significantly lower levels than those in the monographs. Water distribution systems need to be designed to prevent contamination by materials of construction or by cross-contamination from waste systems. Drinking water may be used for the synthesis of active ingredients. It is also used for cleaning of equipment and facilities.

Purified Water

Purified Water monographs identify quality attributes that include ionic and organic contaminants, and limit the level of microbiological contamination. This water is intended to be used in the preparation of nonparenteral dosage forms, such as tablets, capsules, syrups, and ointments. Sterilized Purified Water may be used for sterile ophthalmic preparations and some topical preparations. The water is of the minimum grade for performing the official test method. Preparation of the active ingredients also requires purified water.

Water for Injection

Water for Injection monographs generally include the same chemical attributes as Purified Water. Additionally, they include attributes for bacterial endotoxins and lower levels of microbiological contamination. All pharmacopoeias limit the method of preparing the water to distillation, reverse osmosis, and ultrafiltration (Table 6).

Non-Compendial Water

Water used for the preparation of pharmacopeial articles must be manufactured using Purified Water, Water for Injection, or other compendial forms of water. Other uses of water include washing of equipment and packaging components, autoclave cooling, and facility cleaning. There are no regulatory requirements that define the quality of water that may be used for these purposes.

The selection of a water quality for these uses must take into consideration the application in which the water will be used, subsequent treatment of the object or area that is in contact with it, and the relationship to the finished product. The accepted practice for equipment and component washing has been, at a minimum, to perform a

TABLE 6 Methods of Manufacture for Water for Injection

Method	EP	JP	USP
Distillation	X	X	X
Reverse osmosis		X	X
Ultrafiltration		X	

Water for Pharmaceutical Use

final rinse with the same water quality that is used for preparation of the product. This practice is based on the assumption that surface contaminants will be removed to the same quality level present in the water. Preparing compendial water for washing applications is at times not feasible, and the user defines and employs other, non-compendial forms of water.

User-defined water includes specifications for inorganic and organic contaminants, microbial quality, and possibly bacterial endotoxins levels. Non-compendial water must be evaluated and determined to be appropriate for the application. It must be validated, monitored, and controlled in the same manner as a compendial water system.

The USP permits drinking water to be used for preparation of drug substances or active ingredients. There are also no regulatory requirements that define the quality of water that may be used for drug substance preparation. The concern with such water is that the chemical and microbiological contaminants introduced during manufacture cannot be removed during the preparation of the finished dosage form and become a contaminant in the finished drug.

Water that is used for the preparation of drug substance must be of appropriate quality in order not to interfere with the drug synthesis or purification. The chemical contaminants should not produce impurity by-products. The microbiological impurities, viable organisms and bacterial endotoxins need to be adequately controlled in order not be a source of microbial contamination in the finished drug.

A decision tree can be used to identify the criteria that need to be evaluated for selecting water quality attributes in pharmaceutical applications (Fig. 2).

Clean Steam

Steam is a form of water that may be used in pharmaceutical applications for the sterilization of components, equipment, and product, and as a heating utility for distillation operations, heat exchangers, and humidification. Steam in contact with the product, components, or equipment may introduce contaminants from the additives used in steam boilers. Steam used for pharmaceutical sterilization operations should be free of additives. It is generally prepared from deionized water and referred to as clean steam, pure steam, or additive-free steam. Water for Injection distillation columns are at times used to clean steam.

Design of Water Systems

The preparation of pharmaceutical water involves many treatment operations. Water systems consist of treatment operations and sections to store the water and to distribute it to the points of use.

The process begins with water that meets drinking water quality attributes. Water that does not meet these attributes may be treated to remove impurities to drinking water levels. The water is treated to remove ionic, organic, and microbiological contaminants to meet the quality attributes of the Purified Water or Water for Injection monograph.

The treatment-system unit operations sequentially remove contaminants to improve the quality of the water or to ensure the proper operation of subsequent steps. A series

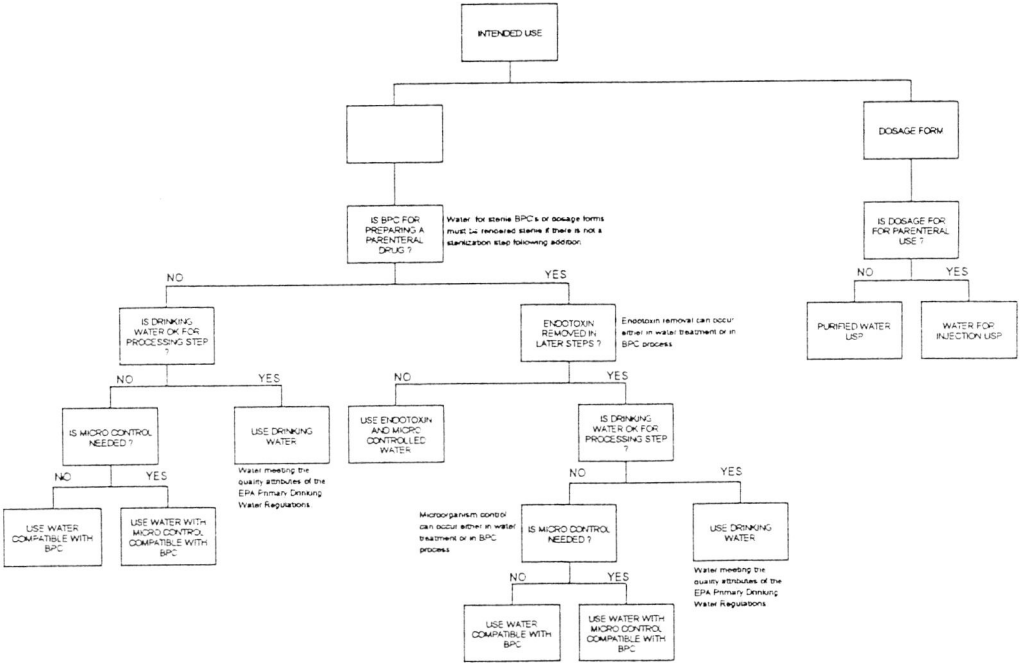

FIG. 2. Selection of water quality for pharmaceutical applications. Adapted from USP 23, <1231> Water for Pharmaceutical Purposes. (Courtesy of PhRMA Water Quality Committee.)

of typical treatments steps is shown in Fig. 3, including particulate filtration, carbon filters, deionization, reverse osmosis, ultrafiltration, and distillation.

Particulates are removed by mechanical filtration through multimedia or cartridge filters which consist of several layers of fine sand and quartz media. Levels of approximately 10 µ are nominally achieved. This step is performed to remove silt and debris that can obstruct water flow in later operations. The multimedia filters need to be periodically backwashed to remove the accumulated debris.

Activated carbon beds remove some organic compounds, chlorine that is generally present as an antimicrobial agent, and other particles. Removal of the chlorine is recommended because further treatment steps such as deionization, reverse osmosis, and distillation are affected by its presence. Carbon beds provide a nutrient-rich environment for microbial proliferation and the absence of an antimicrobial agent makes the water susceptible to contamination. Maintenance of a carbon bed must include periodic sanitization to control the microbial levels and replacement of carbon that no longer retains organic compounds.

Ionic compounds are removed by various deionization processes. Anion and cation resin may be used in series as a dual-bed deionizers or combined in a mixed-bed deionizer. Salts, some organic compounds, and bacterial endotoxins are retained by the resin media. The performance of the deionizer is monitored by evaluating the ionic quality of the water by conductivity measurement. The resin is periodically recharged to remove the accumulated ions with the help of strong acids and bases. Deionizers are also a source of microbial growth and contamination. Regeneration of the resin based on time and microbial levels prevents microbial growth before the product water is contaminated beyond control.

Water for Pharmaceutical Use

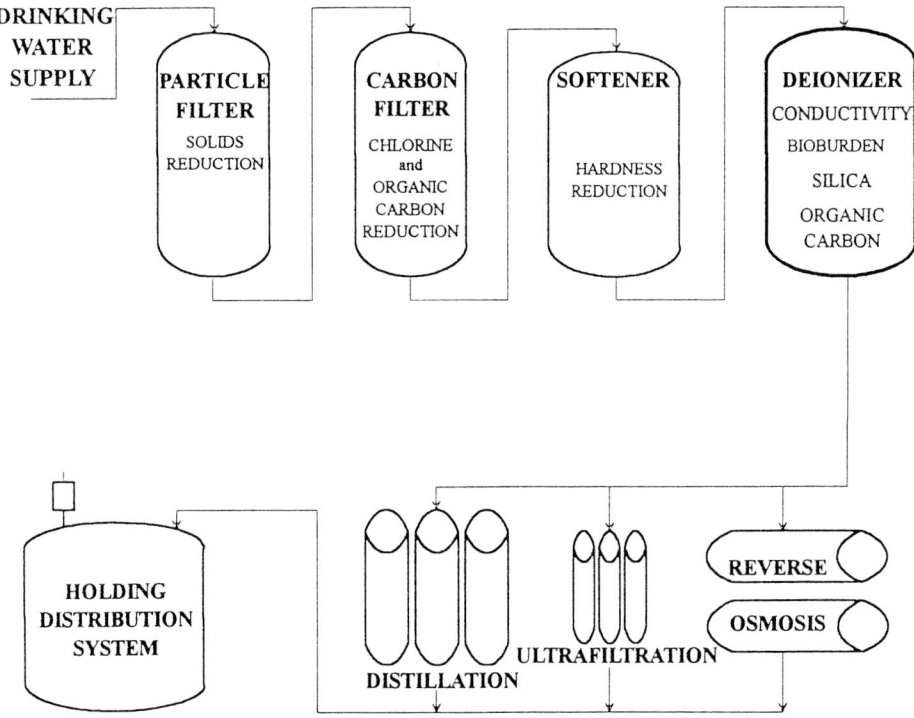

FIG. 3. Water treatment unit operations. (Courtesy of R. Slabicky.)

Reverse osmosis membranes purify the water by physical separation of the impurities. This process is capable of removing ions, organic compounds, bacterial endotoxins, and microorganisms. The membrane material and the construction of the unit make the technology sensitive to mechanical and chemical stress. The unit can be fouled by organic matter, degraded by chemical attack, or ruptured because of pressure fluctuation. Proper maintenance is required to ensure its proper operation. Reverse osmosis can be used for the production of Water for Injection. Often two units are placed in a series to provide a higher level of assurance in the integrity of the membrane.

Ultrafiltration is another mechanical separation process capable of removing large organic molecules, microorganisms, and bacterial endotoxins. The material and construction of the membranes are very robust, typically polysulfone or even ceramics. The membranes are susceptible to plugging and fouling, but can be easily cleaned and sanitized by chemicals, heat, and water pressure. Ultrafilters are capable of reliably producing water that meets the microbial and bacterial endotoxin attributes of Water for Injection. However, their use for this application is not permitted by some pharmacopeias.

The classic method for producing Water for Injection is distillation. It is capable of removing ionic and organic chemicals, bacterial endotoxins, and inactivating microorganisms. The processes involved include phase change, mechanical separation, and in some designs, centrifugal separation. Water is evaporated and the steam is condensed into WFI. A portion of the feed water is discharged with the concentrated contaminants. The process is tolerant of feed water quality fluctuations and is easy to operate and maintain. However, the simplicity of the operation may become the source of problems, because the system may not receive the appropriate level of monitoring needed to ensure consistent quality.

The holding and distribution system shown in Fig. 4, is designed to provide storage of the treated water and distribute it to individual points of use. The system must protect the water from chemical and microbial contamination. Sources of contamination may include the materials of construction, poor operation, exposure to air or personnel, lack of flow, and cross-connections to other systems. Operational sources of contamination include inadequate sanitization frequency or conditions, lack of maintenance, and improper handling. Frequent sanitization is essential for maintaining the microbial quality of the water. WFI systems are typically maintained hot, with the water temperature above 65°C.

Sanitary Designs

Sanitary design concepts for water systems are used to minimize sources of contamination and permit sanitzation. They generally focus on the microbiological attributes. The concepts call for easy-to-clean, smooth surfaces, nonreactive materials of construction, minimal crevices from poor welds or connections, no threaded connections, proper drainage of components and pipes, and no areas of stagnant or poor flow.

Sanitary design requires piping and components that satisfy the principles of smooth, easy-to-clean surfaces. Lead legs (sections that have a length greater than six times the diameter of the section) or areas of low flow are not permitted. The materials of construction are generally an appropriate grade of stainless steel, such as 316 or 316L, or plastic, such as polyvinylidene fluoride (PVDF) or polytetrafluoroethylene (PTFE). Flow rates in piping are designed to be turbulent and flowing with minimal interruption.

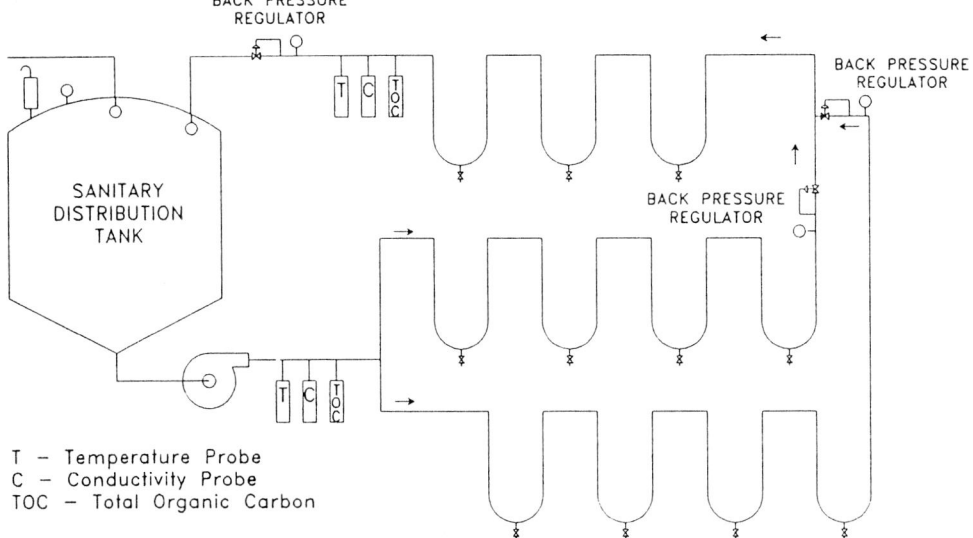

FIG. 4. Holding and Distribution System. (Courtesy of R. Slabicky.)

Validation

Validation is defined as "establishing documented evidence which provides a high degree of assurance that a specific process will consistently produce a product meeting its predetermined specifications and quality attributes."

Validation is a program for assuring that the product is acceptable by systematically verifying the installation, operation, and performance of the water treatment and distribution process.

Validation Life Cycle

The validation life cycle comprises documentation and verification of the water system from the initial design concept, through installation and start-up and its complete operational life. Major components include installation qualification, operational qualification, performance qualification, and validation maintenance. A validation protocol identifies all the specific tests and acceptance criteria used to evaluate the system. The elements that may be included in the protocol are shown below.

- Installation Qualification
  Component list
  List and verification of drawings
  Operating and maintenance manuals
  System specifications
  Installation verification
  Operating procedures
  Control sequences
  Monitoring and alarm points
  Input–output signals
  Instrument calibration
  Preventive maintenance procedures
- Operational Qualification
  Functional verification of components
  Functional verification of control sequences
  Monitoring and alarm function verifications
  Operating range verification
- Performance Qualification
  Process control tests
  Chemical tests
  Microbial tests
  Effect of process dynamics on system performance and water quality

Installation Qualification

Installation qualification (IQ) verifies and documents that the system has been properly installed. Operating procedures, instrument calibration, and preliminary operating range should be established prior to implementation of the test protocol.

Operational Qualification

Operation qualification (OQ) tests and documents that the system functions properly and ensures that the control sequences for equipment function in the correct order.

Performance Qualification

Performance qualification (PQ) generates data to characterize the ability of the system to repeatably produce, hold, and distribute water over an extended period of time. The water is tested for a period of time prior to being used for pharmaceutical production. This period ranges from two to six weeks, normally four weeks. After this test period, the data are evaluated and a decision is made to proceed with the use of the water for drug production. Monitoring the chemical and microbial attributes of the water continues for the life of the system.

Validation Maintenance

Validation of water systems is an ongoing activity that ensures that the system continuously produces water which meets the quality standards. Numerous programs are established to maintain and monitor proper operation, including preventive maintenance, calibration, change control, monitoring, and other procedures.

Bibliography

National Primary Drinking Water Regulations, U.S. Code of Federal Regulations, Title 40, Part 141 (current edition), Govt. Printing Office, Washington.

National Secondary Drinking Water Regulations, U.S. Code of Federal Regulations, Title 40, Part 143 (current edition), Govt. Printing Office, Washington.

Pharmaceutical Manufacturers Association Water Quality Committee, Updating requirements for pharmaceutical grades of water : conductivity, *Pharmacopeial Forum* 17(6, Nov–Dec): 2669–2675 (1991).

Pharmaceutical Manufacturers Association Water Quality Committee, Updating requirements for pharmaceutical grades of water : proposed revisions, *Pharmacopeial Forum*, 20 (3, May–June): 7526–7544 (1994).

Pharmaceutical Manufacturers Association Water Quality Committee, Updating requirements for pharmaceutical grades of water : rationale for changes to conductivity, pH, and TOC test proposals, *Pharmacopeial Forum* 22 (1, Jan.–Feb.): 1934–1939 (1996)

Slabicky, R. O., Pharmaceutical Water Systems: Design and Validation. In: *Bioprocess Engineering Systems, Equipment, and Facilities* (B. K. Lyderson, N. A. D'Elia, and K. L. Nelson, eds.), Wiley, New York, 1994.

The Pharmacopoeia of Japan, 12th ed., Japan Ministry of Health and Welfare, Tokyo

The United States Pharmacopeia 23 and Supplements, The United States Pharmacopeial Convention, Rockville, MD, 1995.

ROSTYSLAW O. SLABICKY

Water Sorption of Drugs and Dosage Forms

Introduction

The physical, chemical, and mechanical properties of pharmaceutical drugs and dosage forms are critically dependent on the presence of moisture. Pharmaceutical scientists can cite numerous examples of desirable and undesirable properties that result from varied levels of moisture associated with a particular solid or formulations consisting of mixtures of solids. Flow, compaction, caking, disintegration, dissolution, hardness, and chemical stability are just some of the properties influenced by moisture. Since water is present in bulk liquid form or as vapor at some relative humidity in virtually all stages of solid manufacture (active ingredient and excipients), storage, processing into formulations, and final product packaging, a fundamental understanding of the role of water in affecting solid properties (and vice versa) is necessary.

Though the properties of individual solids and the performance of solid dosage forms are dependent on moisture, characterization of the underlying water–solid interaction is often nebulous. For example, many solids are described as "hygroscopic" without further reference to whether and how this relates to the rate and amount of moisture uptake as a function of relative humidity and temperature [1]. To illustrate this ambiguity, consider that water-soluble, nonhydrating crystalline substances such as sodium chloride sorb very low levels of moisture (e.g., less than 0.1%) below their critical relative humidities, yet sorb significant quantities of moisture above their critical relative humidities, where the solid actually dissolves in the sorbed moisture. On the other hand, some typical excipient materials used in solid dosage forms, such as starches, celluloses, and gelatin capsules, sorb significant quantities of moisture (e.g., 25-50%), and even though they do not dissolve, they do undergo significant morphological changes at high relative humidities (i.e., swelling). For these substances, the moisture-uptake rate depends on the relative humidity of the environment and the time-dependent moisture content of the solid. On the other hand, sodium chloride has a very low moisture uptake–loss rate that falls to zero if the environmental relative humidity is kept below its critical relative humidity. However, if the relative humidity is above the critical value, the uptake rate is much higher and continuous, until all the solid is dissolved. For situations in which the environmental relative humidity is significantly different from the relative humidities at which the starch, cellulose, or gelatin were previously equilibrated, the initial uptake–loss rate is significant, but approaches zero over time (i.e., a constant amount of sorbed moisture is attained at a given relative humidity). Obviously, very different mechanisms of water sorption–desorption occur for the different samples. In this light, describing sodium chloride and/or starch as hygroscopic offers very little toward understanding the water–solid interactions that might affect their physical-chemical properties. These examples illustrate the need to understand the underlying mechanism(s) of uptake for a particular solid. In this regard, therefore, addressing the following questions provides a basis for studying the various mechanisms of water-solid interaction:

1. How much water is present and what is the corresponding water activity (approximated by relative pressure or percent relative humidity/100)?
2. What are the kinetics of moisture uptake or loss, and is the rate constant or changing over time?
3. Where is the water located (i.e., adsorbed to the external surface of crystals, absorbed into crystals as specific or nonspecific water of hydration, absorbed into amorphous regions, condensed into pores, etc.)?
4. What is the state of the moisture associated with the solid (i.e., bulk water, water of hydration, "physisorbed" water, etc.)?
5. In what form is the solid present (i.e., particle morphology, polymorphic species, degree of crystallinity, anhydrate), and is this form thermodynamically stable over the temperature and relative humidity range that the solid is expected to encounter?

It is the objective of this article to discuss the various mechanisms whereby water can interact with solid substances, present methodologies that can be used to obtain the necessary data, and describe moisture uptake for nonhydrating and hydrating crystalline solids below and above their critical relative humidities, for amorphous solids and for pharmaceutically processed substances. Finally, transfer of moisture from one substance to another will be discussed.

The Water Sorption Isotherm

The most fundamental manner of demonstrating the relationship between sorbed water vapor and a solid is the water sorption–desorption isotherm. It describes the relationship between the equilibrium amount of water vapor sorbed to a solid (usually expressed as amount per unit mass or per unit surface area of solid) and the thermodynamic quantity, water activity (a_w), at constant temperature and pressure. At equilibrium, the chemical potential of water sorbed to the solid must equal the chemical potential of water in the vapor phase. Water activity in the vapor phase is related to chemical potential by Eq. (1),

$$\mu = \mu^0 + RT \ln a_w \qquad (1)$$

where μ is the chemical potential of water in the system at equilibrium, μ^0 is the standard chemical potential of water at a specific reference temperature and pressure, R is the gas constant, and T is absolute temperature. Lewis et al. [2] defined the relative activity of any pure substance or component (such as water) as a ratio of fugacities shown by Eq. (2),

$$a_w = \frac{f_w}{f_w^0} \qquad (2)$$

where f_w is the fugacity of water in the system at equilibrium and f_w^0 is the fugacity of pure water at a standard temperature and pressure. For all practical purposes, the fugacity (or "escaping tendency") of water vapor can be approximated by the water vapor pressure in the system. This assumption is valid as long as the water vapor behaves as an ideal gas. For the water pressure range of usual interest at temperatures less than 50°C, this approximation is excellent (<0.2% relative error) [3]. Thus, the relative pressure of water vapor, P/P^0, is usually employed as an estimate of the relative water activity in the system, as expressed by Eq. (3),

$$a_w \sim \frac{P}{P^0} \qquad (3)$$

where P is the water vapor pressure in the system and P^0 is the vapor pressure above pure water at the temperature of interest. Relative humidity (RH) is defined as the relative pressure expressed on a percentage basis as in Eq. (4).

$$RH = 100 \times \frac{P}{P^0} \qquad (4)$$

The sorption branch of the isotherm is obtained experimentally by measuring the equilibrium amount of water sorbed to a solid at known relative pressure, beginning with a known mass of absolutely dry solid and progressively increasing the relative pressure in the system. Drying the solid sample under heat, possibly using vacuum to facilitate the removal of desorbed water vapor, is usually necessary to eliminate residual moisture. One must be aware, however, of the effects of such conditions on the chemical and physical stability of the solid. The desorption portion of the isotherm is obtained by progressively decreasing the relative pressure in the system from a relative pressure of approximately unity, again monitoring the equilibrium amount of moisture sorbed at each relative pressure. Generation of water sorption–desorption isotherms for a particular solid can lend considerable insight into the nature of the water–solid interaction, as well as the surface characteristics of the solid. This information is readily obtained from the amounts of moisture sorbed at lower relative humidities in comparison with the specific surface area of the sample; from the general shape of the isotherm; from whether the water uptake is a completely reversible process (i.e., whether hysteresis is observed between sorption and desorption); and from the shape of the hysteresis loop if present. With knowledge of the aforementioned, one can usually obtain an indication of the mechanism of moisture sorption for the material of interest. For example, a material is most likely absorbing water into its internal structure if it exhibits sorption at lower relative humidities in much greater amounts than one might expect based on the specific surface area of the sample, and if it exhibits hysteresis over the complete range of relative humidities. On the other hand, a material is probably porous in nature if it exhibits a closed hysteresis loop over the higher relative humidity range while sorbing moisture over the lower relative humidity range similar to what might be expected based on its specific surface area. This material is most likely sorbing water via capillary condensation over the higher relative humidity range.

Models Describing Vapor Adsorption

The Brunauer, Emmett, and Teller Equation

The model most commonly referred to in the literature describing vapor adsorption onto solid surfaces was put forth in 1938 by Brunauer, Emmett, and Teller [4]. The so-called

BET model was originally derived using kinetic arguments in a manner very similar to those used by Langmuir [5]. The BET model has since also been derived using statistical mechanics [6–8]. It assumes that vapor molecules, behaving as an ideal gas, exist in a state of equilibrium with a solid that consists of identical, homogeneous adsorption sites. The first vapor molecule absorbed to an adsorption site on the solid is proposed to be bound, whereas molecules adsorbing beyond the first layer are assumed to have the properties of bulk liquid. Furthermore, adsorption is proposed to occur in such a way that the adsorbed molecules do not interact laterally. The linear form of the BET equation is given by Eq. (5),

$$\frac{1}{W[P^0/P)-1]} = \frac{(C_b - 1)(P/P^0)}{W_m C_b} + \frac{1}{W_m C_b} \quad (5)$$

where W is the mass of vapor adsorbed per gram of solid at a particular relative pressure, P/P^0; W_m is the theoretical quantity of vapor adsorbed when each adsorption site has one vapor molecule adsorbed to it; and C_b is expressed by Eq. (6),

$$C_b = k \exp \frac{H_1 - H_L}{RT} \quad (6)$$

where H_1 is the heat of adsorption of the first vapor molecules adsorbed to a site, H_L is the heat of condensation of bulk adsorbate, R is the universal gas constant, T is absolute temperature, and k is a constant, usually assumed to be close to unity. The two BET constants, W_m and C_b, can easily be obtained from the linear plotting form of the BET equation given in Eq. (5). Plotting the quantity $1/[W\{(P^0/P) - 1\}]$ versus P/P^0 gives a slope equal to $(C_B - 1)/W_m C_B$ and an intercept equal to $1/W_m C_B$. Algebraic manipulation gives expressions (7) and (8).

$$W_m = \frac{1}{\text{slope} + \text{intercept}} \quad (7)$$

$$C_b = 1 + \frac{\text{slope}}{\text{intercept}} \quad (8)$$

In general, the BET equation fits adsorption data well over the relative pressure range of 0.05 to 0.35, but predicts considerably more adsorption at higher relative pressures than is experimentally observed. This is consistent with an assumption built into the BET derivation that an infinite number of layers are adsorbed at a relative pressure of unity. The BET equation is frequently applied to nonpolar gas adsorption results to obtain estimates of the specific surface area of solid samples. By assuming a cross-sectional area for the adsorbate molecule, one can use W_m to calculate the specific surface area by the relationship (9),

$$S = \frac{W_m X N_{av}}{M \Sigma} \quad (9)$$

where S is the specific surface area in m²/g, W_m is the mass of adsorbate adsorbed at monolayer coverage, X is the cross-sectional area of an adsorbed adsorbate molecule (assumed to be 0.195 nm² for krypton, 0.162 nm² for nitrogen, and 0.125 nm² for water [9, 10]), N_{av} is Avogadro's number of molecules, M is the molecular weight of adsorbate, and Σ is the mass of the sample. Obviously, calculating surface areas from moisture-uptake data that do not lead to monolayer coverage at W_m (either incomplete coverage or absorption into the solid) results in (incorrect) values that have no physical meaning.

The Guggenheim and deBoer Equation

Many attempts to modify the BET adsorption theory have been made since its original derivation. Its simplicity and ability to fit adsorption data extremely well at lower relative pressures have, however, made it the model of choice for estimating surface areas from nonpolar gas adsorprtion. Most modifications of the BET model, developed to analyze data over the entire range of relative pressures, usually add at least one fitting parameter to the equation. This makes computer fitting a necessity, since only two measurable parameters, W and P/P^0, are available. From a modeling perspective, additional fitting parameters of unknown or undefined physical meaning that arise from such approaches are often a deterrent to the use of multiparameter models because of the consequent difficulty in interpreting results. In this regard, therefore, only a single modification of the BET model, which has been shown to extend the relative pressure range over which vapor adsorption data are able to be fit, will be considered here. This extension of the BET model, independently derived by Guggenheim [11] and deBoer [12], accounts for the adsorption of an intermediate state of vapor between the tightly bound first molecule adsorbing to an adsorption site and the condensed molecules adsorbed at very high relative pressures. Molecules adsorbed in the intermediate range can be considered to interact with the solid, but the interaction is assumed to be considerably less than that of the first molecule sorbed at an adsorption site. This equation is given as Eq. (10),

$$W = \frac{W_m C_G K(P/P^0)}{[1 - K(P^0/P)][1 - K(P/P^0) - C_G K(P/P^0)]} \quad (10)$$

where P, P^0, H_L, W, and W_m are identical to the parameters used in the BET equation, and K is expressed by Eq. (11),

$$K = B \exp \frac{H_L - H_m}{RT} \quad (11)$$

where B is a constant and H_m is the heat of adsorption of vapor adsorbed in the intermediate layer. The constant C_G is defined by Eq. (12),

$$C_G = D \exp \frac{H_L - H_m}{RT} \quad (12)$$

where D is a constant, H_1 is the heat of adsorption of the first molecule adsorbed at a site, and H_m is the heat of adsorption of the intermediately bound molecule.

Water Vapor Absorption by Amorphous Solids

Although water vapor is absorbed into amorphous solids and not simply adsorbed on the surface, it still has been found that such absorption isotherms can be fit to the BET equation up to a P/P^0 of about 0.40 as with vapor adsorption, and over the entire range of P/P^0 using its extension, Eq. (10). Since this was first reported by Anderson [13] to be the case for water absorption, Eq. (10), applied to water vapor absorption, is often call the GAB equation for Guggenheim, Anderson, and deBoer [14]. Since the theoretical basis for the derivation of the original equation does not translate directly to the absorption process, which involves dissolution of water in the amorphous solid, the significance of fit to the GAB equation is somewhat limited. It is, however, a very useful equation since it does allow one to describe the entire isotherm and to draw out some useful parameters (to be discussed later).

Since water vapor dissolves in the solid during absorption, several models based on solution theory, proposing that the sorbate is taken up into the solid as a solid solution, have been derived and used to describe water sorption on polymers (e.g., Flory-Huggins [15] and Hailwood-Horrobin [16]). The development of these sorption theories is based on meaningful physical-chemical principles. As with the many modifications of the BET adsorption model, however, the physical significance of the constants, and the meaning of the values obtained (from computer fitting) from such analyses are often of limited utility in helping to gain a basic understanding of the mechanisms of sorption from a molecular viewpoint. From this perspective, other models based on entirely different theoretical concepts are not considered here. For further reference, the reader is directed to several excellent literature reviews of the many sorption theories that have been proposed [17, 18].

Capillary Condensation

Vapor sorption onto porous solids differs from vapor uptake onto the surfaces of flat materials in that a vapor (in the case of interest, water) condenses to a liquid in a pore structure at a vapor pressure, P_r, below the vapor pressure, P^0, where condensation occurs on flat surfaces. This is generally attributed to the increased attractive forces between adsorbate molecules that occur as surfaces become highly curved, such as in a pore or capillary. This phenomenon is referred to as capillary condensation and is described by the Kelvin equation [19], as in Eq. (13),

$$\ln \frac{P_r}{P^0} = -\frac{2\gamma V_m}{r\,RT} \tag{13}$$

where γ is the surface tension of the adsorbed film (assumed equal to that of the bulk liquid), V_m is the molar volume of the liquid, r is the pore radius, R is the gas constant, and T is temperature. The Kelvin equation has been shown to be applicable to pore radii as small as 5 nm for water adsorption onto mica [20, 21]. As mentioned earlier, capillary condensation results in closed hysteresis loops in the adsorption-desorption isotherms of porous materials. Calculating P_r/P^0 by assuming a surface tension for water of 72.8 ergs/cm^2 and a density of 0.998 g/cm^3 at 293 K, shows that condensation is predicted at relative pressures of 0.998, 0.989, 0.898, and 0.340 for pore radii of 1000, 100, 10, and 1 nm, respectively. In this regard, it is clear that capillary condensation need only be considered for very small pore dimensions. In practical terms, one should be concerned about this mechanism of water uptake for microporous pharmaceutical powders that exhibit a relatively large specific surface area (i.e., >100 m^2/g), as determined from nonpolar gas-adsorption studies.

Methodology
Control of Relative Humidity

Maintenance of constant relative humidity environments is essential for studying water-solid interactions. There are primarily four techniques employed to maintain constant relative humidity:

- Saturated salt solutions
- Sulfuric acid solutions
- Temperature modification of an aqueous solution
- Mixing wet and dry air streams

Saturated salt solutions and sulfuric acid solutions establish relative humidity by reducing the vapor pressure above an aqueous solution (a colligative effect). At controlled temperature, saturated salt solutions maintain a constant relative humidity as long as there is excess salt and bulk water present. As water is added or removed, moisture from the headspace condenses or evaporates with subsequent dissolution or precipitation of salt to maintain the equilibrium vapor pressure. Since the degree of vapor pressure depression depends on the number of species in solution and since the solubility of most salts is dependent on temperature, the relative humidity generated is also temperature dependent. Hence, use of the same salt at different temperatures can result in different relative humidities. References 22–26 can be consulted for specific saturated salt solutions that result in defined relative humidities as a function of temperature. Since relative humidity is dependent on the number of dissolved species, saturation must be attained prior to beginning experimentation. Furthermore, preparing the salt solutions several days before beginning a sorption study is recommended.

Sulfuric acid solutions of varying concentration [26] are also used to establish relative humidity. Addition or removal of water from the solution by desorption of sorption of water to the solid, however, alter the concentration of the sulfuric acid (and water) and thus change the relative humidity of the headspace. This technique for controlling relative humidity in the headspace is more practical when small amounts of water are sorbed or desorbed from the solid.

Temperature modification of an aqueous solution can also be used to maintain constant relative humidity in the headspace [14]. This technique maintains the solid at one temperature and an aqueous solution connected to the system at another temperature. Due to the strong vapor pressure dependence on temperature, very tight temperature control of both the aqueous solution and the solid are required to maintain constant relative humidity in the vicinity of the solid.

Mixing dry and water vapor-saturated air in defined proportions can also be used to generate constant relative humidity; flow rates and the water vapor content of the dry and saturated air must be strictly controlled [27,28].

Measurement of Relative Humidity

The measurement of relative humidity depends on the system used. Systems employing vacuum are usually evacuated prior to the introduction of water vapor [29]. In the absence of gas-forming reactions, measurement of total pressure in the system can be used as a measure of water vapor pressure. Systems under normal air pressure require specific measurement of water vapor pressure. Caution should be taken to ensure that the relative humidity source is in close proximity to the solid, since the diffusion of water vapor through air to the solid is required to maintain a constant relative humidity in the immediate vicinity of the solid. A wide variety of pressure-measuring instrumentation is commercially available with varying accuracy, precision, and cost.

Measurement of the Critical Relative Humidity, RH_0

The relative humidity at which a solid begins to deliquesce, RH_0, can be determined:

- Directly, by measuring the relative humidity above a saturated solution of the substance or the relative humidity at which significant moisture uptake and simultaneous dissolution occurs, or
- Indirectly, by measuring the steady-state moisture-uptake rate at relative humidities above RH_0 and extrapolating to the relative humidity at which the moisture-uptake rate is zero [1, 30, 31].

Although other techniques can be used to measure the relative humidity above a saturated solution, one relatively simple procedure is to utilize a vacuum system to remove air from the headspace (by vapor-phase expansions) and then, with the vacuum pumps isolated and the saturated solution maintained at a constant temperature, measure the water vapor pressure, which can be converted to relative humidity by dividing by P^0, the vapor pressure above pure water at the temperature of interest [33].

Measurement of Moisture Uptake (Kinetics of Deliquescence)

The rate of moisture uptake above RH_0 requires maintenance and measurement of a range of relative humidities, and the capability of measuring the moisture content of the solid over time. Use of a vacuum system can minimize vapor diffusion through the headspace, thus maintaining constant relative humidity in the vicinity of the sample. Furthermore, since the estimate of the steady-state moisture-uptake rate is most reliable when the integrity of the solid is intact and the film of sorbed moisture is thin (and saturation most likely), it is advisable to determine the moisture-uptake rate early. It is also helpful to be able to view the solid during the experiment to verify that integrity is maintained and excess solid remains [31, 34].

Water Sorption of Drugs and Dosage Forms

Measurement of Equilibrium Moisture Sorption

Water sorption–desorption isotherms in a controlled relative humidity environment can be generated gravimetrically or volumetrically. Gravimetric methods require:

1. A dry sample weight,
2. Constant sample temperature,
3. Maintaining predetermined constant relative humidities in the headspace, and
4. Attaining and measuring an equilibrium weight of sorbed water vapor.

Gravimetric measurement of moisture uptake can be taken continuously or discontinuously. In continuous measurement a sample is placed on a balance in a temperature- and relative humidity-controlled environment. Microbalances in closed systems have been used successfully for this purpose [27–29, 32], and commercial systems are now available that can accurately and precisely control relative humidity and simultaneously monitor sample weight.

Volumetric methods require, in addition to points 1 and 2 above, water vapor pressure measurement in a dosing volume and, later, in the headspace above the equilibrated sample, and measuring dead volumes of the individual chambers, including the sample chamber.

In essence, volumetric methods equilibrate a known headspace dosing volume at a given (measured) water vapor pressure, followed by exposure of the pre-equilibrated sample to this water vapor, with subsequent measurement of the water vapor pressure after equilibration. The mass of water sorbed, Δn (in moles), at the final pressure in the system, P_f, is obtained from the difference, ΔP, between P_f^{calc}, the calculated water vapor pressure at equilibrium, and P_f^{meas}, the final measured water vapor pressure, as expressed by Eq. (14),

$$\Delta n = \frac{\Delta P V}{RT} \tag{14}$$

where V is the final volume, R is the gas constant, and T is absolute temperature [29].

Water Sorption by Crystalline Solids

General Model

Figure 1 schematically describes the important steps in the uptake of water vapor by crystalline water-soluble solids. At low relative humidities, water is adsorbed to the surface of a nonhydrate-forming solid. As the relative humidity is increased, some tendency for multilayer sorption is expected. At some relative humidity (characteristic for a given substance), the solid begins to dissolve in the sorbed film of water. A saturated solution of solute most likely exists, and this causes the vapor pressure over the sorbed film of water to be depressed relative to that over pure water and to be constant and equal to that above a saturated solution of the substance. This vapor pressure may be expressed as the critical relative humidity, RH_0. If the relative humidity in the atmosphere is greater than that over the saturated solution (RH_0), water condenses spon-

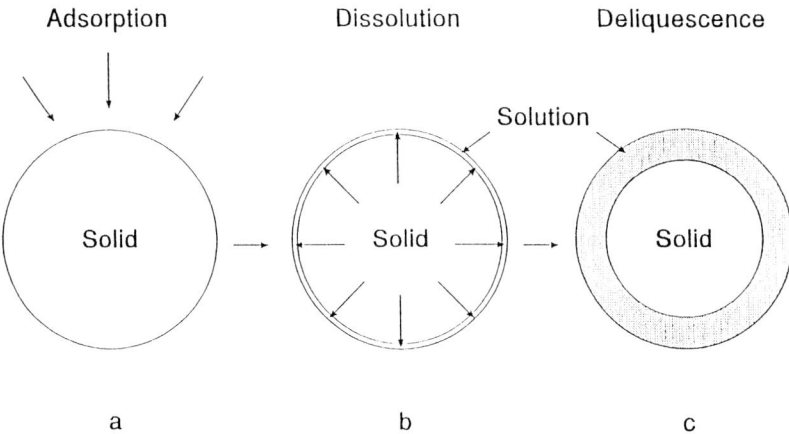

FIG. 1. Water vapor adsorption and deliquescence of a water-soluble solid. (a) Atmospheric relative humidity, $RH_i < RH_0$; (b) $RH_i = RH_0$; and (c) $RH_i > RH_0$.

taneously on the aqueous film. This dilutes the film, allowing more solid to dissolve, which, in turn, maintains the pressure gradient. The process of water vapor uptake continues until all the solid has dissolved and the solution is diluted further. Only when the relative humidity above the solution is raised to that of the atmosphere will this process terminate. This phenomenon is called deliquescence. Although hydrates undergo solid-state transitions in transforming from the anhydrate to the hydrate, as well as from one hydrate species to another, behavior similar to that previously described for nonhydrates is also noted at and above RH_0 for hydrates. In pharmaceutical systems, water-soluble species are frequently encountered in solid dosage forms. Thus, it is important to understand the conditions responsible for deliquescence and the molecular events occurring at relative humidities below the deliquescence point.

Water Sorption onto Nonhydrates Below RH_0

The sorption of water vapor onto nonhydrating crystalline solids below RH_0 depends on the polarity of the surface(s) and is proportional to the surface area. For example, water exhibits little tendency to sorb to nonpolar solids like carbon or polytetrafluorethylene (Teflon) [21], but it sorbs to a greater extent to more polar materials such as alkali halides [35–38] and organic salts like sodium salicylate [38]. Since water is only sorbed to the external surfaces of these substances, relatively small amounts (i.e., typically less than 1 mg/g) of water are sorbed compared with hydrates and amorphous materials that absorb water into their internal structures.

Unfortunately, the literature is relatively sparse with examples of water uptake profiles onto crystalline, nonhydrating substances below RH_0. This is most likely due to the difficulty in accurately measuring the small amounts of water that are sorbed. Alkali halides are an exception, however, likely due to their well-characterized particle morphologies [35–38]. Figure 2 shows a water uptake isotherm onto recrystallized sodium chloride [38]. Note that the amount of water sorbed as a function of relative humidity is normalized to the specific surface area of the sample. Since water is sorbed

Water Sorption of Drugs and Dosage Forms

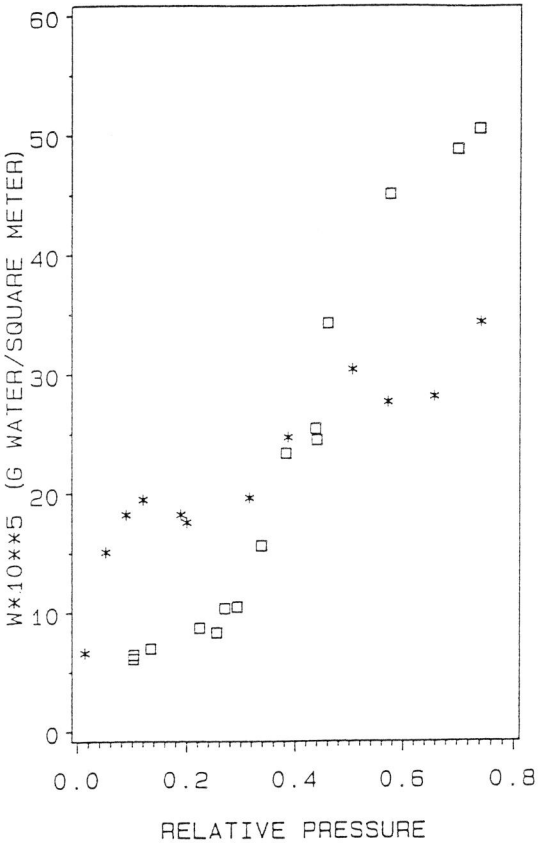

FIG. 2. Water vapor sorption for recrystallized (□) and ground (*) sodium chloride at 20 °C. (From Ref. 38.)

only to the external surface of this material, this allows comparison of water uptake data from different lots of material, whereas plotting these data on a "per-gram" basis would have little or no meaning. For the sodium chloride sample in Fig. 2 (specific surface area = 0.0875 m^2/g, from krypton adsorption studies), only 5×10^{-4} g water per m^2 of sodium chloride is sorbed, even up to 70% relative humidity. Also note the apparent steplike nature of the isotherm. From BET analysis of the sorption data at the lower relative humidities, a W_m value of 7.6×10^{-5} g/m^2 is obtained. This value is only about 0.32 that of the predicted value for monolayer coverage assuming an area per water molecule of 0.125 nm^2. This suggest that it is meaningless to refer to the number of layers of sorbed water as multiples of W_m, except as a point of reference. Interestingly, the second step plateau in Fig. 2 occurs at about three times the moisture content corresponding to W_m, suggesting that for sodium chloride the monolayer is actually completed during the second step of the isotherm. Isosteric heat-of-sorption results for sodium chloride from Barraclough and Hall [35] suggest that the heat of sorption of water up to W_m is invariant, whereas the heat of sorption decreases and becomes constant at about two times W_m. Considering the experimental error involved in obtaining

W_m and the isosteric heats of sorption, this suggests that water is sorbed with a homogeneous binding energy up to W_m and then interacts to a lesser extent until the monolayer is complete.

As shown in Fig. 2 [38], and also by the work of Barraclough and Hall [35], moisture uptake onto sodium chloride as a function of relative humidity is reversible as long as RH_0 is not attained. This is evidence that actual dissolution of water-soluble crystalline substances does not occur below RH_0. This is consistent with the thermodynamic rationale that dissolution below RH_0 would require a supersaturated solution (i.e., an increased number of species in solution would be necessary to induce dissolution at a relative humidity below that of the saturated solution, RH_0). In this regard, one should only need to consider the solid-state properties of a purely crystalline material below RH_0. As described later, other considerations may be warranted for a substance that exists in multiple polymorphic forms or contains amorphous material.

Water Sorption onto Hydrates Below RH_0

Many drugs (cephalexin monohydrate, quinidine sulfate dihydrate, ampicillin trihydrate, codeine sulfate trihydrate, morphine sulfate dihydrate, dicalcium phosphate dihydrate) utilize water as an integral part of their crystal structure. Solids that form specific crystal hydrates tend to sorb relatively small amounts of water to their external surface below a characteristic relative humidity, when initially dried to an anhydrous state. Below this characteristic relative humidity, these materials behave similarly to nonhydrates. Once the characteristic relative humidity is attained, addition of more water to the system does not result in a further increase in relative humidity. Rather this water is sorbed so that the anhydrate crystal is converted to the hydrate. The strength of the water–solid interaction depends on the level of hydrogen bonding possible within the lattice [21,39]. In some hydrates (e.g., caffeine and theophylline) where hydrogen bonding is relatively weak, water molecules can aid in hydrate stabilization primarily due to their space-filling role [21,39].

Since water molecules occupy regular positions within the lattice of a hydrate with a specific stoichiometry (e.g., 1:1 monohydrate, 2:1 dihydrate, 5:1 pentahydrate) to the solid, relatively large quantities of water are sorbed. Figure 3 shows a moisture uptake isotherm for ipratropium bromide [40]. This substance undergoes an apparent hydration of the crystal between 63 and 75% relative humidity. Above 75% relative humidity, approximately 4.6% water is sorbed (theoretical value for monohydrate is 4.4 g/g). Interestingly, as anhydrous ipratropium bromide is equilibrated for extended time periods (e.g., 2 and 5 months, respectively, as shown in Fig. 3), hydration of the crystal appears to occur at 53 and 63% relative humidities. This example clearly shows that time periods of many months may be required to attain a reliable estimate of the equilibrium uptake at selected relative humidities. Characteristic of many hydrates, ipratropium bromide exhibits significant hysteresis between the sorption and desorption isotherms. This is attributed to the degree of binding and the physical fit of water in the hydrated lattice.

Nonspecific hydration, or hydration of the lattice without a first-order phase transition, must also be considered. Cox et al. [41] reported the moisture uptake profile of cromolyn sodium, and the related effects on the physical properties of this substance. Although up to nine molecules of water per molecule of cromolyn sodium are sorbed into the crystalline lattice at 90% relative humidity, the sorption profile does not show

Water Sorption of Drugs and Dosage Forms

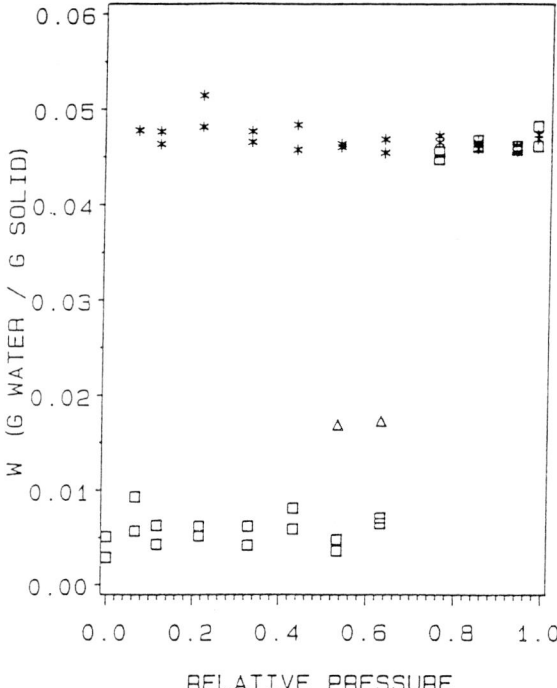

FIG. 3. Water vapor sorption and desorption isotherms for ipratropium bromide at 20 °C. Key: (□), 2-months sorption; (Δ), 5-months sorption; (*), 2- and 5-months desorption. All 2-month sorption results, except at 53 and 63% relative humidity, were verified at 5 months.

any sharp plateaus corresponding to fixed hydrates. Rather, the uptake profile exhibits a gradual increase in moisture content as relative humidity increases, which results in marked changes in x-ray diffraction patterns, density, and other physical properties. For this example, moisture uptake onto cromolyn sodium was correlated with expansion of the lattice in the b crystallographic direction, which was shown to be reversible on dehydration.

A thorough understanding of the hydration profile for a solid forming a crystalline hydrate is important for several reasons. First, since an anhydrate and hydrate(s) are distinct thermodynamic species, they have different physical-chemical properties (e.g., solubility) that may affect dissolution and bioavailability. Second, a desired hydrate species can be formed and used (and retained) simply by controlling the established environmental conditions. Third, since significant quantities of water can be sorbed and liberated as a hydrate becomes hydrated and dehydrated, the physical-chemical properties of the immediate system (including other nearby solids) can be markedly affected.

The Critical Relative Humidity, RH_0

Knowledge of RH_0 for each component in a formulation and for the entire system is extremely important for predicting relative humidities where gross physical changes of the system are expected due to dissolution of the water-soluble components. The value of RH_0, as a colligative property, is significantly influenced by the number of species in solution. As a rule of thumb, two general comments can be made. First, compounds exhibiting poor water solubility typically have RH_0 values in the high 90% range. Second, as solubility increases, RH_0 decreases. Since nonidealities are introduced as solutions become more and more concentrated, however, it is not usually possible to use dilute solution models (e.g., Raoult's law) to predict the expected RH_0 for a solute of significant aqueous solubility. Hence, RH_0 should be measured for individual solids. Examples of RH_0 values for single-component systems are shown in Table 1.

Values of RH_0 for mixtures, on the other hand, can be calculated from the RH_0 values of single components using Eq. (15), developed by Ross [43],

$$\frac{(RH_0)_{mix}}{100} = \frac{(RH_0)_1}{100} \cdot \frac{(RH_0)_2}{100} \cdot \frac{(RH_0)_3}{100} K \qquad (15)$$

where $(RH_0)_{mix}$ is the relative humidity above a saturated solution of the mixture and $(RH_0)_i$ represents the relative humidities of the individual saturated salt solutions. The Ross equation was derived assuming dilute solutions and negligible interaction between components in solution. The results presented in Table 2 compare RH_0 values obtained by calculating RH_0 values for mixtures from the Ross equation and those obtained experimentally. Agreement is very good, especially considering the high concentrations of dissolved solute(s) that are attained, (estimated as high as 50 molal for the tetrabutylammonium bromide–choline bromide system [34].

TABLE 1 RH_0 Values for Single-Component Systems at 25°C

Compound	RH_0	Reference
Potassium chloride	84	31
Potassium bromide	81	31
Potassium iodide	68	31
Sodium chloride	75	31
Choline iodide	72	31
Choline bromide	41	31
Choline chloride	23	31
Tetrabutylammonium bromide	61	31
Potassium acetate	23	22
Potassium carbonate	43	22
Sucrose	84	31
Fructose	64	31
Glucose	87	31
Sodium salicylate	79	29
Sodium benzoate	88	29
Salicylic acid	>99	42
Benzoic acid	>99	42
Malic acid	78	42
Tartaric acid	93	42
Fumaric acid	98	42
Succinic acid	95	42

TABLE 2 Calculated and Experimental Values of RH_0 for Mixtures

Mixture	RH_0 Calculated	RH_0 Experimental
Sodium chloride–potassium bromide	61	64
Potassium chloride–sodium chloride	64	67
Potassium chloride–potassium bromide	68	73
Sucrose–potassium bromide	68	66
Sucrose–dextrose monohydrate	69	68
Sucrose–sodium chloride–potassium bromide	51	57
Choline bromide–potassium bromide	33	40
Tetrabutylammonium bromide–potassium bromide	49	57
Tetrabutylammonium bromide–choline bromide	25	34

The Kinetics of Deliquescence Above RH_0

Initial work by Edgar and Swan [44], Adams and Merz [45], Prideaux [46], Markowitz and Boryta [47], and Carstensen [1] suggested that the rate of moisture uptake onto water-soluble solids above RH_0 should depend on the temperature, the exposed surface area of the solid, the velocity of movement of the moist air, a specific reaction constant that is characteristic of the individual solid, and the difference between the partial pressure of water in the environment and that of the partial pressure of water above a saturated solution of a water-soluble substance.

Van Campen et al. [31] developed models describing the rate of moisture uptake above RH_0 that consider both the mass transport of water to the solid substance and the heat transfer away from the surface. For the special case of an environment consisting of pure water (i.e., initial vacuum conditions), the Van Campen model is greatly simplified since vapor diffusion need not be considered. Here, only the rate at which heat is transported away from the surface is assumed to be an important factor in limiting the sorption rate, W'. For this special case, an expression was derived to base the rate of moisture uptake solely on RH_i, the relative humidity of the environment, and RH_0.

This model was shown to be applicable for describing moisture uptake kinetics (in vacuum) above RH_0 for single-component systems of alkali halides, sugars, and choline salts [31]. The model was later extended to consider the moisture uptake kinetics above RH_0 for multicomponent systems of these substances [34].

Water Sorption by Amorphous Solids

Isotherm Analyses at Ambient Temperatures

The amount of moisture sorbed by amorphous solids is typically much greater than that sorbed by nonhydrating crystalline substances below their critical relative humidities. Typical substances of pharmaceutical interest in this class of solids include celluloses, starches, polyvinylpyrrolidone, gelatin, and some lyophilized proteins. Though some of these substances exhibit partially crystalline character, they generally contain significant fractions of amorphous material and, thus, fall into this class of solids. A typical isotherm for microcrystalline cellulose is shown in Fig. 4. Significant amounts of water are sorbed over the entire relative humidity range, and both the sorption and desorption isotherms are characterized by the classical sigmoidal shape often observed with the physical adsorption of gases. Also apparent is the hysteresis between the sorption and desorption portions of the isotherm (i.e., the amount of water associated with the solid is greater for the desorption isotherm than for the sorption isotherm for a given relative pressure). This is typical for these types of materials and is generally attributed to kinetic effects or to a change in the polymer-chain conformation caused by the plasticization effects of sorbed water [14,48–50].

Figure 4 also shows the excellent fit to the GAB equation (Eq. 10) of the sorption and desorption isotherms for microcrystalline cellulose. In this regard, this equation offers considerable practical utility in fitting isotherms for these types of materials over the entire relative humidity range, especially in contrast to the BET equation, which usually only fits uptake data up to about 40% relative humidity. As previously mentioned, however, this does not in itself confirm the validity of the GAB model for

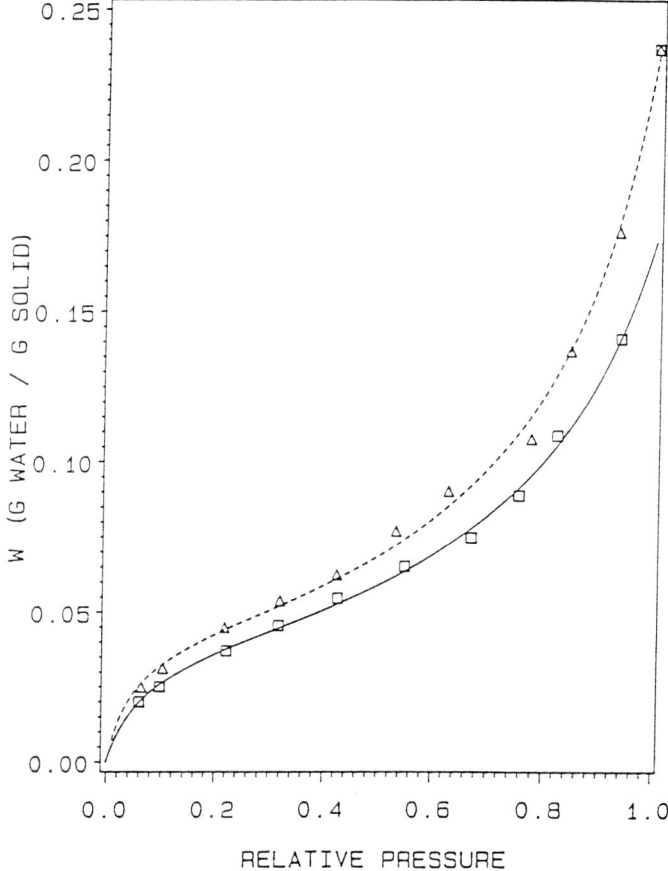

FIG. 4. Water vapor sorption (□) and desorption (Δ) isotherms for microcrystalline cellulose at 20°C. Key: —, GAB fit to sorption data; - - - -, GAB fit to desorption data.

describing moisture sorption data on these materials. Rather, independent confirmation of the physical meaning is necessary.

Considerable physical insight has been gained into the primary binding mechanism of water onto starches and celluloses from isotherm analyses that yield values for W_m (Eqs. (5), (7), and (10)). This is illustrated in Table 3, which gives W_m values for three types of starches [50]. Table 3 shows that despite significant morphological differences between the various starches, the values for W_m are quite constant. One value of W_m, taken from a fit of desorption data, appears to be slightly higher than values obtained from sorption data. This might be expected if the availability of primary sorption sites had been increased by previous exposure to elevated relative humidities, with subsequent increased levels of water sorption. As shown by Van den Berg et al. [14,48,49], these values of W_m are all close to the value of 0.11 g of water per g of starch, calculated by assuming that one water molecule sorbs per anhydroglucose unit. Since this calculation assumes that all anhydroglucose units are available for primary binding, and since this is not likely to be precisely the case, it is not surprising that the values measured for W_m are slightly less than 0.11 g/g.

Zografi et al. [50, 52] have extended this analysis to the sorption of water vapor by various celluloses. For celluloses, corrections are necessary because only the amorphous regions of cellulose take up water vapor. Table 4 shows the W_m values obtained from isotherm analyses of several cellulosic materials after accounting for the degree of crystallinity. As expected, celluloses with different degrees of crystallinity exhibit different values of W_m without correction for crystallinity, and all are considerably lower than those for the starches. When corrected, however, for the degree of crystallinity, all of the values are in reasonable agreement with each other and with the W_m values obtained for the starches. Especially interesting are the results in Table 4 for microcrystalline cellulose samples having different degrees of crystallinity due to grinding [54]. These results suggest that a similar mechanism of water uptake is occurring in starches and the noncrystalline regions of celluloses.

Similar analyses of moisture-uptake data are available in the literature for other cellulose and starch derivatives used as pharmaceutical excipients (Table 5). Considering the uncertainties associated with estimating the moisture uptake values from published graphs, the values of W_m are all rather consistent with each other and with a stoichiometry of one water molecule per anhydroglucose unit. It is interesting that the two samples derived from cellulose, sodium carboxymethylcellulose and sodium cro-

TABLE 3 Starch W_m Values Based on BET Analysis of Moisture-Uptake Isotherms[a]

Starch	W_m (g/g)	Reference
Corn	0.095[b]	29
Corn	0.083	51
Potato	0.085	14
Wheat	0.080	14

[a]Data from Ref. 50.
[b]This value is taken from the desorption isotherm. The others are from sorption isotherms.

TABLE 4 Cellulose W_m Values Based on BET Analysis of Moisture-Uptake Isotherms Corrected for Degree of Crystallinity[a]

Cellulose	% Crystallinity	W_m, corr (g/g)	Reference
Cotton	70	0.093	53
Cellophane	40	0.098	53
MCC[b]	63	0.095	54
MCC[c]	49	0.076	54
MCC[c]	38	0.107	54
MCC[c]	0	0.086	54

[a]Data from Ref. 50.
[b]Microcrystalline cellulose.
[c]MCC ground in a ball mill [54].

scarmellose, did not require any correction for the degree of crystallinity to conform close to a 1:1 stoichiometry. It appears quite likely, therefore, that the change in chemical structure and the processing of these materials essentially eliminates the crystallinity of cellulose.

The preceding analysis suggests that water, indeed, penetrates throughout the amorphous regions of these materials and undergoes a specific interaction with available sorption sites, most likely the available hydroxyl groups on the anhydroglucose units. Differential heat of sorption results for various starches [14, 51] and celluloses [10, 56] support this model. Figure 5 is an example of a pattern that is obtained for all these materials and that supports a model where there is a specific water–solid interaction to a moisture content of at least the equivalent three times W_m. This means that water is in a more structured state (i.e., reduced mobility) than bulk water in this range. Interestingly, the heats of sorption exhibit discreet breaks corresponding to stoichiometries of one and two water molecules per anhydroglucose unit. Some differential-heat-of-sorption results are nearly constant over the W_m range, suggesting that binding is homogenous over this range [10,14]. This is, however, not always the case.

Other supportive evidence for a specific water–solid interaction is available from thermal studies showing the amount of nonfreezable water [58–60], nuclear magnetic resonance [29, 61–67], and diffusion studies [68, 69]. The evidence is less clear, however, concerning the presence of distinct binding of water to sorption sites with discrete

TABLE 5 W_m Values for Pharmaceutical Excipients Based on BET Analysis of Moisture-Uptake Isotherms[a]

Excipient	W_m (g/g)	Reference
Starch 1500	0.074	51
Sodium starch glycolate (Explotab)	0.081	55
Sodium starch glycolate (Primogel)	0.092	55
Cross-linked dextrose (CLD-2)	0.098	56
Croscarmellose, sodium (Ac-Di-Sol)	0.094	56
Sodium carboxymethylcellulose	0.103	57

[a]Data from Ref. 50.

Water Sorption of Drugs and Dosage Forms

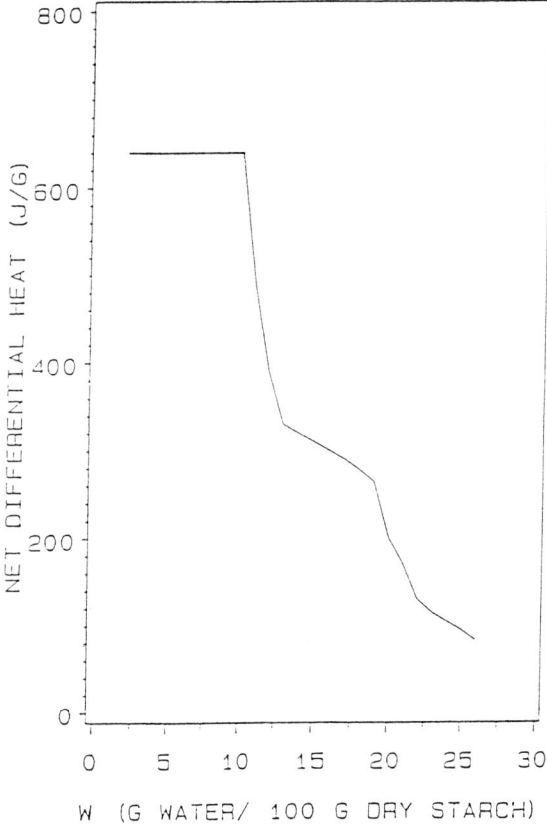

FIG. 5. Net differential heat of sorption for water vapor by native potato starch at 20 °C as a function of amount of water sorbed per mass of dry starch. (From Ref. 14.)

energy levels or of a continuum of states where water interacts to a lesser extent with increasing amount sorbed [50,70].

Isotherm Analyses as a Function of Temperature

Generally speaking, the absorption of water vapor into amorphous solids as a function of relative humidity decreases as the temperature increases, reflective of an overall exothermic process, normally expected with vapor adsorption processes. Such behavior has been observed with cellulose [71], starch [14], polyvinylpyrrolidone [72], and polymethyl methacrylate [73]. In such cases, it is often assumed that the dominant factor is the negative heat of absorption arising from the change in extent of water binding. The process, however, is much more complex than this because of the changing morphology of the solid and, hence, an entropy change as well. The complexity of the effects of temperature on water vapor absorption and the possible links to the plasticizing effects of water may be observed in the work of Oksanen and Zografi [72], who have reported that the W_m values for polyvinylpyrrolidone over the temperature range of −40 to 60°C decrease by a factor of three, suggesting that W_m does not reflect the absolute number of available binding sites on the polymer for directly "bound" water. Rather, W_m appears to be related to $W_{Tg\,=\,T}$, the amount of water sorbed that reduces the glass transition temperature, T_g to the temperature of the sample, as the ratio of $W_{Tg\,=\,T}$ to W_m remains nearly constant at 3.0 over the entire temperature range.

In summary, it is clear that water absorbs into amorphous polymers to a significant extent. Interaction of water molecules with "available" sorption sites likely occurs via hydrogen bonding in such a way that the mobility of the sorbed water is reduced and the thermodynamic state of this water is significantly altered relative to bulk water. Yet accessibility of the water to all potential sorption sites appears to be dependent on the previous history and physical-chemical properties of the solid. In this regard, the water–solid interaction in amorphous polymer systems is a dynamic relationship depending strongly on water activity and temperature.

The Meaning of Specific Surface Areas Calculated from Water Absorption Studies

Simply calculating specific surface areas from the W_m values in Tables 3–5 leads to "apparent" specific surface areas of approximately 300-500 m^2/g [50, 52]. Specific surface areas obtained from similar analyses of nonpolar gas (nitrogen or krypton) adsorption studies, however, are typically in the range of 1 m^2/g, independent of sample pretreatment.

Interestingly, the ball-milling studies of microcrystalline cellulose by Nakai (Table 4 [54]) have shown that the W_m values obtained from water sorption studies increase to a much greater extent than the increase in surface area due to comminution of the sample. In fact, as discussed earlier, moisture sorption was shown to be proportional to the degree of amorphous character, suggesting that water is being absorbed throughout the amorphous regions of MCC. In this regard, artifactual specific surface areas can be calculated from water absorption data [52] for these types of substances.

The Role of Water as a Plasticizer

Absorption of significant amounts of water into the internal structure of a solid has been shown to influence the properties of the solid. This is apparent, for example, in the hysteresis observed between the sorption and desorption isotherms in Fig. 4. This phenomenon becomes exaggerated to a greater extent for materials that contain higher proportions of amorphous material. Levine and Slade [74, 75], have demonstrated that water, with a very low glass transition temperature, can act as a plasticizer, thereby lowering the glass transition temperature, T_g, of amorphous polymers. Recognizing that the viscoelastic properties of the solid are altered significantly above (rubbery state) T_g, compared to below (glass or vitreous state) T_g, it is likely that the solid undergoes changes of its physical properties at distinct moisture contents and defined temperatures as a result of this phenomenon [72, 74]. Oksanen and Zografi [72] have shown with polyvinylpyrrolidone that the moisture content at which the moisture sorption isotherm begins to increase significantly correlates well with the moisture content that reduces T_g to the temperature of the isotherm. This is illustrated in Fig. 6, which shows water absorption isotherms for polyvinylpyrrolidone over the temperature range of –40 to 60°C [72, 79].Clearly, the inflection point at which the isotherm begins to turn markedly upward shifts to a higher moisture content as the temperature is reduced. To illustrate

Water Sorption of Drugs and Dosage Forms

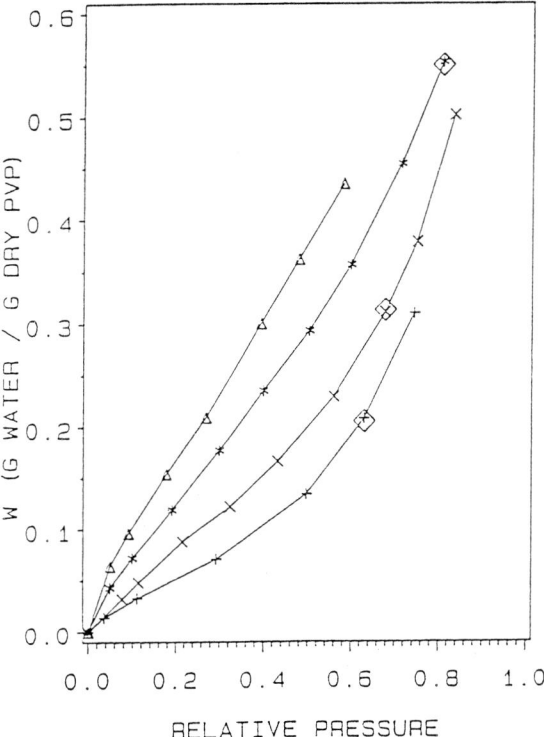

FIG. 6. Water vapor sorption isotherms for polyvinylpyrrolidone at 60 °C (+); 30 °C (x); −20 °C (*); and −40 °C (△). Data were taken from Oksanen and Zografi [63, 65]. A rectangle (◇) represents the calculated water contents necessary to depress T_g to the temperature of the isotherms.

this, note that the moisture content (0.674 g/g) necessary to reduce T_g to −40°C has not yet been attained in Fig. 6, and the isotherm appears linear over the relative humidity range shown. To further clarify, the moisture contents [$W_{T_g=T}$] corresponding to T_g at 60, 30, −20, and −40°C were shown to be about 0.205, 0.313, 0.553, and 0.674 g/g, respectively. Oksanen and Zografi [72] reported that cellulose and elastin (a protein) exhibit similar relationships, where the glass-to-rubber transitions correspond to the upward inflections in their respective isotherms.

Subsequent studies by Hancock and Zografi [76] demonstrated that the glass transition temperatures for PVP, hydroxypropyl methylcellulose and polymethyl methacrylate were linearly depressed by the weight fraction of sorbed water, according to a simplified Gordon-Taylor-Kelly-Bueche Eq. (16),

$$\frac{1}{T_g(\text{mix})} = \left(\frac{W_1}{T_{g1}} + \frac{W_2}{T_{g2}} \right) \quad (16)$$

where W_1 and W_2 are the weight fractions of components with T_g values T_{g1} and T_{g2} [77]. The results clearly indicate that the viscoelastic properties of amorphous materials can undergo significant changes such as the solid transitions from the glassy to rubbery state. Furthermore, these changes can occur due to elevation of temperature at fixed moisture content, or to an increase in moisture content at constant temperature, or to a combination of these effects. For dry amorphous substances, molecular mobility of the solid begins to be enhanced compared to the glassy state as low as 50°C below T_g [78]. Similar increases in molecular mobility due to the plasticizing effects of absorbed water suggest the need to maintain amorphous systems at least 50°C below the system glass transition temperature to avoid physical, chemical, and/or mechanical property changes over the product shelf life. Properties that are likely to be affected include tablet compaction [80, 81], gelatin capsule brittleness [74, 82], collapse of lyophilized amorphous powders [79, 83], protein stability [84], and the stability of low molecular weight, moisture-sensitive drugs mixed with amorphous polymeric substances [85].

Water Sorption by Pharmaceutical Solids Subjected to Processing

Understanding the mechanisms of moisture sorption by solids existing in either the crystalline or amorphous states allows a conceptual estimation of critical points where major changes in physical or chemical properties occur (e.g., RH_0, a crystal hydration relative humidity, glass transition temperature). Processing (i.e., milling, spray drying, compaction, lyophilization, etc.) of pharmaceutical solids, however, often induces at least a partial conversion of most substances to a high energy form [86–92]. Such local disorder has been associated with enhanced chemical reactivity [87–93] and increased solubility [94] relative to the thermodynamically favored crystalline state. These regions have been referred to as "hot" spots of the bulk solid and, when present, leave the solid in an "activated state" [86–99].

This nonhomogeneity in processed solids complicates the study of moisture-sorption phenomena in these materials, as more than one mechanism of uptake must be considered. This is especially difficult, and often frustrating, for cases in which only a small amount of amorphous material is present, as experimental techniques are not readily available to measure small amounts of amorphous material in the presence of a mostly crystalline substance [100]. Yet, relatively low percentages of amorphous material can absorb considerable amounts of water into their structure and act as the regions that undergo considerable change and affect the overall properties of the bulk substance [86]. This is especially important for low molecular weight substances that have the ability to readily recrystallize due to their overall greater mobility compared to that of higher molecular weight polymeric materials. This has been demonstrated for sodium chloride and sodium salicylate ground for 15 min with a mortar and pestle [38]. Whereas recrystallized materials exhibited no changes in specific surface areas with increasing relative humidities, the ground samples exhibited significant reductions in specific surface areas as relative humidities were increased. Figure 2 illustrates the differing moisture uptake profiles for the recrystallized and ground sodium chloride samples, normalized for specific surface area [38]. Whereas the ground material sorbed significantly more water at lower relative humidities than the recrystallized sample, the recrystallized material sorbed greater amounts at higher relative humidities. This relative reduction in sorption capacity of the ground sample is attributed to a reduction in surface area as relative humidity increased, due to the consequent recrystallization of the disordered surface material [38]. Fukuoka et al. [101] have demonstrated that a variety of pharmaceutical substances can be made amorphous and, furthermore, exhibit glass transition temperatures over a range of 243 to 354 K. For example, aspirin, progesterone, phenobarbital, and sulfadimethoxine exhibit T_g values of 243, 279, 321, and 339 K, respectively.

Similar to amorphous polymeric systems, low molecular weight amorphous substances also exhibit a reduction in T_g as moisture content increases [102], thereby leading to favorable conditions for recrystallization. Unfortunately, recrystallization of nonhydrating, low molecular weight amorphous systems can lead to the liberation of significant amounts of water to the headspace. Such "moisture dumping" can have additional impact on the physical, chemical, and mechanical properties of the system.

This is illustrated more quantitatively, by the hypothetical sucrose example discussed by Ahlneck and Zografi [86]. Assuming that all the sorbed water is taken up by the amorphous portion of the material, 0.1% total moisture would correspond to approximately 20, 10, 4, and 2% moisture content in the amorphous material, respectively, for 0.5, 1, 2.5, and 5% of amorphous solid. The glass transition temperatures for the amorphous portions of these systems range from 9 to 49°C, respectively [75, 86]. Hence, significant changes in the solid-state properties are expected at room temperature if relatively small amounts of amorphous material (i.e., <1%) are initially present. This example illustrates that even for low moisture content materials, significant changes can occur in certain regions of a solid, which may affect properties of the material influenced by molecular mobility [86].

Events resulting from increased molecular mobility due to increased moisture absorption and a subsequent reduction in T_g can be prevented by formulating such materials with amorphous substances of higher T_g. The net effect is to raise the system Tg to a level where molecular mobility is again sufficiently low (high viscosity) that the undesired property changes do not occur [93,103].

Transfer of Water Between Solid Components via the Headspace

Combining solids that have previously been equilibrated at different relative humidities results in a system that is thermodynamically unstable, since the moisture will tend to distribute in the system so that a single relative humidity is attained in the headspace. As shown in Fig. 7, moisture desorbs into the headspace from the component initially equilibrated at a higher relative humidity and sorbs to the component initially equilibrated at a lower relative humidity. This process continues until both solids have equilibrated at the final relative humidity. It can be predicted a priori by the sorption–desorption moisture transfer (SDMT) model [104] based on the moisture-uptake isotherms for each of the solid components, their initial moisture contents and dry weights, headspace volume, and temperature. Final moisture contents for each solid can easily be estimated from the isotherms for the respective solids.

The SDMT model has practical utility in aiding the rational optimization of the initial moisture contents of individual components in a system to attain the final desired relative humidity. Practical applications to date have included adjustment of the initial formulation LODs (loss on drying) prior to gelatin capsule filling to avoid brittleness [82,

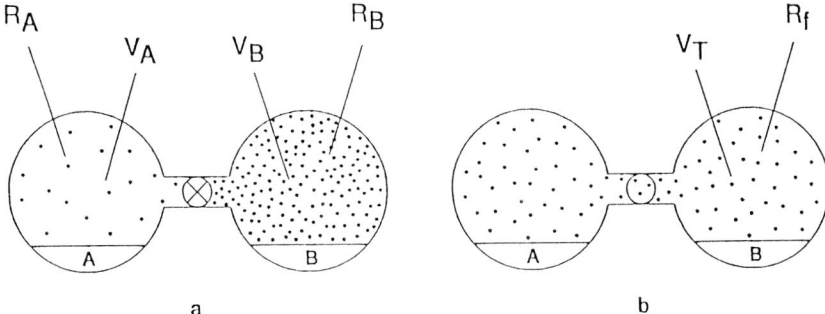

FIG. 7. Schematic representation of moisture transfer between solid components A and B. (a) Headspaces isolated from one another; (b) headspaces allowed to equilibrate. R_A and R_B = initial relative humidities above A and B, V_A and V_B = headspace volumes above A and B; R_f and V_T = final relative humidity and headspace volume above A and B. (From Ref. 104.)

105], choosing the appropriate formulation moisture content and amount of desiccant to maintain the relative humidity inside a container below a defined value [106], and selection of appropriate dry powder inhaler design and packaging conditions for optimal stability [107].

Summary

Moisture is present in all solid pharmaceutical drugs and dosage forms and in most processing techniques. Understanding where the water resides, its state, and the manner in which it affects the properties of individual materials, their mixtures, and ultimately, final product performance and integrity are essential for the developmental scientist to better understand the role of water in a particular system. Especially important are the kinetics of moisture uptake or loss, "equilibrium" uptake values as a function of relative humidity, whether the water resides externally or is absorbed into the material, its degree of binding with the solid, and the tendency for water to redistribute in a system consisting of more than one solid. Although water–solid interactions can be extremely complex in pharmaceutical systems, application of these fundamental concepts to product development can greatly aid in understanding the role of moisture in affecting the physical-chemical properties of solid materials.

Acknowledgments

This work was taken in part from the chapter Sorption of Water by Solids. In:*Physical Characterization of Pharmaceutical Solids* (H. Brittain, ed.), Marcel Dekker, Inc., 1995. The author would like to thank Professor George Zografi, Dr. Cindy Oksanen, and Mr. James Conners for their technical contributions to this chapter, Mr. Conners and Ms. Linda Schweikardt for their graphical support, and Ms. Alice Johnson-Cress for typing and editing this work.

References

1. Carstensen, J. T. In: *Pharmaceutics of Solids and Solid Dosage Forms*, J. Wiley & Sons, New York, 1977, pp. 11-15.
2. Lewis, G. N., Randall, M., Pitzer, K. S., and Brewer, L. In: *Thermodynamics*, 2nd rev. ed., McGraw-Hill, New York, 1961.
3. Gal, S. In: *Vapor Sorption Equilibria and Other Water-Starch Interactions: A Physico-Chemical Approach* (C. Van den Berg, Ph.D. Thesis), Agricultural University, Wageningen, The Netherlands, 1981, p. 10.
4. Brunauer, S., Emmett, P.H., and Teller, E., *J. Am. Chem. Soc.*, 60:309 (1938).
5. Langmuir, I., *J. Am. Chem. Soc.*, 40:1361 (1918).
6. Fowler, R., and Guggenheim, E. A. In: *Statistical Thermodynamics*, Cambridge University Press, Cambridge, UK, 1939.
7. Hill, T. L., *J. Chem. Phys.*, 14:263 (1946); *J. Am. Chem. Soc.*, 68:535 (1946).
8. Cassie, A. B. D., *Trans. Faraday Soc.*, 41:450 (1945); 41:458 (1945).
9. Lowell, S. In: *Introduction to Powder Surface Area*, J. Wiley & Sons, New York, 1979.
10. Hollenbeck, R. G., Peck, G. E., and Kildsig, D. O., *J. Pharm. Sci.*, 67:1599 (1978).
11. Guggenheim, E. A. In: *Applications of Statistical Mechanics*, Clarendon Press, Oxford, 1966.
12. deBoer, J. H. In: *The Dynamical Character of Adsorption*, 2nd ed., Clarendon Press, Oxford, 1968.
13. Anderson, R. B., *J. Am. Chem. Soc.*, 68:686 (1946).
14. Van den Berg, C. In: *Vapor Sorption Equilibrim and Other Water-Starch Interactions: A Physico-Chemical Approach*, Ph.D. Thesis, Agricultural University, Wageningen, The Netherlands, 1981.
15. P. J. Flory. In: *Principles of Polymer Chemistry*, Cornell University Press, Ithaca, New York, 1953.
16. Hailwood, A. J., and Horrobin, S., *Trans. Faraday Soc.*, 42B:84 (1946).
17. Van den Berg, C., and Bruin, S. In: *Water Activity: Influences on Food Quality* (L. B. Rockland and G. F. Stewart, eds.), Academic Press, New York, 1981.
18. Venkateswaren, A., *Chem. Rev.*, 70:619 (1970).
19. Martin, A., Swarbrick, J., and Cammarata, A. In: *Physical Pharmacy*, 3rd ed., Lea & Febiger, Philadelphia, 1983, pp. 510-512.
20. Fisher, L. R., and Israelachvili, J. N., *Chem. Phys. Letters,* 76:325 (1980).
21. Zografi, G., *Drug Devel. Ind. Pharm.*, 14:1905 (1988).
22. Greenspan, L., *J. Res. N.B.S.*, 81A: 89 (1977).
23. Rockland, L. B., and Nishi, S. K., *J. Food Technol.*, 34:43 (1980).
24. Winston, P. W., and Bates, D. H., *Ecology*, 41:232 (1960).
25. Stokes, R. H., and Robinson, R. A., *Ind. Eng. Chem.*, 41:2013 (1949).
26. *Handbook of Chemistry and Physics*, 67th ed. (R. C. Weast, ed.), Chemical Rubber Co., Cleveland, 1986-1987, p. E-42.
27. Bergren, M., *Water-Solid Interactions*, AAPS Shortcouse, Orlando, FL, 1993.
28. Spancake, C.W., Hastedt, J. E., and Venero, A. F., *Pharm. Res.*, 10:S-280 (1993).
29. Kontny, M. J. In: *Water Vapor Sorption Studies on Solid Surfaces*, Ph.D. Thesis, University of Wisconsin-Madison, 1985.
30. Van Campen, L., Zografi, G., and Carstensen, J. T., *Int. J. Pharm.*, 5:1 (1980).
31. Van Campen, L., Amidon, G. L., and Zografi, G., *J. Pharm. Sci.*, 72:1381, 1388, 1394 (1983).
32. Bergren, M., *Int. J. Pharm.*, 103:103 (1994).
33. *Handbook of Chemistry and Physics*, 67th ed. (R. C. Weast, ed.) Chemical Rubber Co., Cleveland, 1986-1987, pp. D-189-190.

34. Kontny, M. J., and Zografi, G., *J. Pharm. Sci.*, 74:124 (1985).
35. Barraclough, P. B., and Hall, P. G., *Surface Sci.*, 467:393 (1974).
36. Walter, H. U., *Zeitschr. Physik. Chem. Neue Folge Bd.*, 75:S.287 (1971).
37. Ladd, R. A., *Surf. Sci.*, 12:37 (1968).
38. Kontny, M. J., Grandolfi, G. P., and Zografi, G., *Pharm. Res.*, 4:104 (1987).
39. Byrn, S. R. In: *Solid State Chemistry of Drugs*, Academic Press, New York, 1982, p. 149.
40. Conners, J., Boehringer Ingelheim Pharmaceuticals, Inc., personal communications, 1991.
41. Cox, J. S. G., Woodard, G. D., and McCrone, W. C., *J. Pharm. Sci*, 60:1458 (1971).
42. Kontny, M. J., unpublished data.
43. Ross, K. D., *Food Technol.*, 29:26 (1975).
44. G., Edgar, and W. O., Swan, *J. Am. Chem. Soc.*, 44:570 (1922).
45. Adams, J. R., and Merz, A. R., *Ind. Eng. Chem.*, 21:305 (1929).
46. E. B. R., Prideaux, *J. Soc. Chem. Ind.*, 39:182 (1920).
47. Markowitz, M. M., and Boryta, D. A., *J. Chem. Eng. Data*, 6:16 (1961).
48. Van den Berg, C., Kaper, F. S., Weldring, J. A. G., and Wolters, I., *J. Food Technol.*, 10:589-602 (1975).
49. Van den Berg, C. In: *Water Activity: Influences on Food Quality* (L. B. Rockland and G. F. Stewart, eds.), Academic Press, New York, 1981, pp. 1-61.
50. Zografi, G., and Kontny, M. J., *Pharm. Res.*, 3:187 (1986).
51. Wurster, D. E., Peck, G. E., and Kildsig, D. O., *Starch*, 36:294 (1984).
52. Zografi, G., Kontny, M.J., Yang, A. Y. S., and Brenner, G. S., *Int. J. Pharm.*, 18:99 (1984).
53. Stamm, A. J. In: *Wood and Cellulose Science*, The Ronald Press Co., New York, 1964.
54. Nakai, Y., Fukuoka, E., Nakajima, and Hasegawa, J., *J. Chem. Pharm. Bull.*, 25:96 (1977).
55. Mitrevej, A., and Hollenbeck, R. G., *Pharm. Tech.*, 6:48 (1982).
56. Gordon, R. E., Peck, G. E., and Kildsig, D. O., *Drug Devel. Ind. Pharm.*, 10:833 (1984).
57. Callahan, J. C., Cleary, G. W., Elefant, M., Kaplan, I., Kensler, T., and Nash, R. A., *Drug Dev. Ind. Pharm.*, 8:355 (1982).
58. Rupley, J. A., Yank, P. H., and Tollin, G. In:*Water in Polymers* (S. P. Rowland, ed.), ACS Symposium 127, American Chemical Society, Washington, DC, 1980, pp. 111-132.
59. Nagashima, N., and Suzuki, E.-I., *Appl. Spectroscopy Rev.*, 20:1 (1984).
60. Duckworth, R. B., *J. Food Technol.*, 6:317 (1971).
61. Hennig, H. J., and Lechert, H., *J. Coll. Interf. Sci.*, 62:199 (1977).
62. Mousseri, J., Steinberg, M. P., Nelson, A. I., and Wei, L. S., *J. Food Sci.*, 39:114 (1974).
63. Tait, M. J., Ablett, S., and Wood, F. W., *J. Coll. Interf. Sci.*, 41:594 (1972).
64. Tait, M. J., Ablett, S., and Ranks, F. In: *Water Structure at the Water-Polymer Interface* (H. Jellinek, ed.), Plenum Press, New York, 1972, pp. 29-38.
65. Carles, J. E., and Scallan, A. M., *J. Appl. Poly. Sci.*, 17:1855 (1973).
66. Hsi, E., Voight, G. J., and Bryant, R. G., *J. Coll. Interf. Sci.*, 70:338 (1979).
67. Froix, M. F., and Nelson, R., *Macromolecules*, 8:726 (1975).
68. Fish, B. P. In: *Fundamental Aspects of the Dehydration of Foodstuffs*, Society of Chemistry and Industry (S.C.I.), London, 1958, pp. 143-157.
69. Duckworth, R. B., and Smith, G. M. In: *Recent Advances in Food Science*, Vol. 3 (J. M. Leitch and D. N. Rhodes, eds.), Butterworths, London, 1962, pp. 230-238.
70. Etzler, F. M., *J. Coll. Intef. Sci.*, 92:43 (1983).
71. Urquart, A. R., and Williams, A. M., *J. Textile Inst.*, 15:550 (1924).
72. Oksanen, C. A., and Zografi, G., *Pharm. Res.*, 7:654 (1990).
73. Smith, L. S. A., and Schnitz, V., *Polymer*, 29:1871 (1988).
74. Levine, H., and Slade, L. In: *Water Science Reviews*, Vol. 3 (F. Franks, ed.), Cambridge University Press, Cambridge, MA, 1987, pp. 79-185.
75. Slade, L., and Levine, H., *Pure Appl. Chem.*, 60:1841 (1988).

76. Hancock, B. C., and Zografi, G., *Pharm. Res.*, 11:471 (1994).
77. Gordon, M., and Taylor, J. S., *J. Appl. Chem.*, 2:493 (1952).
78. Hancock, B. C., Shamblin, S. L., and Zografi, G., *Pharm. Res.*, 12:799 (1995).
79. Mackenzie, A. P., and Rasmussen, D. H. In:*Water Structure at the Water-Polymer Interface* (H. H. G. Jellineck, ed.), Plenum, New York, 1972, pp. 146-172.
80. Shukla, A. J., and Price, J. C., *Pharm. Res.*, 8:336 (1991).
81. Amidon, G. E., and Houghton, M. E., *Pharm. Res.*, 12:923 (1995).
82. Kontny, M. J., and Mulski, C. A., *Int. J. Pharm.*, 54:79 (1989).
83. Mackenzie, A. P. In:*Freeze Drying and Advanced Food Technology* (S. A. Goldblith, L. Rey, and W. Rothmayr, eds.), Academic Press, New York, 1975, pp. 277-307.
84. Hageman, M. J., *Drug Devel. Ind. Pharm.*, 14:2047 (1988).
85. Kararli, T. T., and Catalano, T., *Pharm. Res.*, 12:923 (1990).
86. Ahlneck, C., and Zografi, G., *Int. J. Pharm.*, 62:87 (1990).
87. Vadas, E. B., Toma, P., and Zografi, G., *Pharm. Res.*, 8:148 (1991).
88. Levine, H., and Slade, L., *J. Chem. Soc. Faraday Trans. I*, 84:2619 (1988).
89. Huttenrauch, R., *Acta Pharm. Technol.*, 34:1 (1988).
90. Huttenrauch, R., Frike, S., and Zielke, P., *Pharm. Res.*, 2:302 (1985).
91. Otsuka, M., and Kaneniwa, N., *Int. J. Pharm.*, 62:65 (1990).
92. Hersey, J. A., and Krycer, I., *Int. J. Pharm. Technol. Prod. Manuf.*, 1:18 (1980).
93. Hancock, B. C., and Zografi, G., *J. Pharm. Sci.*, In Press, 1996.
94. Makower, B., and Dye, W. B., *Agr. Food Chem.*, 4:72 (1956).
95. Carstensen, J. T., and Van Scoik, K., *Pharm. Res.*, 7:1278 (1990).
96. Waltersson, J.-O, and Lundgren, P, *Acta Pharm. Suec.*, 22:291 (1985).
97. Prout, E. G., and Tompkins, F. C., *Trans. Faraday Soc.*, 40:489 (1944).
98. Ng, W.-L., *Aust. J. Chem.*, 28:1169 (1975).
99. Hasegawa, J., Hanano, M., and Awazu, S., *Chem. Pharm. Bull.*, 23:86 (1975).
100. Saleki-Gerhardt, A. In:*Estimation of Percent Crystallinity in Milled Samples of Sucrose*, M.S. Thesis, University of Wisconsin, Madison, 1991.
101. Fukuoka, E., Makita, M., and Yamamura, S., *Chem. Pharm. Bull.*, 37:1047 (1989).
102. Saleki-Gerhardt, A., and Zografi, G., *Pharm. Res.*, 11:1166 (1994).
103. Yoshioka, M., Hancock, B. C., and Zografi, G., *J. Pharm. Sci.*, 84:983 (1995).
104. Zografi, G., Grandolfi, G. P., Kontny, M. J., and Mendenhall, D. W., *Int. J. Pharm.*, 42:77 (1988).
105. Kontny, M. J., *Drug Devel. Ind. Pharm.*, 14:1991 (1988).
106. Kontny, M. J., Koppenol, S., Graham, E. T., *Int. J. Pharm*, 84:261 (1992).
107. Kontny, M. J., Conners, J. J., and Graham, E. T., *Proceedings of Respiratory Drug Delivery IV*, Interpharm Press, Richmond, VA, 1994.

MARK J. KONTNY

Waxes

Introduction

The term wax generally refers to a substance which is a plastic solid at room temperature and a liquid of low viscosity above its melting point. Strictly speaking, a wax is chemically defined as an ester of a monohydric long-chain fatty alcohol and a long-chain fatty acid. However, generally the term wax has been applied to a broad group of chemically heterogeneous materials. Waxes usually contain a wide variety of materials including glycerides, fatty alcohols, and fatty acids and their esters. In the pharmaceutical literature, the terms waxes, fats, or lipids have often been used interchangeably and no consistent terminology has been established. These substances have in common their lipophilic character, insolubility in water, and solubility in nonpolar solvents. Besides natural materials, many semisynthetic products such as fatty acids or alcohols or surfactants are derived from lipids.

Waxes have been used by the pharmaceutical industry for many years. Their applications in semisolid preparations including ointments, creams or lotions, and suppositories are well known and numerous publications exist on this topic. Because of their lipophilic properties, waxes are used in sustained-release single- or multiple-unit solid dosage forms. This article reviews the different uses of waxes as sustained-release carriers or coating materials.

Waxes in Pharmaceutical Dosage Forms

Waxes are obtained from various sources and are generally classified into animal, insect, vegetable, mineral, and synthetic waxes [1–7].

The most familiar animal wax is probably lanolin, which is obtained from the wool of sheep. It consists primarily of esters of C_{18}–C_{26} alcohols and fatty acids, sterols (cholesterol), and terpene alcohols. It is frequently used in topical preparations. Until recently, spermaceti was another commonly used animal wax. Spermaceti is obtained by precipitation of the head oil from the sperm whale upon cooling. It consists primarily of cetyl palmitate. Because of public concerns with animal-derived products, spermaceti has been replaced with other natural or synthetic products.

The most commonly used insect wax is beeswax. It is obtained from the honeycomb of the bee. White and yellow beeswaxes are GRAS-listed (Generally Recognized as Safe) and consist of mixtures of various esters of straight-chain monohydric alcohols with even-number carbon chains (C_{24}–C_{36}) esterified with straight-chain fatty acids. The principal ester constituent is myricyl palmitate. Beeswax also contains free acids and carbohydrates. White beeswax is obtained by bleaching yellow wax with oxidizing agents or sunlight. The *National Formulary* 18 (NF18) [8] specifications list a melting range of 62–65°C, an acid value of 17–24 and an ester value of 72–79. White beeswax is practically insoluble in water, sparingly soluble in ethanol, and soluble in chloroform and various oils. Beeswax is used as a stiffening agent in topical preparations, as a stabilizer of water/oil (w/o) emulsions, and as a polishing agent in sugar coating.

Most plants are covered with a protective layer of wax, in particular in arid climates. Carnauba wax is plant derived and obtained from the carnauba palm tree, indigeneous to Brazil. The wax is obtained from the surface of dried leaves. It is widely used in food, cosmetic, and pharmaceutical products. It consists of a complex mixture of high molecular weight esters of acids and hydroxyacids. Carnauba wax is very hard and brittle, and has a high melting point. The NF18 specifications list a melting range of 81–86°C, an acid value of 2–7, and a saponification value of 78–95. It is insoluble in water, slightly soluble in boiling ethanol, and soluble in warm chloroform. Besides the sustained-release applications described below, it is used in topical preparations and, because of its high gloss, as a polishing agent in sugar coating. The availability of carnauba wax is controlled by the Brazilian government. Other, less used vegetable-derived waxes include candelilla wax and castor wax.

Hydrogenated vegetable oils are prepared by the hydrogenation of refined vegetable oils. Hydrogenated vegetable oil consists of mixtures of triglycerides, with two types being defined in the *USP* 23 [8]. Type II includes partially hydrogenated vegetable oils and has a lower melting range and a higher iodine value than type I. Type I melts in the range of 57–70°C and has an iodine value of 0–5, whereas Type II has a melting range of 20–50°C and an iodine value of 55–80. They are used as lubricants, as sustained-release matrix materials, as viscosity modifiers in semisolid formulations, to enhance the solidification of suppositories, and to minimize the sedimentation of dispersed drug. Trade names include Lubritab (hydrogenated cottonseed oil), Dynasan P60, Softisan 154 (hydrogenated palm oil), and Sterotex (hydrogenated soybean oil).

Commonly used mineral-derived waxes include petroleum wax, which is microcrystalline, and paraffin wax, which is crystalline; both are obtained from petroleum. Quality and yields depend on the source of the crude oil and the refining process.

Microcrystalline wax (petroleum ceresin or wax) consists of straight-chain and branched saturated alkanes with a chain length range from C_{41} to C_{57}. The NF18 specifications list a melting range of 54–102°C; it is available in plastic and hard grades. It is insoluble in water, slightly soluble in ethanol, and soluble in chloroform. In addition to its application as a sustained-release carrier, it is used as a stiffening agent in topical preparations. Because of its high viscosity and melting point, it increases the consistency of creams and ointments. It also minimizes sweating and bleeding of oil-wax blends.

Paraffin and petroleum waxes can be differentiated by their refractive index and congealing point. Paraffin wax (hard paraffin) is a mixture of solid straight-chain alkanes. It is used in ointments or creams as a base or stiffening agent, and congeals between 47 and 65°C. Various grades with different melting ranges are available. It is insoluble in acetone, ethanol, and water and soluble in chloroform and most warm fixed oils. Low molecular weight polyethylenes (MW < 10,000) have wax-like properties and are used in topical preparations, for example, as gelling agents in Plastibase.

Characterization

Since the harvesting of vegetable or insect waxes is often from wild, noncultivated sources and because of their complex composition, it is important to characterize their chemical and physical properties [1–6]. The composition of natural materials often varies with location, weather, season of harvesting, and age. A good quality control of the raw materials is of upmost importance in order to obtain pharmaceutical products of high quality. As with all natural products, the constant availability of waxes from reliable sources with a reproducible quality has to be assured.

The chemical methods to characterize waxes include the determination of the acid, saponification, iodine, hydroxyl, and peroxide values. The acid value is a measure of the total free acid. The amount of fatty acids could affect the drug release from sustained-release matrices, resulting, for example, in a pH-dependent drug release at higher amounts of acids or in the formation of insoluble salts with cationic drugs. The type of fatty acids present can be identified by gas chromatography after converting the fatty acids into their methyl esters. With regard to the stability of the material, the iodine and peroxide values are important. The iodine value is a measure of the degree of unsaturation whereas the peroxide value indicates the extent of oxidation within the sample.

Various tests, often yielding different values, are available to measure the melting point of waxes. Since they are nonhomogeneous in chemical composition, a melting range rather than a clear melting point is usually observed. The melting point of glycerides increases with increasing hydroxyl number, decreasing degree of unsaturation, and increasing molecular weight of the fatty acid. The melting point of many waxes can be determined in capillary tubes. The slip point is defined as the temperature at which a column of the testing material starts raising in an open-ended capillary tube, which is dipped in a water-filled beaker and heated under specific conditions. The drop-point test can be used, although it is not reliable for the more viscous waxes. The congealing point of a wax is the temperature at which the molten wax stops to flow upon cooling. Thermal methods such as differential scanning calorimetry (DSC) are widely used to characterize the heating and cooling profiles of waxes in a qualitative and quantitative manner. The physical state of the drug in the wax base can be determined. Potential polymorphic transitions and recrystallization during processing can be simulated by running different temperature profiles.

The contraction of suppository bases during cooling within the mold is a well-described phenomenon. The expansion or contraction of waxes is also important during the processing of wax melts, for example during the preparation of microparticles by spray congealing, hot-melt coating, or hot-melt filling of hard gelatin capsules. The dilatation of waxes or thermal expansion during the transition from the solid to the liquid state can be measured with a dilatometer. The hardness of a wax is measured with a penetration test, whereby the depth of penetration of a needle under a given weight is measured, preferably at different temperatures. The viscosity of the molten wax is an important parameter, especially for processes such as hot-melt coating or spray congealing, where wax melts are processed. The time which a certain quantity of molten wax requires to flow through an orifice of specified dimensions is measured in ASTM D-88.

The color of the wax affects the color of a finished product and is an important indication of the quality of the material. A Lovibond Tintometer is often used to compare the color of the raw material against a series of colored standard glasses under a standard light source. The color of the solidified wax of the same sample may be different, depending on the amount of occluded air, the rate of cooling, or the surface finish. Therefore, the color of many waxes is best measured in the molten state. Two ASTM color standards are used to measure dark-brown to off-white color and off-white to pure white. The refractive index and the specific gravity are other parameters often determined.

The structural and physical properties, in particular, the solid- and liquid-state behavior of lipids, and the optical and spectral characteristics of waxes have been described in detail [4].

Pharmaceutical Applications

Waxes in Matrix-Type Drug Delivery Systems

The incorporation of drugs into inert matrices is a popular approach to prolong drug release. Numerous carrier materials are available for the preparation of matrix-type sustained-release systems. Water-insoluble polymers such as cellulosic (ethylcellulose, cellulose acetate) or acrylic derivatives (polymethyl methacrylate, Eudragits) mostly result in insoluble, nondisintegrating matrices, from which the drug is released primarily by diffusion through aqueous channels. Matrices prepared from water-soluble polymers such as hydroxypropyl methylcellulose release the drug by erosion of or diffusion through the gelled polymer layer.

Waxes, although not as frequently used as polymers, represent another class of carrier materials with lipophilic properties, which are able to sustain the drug release. Sustained-release wax-matrix drug delivery systems include wax granules or beads prepared by granulation or extrusion–spheronization, tablets, and wax-filled hard gelatin capsules. The drug release from wax matrices is analyzed using the diffusion-controlled model with square root of time release profiles rather than with first-order kinetics [9]. A correlation exists between the drug release and the fluid penetration; the volume penetrated is also proportional to the square root of time [10].

Wax Granules and Beads

Drug-containing wax granules were prepared by melt congealing, congealing in chloroform, granulation, and aqueous dispersion [11–13]. In the congealing method, the drug was suspended in the molten wax. This suspension was cooled gradually while stirring until a solid mass formed, which was comminuted into granules. Granules made by congealing in chloroform were prepared similarly, the drug being suspended in a chloroform solution of the wax. This mixture was agitated until the solvent evaporated, and was then comminuted into granules. In the granulation method, the powdered wax and drug were granulated with chloroform. Hot water was added to the molten drug-wax mixture until phase inversion occurred. The emulsion was cooled and the particles were separated from the aqueous phase by filtration. The lowest drug-release rate was obtained by the melt-congealing method, probably because of the denser structure of the granules when compared to granules prepared by the other methods. The effect of enzymes such as pepsin and pancreatin as well as of bile and ionic concentration on the drug release from different wax granules was described. With most waxes, the effect was not strong.

Sustained-release nitrofurantoin granules containing stearic acid and glycerol monostearate as matrix materials were prepared by fusion, solvent evaporation, or melt granulation [14]. Various channeling agents including Aerosil, Avicel, dibasic calcium phosphate dihydrate (Emcompress), and sodium chloride were investigated in order to increase drug release. In the fusion method, the lipid was molten and the drug was added to the melt. After cooling, the congealed mass was granulated through standard sieves. In the solvent evaporation method, the drug and the wax carriers were dissolved in dimethylformamide. The solution was cast and the solvent was evaporated at 70°C. The resulting mass was granulated as described above. In the melt granulation method, the drug and carriers were mixed at high speeds; the temperature increased by friction and granulation occurred by sintering the fatty materials near their melting point. The cooled granules were crushed and sieved. Sustained release could only be obtained with granules prepared by the fusion method. The solvent evaporation method and, surprisingly, melt granulation, resulted in granules with a fast drug release. The amount of drug release is significantly increased by increasing the concentration of the channeling agents. The enhancing effect was of the order of Avicel > Aerosil > Emcompress > sodium chloride. At higher Aerosiol or Avicel levels (20%), the granules eroded completely and no controlled drug release was obtained.

Sustained-release KCl tablets were prepared by melt granulation [15]. This method offers several advantages over solvent granulation, including improved safety because of the absence of solvent hazards and lower cost. The heat required for melt granulation can be supplied by a heated jacket or the friction generated by the mixer blades. After reaching the desired temperature, the vessel jacket was cooled by water and the granulation was further agitated to prevent caking during cooling. Reaching the optimum temperature (granulation end point temperature) was critical to obtain good fusion of the wax within the granules and therefore low dissolution rates. The drug release was dependent on the wax concentration and the amount of extragranular excipients (colloidal silica).

The wax was added in powder or molten form to prepare granules by a melt granulation method [16]. Granulation occurred immediately when the molten wax was added or within 5 min with the wax powder. With decreasing wax content of the granules, the time to reach the granulation endpoint increased, the granule size decreased, and the drug release increased. In the melt granulation process, granulation occurs by a sintering process, wherein the particles aggregate because of local melting of the wax particles surface. In order to investigate the reworkability of granulations (which do not comply to the desired product specification), a batch granulated to the optimum end point was regranulated; no change in dissolution rate was observed.

Drug-containing beads were prepared by the extrusion–spheronization of powder blends containing 10% drug (chlorpheniramine maleate or acetaminophen), 60% Avicel PH-101, and 30% wax [17–19]. The incorporation of the wax without subsequent thermal treatment did not result in the same drug release rate as obtained with wax-free beads. Thermally treating the beads at 80°C for 30 min resulted in the melting and recongealing of the wax within the beads and in a decrease in the drug release rate, probably because of a densification and redistribution of the wax within the beads. The drug release was dependent on the treatment temperature and the wax concentration with an increase in both resulting in a decrease in drug release. The use of spermaceti, Precirol, beeswax, and castor wax resulted in sustained release, whereas other fillers resulted in an increase. The beads were subsequently compressed into tablets, which had lower release rates than the beads. Without treatment, compacts disintegrated mainly into the beads, whereas thermal treatment resulted in nondisintegrating matrices.

Wax Matrix Tablets

Wax matrix tablets are prepared by compression of the wax granules or beads described in the previous section, or, with the higher melting waxes available in powder form, by direct compression of powder blends. Compared to polymeric matrix materials, the amount of waxes within the tablet is limited because of fusion and sticking to the punches at higher wax concentrations. This problem could possibly be overcome by compression at lower temperatures.

Matrix tablets containing ephedrine hydrochloride and hydrogenated castor oil were prepared by compression of a physical mixture or a congealed melt [20–22]. In the second method, the drug was added to the molten hydrogenated castor oil at 100°C, and this molten mass was poured onto a glass plate, congealed, comminuted, and finally compressed into a matrix. A surfactant (0.1% alkyltrimethylammonium bromide) was added to the dissolution medium to enhance the wetting of the wax matrix. The drug release increased with increasing amounts of drug in the matrix because of an increased porosity, following the square root of time relationship (Fig. 1). The release was slower from the matrix prepared by the melt method because of a higher tortuosity and lower porosity of the melt matrix compared to the matrix prepared from the physical mixture. Increasing the pressure reduced the release rate with both preparation processes, although the effect was much more pronounced for the matrix prepared from the physical mixture (Fig. 2). The total porosity of the matrices decreased with increasing pressure from 45 to 35.5% at a compression up to 350 MPa (2413 × 10^3 psi). The porosity was lower for the tablets prepared by the melt process. The processing method also affected the mechanism and release rate. A matrix diffusion mechanism was dominant with the melt process, whereas a boundary-layer diffusion was effective with matrices prepared by the compression of physical mixtures. In the first case, the drug release was independent of stirring speed, but it was dependent in the second case.

Ishino, et al. investigated the effects of the internal structure of hydrogenated castor oil matrix tablets prepared by melt granulation and of the compression force on the drug release [23,24]. They compared the release rates of tablets containing different amounts of drug and wax with the water penetration rates from the compressed and the lateral surfaces of the tablets. The penetration rates from the lateral surface were much higher than those from the compressed surface. This was explained with the higher

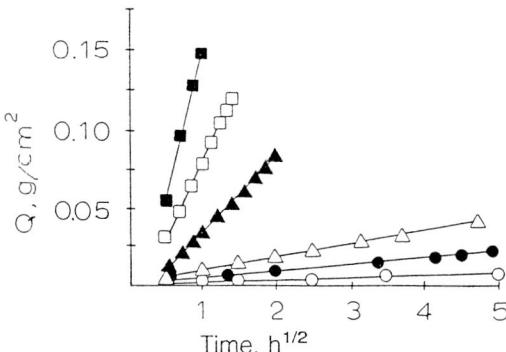

FIG. 1. Effect of concentration of ephedrine hydrochloride on release from matrixes compressed at 7 MPa (48,265 psi). (○) 5%; (●) 10%; (△) 20%; (▲) 30%; (□) 40%; (■) 50%. (Reproduced with permission from Ref. 21.)

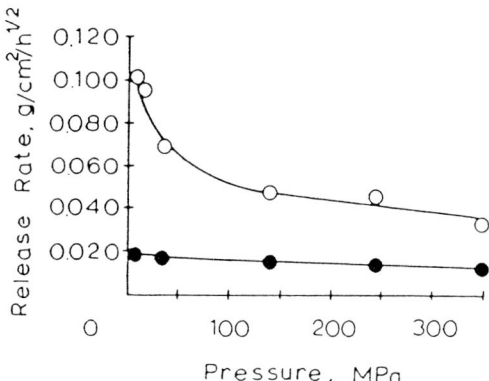

FIG. 2. Effect of applied pressure on release flux from matrixes prepared by (○) compression of a physical mixture and (●) the melt process. (Reproduced with permission from Ref. 20.)

tortuosity of the water channels in the vertical than in the horizontal direction; the drug granules were elongated in the horizontal direction by compression. Surprisingly, the drug release rate increased with increasing compression force. This discrepancy was attributed to the poor wettability of the matrix materials. After compression, the void space left in the tablet did not act as an effective channel for water penetration because of the poor wettability of the wax. The addition of surfactants to the dissolution medium could probably have clarified this phenomenon.

Sustained-release nifedipine tablets based on Gelucires were developed [25,26]. A drug–PVP coprecipitate was added to a solution of Gelucire in chloroform which was subsequently removed or it was added to the molten Gelucire and the paste was subsequently cooled. The mixtures were granulated through a 0.5-mm sieve and tableted. No difference in the release profiles from the two granulates was observed. However, the melting method was preferred because of the absence of organic solvents. Gelucire 53/10 gave the desired release profiles and in vivo studies on the tablets showed similar results as a commercial nifedipine product, Adalat Retard. Accelerated stability studies on the tablets as a function of temperature and relative humidity revealed no changes in chemical stability; however, the dissolution profiles changed. Changes occurring after storage at high humidities and temperatures were attributed to the formation of nifedipine microcrystals and to structural changes in the wax vehicle.

A combination of ethylcellulose and paraffin wax or hydrogenated castor oil was used as carrier material in sustained-release aminophylline tablets [27]. The tablet granulation was prepared by a wet granulation procedure with hot ethanol. The tablets were further coated with Eudragit RL-RS or HPMC-ethylcellulose. An annealing step at 70°C significantly reduced drug release due to fusion within the tablet core. Hydrogenated castor oil was superior to paraffin wax. Increasing the wax content and decreasing the amount of ethyl cellulose or increasing the drug content accelerated the drug release. Picking and sticking problems during compression increased with increasing wax concentration and could be eliminated or reduced by including ethylcellulose.

In order to overcome the disadvantage of hydrophilic matrices of uncontrollable erosion of the hydrated polymer gel on the tablet surface, a combined polymer–wax carrier material was evaluated by Huang, et al. [28]. Carnauba wax was combined with the enteric acrylic polymer, Eudragit L 100, and investigated as a carrier material for diphenhydramine HCl, a cationic drug with a pKa of 9.1. The drug is positively charged at the pH of the GI tract and interacts with the anionic polymer. A mixture of drug and Eudragit L100 was added to the molten wax, followed by compression of the congealed granules. The polymer provided an insoluble structure for the wax. The drug release was significantly retarded with increasing amounts of the anionic polymer. The cationic drug, diphenhydramine HCl, interacted with Eudragit L within the wax matrix and formed a complex after water penetration. The drug release from tablets prepared from only the drug and the enteric polymer was highly dependent on the pH of the dissolution media. However, it was almost independent of pH after the inclusion of carnauba wax in the matrix. At low pH, the release was retarded by the enteric polymer, and at high pH, the drug formed a less-soluble complex with the enteric polymer, thus negating the effect of pH on the drug release. With neutral drugs, a faster release is expected in a pH-7.4 buffer because of the solubility of the enteric polymer in this medium [29]. The release of phenacetin from a carnauba wax matrix increased with increasing amount of an acrylic acid polymer, which formed channels and pores after leaching. Because of the acidic character of the polymer, the addition of this polymer to wax matrices may be useful in preparing drug delivery systems, which release most of the drug in the intestinal tract.

Surfactants were incorporated into wax matrices in order to increase drug release [30]. The drug and surfactant were added to a molten mixture of carnauba wax and stearyl alcohol. This mixture was granulated after congealing the melt on a glass plate and was compressed into cores. Water-insoluble surfactants such as glycerol monostearate had no effect on the dissolution rate, slightly soluble surfactants such as sodium stearate or dioctyl sodium sulfosuccinate moderately increased the drug release, and polyoxyethylene 23 lauryl ether significantly increased the drug release. This was attributed to the hydrophilic nature of the surfactant and its wetting action in the aqueous environment. The drug release occurred via a leaching mechanism; drug diffusion through the matrix did not occur. It was speculated that the surfactant created more channels for the drug to leach into the dissolution medium by increasing the porosity of the matrix. In a related study, povidone was used as a channeling agent increasing the dissolution rate [31]. The same authors showed by DSC-studies that no interactions occurred between the drugs tripelenamine HCl and tolazoline HCl and carnauba or castor wax [32]. Phase diagrams constructed by plots of the melting point of each compound vs. concentration suggested that the drug–wax combinations were strictly physical.

Although the drug release from wax matrix tablets followed the square root of time relationship, approximately zero-order release of ephedrine hydrochloride and procaine hydrochloride could be obtained with multiple-layered matrices of hydrogenated castor oil containing different concentrations of the active compound in each layer [33]. With matrix tablets, the diffusional path length increases with time and the amount of drug release decreases. The amount of drug release therefore has a square root of time dependency. Zero-order or constant drug release can be achieved with matrix systems by offsetting the increase in diffusion path length with an increase in drug concentration. A constant rate of release was obtained with wax multiple-layer tablets consisting of two or three layers with different drug concentrations. The layered matrix tablets were coated with paraffin so that only one surface of the outer layer was exposed to the dissolution medium.

A bioadhesive lozenge containing cetylpyridinium chloride was developed based on a multilayered tablet [34]. One layer contained the bioadhesive polymer carbopol, and the other contained the drug and a wax (spermaceti or Precirol ATO-5).

Wax Implants

Like polymers such as polylactides, waxes have the potential as biocompatible–biodegradable carriers in implants. Standard tableting equipment can be used to prepare wax compacts.

Various lipids including triglycerides (e.g., trilaurin, trimyristin, tripalmitin, and tristearin) and fatty acids were evaluated as carrier materials in sustained-release insulin implants [35]. The drug–wax powder blend was compressed into a disk and implanted subcutaneously into Wistar rats. The monoglycerides eroded too fast and were not suitable. The triglycerides sustained the insulin release only briefly. Palmitic and stearic acid carrier material imparted the best sustained-release properties.

The drug release of the model protein, bovine serum albumin (BSA), from compressed stearic acid pellets was investigated as function of drug loading, drug and carrier particle size, and compression force [36]. At low loadings (5%), the drug release increased with increasing BSA particle size irrespective of the particle size of stearic acid. At high loading (20%), the drug-release rate was higher with large stearic acid particles. More BSA was released with increasing BSA particle size only with small stearic acid particle size. The compression force was not relevant in the range investigated. The pellets increased in size during dissolution studies, probably because of the relaxation of the compacted stearic acid particles. It was proposed that the drug release occurred via diffusion through an interconnected pore network, created not only by BSA particles, but also by the void space between the stearic acid particles. In a series of papers, the same research group investigated cholesterol–lecithin implants as a delivery system for antigens [37–39].

The mechanical properties of waxes are inferior to those of polymeric implants. The handling of the matrix may be difficult because of the softness or brittleness of waxes. This problem could be overcome with injectable microspheres. Suspensions of growth hormone-containing beeswax and glyceryl di- and tristearate microspheres in aqueous or oily vehicles were prepared for injection into cattle [40].

Hard Gelatin Capsules Filled with Waxes

At high concentrations, waxes are difficult to compress. The energy imparted during compaction causes melting, resulting in sticking and picking of the formulation, and the drug-wax granules require inert fillers. High-dose drugs need large amounts of wax to acquire sustained-release properties and are therefore difficult to formulate into tablets. As an alternative to compressed tablets, hard gelatin capsules have been filled with solutions or dispersions of drugs in molten waxes. Upon cooling, drug–wax plugs are obtained. The drug could be protected against moisture or oxygen and its release could be sustained or increased, depending on the solubility properties of the carrier material. Some of the advantages of filling hard gelatin capsules with liquid compared to filling with solids, include a better weight uniformity and the elimination of dust hazards and cross-contamination via airborne particles. In addition, no other excipients, such as binders, lubricants, glidants, disintegrants, etc., commonly used in tableting or powder filling of hard gelatin capsules, are needed and therefore more concentrated systems can be processed. The drug-carrier system should not interact with the gelatin shell in the molten as well as in the congealed state and the physical state of the drug and wax should not change during storage. The melting point of the wax has to be low enough to avoid degradation of the drug and damage to the capsule shell.

A Zanasi hard gelatin powder filling capsule machine (model LZ64) was modified in order to allow the filling of molten or thixotropic formulations into hard gelatin capsules [41,42]. This technique resulted in excellent fill weight uniformity and many of the problems frequently associated with the filling of conventional capsules were avoided.

The release of liquid or deliquescent drugs (benzonatate, nicotinic acid, chloral hydrate, and paramethadione) incorporated into Gelucire bases within hard gelatin capsules were related to the behavior of the carriers in simulated gastric fluid [43]. Gelucires are semisynthetic glycerides with varying amphiphilic properties, and are derived from natural hydrogenated food-grade fats and oils. They are characterized by their melting point range (33–64°C) and HLB (hydrophilic-lipophilic balance range = 1–13). The drugs were released faster from the Gelucires with the higher HLB value and with lower melting points. The Gelucires dissolved completely or remained intact but softened; the degree of softening in the dissolution fluids depended on the melting point (Table 1). Except for chloral hydrate-containing capsules, the drug release from the capsules did not change after storage for more than two years. The expected relationship between the HLB of the Gelucire samples and the release of salicylic acid from melt-filled hard gelatin capsules was established [44]. The drug release occurred by diffusion or erosion, depending on the HLB value and melting point of the vehicle.

It is well-known that wax-based dosage forms may be unstable. Suppository bases often show an increase in melting point, accompanied by a hardening process. This hardening can result in a reduced release rate, which could also affect the in vivo performance. Melt-filled hard gelatin capsules were evaluated by DSC, dissolution, and hardness properties as expressed by a relative penetration [45]. Ketoprofen dissolved in the wax, Gelucire 50/13, and apparently formed a solid solution at room temperature as indicated by the absence of crystalline drug by DSC and microscopy. The melting point of the wax increased during storage and was accompanied by a hardening process. However, the release rate increased, which was attributed to an increased rate of matrix erosion. The observed in-vitro changes did not affect the in-vivo performance of the wax matrix.

Hawley, et al. evaluated the suitability of various carrier materials for a hot-filling process by studying the influence of thermal effects on the crystal structure of the carriers, the rheology of the wax with regard to filling, and the drug release from model drug–carrier formulations [46]. Possible changes in the crystalline state of the carrier and drug during the melting, cooling, and recrystallization cycle were followed by hot-stage microscopy and DSC analysis. With PEG-10,000 and 20,000, Dynafill (a polyethylene oxide–polypropylene oxide block copolymer with palmitic acid end groups), and Lutrol-F68 (poloxamer), there was no evidence of polymorphic transitions after temperature cycles, which simulated the hot-melt filling process. On the contrary, one or more metastable polymorphic forms were observed with Dynasan-114 (a myristic acid triglyceride), depending upon the cooling rate. During storage, the polymorphic form converted back to the original form; the conversion took less than 24 h at 37°C and one month at room temperature. The phase diagram of ibuprofen–Lutrol-F68 revealed an eutectic point between 30 to 35% w/w ibuprofen. Ibuprofen did not have a significant solubility in the base, as indicated by the separate crystallization of the drug and base. The filling of capsules with molten carriers depends on their rheological properties. The four bases evaluated had Newtonian flow behavior and only PEG-20,000

TABLE 1 Characteristics of Gelucires[a]

Type of Gelucire (mp/HLB)	Medium[b]	Density[c]	Appearance of the Mass[d]			Observations, Remarks
			5 min	30 min	60 min	
33/01	GJ	F	D+	D+	D+++	Spreads on surface, mucilaginous appearance
	GJP	F	D+	D+	D+++	
	GJS	F	D+	D+	D++	
35/10	GJ	F	D−	D−	D+	Softens
	GJP	F	D−	D−	D+	Softens
	GJS	F	D−	D−	D+	Softens
37/02	GJ	F	D+	D++	D+++	
	GJP	F	D++	S++/D+++	S++/D+++	
	GJS	F	D++	S++/D+++	S++/D+++	
42/12	GJ	U	D+	D++	D++	Transparent mass spreads at bottom of beaker
	GJP	U	D−	D+	D+	Transparent mass deforms
	GJS	U	D−	D+	D+	
44/14	GJ	U	S+	S++	S++	Remains a transparent mass
	GJP	U	S+	S++	S+++	
	GJS	U	S+	S+++	S+++	
46/07	GJ	F	D−	D−	D−	
	GJP	F	D−	D−	D−	
	GJS	F	D−	D−	D−	
48/09	GJ	F	D−	D−	D−	Remains intact, but softens
	GJP	F	D−	D−	D−	
	GJS	F	D−	D−	D−	
50/02	GJ	F	D−	D−	D−	Remains intact, but softens
	GJP	F	D−	D−	D−	
	GJS	F	D−	D−	D−	
50/13	GJ	U	D−	D−/S+	D−/S++	Entire mass sinks to bottom of beaker; softens, becomes plastic
	GJP	U	D−	D−/S++	D−/S++	
	GJS	U	D−	D−/S++	D−/S++	
53/10	GJ	U	D−	D−	D+	
	GJP	U	D−	D−	D−	
	GJS	U	D−	D−	D−	
62/05	GJ	F	D−	D−	D−	
	GJP	F	D−	D−	D−	
	GJS	F	D−	D−	D−	

[a]Reproduced with permission from Ref. 43.
[b]GJ = Simulated gastric juice (Ph.Helv.VI).
GJP = Simulated gastric juice with 0.1% polysorbate 80.
GJS = Simulated gastric juice with 0.1% sodium laurylsulfate.
[c]F = Mass floats.
U = Mass sinks.
[d]D = Degree of disintegration/deformation: none(−) to complete (+++).
S = Degree of solubilization: none(−) to complete (+++).

caused difficulties during filling because of its high viscosity. However, the viscosity of molten drug-containing bases could be significantly higher, especially with drug dispersions of high drug loadings. The dissolution of melt-filled hard gelatin capsules was studied with various model drugs, including ibuprofen, theophylline, quinidine sulfate, indomethacin, and acetohexamide. Only ibuprofen, a drug with a low melting point of 76°C, dissolved in all molten bases; the other drugs had to be dispersed. The drug release was slowest from Dynasan-114-filled capsules.

As an alternative to holt-melt filling of capsules, sustained-release wax matrices were formed in a novel way within hard gelatin capsules through fluidization in a heated air stream within a fluidized bed [47]. A drug–wax powder blend was filled into hard gelatin capsules, which were suspended in an upward-moving, heated airstream and circulated within the chamber of a fluidized-bed unit. The capsules rotated during fluidization at temperatures above the melting point of the wax and centrifugal forces caused the drug–wax melt to flow into the ends of the capsules. The molten mixture solidified after ending the heating and two solid wax matrices with dissolved dispersed drug were obtained in the ends of the capsules. A thin film formed between the two wax plugs on the inner surface of the capsules, sealing them hermetically. During dissolution studies, the capsule shell dissolved rapidly. The wax matrix broke into the two plugs at stirring speeds above 100 rpm. The force necessary to break the thin film between the two plugs was minimal. The mechanical stresses exerted on solid dosage forms during the passage through the gastrointestinal (GI) tract would rupture the thin film under in vivo conditions. Although hydrophilic substances have been used to increase the drug-release rate from wax matrices, good control was obtained with blends of waxes with different amphiphilic properties (HLB values). Gelucire 50/13 (melting point, 50°C; HLB = 13) and Precirol ATO-5 (melting point, 53°C; HLB = 2) were selected as the drug carriers. As shown in Fig. 3, the drug-release rate increased with increasing proportion of the more hydrophilic wax. The drug release was independent of the pH of the dissolution medium. After cooling of the drug–wax melt, the drug could be dispersed, dispersed–dissolved, or dissolved in the wax matrix. The physical state of the drug after formation of the

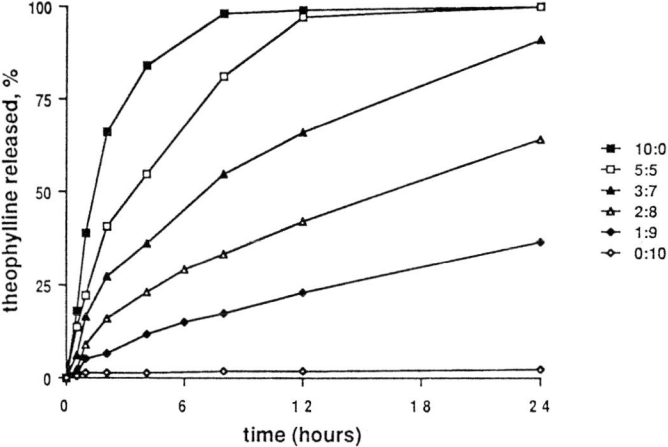

FIG. 3. Effect of the ratio of Gelucire 50/13 to Precirol ATO-5 on the release of theophylline (33% w/w) from the wax matrices in 0.1M HCl. (Reproduced with permission from Ref. 47.)

Waxes

wax matrix was studied by DSC. A linear relationship was established between the heat of fusion and the amount of drug in the wax matrix (Fig. 4). The solubility of the drug in the matrix at its melting point corresponds to the intercept of the line. As sometimes observed with suppositories, the drug may crystallize over time, if the amount of drug dissolved in the matrix during the melting process exceeds the solubility of the drug at storage temperature. Propranolol HCl was insoluble and dispersed in the Precirol ATO-5 matrix, whereas theophylline was partially dissolved in the wax. The DSC thermograms of wax matrices prepared from blends of Gelucire 50/13 and Precirol ATO-5, showed no melting transition of Gelucire 50/13 after dissolution studies. The hydrophilic wax leached out, leaving an exhausted matrix of Precirol ATO-5.

Coating with Waxes

Besides their predominant application in matrix preparations, waxes have also been used as coatings for granules and pellets. Solid dosage forms are often coated to sustain drug release, improve the stability, or mask the taste of poorly tasting drugs. Solid dosage forms are generally coated with polymer solutions or aqueous colloidal polymer dispersions. Wax coatings have various advantages over coating with polymer solutions or dispersions. The waxes can be applied without organic solvents, and, in the case of hot melts, at a high application rate and therefore shorter processing time. Many food-grade natural or semisynthetic waxy materials are available. Waxes are frequently used as barrier coatings in the food industry or as polishing agents with sugar-coated tablets, but little information on waxes as primary coatings can be found in the pharmaceutical literature.

Waxes can be applied onto solid dosage forms in the forms of hot melts, hot emulsions, aqueous suspensions (colloidal wax particles), or organic solutions. Coating processes include dip coating, pan coating, and fluidized-bed coating. The coating of drug particles by spray congealing is discussed in the section on microencapsulation with waxes.

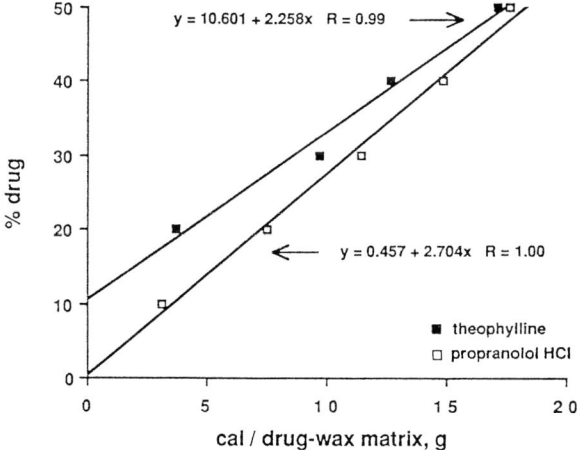

FIG. 4. Relationship of propranolol HCl and theophylline loading and the heat of fusion. (Reproduced with permission from Ref. 47.)

Coating with Hot Melts

With regard to coating processes, various fluidized-bed techniques and their modifications were evaluated for hot-melt coating [48,49]. The fluidized-bed techniques include the top, bottom, and tangential spray or rotary fluidized-bed modes. The particles to be coated are suspended in a heated, high-velocity air stream, and the molten wax is applied in the form of atomized liquid droplets.

The top-spray mode is the system of choice for hot-melt coating. The wax melt is sprayed downward on upward-moving particles (Fig. 5). The product temperature can be kept closest to the congealing temperature of the wax compared to the two other spray modes. The wax has to be kept in a molten state in order to be atomized into the fluidized bed. A special nozzle had to be developed. Its wand has a triaxial structure with a center tube for the molten liquid, which is surrounded by a small air space for the delivery of high-pressure, low-volume air to control the nozzle valve which opens when the pump is running. Both of these tubes were surrounded by a larger air space through which the heated atomization air was supplied. The nozzle should be placed as closely as possible to the substrate bed in order to minimize the distance which the molten droplets had to travel before contacting the substrate surface. The nozzle wand must be insulated with a nonconductive material in order to avoid remelting of the coated product on the wand.

For substrates with poor fluidization characteristics such as larger particles and/or particles of higher density the bottom-spray mode is preferred. In the Wurster bottom-spray coating mode the melt is sprayed on the upward-moving particles. Various modifications allow the coating of solid dosage forms with molten materials. These modifications depend on the fluidization conditions in order to ensure an even application of the coating and avoid agglomeration. With the tangential-spray process, one of the latest developments in fluidized-bed technology, the process considerations concern the spray nozzle and the tacky nature of the bed during spraying. The product temperatures have to be maintained lower than with the top-spray technique in order to avoid adherence

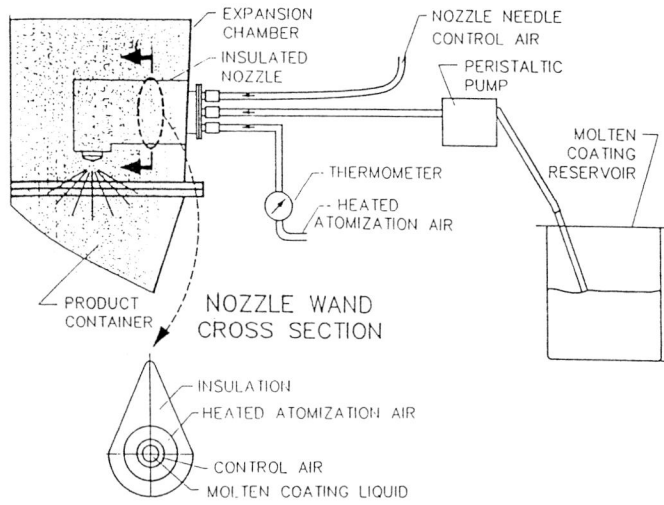

FIG. 5. Insulated nozzle and wand for top-spray hot-melt coating. (Reproduced with permission from Ref. 48.)

of the coated particles to the product container. The tangential-spray method strains the substrates more than the other two techniques. Besides the substrate, the coated product also has to be mechanically resistant. Some coatings, especially those of certain waxes, are brittle and could crack during the coating process, resulting in the loss of protective properties.

Important process and formulation variables include the product bed temperature, the atomization conditions, the type of substrate, the properties of the coating materials, and the desired release rates (immediate or sustained release). For good coatings, the atomization air has to be heated to the same temperature as the molten wax in order to avoid premature congealing. The droplets must remain in a liquid state until they hit the substrate surface. The product bed temperature is highly critical to the successful coating of solid dosage forms with molten materials. At low product temperatures, premature congealing of the molten droplets results in poor spreading of the coating on the substrate surface and, in the extreme case, in the failure of the coating to adhere. Rough and porous surface structures are obtained, resulting in faster drug release compared to substrates with smooth coatings. At too high product temperatures, excessive particle agglomeration or clogging of the outlet filter bags is a result of inadequate congealing and hardening of the coating. An outlet filter should not be employed with larger particles, in order to use process temperatures as close as possible to the congealing temperature. The product bed temperature can be regulated by the fluidization air temperature. The temperatures of the molten wax and of the atomizing air have to be optimized to allow proper spreading of the molten droplets on the substrate surface. Inlet air temperatures should be 10–15°C below the melting piont of the coating, and temperatures for the atomization air and the molten wax should be 40–60°C above the melting point.

Droplet size and uniformity are also critical for a successful coating process. The size of the molten droplet is dependent on the viscosity of the melt and the atomization air pressure. Smaller particles require smaller droplet sizes and therefore higher atomization air pressures in order to minimize agglomeration or granulation. In order to obtain small droplets, the viscosity of the molten material can be decreased by increasing the temperature of the melt. At the same atomization conditions, low feed rates result in smaller droplets. The spray rate of melts is generally much lower than that of the coating solutions or dispersions. The lower spray rate, however, is offset by the application of pure coating material. The application rate is therefore still higher compared to polymer solutions or dispersions, which require solvent evaporation. In general, lower feed rates result in less agglomeration of the coated particles and more uniform coatings.

After the application of the melt, the fluidization is reduced and the product bed is cooled. The cooling period should be short in order to avoid attrition of the coated product. Rapid cooling, however, may result in cracks in the coating because of contraction and in unstable polymorphic forms of the wax.

The ideal substrate is spherical with a mean particle size between 100 and 2000 μm and a smooth surface. The coating of small particles is difficult because of the agglomeration into larger aggregates. Larger particles or pellets are generally coated as single particles.

The important variables for the selection of the waxes include the melting point, melting range, and melt viscosity. The wax should have a melting point below 85°C because the melt is usually kept 40–60°C above its melting point. The coating material has to be delivered to the spray nozzle in a molten state, which presents some challenges to the equipment design. Materials with a broad melting point range can become tacky during spraying because of the broad range of product temperatures and the presence of low-melting fractions. The coating materials include various hydrogenated vegetable oils, beeswax, paraffin wax, carnauba wax, and polyethylene glycol (Table 2).

The drug release from the coated pellets depends on several variables. Besides drug properties (e.g., solubility, etc.), the particle size of the coated product, the type of the coating material, and the coating level primarily affect the drug release. At the same solids content, the quality of the coating (smooth vs. regular coating) also affect drug release. The structure or porosity of the coating have a significant effect on drug release, with more irregular coatings resulting in faster release. Irregularily shaped particles generally release the drug faster than spherical particles because of a higher surface area and therefore thinner coatings. Examples of optimized process conditions for the hot-melt coating of particles with hydrogenated cottonseed oil by the top, bottom, and rotor spray mode with a Glatt GPCG 5 unit and the resulting release properties of the coated spheres are given in Ref. 48.

Coating with Hot Emulsions, Aqueous Suspensions, or Organic Wax Solutions

The coating with hot emulsions has various advantages over the hot-melt process [50,51]. The wax remains in the molten state and premature congealing can be avoided because of the presence of hot water. This facilitates the transport of the wax to the spray nozzle and improves the experimental setup. In addition, the temperatures of the wax emulsion are lower than those of the comparable wax melts. Oil/water (o/w)

TABLE 2 Types of Coating Materials[a]

Material	Trade Name	Melting point (°C)	Color
Partially hydrogenated cottonseed/soybean oil	Van Den Bergh Foods K.L.X.	51–55	White
Partially hydrogenated palm oil	Van Den Bergh Foods 27 Stearine	58–63	White
Partially hydrogenated cottonseed oil	Van Den Bergh Foods 07 Stearine	61–65	Off-white to tan
Partially hydrogenated soybean oil	Van Den Bergh Foods 17 Stearine	67–71	White
Beeswax		62–65	Light tan
Paraffin wax[b]	Frank B. Ross Co. 130/135 AMP	55	White
Carnauba wax	Frank B. Ross Co. No. 1 Yellow	84 (min.)	Yellow
Partially hydrogenated castor oil	Cas Chem Castor Wax	85–88	White
Polyethylene glycol[a]	Union Carbide Carbowax 3350	54–58	White

[a]Reproduced with permission from Ref. 48.
[b]Various types and melting points available.

emulsions of various waxes (e.g., glyceryl behenate-Compritol-888 and glyceryl palmitostearate-Precirol-ATO 5) with a solids content of up to 50% were prepared. The emulsions were passed through a microfluidizer to further reduce the particle size of the oil phase. The hot emulsion was either sprayed directly on the beads or cooled to form a "wax pseudolatex" prior to the coating process. The disadvantages, compared to hot-melt coating, include the amount of water to be evaporated and therefore longer processing times, and the presence of surfactants in the wax coating. The surfactants needed to stabilize the emulsions could affect the drug release. The use of liquid surfactants such as various Tween/Span combinations resulted in sticky beads. Sodium lauryl sulfate, a solid surfactant, was more suitable. The guaifenesin release from coated pellets decreased with increasing hydrophobicity of the wax and increasing coating level. The coating conditions (e.g., temperature, spray rate, curing) and the particle size of the emulsion–suspension primarily influenced the microstructure of the wax coatings and hence the drug release. Thicker coatings must be applied with waxes to obtain the same sustained-release profiles as with polymer coatings.

Bagaria prepared emulsions with waxes including carnauba, paraffin, ceresin, and beeswax and hydrogenated castor, soybean, or cottonseed oil, which were coated onto drug-containing nonpareil beads [52]. The term emulsions was actually misleading because the final products were aqueous suspensions of the waxes of partially submicron particle size ("wax pseudolatex"). Similar to aqueous polymer dispersions, the wax dispersions were converted into powders by spray drying. The release from beads coated with the redispersed spray-dried powder was compared to that from beads coated with the original dispersion. With almost all preparations, 100% drug was released within 2–4 h.

Like organic polymer solutions, the wax can be dissoved in an organic solvent and sprayed onto the solid dosage form. The wax film around the solid substrate forms upon solvent removal. In most studies, waxes such as beeswax, hydrogenated castor oil, microcrystalline wax, or glyceryl mono- or distearate were dissolved in chlorinated organic solvents such as chloroform, carbon tetrachloride, or trichlorethane and applied in coating pans at elevated temperatures [53–57]. Mixtures of ethylcellulose with different waxes such as castor, carnauba, or paraffin wax in chloroform were evaluated as sustained-release coatings [58]. A lower ratio of ethylcellulose to wax was used with drugs of higher molecular weight and/or low solubility and a higher ratio for drugs of low molecular weight and/or high solubility to achieve the desired release properties at a 10% coating level. As the date of the references indicates, coating with organic solutions is obsolete because of the undesirability of organic solvents.

Other Coating Procedures

Potassium chloride disks can be coated with stearic acid by sublimation or solvent coating [59]. In the sublimation technique, the stearic acid is vaporized at 126°C followed by condensation onto the cooled disk. Scanning electron micrographs revealed uneven coatings with large stearic acid flakes (100 μm) on disks coated by solution coating; small globules, 2.5 μm in diameter, were visible on disks coated by sublimation.

A pulsatile drug delivery system is based on a dry-coated wax matrix tablet [60,61]. The plain wax matrix tablet, based on behenic acid, did not disintegrate during the dissolution test. A disintegrant, partly pregelatinized starch, promoted disintegration of the tablet core. The tablets were dry-coated with a wax-containing layer by compression. Drug can also be incorporated into the coating layer. Dry-coated tablets keep their form for a relatively long period until the dissolution medium penetrates into the core. The drug release increased rapidly because of the disintegration of the tablet core; the release profiles are of sigmoidal shape. Before disintegration, the drug is released from the outer layer. The disintegration time can be controlled by the thickness of the coating layer and by drug concentration and core weight. The contact angle of the wax matrix decreases with an increase in drug concentration and, therefore, the fluid penetration into the wax matrix and drug release increased with increasing concentration.

Microencapsulation with Waxes

The trend toward multiparticulate dosage forms makes the incorporation of drugs into microparticles an attractive alternative to conventional single-unit sustained-release dosage forms such as tablets or capsules. Only a few dozen papers have described the application of waxes in the area of microencapsulation, in contrast to the numerous papers published on the preparation of microparticles using polymers as carriers. The major advantage of waxes over polymers is the easy processability of low-viscosity melts, obviating the need for organic solvents. Most microencapsulation techniques based on water-insoluble polymers (e.g., solvent evaporation, organic phase-separation methods) require organic solvents to dissolve the polymer. Wax microparticles are prepared primarily by aqueous and nonaqueous melt dispersion techniques or spray congealing and drying. These techniques are briefly reviewed below.

Microparticles Prepared by Melt-Dispersion Techniques

In the melt-dispersion technique, the drug-containing molten-wax phase is emulsified into a heated, emulsifier-containing external phase. Depending on the solubility of the drug, the external phase can be aqueous (for water-insoluble drugs) or nonaqueous (for water-soluble drugs). Upon cooling the emulsion, the liquid droplets congeal and a suspension of the wax microparticles is formed. The microparticles are separated, mostly by filtration or centrifugation, sometimes washed to remove free drug crystals and surfactants, dried, and sized.

Ibuprofen–wax (carnauba, paraffin, beeswax, Gelucire 64/02, or Precirol ATO5) microparticles were characterized with respect to drug loading and morphological and release properties [62]. Microparticles of the more hydrophilic waxes, Gelucire 64/02 and Precirol ATO5, can be prepared without surfactants, whereas the other waxes rapidly coalesce and form big lumps upon cooling. With these waxes, increasing the amount of sodium lauryl sulfate in the external aqueous phase decreased the drug loading because of drug solubilization. This was not the case, however, with polyvinyl alcohol as stabilizer. During emulsification, the drug partitions into the external aqueous phase until its solubility at the emulsification temperature is reached. Upon cooling of the emulsion, the drug can precipitate in the aqueous phase because of reduced solubility. The ibuprofen crystals were removed from the microparticles by washing with pH-7.4 buffer during filtration or by raising the pH of the aqueous phase with diluted sodium hydroxide solution prior to filtration. This washing step has to be optimized in order not to extract encapsulated drug from the microparticles. With other drugs, the crystals could possibly be separated by centrifugation or washing with organic solvents. The type of wax, the rate of cooling, the stirring time, and the temperature of the aqueous phase have no significant effect on the drug loading because of the low solubility of ibuprofen in the external aqueous phase. Actual drug loadings close to 60% can be achieved. All microparticles in this study were spherical and nonagglomerated, but had different surface morphologies. Gelucire 64/02 and Precirol ATO5 microparticles had a porous surface, probably because of the more hydrophilic character of the waxes. The surfaces of carnauba, paraffin, and beeswax were nonporous with indentations, especially those of paraffin wax. These depressions could have been caused by the rapid contraction of the wax during cooling of the emulsion in an ice bath. The drug release was controlled by the hydrophobicity of the wax (Gelucire 64/02 > Precirol ATO5 > beeswax > carnauba wax > paraffin wax, Fig. 6). These microparticles could be formulated into aqueous sustained-release oral suspension-dosage forms because of the low solubility of the drug.

A modified USP method using minibaskets was used to study the effect of formulation variables, such as type of wax, type of modifier, drug loading, and particle size, on the ibuprofen release from wax microspheres [63]. The drug release was on the order of beeswax > ceresine wax > refined paraffin wax and microcrystalline wax. After an initial burst of release, the drug release was slow from microparticles prepared with the last two waxes. The dissolution studies were performed in simulated intestinal fluids because sink conditions could not be maintained in simulated gastric fluids due to the drug solubility. To increase drug release, glycerol monostearate or stearyl alcohol were added prior to the preparation of the microparticles. Their addition also reduced the tendency of the waxes to agglomerate [64]. Ibuprofen dissolved in the molten wax and did not crystallize during congealing and microsphere formation, as indicated by DSC studies. However, with waxes that melt at lower temperatures than the drug, the drug could be present in the crystalline state but dissolve in the wax melt during the DSC run. This could result in the misinterpretation of the drug being soluble in the wax; hot stage microscopy or other methods have to be used to prove beyond doubt the absence of the crystalline drug.

In a modified melt-dispersion method, sulfamethoxazole particles were dispersed in hot water and powdered beeswax was added. The molten wax droplets collected the drug

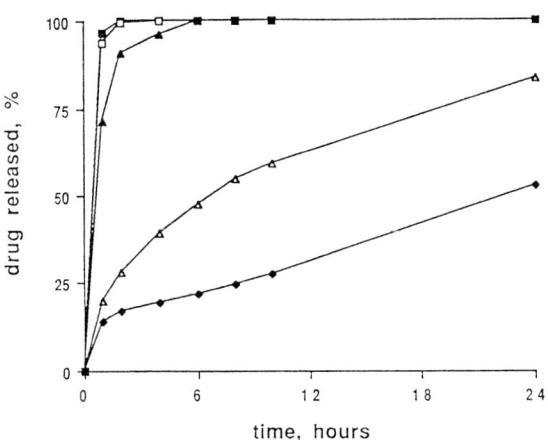

FIG. 6. Ibuprofen release from different wax microparticles (actual drug loading): (■) Precirol ATO5 (35.3%), (□) Gelucire 64/02 (35.4%), (▲) beeswax (37.7%), (△) carnauba wax (37.3%), (♦) paraffin wax (35.0%). (Reproduced with permission from Ref. 62.)

particles, and spherical agglomerates with sustained-release properties were obtained after cooling. The agglomerates can also be formed at room temperature by using solutions of the wax in a water-immiscible solvent [65].

Water-soluble drugs cannot be encapsulated by the o/w-emulsion technique because the drug would be lost to the external aqueous phase. Two methods have been described for the encapsulation of hydrophilic drugs; one is based on an external oil phase and the other on the formation of the microparticles by a w/o/w-melt dispersion technique.

Carnauba wax microspheres containing 5-fluorouracil for chemoembolization were prepared by a melt-dispersion process with an external silicone oil phase [66]. The drug was dispersed in the molten carnauba wax and emulsified into silicone oil at temperatures above the melting point of carnauba wax (85°C). The resulting emulsion was cooled by adding cold silicone oil and immersion in an ice-water bath. After solification, the microspheres were separated from the oil phase by centrifugation and washed with cyclohexane to remove the silicone oil. 5-Fluorouracil is a hydrophilic drug; an external aqueous phase would have resulted in drug partitioning and therefore low encapsulation efficiencies. However, even with silicone oil, an external phase in which the drug was insoluble, only up to 5% of the drug could be encapsulated within the carnauba wax microspheres. This was attributed to the poor wetting of the drug crystals by the molten wax and therefore the loss of drug crystals to the external silicon oil phase. Various surfactants were added to the wax phase in order to improve the wettability of the drug by the molten wax. Surfactants with an HLB value of 15–16, such as polysorbate 40, macrogol ester, and poloxamer, were able to wet the drug and substantially increased the encapsulation efficiencies. Lipophilic surfactants with low HLB values did not increase the encapsulation efficiency. The surfactants had to be used at concentrations of at least 5% to improve drug loading. The drug release was independent of pH and followed first-order kinetics.

A technique based on the formation of a multiple emulsion with an external aqueous phase was developed for the encapsulation of water-soluble drugs in order to replace the external oil phase [67]. Possible unwanted interactions between the oil and the emulsified wax resulting in swelling or dissolution of the wax, cleaning of the final product, and recovery of the oil phase can be eliminated. Like with the encapsulation of water-soluble drugs within polymeric microparticles by a w/o/w-solvent evaporation method, a molten wax phase was used instead of an organic polmer solution. A hot aqueous solution of pseudophedrine·HCl was emulsified into the molten carnauba wax, followed by emulsification into a hot external aqueous phase. The temperature of the internal and external aqueous phases had to be kept above the melting temperature of the wax in order to avoid premature congealing and to ensure the formation of an emulsion. The microparticles formed after congealing of the wax. A key for high encapsulation efficiencies was the formation of ultrafine internal aqueous phase droplets by sonication. The wax acted as a diffusion barrier between the internal and the external aqueous phase and therefore minimized drug partitioning into the external aqeous phase. Scanning electron micrographs revealed drug crystals embedded in the wax matrix; the drug precipitated within the wax microparticles when the internal water was removed by vacuum drying. Important process variables affecting the drug loading included the cooling rate and contact time with the external phase and the volume of the internal aqueous phase. Because of the high solubility of the drug in the external aqueous phase, the contact time of the droplets and microparticles with the continuous aqueous phase had to be minimized in order to avoid drug loss; the microparticles were separated from the aqueous phase within minutes after formation. The cooling rate and the contact time with the external phase are not critical with respect to the drug loading with drugs that are not soluble in the external phase, as described above for ibuprofen microparticles. Increasing the volume of the internal aqueous phase decreased the drug loading because more drug-containing droplets came in contact with the external aqueous phase. Dispersing micronized pseudoephedrine·HCl crystals rather than the drug solution into the wax prior to emulsification into the aqueous phase resulted in a complete loss of drug. The drug crystals were probably still too large and were not preferentially wetted by the wax phase.

Generally, the wax phase is emulsified into a hot external phase to avoid premature congealing. However, sulfamethazine–Japanese synthetic wax particles were prepared by dispersing the drug in the molten wax, followed by slowly pouring the wax phase into a precooled external aqueous phase [68]. The microparticles were separated by filtration after 3 min. Beeswax microparticles were prepared by a phase-inversion technique, whereby an aqueous solution of sorbitan monooleate and polysorbate 80 was added to the drug-containing molten wax phase to form a w/o emulsion prior to phase inversion. Smaller microparticles were obtained at higher temperatures, with increased amounts of continuous phase, lower rates of cooling, and higher speeds of mixing [69].

Suspensions of lipid nanoparticles can be prepared by reducing the size of the molten or dissolved drug containing the lipid phase into the colloidal size range by high pressure homogenization [70,71]. After cooling or solvent evaporation, nanoparticles are obtained. These suspensions can be converted into powders by freeze drying or spray drying. The nanoparticles act as carriers for poorly water-soluble drugs and apparently can result in controlled release over longer periods of time. However, because of the small size and therefore high surface area of the particles, an increase in dissolution rate would be expected, unless very low loadings are used.

Microparticles Prepared by Spray Drying and Spray Congealing

Similar to organic polymer solutions, drug-containing organic wax solutions were spray dried to give sustained-release microparticles [72]. The drug could be dissolved or dispersed in the organic wax solutions. Spray drying is a single-step, rapid drying process which can be scaled up and used for heat-sensitive drugs. The use of organic solvents, however, is undesirable because of hazards, residuals, and cost. Because of their low melt viscosity, wax microparticles can also be prepared without organic solvents by spray congealing drug-containing wax melts.

Sulfaethylthiadiazole–hydrogenated castor oil particles were prepared by spray congealing using a centrifugal wheel atomizer [73]. The wax powder was suspended in water to give an oral sustained-release suspension. In a subsequent paper, the effect of various process and formulation variables on the particle size using a centrifugal wheel atomizer was investigated [74]. The particle size was directly proportional to the feed rate and inversely proportional to the feed viscosity and the wheel velocity. The particle size was related to each variable through simple exponential equations and the predicted particle sizes closely agreed with the experimentally obtained particle sizes.

In a series of publications, sulfaethylthiadiazole–wax microparticles prepared by spray congealing were evaluated. Most important for drug release was the type of wax used [75]. The effect of surfactant on the drug release from spray-congealed wax microparticles was investigated by John and Becker [76]. White wax USP, a synthetic wax-like ester, and 1:1 combinations of these two waxes were used as sustained-release matrices. The particle size of the microparticles could be controlled by the nozzle size, with larger nozzles resulting in larger particles and lower dissolution rates. Up to 4% sorbitan monooleate apparently softened the particles and promoted wetting, resulting in an increase in drug release. However, at a surfactant level of 10%, the lowest release rate was observed. This was partly attributed to the tackiness of the particles, which resulted in agglomeration and a reduction in total surface area available for drug release. The addition of the surfactant allowed the compression of the microparticles into tablets, which was difficult in the absence of surfactant [77]. The surfactant-free microparticles adhered or stuck to the punch surface, and resulted in a high friability of the finished tablets. If no additives were incorporated, nondisintegrating wax matrix tablets were obtained. The amount of drug released in alkaline pancreatin medium was greater than in acidic pepsin medium. This was attributed to the higher solubility of the drug in the alkaline medium, the more rapid emulsification, disintegration, or solubilization of the wax particles, and to the higher solubility of fatty acids in the alkaline medium.

The effect of the inclusion of lipase into triglyceride spray-congealed particles on the dissolution rate was investigated by Javaid, et al. [78]. The drug release from compressed particles increased with increasing lipase activity because of the hydrolysis of the triglyceride. The addition of lipase accelerators such as calcium ions further increased the drug release.

A palatable suspension of the bitter-tasting drug, remoxipride, was developed based on microparticles prepared by spray congealing [79]. Because of the high water solubility of the drug, the microparticles were formulated into an external oil phase. Unfortunately, neither the nature of the wax nor of the oily vehicle was revealed.

With lipid drug delivery systems, polymorphic transformations may occur during the preparation of the dosage form and subsequent storage. The polymorphic behavior of lipid micropellets prepared from glycerides and phospholipids by spray drying or spray congealing and their surface structure were evaluated by differential scanning calorimetry and scanning electron microscopy [80–82]. The rapid solvent evaporation during spray drying can influence the crystallization of the lipid carrier and different polymorphic structures could be obtained. Similarly, during spray congealing and solidification of the melt, the lipid can crystallize in different polymorphic forms depending on its composition and the cooling rate. The major polymorphic forms of the glycerides are the α, β, and β' forms. Rapid cooling rates generally result in the unstable α form. The transition of the melt to the α, β', and then the β form represents the transformation of triglycerides into the most stable form.

The spraying process, especially spray congealing, was simulated by cooling the molten samples rapidly at 320°C/min. A DSC thermogram of pure tristearin heated at 10°C/min revealed a single endothermic peak representing the β form. After rapid cooling of the melt and reheating, an endothermic peak for the α form and an exothermic peak indicating the recrystallization of the α into the β form, followed by the endothermic peak for the β form were detectable. The DSC thermogram of spray-dried tristearin micropellets was similar to the one of the melt-quenched sample. A crystalline modification took therefore place during spray drying caused by the rapid solvent removal. The micropellets were stored at different temperatures to investigate the effect of storage temperature on the polymorphic transitions. Increasing the storage temperature to 37°C resulted in a complete transformation of the unstable polymorphic form into the stable polymorphic form. The melting endotherm of the α form disappeared.

Waxes

The effect of various emulsifiers such as lecithin or monoglycerides was investigated in order to prevent or delay the transformation of the unstable form into the stable β form. Adding lecithin to the formulation resulted in a delay of the transformation. The type of glyceride (composition and chain length), solvent, and drugs encapsulated affected the polymorphic transformation and its rate, and also the surface structure of the microparticles. Spray-congealed lipid micropellets showed a similar thermal behavior as the spray-dried pellets. The smooth surface of the sprayed lipid micropellets was attributed to the unstable polymorphic form. The unstable α form has various thin and small crystals, resulting in a smooth surface of the crystallized sample. The β and β' forms have larger crystals, causing irregular structures of the micropellets. During aging at elevated temperatures, the lipid micropellets lost their smooth surface structures because of polymorphic transformations.

Novel oral controlled-release microspheres using polyglycerol esters of fatty acids and hydrogenated cottonseed oil (HCSO), stearic acid, stearyl alcohol, or glycerol monostearate as carriers were prepared by spray chilling with a rotating disk [83]. A linear relationship existed between the particle size and the inverse of the rotation speed. The drug release was related to the hydrophobicity of the wax; the release rate decreased in the following order: stearyl alcohol > stearic acid > glycerol monostearate > carnauba wax > hydrogenated cottonseed oil. Adding increasing amounts of lactose to the HCSO raised the drug release as a result of the leaching of lactose. Morphological changes in the HCSO microspheres were attributed to polymorphic transformations (Fig. 7); the theophylline release changed after storage of only one day at 40°C. The HCSO

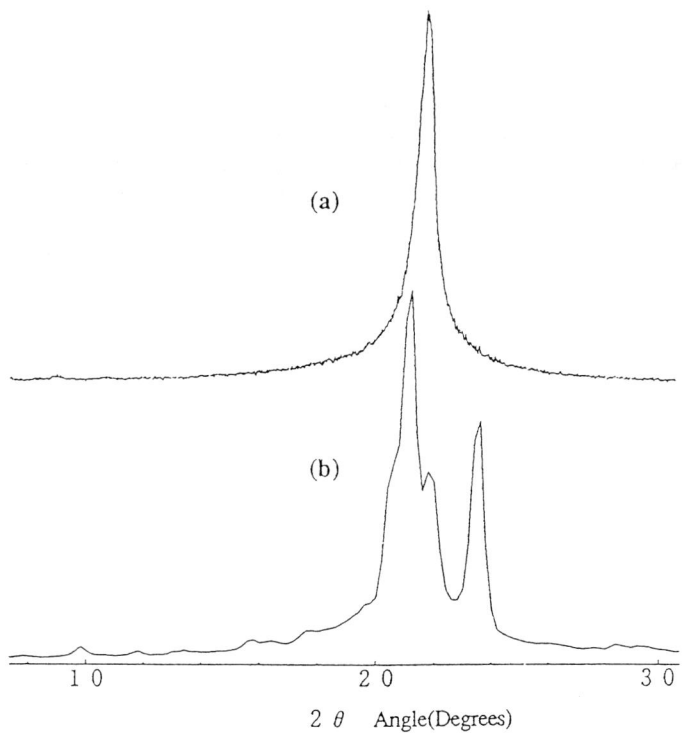

FIG. 7. X-Ray diffraction patterns of HCSO-based microspheres immediately (a) after preparation and (b) after storage at 40°C for 1 day. (Reproduced with permission from Ref. 83.)

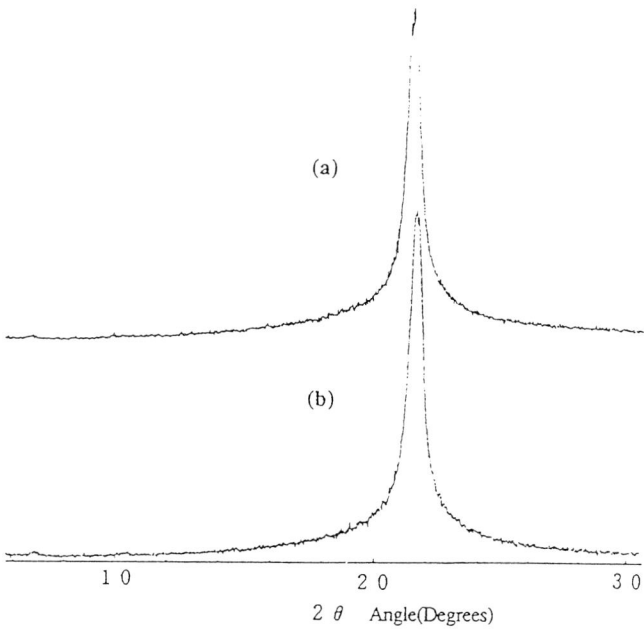

FIG. 8. X-Ray diffraction patterns of tetraglycerol pentastearate (TGPS)-based microspheres immediately (a) after preparation and (b) after storage at 40°C for 6 months. (Reproduced with permission from Ref. 83.)

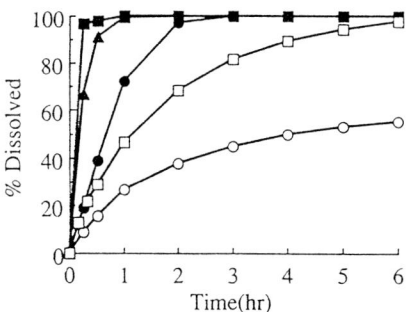

FIG. 9. Effect of HLB on the theophylline release profile from polyglycerol ester of fatty acids (PGEF)-based microspheres. HLB: (■), 8.4; (▲), 5.5; (●), 4.5; (□), 3.8; (○), 2.6. (Reproduced with permission from Ref. 83.)

microspheres therefore did not result in a stable controlled release. The polyglycerol esters gave microspheres with stable release patterns without changes in morphology or x-ray diffraction pattern, indicating the absence of polymorphic transitions (Fig. 8). The HLB value of the esters can be controlled by the degree of glycerol polymerization and esterification. The drug release is controlled by using esters with different HLB values (Fig. 9); no external additives such as lactose had to be used.

References

1. Bennett, H., *Industrial Waxes*, Vol. 1, Natural and Synthetic Waxes, Vol. II, Compound Waxes and Technology, Chemical Publishing Company, New York, 1975.
2. Wade, A., and Weller, P. J., *Handbook of Pharmaceutical Excipients,* American Pharmaceutical Association, Washington, The Pharmaceutical Press, London, 1994.
3. Lechter, C. S., Waxes. In: *Encyclopedia of Chemical Technology*, 3rd ed., Vol. 24 (M. Grayson, ed.), John Wiley & Sons, New York, 1984, pp. 466-481.
4. Gunstone, F. D., Harwood, J. L., and Padley, F. B., *The Lipid Handbook*, Chapman and Hall, London, 1986.
5. Knowlton, J., and Pearce, S., *Handbook of Cosmetic Science and Technology*, Elsevier, Amsterdam, 1993, pp. 21-32.
6. Warth, A. H., *The Chemistry and Technology of Waxes*, Reinhold Publishing Corporation, New York, 1956.
7. Kolattukudy, P. E., *Chemistry and Biochemistry of Natural Waxes*, Elsevier, Amsterdam, 1976.
8. *United States Pharmacopeia, USP23 NF18*, The United States Pharmacopeial Convention, Rockville, MD, 1995.
9. Schwartz, J. B., Simonelli, A. P., and Higuchi, W. I., *J. Pharm. Sci.*, 57:275-277 (1968).
10. Goodhart, F. W., McCoy, R. H., and Ninger, F. C., *J. Pharm. Sci.,* 63:1748-1751 (1974).
11. Asker, A. F., Motawi, A. M., and Abdel-Khalek, M. M., *Pharmazie*, 26:170-172 (1971).
12. Asker, A. F., Motawi, A. M., and Abdel-Khalek, M. M., *Pharmazie,* 26:213-214 (1971).
13. Asker, A. F., Motawi, A. M., and Abdel-Khalek, M. M., *Pharmazie,* 26:215-217 (1971).
14. El-Shanawany, S., *J. Control. Rel.*, 36:11-19 (1993).
15. Flanders, P., Dyer, G. A., and Jordan, D., *Drug Dev. Ind. Pharm.,* 13:1001-1022 (1987).
16. McTaggert, C. M., Ganley, J. A., Sickmueller, A., and Walker, S. E., *Int. J. Pharm.,* 19:139-148 (1984).
17. Ghali, E. S., Klinger, G. H., and Schwartz, J. B., *Drug Dev. Ind. Pharm.,* 15:1311-1328 (1989).
18. Schwartz, J. B., Ghali, E. S., and Klinger, G. H., *Proc. Intern. Symp. Control. Rel. Bioact. Mater.,* 14:192-193 (1987).
19. Klinger, G. H., Ghali, E. S., and Schwartz, J. B., *Proc. Intern. Symp. Control. Rel. Bioact. Mater.,* 15:119-120 (1988).
20. Foster, T. P., and Parrott, E. L., *Drug Dev. Ind. Pharm.,* 16:1309-1324 (1990).
21. Foster, T. P., and Parrott, E. L., *J. Pharm. Sci.,* 79:806-810 (1990).
22. Foster, T. P., and Parrott, E. L., *J. Pharm. Sci.,* 79:938-942 (1990).
23. Ishino, R., Yoshino, H., Hirakawa, Y., and Noda, K., *Chem. Pharm. Bull.,* 38:3440-3445 (1990).
24. Ishino, R., Yoshino, H., Hirakawa, Y., and Noda, K., *Chem. Pharm. Bull.,* 39:3318-3322 (1991).
25. Vila Jato, J. L., Remunan, C., and Martinez, R., *S.T.P. Pharma,* 6:88-92 (1990).
26. Remunan, C., Bretal, M. J., Nunez, A., and Vila Jato, J. L., *Int. J. Pharm.,* 80:151-159 (1992).
27. Boles, M. G., Deasy, P. B., and Donnellan, M. F., *Drug Dev. Ind. Pharm.,* 19:349-370 (1993).
28. Huang, H.-P., Mehta, S. C., Radebaugh, G. W., and Fawzi, M. B., *J. Pharm. Sci.,* 83:795-797 (1994).
29. Emori, H., Ishizaka, T., and Koishi, M., *J. Pharm. Sci.,* 73:910-915 (1984).
30. Dakkuri, A., Schraeder, H. G., and DeLuca, P. P., *J. Pharm. Sci.,* 67:354-357 (1978).
31. Dakkuri, A., Butler, L. D., and DeLuca, P. P., *J. Pharm. Sci.,* 67:357-360 (1978).
32. Schraeder, H. G., Dakkuri, A., and DeLuca, P. P., *J. Pharm. Sci.,* 67:350-353 (1978).

33. Foster, T. P., and Parrott, E. L., *Drug Dev. Ind. Pharm.*, 16:1633–1648 (1990).
34. Collins, A. E., and Deasy, P. B., *J. Pharm. Sci.*, 79:116–119 (1990).
35. Wang, P. Y., *Int. J. Pharm.*, 54:223–230 (1989).
36. Kaewvichit, S., and Tucker, I. G., *J. Pharm. Pharmacol.*, 46:708–713 (1994).
37. Khan, M. Z. I., Tucker, I. G., and Opdebeek, J. P., *Int. J. Pharm.*, 76:161–170 (1991).
38. Khan, M. Z. I., Tucker, I. G., and Opdebeek, J. P., *Int. J. Pharm.*, 90:255–262 (1993).
39. Opdebeek, J. P., and Tucker, I. G., *J. Control. Rel.*, 23:271–279 (1993).
40. Cady, S. M., Fishbein, R., and San Filippo, M., *Proc. Int. Symp. Control. Rel. Bioact. Mater.*, 16:22–23 (1988).
41. Walker, S. E., Ganley, J. A., Bedford, K., and Eaves, T., *J. Pharm. Pharmacol.*, 32:389–393 (1980).
42. McTaggert, C., Wood, R., Bedford, K., and Walker, S. E., *J. Pharm. Pharmacol.*, 36:119–121 (1984).
43. Doelker, C., Doelker, E., Buri, P., and Waginaire, L., *Drug Dev. Ind. Pharm.*, 12:1553–1565 (1986).
44. Howard, J. R., and Gould, P. L., *Drug Dev. Ind. Pharm.*, 13:1031–1045 (1987).
45. Dennis, A. B., Kellaway, I. W., and Davidson, R., *Proc. Intern. Symp. Control. Rel. Bioact. Mater.*, 15:390–391 (1988).
46. Hawley, A. R., Rowley, G., Lough, W. J., and Chatham, S., *Proc. 10th Int. Pharm. Tech. Conf.*, 2:275–288 (1991).
47. Bodmeier, R., Paeratakul, O., Chen, H., and Zhang, W., *Drug Dev. Ind. Pharm.*, 16:1505–1519 (1990).
48. Jones, D. M., and Percel, P. J., Coating of Multiparticulates Using Molten Materials. In: *Multiparticulate Oral Drug Delivery* (I. Ghebre-Sellassie, ed.), Marcel Dekker, Inc., New York, 1994, pp. 113–142.
49. Jozwiakowski, M. J., Jones, D. M., and Franz, R. M., *Pharm. Res.*, 7: 1119–1126 (1990).
50. Bhagwatwar, H., and Bodmeier, R., *Pharm. Res.*, 6:S–73 (1989).
51. Bhagwatwar, H., M. S. Thesis, The University of Texas at Austin, Austin, 1991.
52. Bagaria, S. C., Ph.D. Dissertation, Rutgers University, The State University of New Jersey, New Brunswick, 1986.
53. Blythe, R. H., U.S. Pat. 2,738,303 (1956).
54. Rosen, E., and Swintosky, J. V., *J. Pharm. Pharmacol.*, 12:237T–244T (1960).
55. Greif, M., U.S. Pat. 3,078,294 (1963).
56. Shephard, M., U.S. Pat. 3,080,294 (1963).
57. Heimlich, K. R., and MacDonnell, D. R., U.S. Pat. 3,119,742 (1964).
58. Peters, D., Goodhart, F. W., and Lieberman, H. A., U.S. Pat. 3,492,397 (1970).
59. Fee, J. V., Grant, D. J. W., and Newton, J. M., *J. Pharm. Sci.*, 65:182–187 (1976).
60. Otsuka, M., and Matsuda, Y., *Pharm. Res.*, 11:351–354 (1994).
61. Otsuka, M., and Matsuda, Y., *J. Pharm. Sci.*, 84:443–447 (1995).
62. Bodmeier, R., Wang, J., and Bhagwatwar, H., *J. Microencaps.*, 9:89–98 (1992).
63. Adeyeye, C. M., and Price, J. C., *Pharm. Res.*, 11:575–579 (1994).
64. Adeyeye, C. M., and Price, J. C., *Pharm. Res.*, 8:1377–1383 (1991).
65. Kawashima, Y., Ohno, H., and Takenaka, H., *J. Pharm. Sci.*, 70:913–916 (1981).
66. Benita, S., Zouai, O., and Benoit, J.-P., *J. Pharm. Sci.*, 75:847–851 (1986).
67. Bodmeier, R., Wang, J., and Bhagwatwar, H., *J. Microencaps.*, 9:99–107 (1992).
68. Kowarski, C. R., Volberger, B., Versanno, J., and Kowarski, A., *Am. J. Hosp. Pharm.*, 21:409–410 (1964).
69. Draper, E. B., and Becker, C. H., *J. Pharm. Sci.*, 55:376–380 (1966).
70. Lucks, S., and Müller, R., PCT Application WO93/05768 (1993).
71. Westesen, K., and Siekmann, B., PCT Application WO94/20072 (1994).
72. Asker, A. F., and Becker, C. H., *J. Pharm. Sci.*, 55:90–94 (1966).
73. Robinson, M. J., and Swintosky, J. V., *J. Am. Pharm. Assoc.*, 48:473–478 (1959).

74. Scott, M. W., Robinson, M. J., Pauls, J. F., and Lantz, R. J., *J. Pharm. Sci.,* 53:670–675 (1964).
75. Cusimano, A. G., and Becker, C. H., *J. Pharm. Sci.,* 57:1104–1112 (1968).
76. John, P. M., and Becker, C. H., *J. Pharm. Sci.,* 57:584–589 (1968).
77. Hamid, I. S., and Becker, C. H., *J. Pharm. Sci.,* 59:511–514 (1970).
78. Javaid, K. A., Fincher, J. H., and Hartman, C. W., *J. Pharm. Sci.,* 60:1709–1712 (1971).
79. Sjoqvist, R., Graffner, C., Ekman, I., Sinclair, W., and Woods, J. P., *Pharm. Res.,* 10:1020–1026 (1993).
80. Eldem, T., Speiser, P., and Hincal, A., *Pharm. Res.,* 8:47–54 (1991).
81. Eldem, T., Speiser, P., and Altorfer, H., *Pharm. Res.,* 8:178–184 (1991).
82. Eldem, T., Speiser, P., and Hincal, A., *Proc. Intern. Symp. Control. Rel. Bioact. Mater.,* 15:436–437 (1988).
83. Akiyama, Y., Yoshioka, M., Horibe, H., Hirai, S., Kitamori, N., and Toguchi, H., *J. Control. Rel.,* 26:1–10 (1993).

ROLAND BODMEIER
JOACHIM HERRMANN

Wet Granulation

Introduction

Wet granulation is the most extensively used method of granulation in the pharmaceutical industry. In general, granulation is defined as a process which causes the powdered particles to adhere permanently to each other to form large particles called granules. (See also the article "Granulation" by H. G. Kristensen and T. Schaefer, Vol. 7, pp. 121–160, of this encyclopedia.) In the wet granulation method, in contrast to dry granulation, the aggregation of particles is obtained by using a liquid phase.

Normally, this liquid phase is a solution, suspension, or slurry of a binding agent. This binder solution is added to a homogeneous powdered mixture containing the active ingredient. The binder solution is homogeneously distributed in the powdered mixture by kneading the lumps of the liquid–solid mixture. The solvent evaporates during a drying step.

Products obtained by wet granulation are spherical-like, cylindrical-shaped, free-flowing multiparticular systems with a previously defined particle size (ranging from 0.1 to 2 mm) with constant composition. These products can be used as such as a dosage form or as intermediates in the production of tablets and capsules.

Pharmaceutical granules, made up of small irregular and cylindrical particles, have been used since the 19th century. One of the early references is credited to a professor from Algiers, Dr. Dordant, who proposed the form of granules for administering large amounts of medicinal powders. These granules were obtained by "forming a homogeneous paste of medicinal powder with water containing gum in the 1:20 proportion of powder. The bulk mass was placed over a screen and pressed down with a wooden roller which forced the wet mass to pass through the holes. The granules were then dried in an oven. . . ." [1]. In this reference the profile of different stages of traditional wet granulation is observed. Pharmaceutical granulations attained their highest usage in the first half of the 20th century; thereafter their use started to decline. Nowadays, single-dose specialties with the vermicular-shaped classical granules are used in the pharmaceutical market. Recently, however, suppliers of raw materials have found a new application for wet granulation in the production of granular excipients for direct compression.

The wet granulation method has been used for the longest time in the industrial production of tablets. The two important material properties required to form a compact and reproducible tablet are compressibility and fluidity; both can be obtained by means of granulation. In dry granulation and direct compression methods, compressibility depends on the inherent deformation and cohesive properties of the active substance and diluents. In wet granulation, distribution of binders over the surface of the granules creates an adhesive property in the materials that makes up for the lack of cohesiveness in the drugs and the diluents.

In the pharmaceutical industry, the advantages obtained by using wet granulation procedures in the development of pharmaceutical granules, tablet, and capsule formulations must remain during large-scale production. To assure biopharmaceutical quality, pharmaceutical industries must develop products and machinery resulting in reproducible, controllable quality. Wet granulation has the disadvantage of complexity because it requires several stages. For this reason, recent research has been devoted to the design of equipment that allows to carry out several stages in the same unit and to develop control systems that guarantee the characteristics of product from batch to batch. Attempts have also been made to improve the wet granulation process by utilizing fluidized-bed and spray-drying techniques. In practice, by using these techniques the difference between wet granulation and microencapsulation is only based on the particle size of the resultant product. Finally, spherical granules ("pellets") with a narrow particle size distribution can be obtained by means of pelletization techniques, mainly by the use of extruders, as a special method of wet granulation.

Raw Materials

Besides active substances, production of granulations involves different types of excipients. Each is selected according to the nature of the active ingredient, the processing requirements, and the use of the end product [2–5].

Raw materials required for wet granulation can be divided in two categories:

- Dry Powder Constituents. These are the powders which will be granulated. In addition to the active substance, this mixture normally contains diluents and disintegrating agents. These excipients are necessary from the biopharmaceutical or technological view point. Other types like flavors can be added to improve patients' acceptability, and antioxidants or preservatives for maintaining product quality.
- Liquid Constituents. The liquid phase contains binders and solvents which confer adhesion to the dry powder particles; coloring agents are frequently incorporated into this phase.

This classification is general and not rigid. For example, there are formulations in which binders are part of the dry powdery mixture and the granulating liquid contains only solvent. In other formulations, the active substance is dissolved in the granulating liquid and the solution is added to the excipients mixture [2,6]. The formulation shown in Table 1 corresponds to a standard granulation.

TABLE 1 Inert Granulation Prepared by the Wet Granulation Process[a]

Ingredient	Quantity (% w/w)
Lactose (fine powder)	75
Corn starch	25
Gelatin (5% solution)	q.s.

[a]Mix lactose and starch and moisten with the gelatin solution to proper wetness. Granulate by passing the wet mass through a 14 mesh (1.12 mm) screen and dry at 60°C. Pass the dry granulation through a 16 mesh (1 mm) screen.

Wet Granulation

When granulations are an intermediate product during the tableting process, another series of excipients called external additives are added after the drying step. These are different from the additives that constitute the granulations. The external additives may be disintegrants, lubricants, glidants, and antiadherents [7].

Drug Substance

The role of the active ingredients is very important in the development of the formulation. Selection of the types of diluents, disintegrants, binders, and granulating solvents depends on the physicochemical characteristics and stability of the active substance (Table 2). The viability of the wet granulation process also depends on the solubility characteristics of the drug and its stability in aqueous media and under drying temperatures. Therefore the formulation step of any type of granulation should be preceded by a preformulation step in which all of these parameters are considered. Particle size and shape are critical factors in the mixing operation. In the manufacturing of tablets, fluidity and compressibility of the active substance determine the necessity of wet granulation, particularly when the active substance is only moderately potent or of low density. Attention should be paid to the morphological changes during the moistening and drying stages. Solubility and stability in solvents determine the nature of the granulating solvent and binding agent [4,8–10].

Diluents or Fillers

Fillers or diluents are used to increase the bulk mass to be granulated; their proportions are based on the dosage of the drugs. They may constitute 80–90% of the granulation for a highly potent active ingredient. A list of the diluents most frequently used in wet granulation is shown in Table 3. (See also the article "Diluents" by J. L. Czeisler and K. P. Perlman in Vol. 4, pp. 37–84 of this encyclopedia).

TABLE 2 Critical Characteristics of Drug Substance in the Design of Wet Granulation Procedures

Property	Order of Importance
Organoleptic properties	+
Particle shape and crystal properties	++
Particle size	++
Flowability	++++
Absolute and bulk densities	+++
Compressibility	++++
Polymorphism	+++
pH in solution	+
Solubility	+++
Dissolution rate	+
Solid-state stability	+++
Hygroscopicity	+++
Solution stability	+++

TABLE 3 Fillers Commonly Used in Wet Granulation

Soluble Fillers	Insoluble Fillers
Lactose USP (crystalline or powder)	Calcium sulfate NF
Sucrose USP powder	Dibasic calcium phosphate USP
Mannitol USP	Tribasic calcium sulfate NF
Dextrose USP	Calcium carbonate USP
Sorbitol NF	Starch (corn, potato, rice, wheat) NF
Fructose NF	Hydrolyzed starches
Sodium chloride USP	Microcrystalline cellulose NF
	Celluloses floc

Polysaccharides

The most frequently used diluent is crystalline lactose (Table 4). It is available in the α-monohydrate form as an impalpabe powder in a particle size ranges from 200 to 225 mesh (65-75 μm) [3]. After drying, crystalline lactose gives granules with a high moisture content (4-5% compared to 0.1-0.5% with sucrose, dextrose, and mannitol). Traditionally, crystalline lactose has been used as a filler with starch in equal proportions. Sucrose is used generally as a filler in the form of confectioners sugar or in direct compressible form like Di-Pac and Nu Tab to obtain granules with superior hardness. For this reason, its use as chewable tablet constituent has been criticized. Hardness can be reduced by using a mixture of alcohol and water as a granulating liquid instead of only water. Mannitol is the preferred diluent for chewable tablets (Table 5). It requires more granulating solution than sucrose or lactose and approximately the same amount as dextrose. However, mannitol gives softer granules than sucrose and dextrose [2,11].

Calcium Salts

Calcium sulfate is an inexpensive filler and can be used with a wide range of drugs because of its few incompatibilities. Granulated with polymer solutions, the tablets gen-

TABLE 4 Phenobarbital Tablets[a] Made by Wet Granulation[b]

Ingredient	mg per Tablet	Quantity (% w/w)
Phenobarbital	65	49
Lactose (fine powder)	40	30
Starch (as 10% starch paste)	4	3
Starch (dry)	10	7.5
Talc	10	7.5
Mineral oil, 50 cP	4	3

[a]Data from Ref. 2.
[b]Mix the phenobarbital and lactose and moisten with the starch paste. Granulate by passing the wet mass through a 14 mesh (1.12 mm) screen and dry at 60°C. Pass the dry granulation through a 20 mesh (0.8 mm) screen. Mix with the dry starch and talc. Finally, add the mineral oil and mix again. Compress using 9/32-in. standard cup punches.

TABLE 5 Chewable Antacid Tablets[a] Made by Wet Granulation[b]

Ingredient	mg per Tablet	Quantity (% w/w)
Aluminum hydroxide (dried gel)	400	54.85
Magnesium hydroxide (fine powder)	80	10.98
Sucrose, confectioners	20	2.74
Mannitol (fine powder)	180	24.68
Polyvinylpyrrolidone (as 10% solution in 50% ethanol)	30	4.12
Magnesium stearate	15	2.06
Silica aerogel (Cab-O-Sil M-5)	4	0.54
Oil of peppermint	0.2	0.03

[a]Data from Ref. 2.
[b]Mix the first four ingredients and moisten with PVP solution. Granulate by passing through a 14 mesh (1.12 mm) screen. Dry at 60 to 65°C. Size through a 20 mesh (0.8 mm) screen, add the oil of peppermint mixed with the Cab-O-Sil and finally the magnesium stearate; mix well and compress using 1/2-in. flat-face bevel-edge punches.

erally do not harden with time. However, use of sugar solution for granulation gives tablets which may tend to harden with time. Dicalcium phosphate is used in the form of fine powder. Its properties are similar to those of calcium sulfate, but it is more expensive and its use is limited.

Cellulose

Microcrystalline cellulose can be advantageously utilized in a proportion of 5–10%. This is particularly useful in the granulation with some materials, like calcium carbonate, which, when wetted, form a clay-like mass that clogs the screen during the wet milling process and give hard granulations on drying and resists disintegration. The wicking action of microcrystalline cellulose promotes rapid wet massing of the powder mix. Its ability to retain water makes the wet mass less sensitive to overwetting due to excess of the granulating fluid (Table 6). It also possesses binder and disintegrant properties which are, however, lost when in wet granulation [2].

TABLE 6 Improvement of Wet Granulation Procedure by the Addition of Microcrystalline Cellulose (Avicel)[a]

Formula I[b]		Formula II[c]	
Ingredient	Quantity	Ingredient	Quantity
Calcium carbonate	1000 g	Calcium carbonate	1000 g
Water	300 mL	Avicel PH 101	100 g
		Water	300 mL

[a]Adapted from Ref. 2.
[b]Sticky mass, granulation through 12 mesh (1.4 mm) screen is not possible.
[c]Nonsticky mass, granulation through 12 mesh (1.4 mm) screen is possible.

Disintegrants

Disintegrants facilitate the breakup of granules and tablets into fine particles in the gastrointestinal tract. Their function is to counteract the action of binders and physical forces of compression necessary to form tablets.

The three principal mechanisms of disintegrants are swelling, wicking, and breaking. Some disintegrants like clay and veegum act through swelling and lose their properties if previously in contact with aqueous media; for this reason they cannot be used as internal additives in wet granulation [2]. Frequently used disintegrants are listed in Table 7.

Corn starch is the most widely used disintegrant. In wet granulation, it may also be used as diluent or binder (Tables 1 and 4). In association with Avicel it forms an excellent combination of disintegrants. Acid-base systems are used in the manufacture of effervescents tablets (Table 7) [12].

Materials like low-substituted carboxymethyl starches, cross-linked carboxymethyl cellulose, and cross-linked polyvinylpyrrolidone (PVP) represent a new generation of disintegrants which substantially decreased disintegration time. This property is particularly useful in the formulation of tablets containing water-insoluble drugs. These substances are used in lower concentration than traditional starch (2–3% for cross-linked cellulose and crospovidone, and 4–6% for cross-linked starch in wet granulation formulations) [2,13].

Color, Flavor, and Flavor Modifiers

Colors used in granulations designed for oral drug administration are limited to those certified by the FDA as food, drug, and cosmetic colors (FD&C) and drug and cosmetic colors (D&C). These colors are dyes, their lakes, and certain natural and derived colorants. Normally they are added to the formulation in a maximum concentration of 0.05%. Since they are used in very low concentrations, certified dyes are often treated

TABLE 7 Disintegrating Agents

Disintegrant	Concentration in Granulation (% w/w)
Traditional	
Starch (corn, potato)	5–20
Microcrystalline cellulose	5–20
Alginic acid	5–10
Sodium alginate	2–5
Clays (Veegum)	5–15
Cellulose floc	5–15
Ion exchange resins	0.5–5
Effervescent acid–base systems	3–20
Recent	
Modified starch (sodium starch glycolate NF)	1–8
Modified carboxymethylcellulose (Croscarmelose NF)	5–10
Cross-linked polyvinylpyrrolidone (Crospovidone NF)	0.5–5

Wet Granulation

as inert materials. However, dyes can react with various pharmaceutical excipients. For example, sugars like lactose, sucrose, and dextrose increase the fading rate of FD&C Blue No. 2, but this does not occur with mannitol and sorbitol [2].

Colors are incorporated into the granulation by dissolution (in case of soluble dyes) or dispersion (in case of lakes) in the granulating solvent. To avoid the migration problems of soluble dyes during drying they should be first adsorbed on calcium sulfate, tricalcium phosphate, starch, or some other major granulation ingredient.

An improvement in the palatability of granulations can be attained by means of the proper selection of fillers; sugars, for example, impart sweetness. Flavors are mixed with dry powder constituents or, more frequently, distributed in a fine spray over the dried granulation after dissolving in an alcoholic solution. Microencapsulated flavors are one of the most recent forms of incorporating flavors in dried granules just before compression (14).

Granulating Solvents

Solvents used in wet granulation should be nontoxic and volatile, so that they can be removed from the granulation during drying. Water is the most frequently used granulating fluid. Under some circumstances, organic solvents, mainly ethanol and isopropanol, are used neat or in aqueous mixtures [15,16].

Water

Water has the advantage of being nonflammable, and expensive safety precautions, like flameproof equipment, are not needed. Its use may be disadvantageous in some cases, where it may adversely affect the stability of the drug by causing hydrolysis of a water-sensitive product. Furthermore, it may need longer drying times than organic solvents. This may affect the stability of the active ingredients due to prolonged exposure to heat [11].

Organic Solvents

Organic solvents are used for water-sensitive drugs as an alternative to dry granulation. They are also used when fast drying is necessary and in the production of effervescent granulations [12,15]. Ethanol is mostly utilized. It may be used alone or mixed with water in different proportions. Isopropyl alcohol and methylene chloride are alternative solvents. The last trace of the solvent should be carefully eliminated to avoid an odor of alcohol. Another very important disadvantage of the use of organic solvents is the generation of toxic vapors which can affect the workers or cause explosions.

Binders

Binders are substances with cohesive and adhesive properties capable of agglomerating dry powdered particles to form granules after drying. Binders can be added to the dry powder by dissolving in the granulation solvent, or in dry form, as other constituent of dry mixtures, and after moistening with water, alcohol, or water–alcohol mixture to form a binder solution. (See also the article "Binders" by H. G. Kristensen, Vol. 1, pp. 461–464, of this encyclopedia).

A variation of the second method is produced when the granulating solvent used for kneading dry powder dissolves one of the powdery ingredients. During the drying stage, this material may crystallize and the dissolved substance may act as hard binder. Any material soluble in granulating solvent may exhibit this behavior, for example, when sucrose is incorporated in dry powders and granulated with water [15].

In general, binders are more effective when they can be added by dissolution in granulation solvent. This requires less binder than when the binder is added in dry form. In some cases, it is not possible to obtain granulations with suitable hardness using the dry method. However, incorporation in dry form is useful when large amounts of binder are needed giving viscous solutions. The only effective dry binder is microcrystalline cellulose.

The type and quantity of binder added to the formulation play a fundamental role in the uniformity of the particle size, hardness, disintegration, and compressibility of the granulations. A strong binder or a highly concentrated binder solution may result in hard granulations which require excessive compression force during the compaction of tablets. On the other hand, an insufficient quantity of binder may produce fragile granulations which disaggregates easily [11,17–19]. Table 8 indicates how the hardness of griseofulvin granulations varies when prepared with different proportions of PVP as binding agent [20]. The tensile strength of granulations not only depends on the proportion of binder but also on the water content of the granules. In fact, when granulations are stored in environments of different relative humidity, an increase in their deformation capacity is obtained with increasing relative humidity (Fig. 1). Thus the resistance to higher pressures without producing rupture is observed. This is due to the plastic property of binders, a result of absorbed humidity.

High levels of binders, especially cellulosics and natural gums, may interfere with the disintegration and dissolution of tablets by forming a mucilaginous film around the particle surface [21]. In the case of hydrophobic drugs, however, binders can accelerate dissolution (Fig. 2).

Numerous methods are proposed to evaluate the cohesion property of a binder. These methods are based on the characteristics of the binder (Table 9) alone and in the granulating solution, the mixtures of the binder solution with dry powder constituents, and even the dry granulations.

TABLE 8 Breaking Strength of Griseofulvin Granules Containing Polyvinylpyrrolidone (PVP) as binder[a]

PVP Content (%)	Breaking Load (g)	
	Mean	Standard Deviation
0	11	6
0.6	70	8
1	245	55
1.6	340	73
3.6	582	82

[a]Based on Ref. 20.

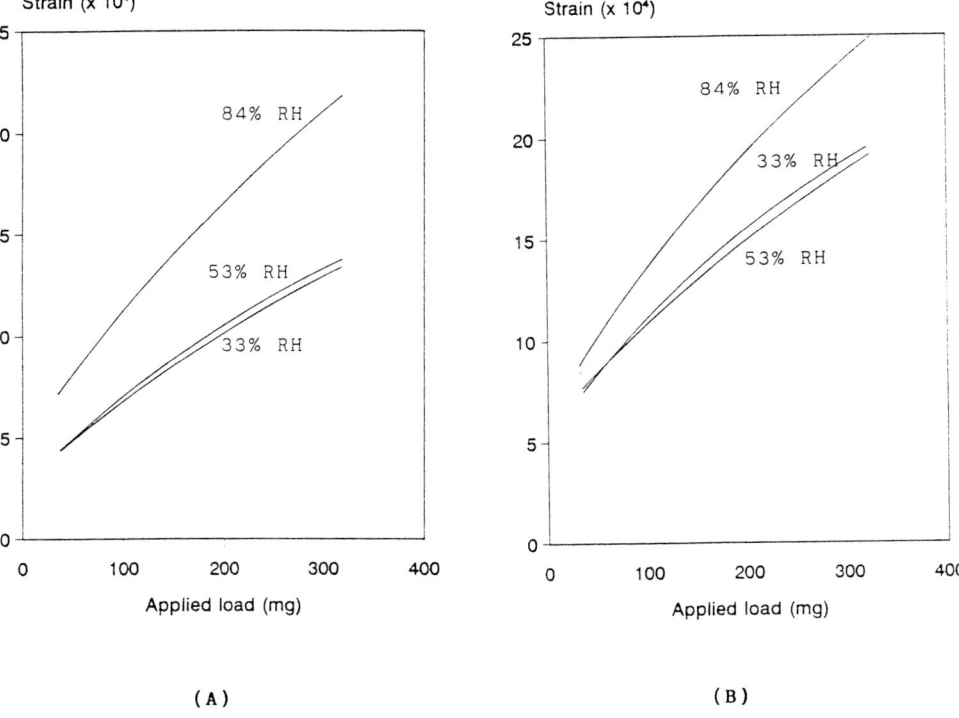

FIG. 1. Effect of relative humidity (RH) of granule storage on the relationship between strain and applied load for granules containing (A) starch and (B) PVP as binding agents. (From Ref. 20.)

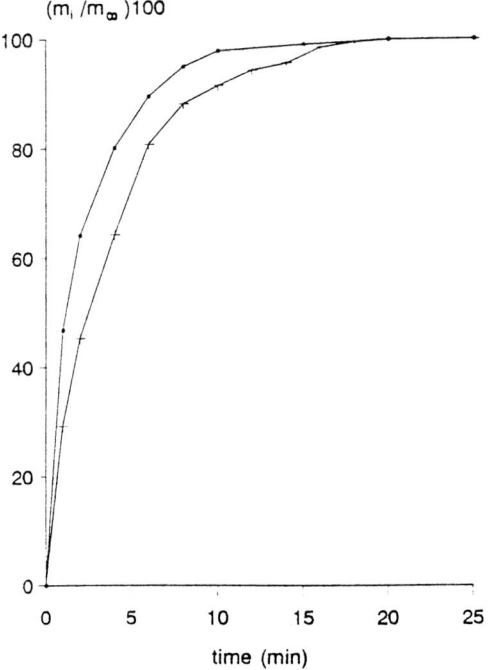

FIG. 2. Increase of dissolution rate of a hydrophobic drug (Mitonafide) during wet granulation; —·— Granulation —+— Drug substance. (Data from the authors.)

TABLE 9 Evaluation of Binder Properties

Indirect Methods	Dry Granulation	Direct Methods
Binder	Size distribution	Torque
Breaking force of binder films	Bulk volume	Conductivity
Reological behavior	Hardness and friability	Power consumption
Surface tension force and contact angle	Porosity	Extruder test
	Compressibility	
	Drug release	

[a]Adapted from Ref. 22.

The binders most widely used in wet granulation are shown in Table 10. Binders can be divided into sugars and polymeric materials. The latter group can be divided into natural polymers such as starch and gums (acacia and tragacanth) and synthetic polymers such as PVP and methylcellulose [2,23].

Natural binders in wet granulation are associated with two difficulties. On the one hand, batch-to-batch variations in the product characteristics make it difficult to standardize the process. On the other hand, binding solutions should be freshly prepared or should contain some preservative. Before using these solutions, straining or centrifugation may also be necessary to eliminate debris.

Starch, in the form of paste, has probably been the most commonly used binder in the past. It gives rise to granulations that disintegrate quickly (Table 4). Its high viscosity is its main disadvantage which makes handling and mixing difficult. To avoid this problem, starch may be added in dry pregelatinized form to the powder mix and

TABLE 10 Binders Commonly Used in the Wet Granulation Process

Binder	Concentration in Granulating Liquid (% w/v)	Granulating Solvent
Starch	5–10	Water
Pregelatinized starch	2–10	Water
Gelatin	2–10	Water
Acacia, tragacanth	5–20	Water
Sugars (glucose, sucrose)	up to 50	Water
Polyvinylpyrrolidone	2–20	Water or alcohol
Methylcellulose (various viscosity grades)	2–10	Water
Sodium carboxymethylcellulose (low-viscosity grade)	2–10	Water
Ethylcellulose (various viscosity grades)	5–10	Alcohol or water–alcohol mixtures
Polyacrylamides	2–8	Water
Polyvinyloxazolidones	5–10	Water or water–alcohol mixtures
Polyvinyl alcohols	5–20	Water

Wet Granulation

later moistened with water. This process needs two to four times more starch to obtain granulations of the same hardness. Pregelatinized starch may also be used in the form of paste. Its binding properties are slightly better and it offers the advantage of being soluble in warm water without boiling [2].

When a stronger binder is needed, gelatin may be a good choice. Gelatin solutions should be used at elevated temperature to avoid gellification. Gelatin produces hard granulations that tend to harden even more with age.

Acacia and tragacanth solutions have been used as binder agents in the past. However, due to bacterial contamination problems, they have been replaced by the recently developed synthetic polymers.

The most widely used binder is probably PVP. It is inert and has the advantage of being soluble in both water and alcohol. It is used in aqueous and dilute alcoholic solutions to granulate insoluble powders and in alcoholic solutions for soluble powders. It may also be added in dry form. It is widely used in anhydrous alcoholic solutions in the manufacture of effervescent tablets. PVP is also an excellent binder for chewable tablets. Although it is a hydroscopic, tablets harden only slightly with age. To avoid hardening, 2–3% of glycerin may be included in the formulation.

Methylcellulose is used as 1–5% aqueous solution, depending on the viscosity grade [3]. Low viscosity grades (10–50 cP) allow higher concentrations than high viscosity grades (1000–10000 cP). With both soluble and insoluble powders, methylcellulose gives granulations that compress easily and produces tablets which do not harden with age. Sodium carboxymethylcellulose (CMC) can also be used to granulate both soluble and insoluble powders. It produces granulations softer than those with PVP, but the tablets have relatively long disintegration times and greater tendency to harden. Ethylcellulose is insoluble in water and is only used in alcoholic solution. Low viscosity grades are used in concentrations of 2 to 10% in ethanol and less frequently in methylene chloride. Tablets prepared with ethylcellulose have relatively short disintegration times without hardening tendency, but dissolution may be delayed due to low solubility of ethylcellulose in water. Hydroxypropyl methylcellulose (HPMC) is soluble in water, aqueous alcohol solutions, and methylene chloride; it is available in various viscosity grades. It competes with methylcellulose and PVP with regard to versatility and inertness.

Polyacrylamides are water-soluble polymers available in various viscosity grades. In a 2–5% solution they produce granulations similar to those produced with starch paste. The tablets are somewhat softer with the disadvantage of having longer disintegration and dissolution times. Polyvinyloxazolidones resemble PVP in practice but with the advantage of nonhygroscopicity. Since some are water soluble and some are soluble in alcohol or in aqueous alcoholic mixtures, they offer a wide range of applicability and utility.

Theory of Granule Formation

Theories explaining the formation of granules can be divided in two groups:

- Theories about the mechanism of bonding among fundamental particles
- Theories about the enlargement mechanism of agglomerates

To understand their real meaning, it should be taken into account that mechanisms involved in producing a specific granule and their participation in obtaining the final product depend greatly on the granulation equipment.

Particle-Bonding Mechanisms

During granulation, particles adhere and agglomerate due to bond formation. These bonds should be strong enough to allow granules to withstand handling without breakdown [15,24]. Rumpf distinguishes five types of particle-bonding mechanisms [25]:

1. Adhesion and cohesion forces in immobile liquid bridges
    Viscous binders
    Thin adsorption layers
2. Interfacial forces and capillary pressure in mobile liquid films
3. Solid bridges
    Crystallization of dissolved substances
    Hardening binders
    Melting
    Sintering and chemical reaction
4. Attractive forces between solid particles
    Molecular forces (van der Waals and valence)
    Electrostatic charges
    Valence forces
5. Mechanical interlocking

Adhesion and Cohesion Forces in Immobile Liquid Bridges

These forces are due to the formation of adsorption layers or the presence of highly viscous binder solutions. The bonds are formed on the outer surface of the particles. Although they are produced in wet granulation, normally they do not contribute greatly to the strength of the final granules.

Adsorption layers of water originate around the outer surface of the slightly wetted powder particles (Fig. 3). This adsorbed humidity reduces the interparticle distance. When this distance is smaller than 3.0 nm, interparticle bonding is favored as it allows the formation of more stable bonds due to the van der Waals forces of attraction.

Although these films of water may remain as liquid residue after the drying of granules prepared by wet granulation, they probably do not contribute significantly to the strength of final granules.

Bonding forces originating among the particles due to highly viscous binder solutions are stronger than those produced by mobile liquid films, which will be discussed later. However, highly viscous binder solutions are not frequently used in wet granulation. Only starch paste can produce this type of film in pharmaceutical granules [27].

Interfacial Forces and Capillary Pressure in Mobile Liquid Films

These forces constitute the most important particle bonding mechanism in wet granulation. They give rise to the formation of liquid bridges that are only temporary struc-

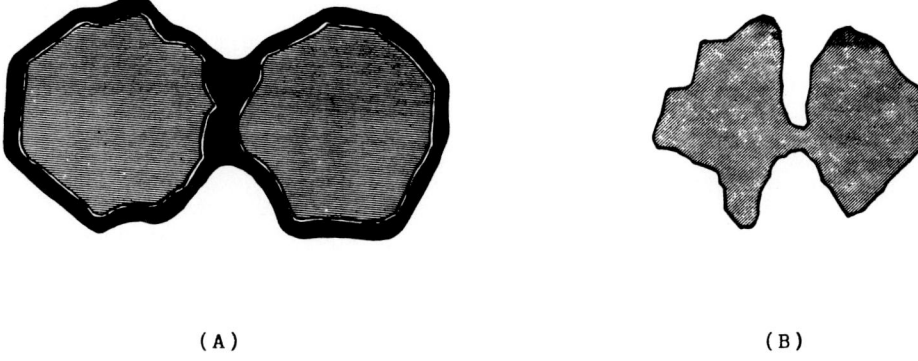

(A)   (B)

FIG. 3. Formal representation of (A) thin adsorption layers, and (B) solid bridges. (From Ref. 24.)

tures because the granulation liquid is later eliminated by drying. However, they are indispensable prerequisites for the formation of solid bridges [28].

When a granulating liquid is added to a powder mixture, it is distributed in such a way that it forms mobile liquid films around the outer surface of the particles and in the interparticle space. Strutures formed between particles and liquid change with the increase in the amount of water added. Newitt and Conway-Jones distinguished three structures of distribution states of water among particles [29]: pendular, funicular, and capillary states (Fig. 4). These states are based on the observation that during the granulation process, the liquid progressively fills the inter- and intraparticle void spaces. Barlow adds the fourth state called droplet or suspension [26,27].

The first state, the pendular state, is produced by low liquid levels. Liquid films are formed on the surface of particles which combine to produce discrete liquid bridges at the contact points of the particles [30]. The surface tension of the concave air–liquid interface and the negative capillary pressure in these liquid bridges gives rise to cohesive forces and causes the particles to stick together [28]. This state has a comparatively low mechanical strength. From geometric considerations supported by Laplace's law, Fisher developed a mathematical expression of the bonding forces in the pendular state [31–33]. This expression is based on the study of the fundamental model shown in Fig. 5 which represents the bonding by a liquid bridge between two spherical particles of same size and character. The interparticle attraction force can be expressed by Eq. (1),

$$F_p = F_T + F_s \tag{1}$$

where F_T is the tensile strength due to surface tension and F_s the negative capillary pressure in the bridges, given by Eqs. (2) and (3),

$$F_T = 2\pi bT \tag{2}$$

$$F_s = \pi b^2 T \left(\frac{1}{c} + \frac{1}{b} \right) \tag{3}$$

where T is the surface tension of the liquid.

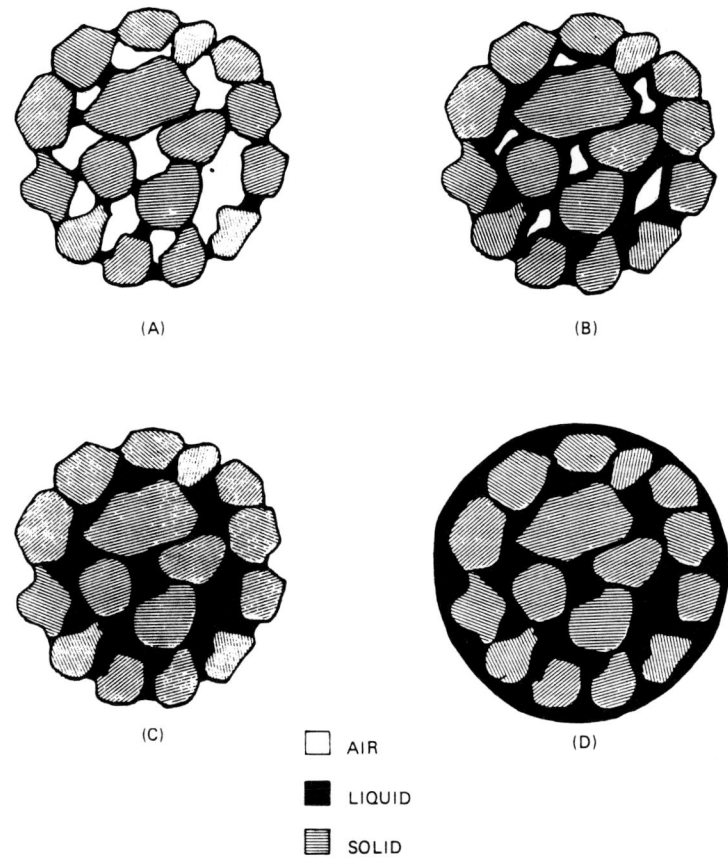

FIG. 4. Interfacial forces and capillary pressure in mobile liquid films. (A) Pendular state, (B) funicular state, (C) capillary state, and (D) droplet state. (From Ref. 24.)

If b and c are expressed as function of r and β, Eq. (4) results.

$$F_p = \frac{2\pi rT}{1 + \tan\beta} \qquad (4)$$

A similar equation was proposed later by Rumpf from a dimensional analysis of the subject.

Funicular state is the intermediate stage between pendular and capillary states. It is attained when the liquid bridges of the pendular state start to coalesce by increasing the liquid content. Consequently, a slight increase in the strength of the wet granules is produced.

The capillary state is reached when intergranule void spaces are totally eliminated due to addition of more liquid and more kneading of the wet mass. In this situation, the particles remain united by the interfacial forces on the granule surface as the void spaces are now completely filled with liquid. This state is also due to the negative

Wet Granulation

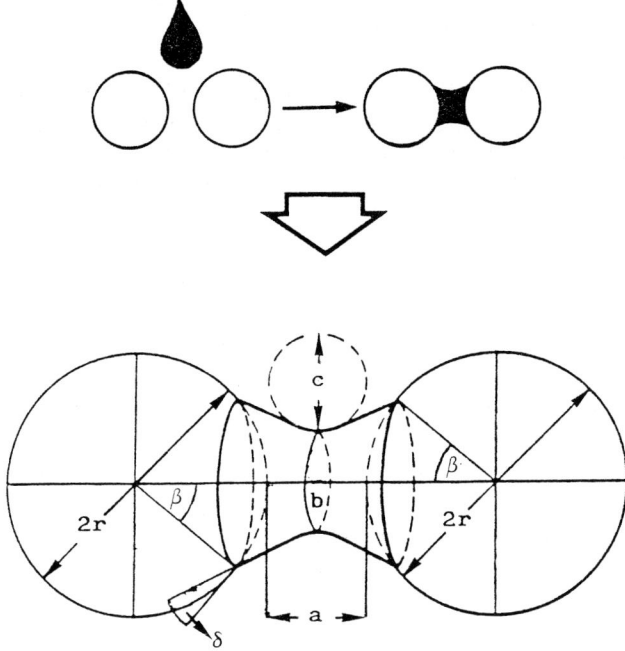

FIG. 5. Fundamental model to study the bonding between two particles by a liquid bridge. (Based on Ref. 31.)

capillary pressure created in every part of the internal side of the space which is filled with liquid [31,32].

Rumpf showed that the strength of the agglomerate as a whole is approximately equal to the mean capillary pressure, P_c, given by Eq. (5),

$$P_c = k \frac{1-\varepsilon}{\varepsilon} \frac{T}{2r} \cos \delta \tag{5}$$

where ε is the porosity, δ the contact angle, and k a coefficient between 6 and 14.5 [25].

The capillary state coincides with the maximum tensile strength of moist granules. This force increases about three times from the pendular to the capillary state. If S is defined as the degree of liquid saturation (volume occupied by the liquid divided by the total pore volume), with a very general consideration, then for the pendular state S is equal to or smaller than 0.25 and for the capillary state S is greater than or equal to 0.8 [31].

According to the above explanation, it may appear that the state of the wet mass depends on its total moisture content but this is not exactly the case. The capillary state may also reach constant volumes of binder liquid but reducing the particle separation by adequate kneading. Shearing and compression forces applied over the wet mass by kneading equipment may densify it, as it passes from the pendular state to funicular or capillary states without addition of more water [27].

The last state represented in Fig. 4 is the droplet state. This state is not attained in the traditional wet granulation method but it is important in the granulation process by spray drying a suspension. As soon as enough liquid is added to the wet mass to completely envelope the solid agglomerates, the concave surfaces are replaced by the convex surfaces of a liquid droplet, and all intergranular capillary bonding forces disappear. However, agglomerated particles are still held together in the droplet by the surface tension of the used liquid.

Solid Bridges

Solid bridges are formed when two or more particles are held together by a solid material which can belong to the solid particles themselves or to another different material (Fig. 3). Solid bridges formed due to hardening binders (PVP, cellulosic products, starch paste) and crystallization of dissolved substances (sucrose) are most important in wet granulation [28]. Upon addition of the granulating solvent to the dry mass, liquid bridges, which agglomerate the particles, are formed. This solvent may contain a binder or may dissolve one of the powder constituents during wet massing. After the granules dry off, the liquid disappears and dissolved material hardens or crystallizes forming solid bridges.

The size and strenght of the crystals not only depend on the quantity of dissolved substance but also on the crystallization rate which determines their structure. The shorter the drying time, the larger the crystal size, and a dramatic increase in the granule strength can occur [28,34].

It may also happen that dissolved substances crystallize at the begining of the drying and form a crust over the granules that are still wet. This phenomenon influences both the drying rate and cohesion force of the granules. Therefore it is desirable to avoid bonding by crystalline bridges in the wet granulation [28].

Attractive Forces Between Solid Particles

In the absence of liquid and solid bridges, there are two basic types of attraction forces that may act among particles to form agglomerates:

- Electrostatic forces can cause powder cohesion during the drying stage but do not contribute significantly to the final strength of the granulation.
- Van der Waals forces are stronger than electrostatic forces but only important in dry granulation where they contribute significantly to the strength of the granules.

Mechanism of Granule Formation

Theories about the mechanisms of enlargement of agglomerates, discussed later, were originally proposed for pan granulators, but they serve as a widespread and useful generalization of the process. The proposed mechanism of enlargement of granules may be divided in three stages [15,24,28,35]:

1. Nucleation. The granulation starts with the adhesion among particles due to liquid bridges and the formation of agglomerates at the capillary state. These structures may act as nucleus for successive enlargement of granules.
2. Transition. The nucleus may be enlarged by two possible mechanisms: individual particles may adhere to the formed nucleus by pendular bridges or two or more

Wet Granulation

nuclei may combine among themselves. The resultant nucleus is reshaped by the continuous agitation in the granulation equipment. The final granulation is characterized by a large amount of smaller granules with a great range of sizes, requiring a narrowing of the size distribution. These granulations, once dried, are usually the best for tablet elaboration or capsule filling.

3. Ball Growth or Enlargement of the Granule. Spherical granules are produced with a mean size that increases with the agitation time. Normally, these granules are too big for pharmaceutical purposes, however, some ball growth is produced in planetary mixers and it is an essential enlargement mechanism for some spheronization equipment. The four possible mechanisms of ball growth are illustrated in Fig. 6.

- *Coalescence.* Two or more granules are united to form a larger granule.
- *Breakage.* Granules break in fragments which adhere to other granules, forming a layer of material over the intact granules.
- *Abrasion Transfer.* The agitation of the granule bed causes attrition of material of the granules by abrasion. This abraded material adheres to other granules, increasing the size of the granules.

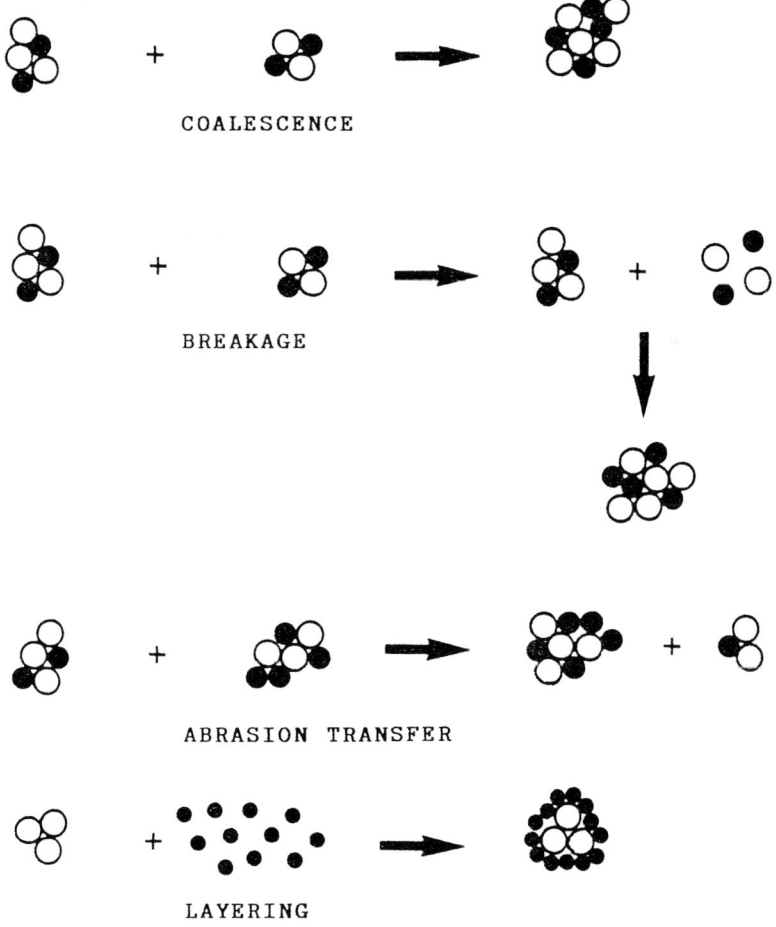

FIG. 6. Mechanisms of ball growth. (Based on Ref. 15.)

- *Layering.* When a second batch of powder mixture is added to the granule bed, it adheres to the already formed granules increasing their size. This mechanism is only important in pelletization for the production of layered granules using spheronization equipment.

Steps in the Traditional Wet Granulation Process

The different steps of traditional wet granulation process are shown in Fig. 7. The process parameters that must be under control during each step depend on the raw material characteristics or the objectives of the granulation process.

Milling and Mixing of Dry Powder Constituents

The dry powder constituents to be granulated should be well mixed to ensure a good distribution of the active ingredient. It is a solid–solid mixing operation [36] which is usually preceeded by a pulverization step to guarantee mix uniformity. An inadequate mixer could give rise to lack of a nonuniform drug content in the end product. These considerations are of special importance for intermediate products in small capsule and tablet manufacturing and when the drug concentration in the mix is relatively low [30,37,38].

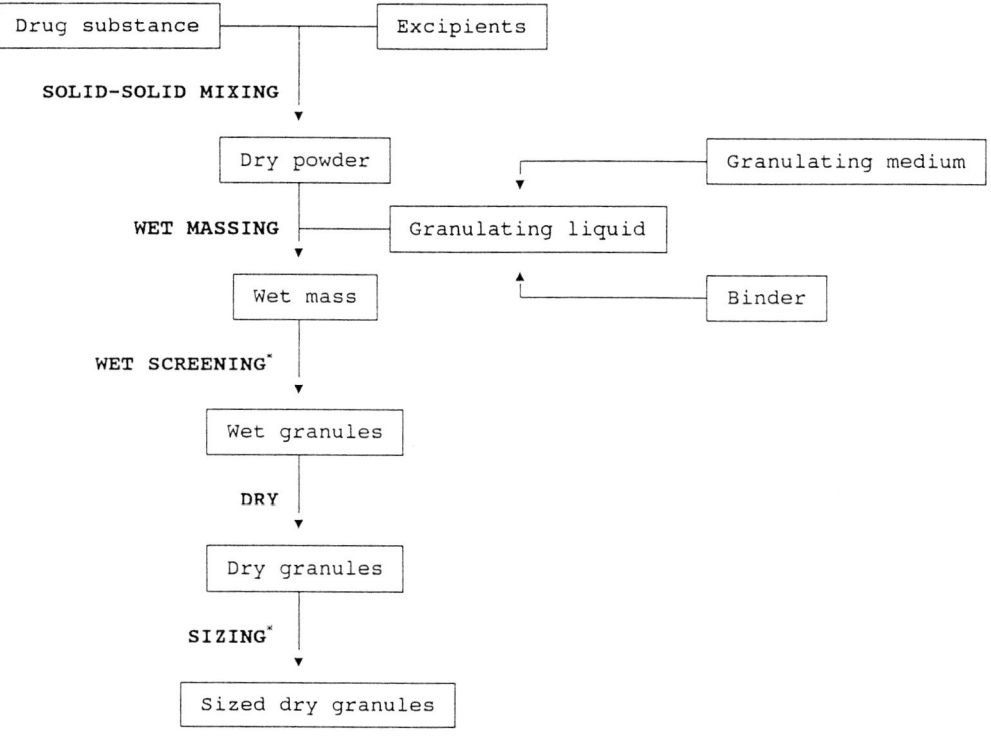

FIG. 7. Steps in the traditional wet granulation process. (*These steps may be omitted.)

Wet Granulation

Wet Massing of the Powders

The granulation liquid is added to the dry powder mixture and uniformly distributed. This is a liquid–solid mixing operation [36].

The process of mixing a liquid with a powder bed in a high shear mixer may be divided into the four steps shown in Fig. 8 [36,39].

In agglomeration, liquid bridges are built up which create agglomerates in the pendular, funicular, and capillary states. A sufficiently low interface tension between the liquid and the solids is needed for good wetting. Otherwise, surface-active agents have to be added.

The agglomeration is broken down when all the liquid has been added. The tensile and shearing strengths of the mixing equipment break the agglomerates and distribute the liquid. At this point, hard agglomerates are not detected and the wet mass is easily crumbled to a powder by hand.

In reagglomeration, as kneading continues and the liquid is completely distributed throughout the dry mix, all the agglomerates reach the capillary state and the growth

1.– AGGLOMERATION

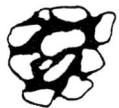

2.–AGGLOMERATION BREAKDOWN

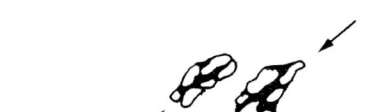

Large agglomerates shear apart by mixer force

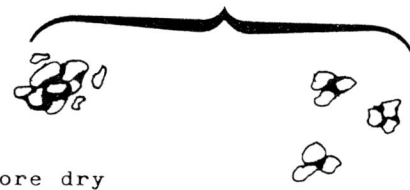

More dry particles contacting agglomerates

Less liquid at particle surface as agglomerates breakdown.

3.– REAGGLOMERATION

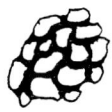

Particle point contact bridged by binder solution and/or solubilized ingredient.

4.– PASTE FORMATION

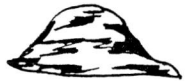

Wet mass with much loss of discrete particle units.

FIG. 8. Steps in the liquid–solid mixing in a high-shear mixer. (Adapted from Ref. 36.)

phenomenon increases (corresponding with the transition stage). The powder mixture changes to a wet mass which offers more resistance to shearing forces, that is, a greater shearing force is required to continue the mixing. Partial solubilization of some of the more soluble formulation ingredients increases resistance to the mixing, due to the increase in the viscosity of the liquid phase, and the end point of the wet massing is reached.

Paste formation follows. If the amount of granulating solution added is excessive ("overwetting") or mixing continues after reaching the final point of the granulation process ("overmassing"), a thick wet mass similar to a paste begins to form. This paste is difficult to granulate and upon drying the granules become extremely hard and are difficult to crush [40].

Addition of Granulation Liquid

The binder solution can be incorporated into the dry powder mixture in one or two steps. First a high concentrated binder solution is added and later additional liquid is incorporated to maintain a standard binder content [11].

The amount of granulation liquid normally needed to reach the capillary state depends, among other factors, on the characteristics of the wetting liquid [39,41]. An example is given in Table 11, where the amount of water and different solutions necessary to granulate 3 kg of filler are shown. Some authors recommend, in a general way, that this quantity ranges from one fifth to one tenth of the quantity of the material to be granulated. Other authors suggest that the tapped density of the dry mixture is related to the amount of water required to reach the capillary state, whenever constituents of the mixture do not absorb water. In this case, the amount of granulating liquid is 90–100% of the void space that exists among the powder particles, as determined by tapping. As it can see in Fig. 9, the higher the volume of the binder liquid, the greater the granule size and the lower the porosity [11,20,42].

Liquids with lower surface tension exhibit a higher wetting capacity, but produce weaker wet agglomerates with slower growth [19]. On the other hand, the higher the surface tension of the binder liquid, the greater the force of the liquid bridges created, that is, the greater the cohesive force of the agglomerates. This behavior is shown in Fig. 10, where the energy required to granulate PVP is higher than that to granulate other binders. The higher surface tension of this binder solution produces stronger ag-

TABLE 11 Granulation Liquid Required for 3000 g of Filler[a]

Granulation Liquid	Filler			
	Lactose	Sucrose	Mannitol	Dextrose
Water, mL	400	300	750	660
Starch paste, 10%, mL	460	285	810	660
Gelatin, 10%, mL	290	200	560	500
PVP in water, 10%, mL	340	260	525	470
Alcohol, 50%, mL	700	460	1000	1000
PVP in alcohol, 10%, mL	650	780	900	825

[a]Adapted from Ref. 2.

Wet Granulation

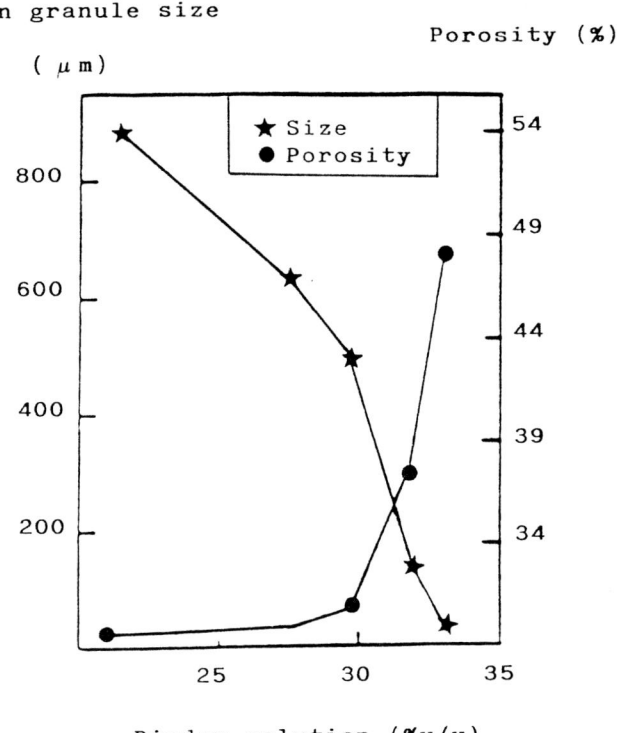

FIG. 9. Intragranular porosity and mean granule size versus volume of PVP solution (Kollidon 90, 3%) added. (Adapted from Ref. 42.)

glomerates, which offer a high resistance to agitation; consequently the energy consumption increases. In the same way, the higher the surface tension of the binder solution, the smaller the volume of it is needed to saturate the granules [42] and a faster granule growth is observed. For most materials, the surface tension/wet particle diameter ratio (T/D) must be higher than 4,600 dynes/cm^2 (460 Pa) for a satisfactory granular growth like capillary granules.

The End Point of Wet Mixing

The granulation end point depends on the characteristics of the formulation and the type of kneading equipment. It may be determined manually when a ball of wet mass can be formed by hand without crumbling. If it is split into two, it gives a clear fracture without sticking or crumbling. If the mass tends to stick or does not clearly break, it is usually overwetted. If it crumbles or breaks into pieces, it is underwetted [2].

In a more practical method, the granulation process is monitored by means of any device which determines the changes in the wet mass resistance produced during the wet massing [34,36]. Amperage, powder consumption, torque, and motor slip have been monitored as effects of the granulation process on the mixer [43–48]. For example, in Fig. 11, the variations in the mixer paddle torque, detected on adding the binder solu-

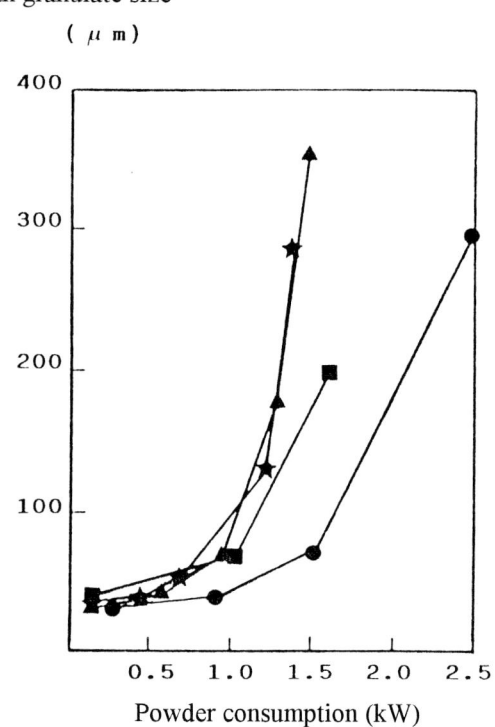

BINDER	Conc. (% w/v)	Surface tension (mN m^{-1}) (25°C)
● PVP (Kollidon 90®)	3	68
▲ PVP-PVA copolymer (Kollidon VA64®)	10	50
■ Hydrolysed gelatine (Protein S®)	10	53
★ HPMC (Methocel E15®)	2	50

FIG. 10. Correlation between mean granule size and powder consumption of an impeller motor (speed 400 rpm). (Adapted from Ref. 42.)

tion over the powder mass in a planetary mixer, are observed [49,50]. In the torque curve, several zones are differentiated:

- Zone 1 corresponds to the pendular bond formation between the binder liquid and the powder particles. The wet mass resistance to stirring is very low.
- In zone 2, funicular structures start to form and the torque begins to increase. At the

Wet Granulation

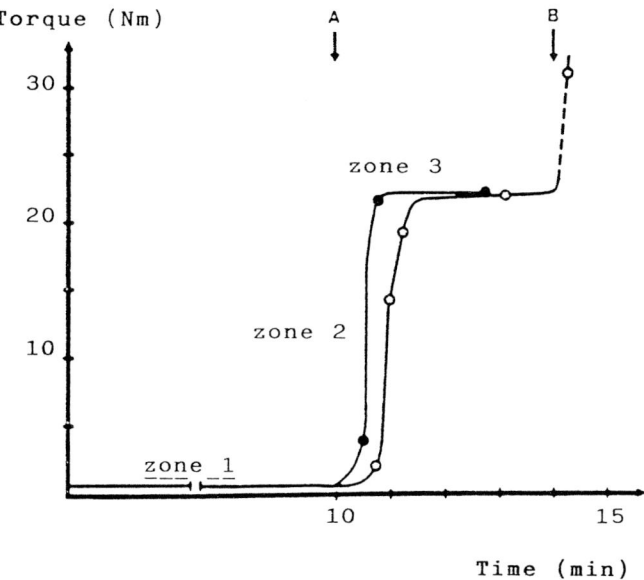

FIG. 11. The torque of the mixer paddle during the granulation of a powder mixture in a planetary mixer; (○) 1.5 kg binding solution added during 60 s; (●) 2.0 kg binding solution added during 5 s; (A) first addition; (B) second addition. (From Ref. 50.)

end of the zone 2 and near the zone 3, the capillary bond granule state is produced; this is the granulation final point.
- In zone 3 overmassing has been produced.

These monitoring devices used in granulation to detect the final point are essential for high speed mixers where the transition from a ungranulated to an overmassed system is very quick.

To guarantee the final product uniformity obtained by an industrial wet granulation process, it is necessary that the wet mixing of every batch of a formulation finishes at the same point.

Wet Screening

The aim of wet screening is to increase the numbers of contact points among the particles for consolidating the granules, and to increase the surface area for facilitating the drying [13]. During this step, the wet mass is forced to pass through a coarse sieve or through a standard perforated plate of 4, 6, 8, or 12 mesh [4.5, 3.15, 2.5, and 1.4 mm), depending on whether the wet mass passes through easily or not.

It is desirable to use the smallest opening possible in order to obtain small granules which facilitate drying because of their greater surface area [2,13,37]. The granulations obtained by sieving are more porous than those obtained by passing through perforated plates.

Wet screening is not always necessary. If the wet mixing has been carried out correctly, the wet mass is dryed directly, and the final granules can be easily crushed to the desired size [7].

Drying

The drying step is essential in all of the wet granulation procedures to eliminate the solvent used during the process of aggregation and reduce the moisture content of the granulation to an optimum value. During the drying step, solid bridges are formed which hold the particles of the aggregated granules. The resultant product is a free-flowing coarse material [13,37,40].

In order to guarantee the stability of the formulation constituents, it is always preferable to dry at the lowest temperature possible. When the formulation contains substances soluble in the granulation liquid which may crystallize during the drying step, slow drying avoids the formation of crusts that impede the internal drying of the granules [39,51].

The granulation must be dryed to an optimum moisture content for binder action since most binders are not effective in the absence of moisture. The friability development of a granulation with its moisture content and the drying time is represented in Fig. 12. As the water content decreases, friability increases, until the binder effect that builds up the solid bridges becomes apparent [52].

Sizing

After drying, the granulation is powdered and sieved again, with the aim of reducing particle size and, more important, of obtaining a uniform size distribution. If the wet granulation is an intermediate step in the tablet manufacturing, the particle size is usually 350–700 μm and presents a narrow distribution so that the tablet weight does not suffer appreciable variations [13,37,39,53].

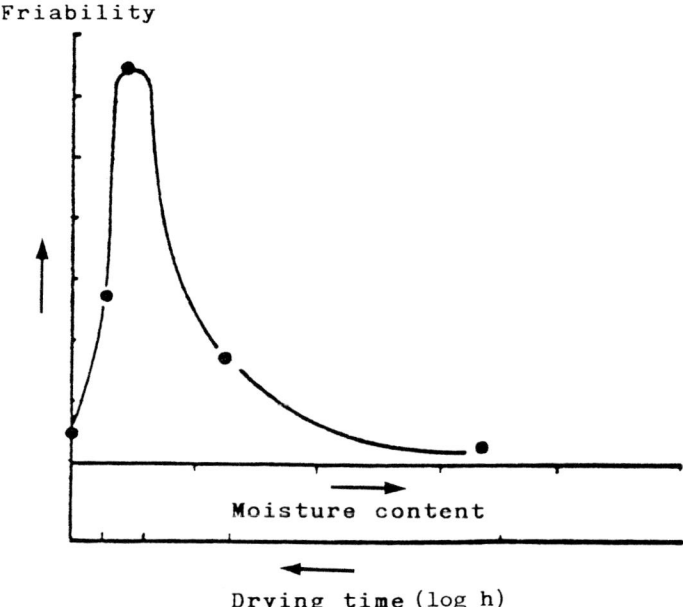

FIG. 12. The effect of moisture content on granule friability. (Adapted from Ref. 52.)

Advantages and Limitations of Wet Granulation

Wet granulation is a size-enlargement procedure of a powder particle, involving improvements in the powder characteristics. It is, however, not free of problems. The most important ones are related to heat- and moisture-sensitive drugs and soluble substances. In spite of these limitations, wet granulation is extensively used in the industrial manufacturing of tablets and pharmaceutical granules. This is partly due to the improvements in the traditional wet granulation method.

Advantages

Granulation increases the particle size and material sphericity. Moreover, the granules are discrete and rigid structures with a very slight tendency to be compacted by vibration or gravity and with a very low cohesive capacity among themselves. The use of a liquid medium can also change the surface free energy of the material. All these properties determine the high flowability of the granulations.

This improvement in the flowability of a granulated material is especially important in the tablet or capsule manufacture of high-dosage drugs which have a poor flow. Wet granulation gives a free-flowing product and guarantees uniform die filling in the tablet machine and of the capsules [2,17,21,54,55].

In spite of the fact that the granulation reduces cohesivity, the capacity of the granule to form a compact mass under pressure, that is, the compressibility, increases substantially. This increase is due to two fundamental facts. First, the granulation reduces the amount of retained air among the particles and thus reduces the possibility of elastic effects of this trapped air during the compression. Second, the binder films distributed inside and around of the granules are plastically deformed during the compression and join to other binder surfaces by hydrogen bonding [54–58]. As shown in Fig. 13, sulfadiazine forms weak tablets when used alone and capping is produced at high compression pressures, whereas with PVP stronger tablets are obtained without capping [20]. The granules with PVP are deformed plastically with the greatest ease and, with the same applied pressure, give rise to the greatest pressures in the die wall of the tablet machine which results in a harder tablet.

The application of lower pressures in the tablet machine to obtain tablets with the same hardness increases tooling life and machine wear.

Wet granulation improves the content uniformity of low-dosage drugs. It adds a liquid phase to the solid constituent mixture in which low-dosage drugs and color additives can be dissolved, giving a more homogeneous distribution. This represents a distinct advantage over direct compression, where content uniformity of drugs and uniform color dispersion can be a problem [2].

Wet granulation prevents segregation of components of a homogenous powder mix during processing, transfer, and handling. The powder mix is constituted normally by particles of different density, size, and shape. All the granules, although of different size, present the same composition, which is the same as, or very nearly, that of the powder mixture at the time of the liquid and binder addition. Segregation has a very small effect on the chemical composition variation of the final pharmaceutical form. The dissolution rate of hydrophobic drugs may be improved by wet granulation employing hydrophilic binders.

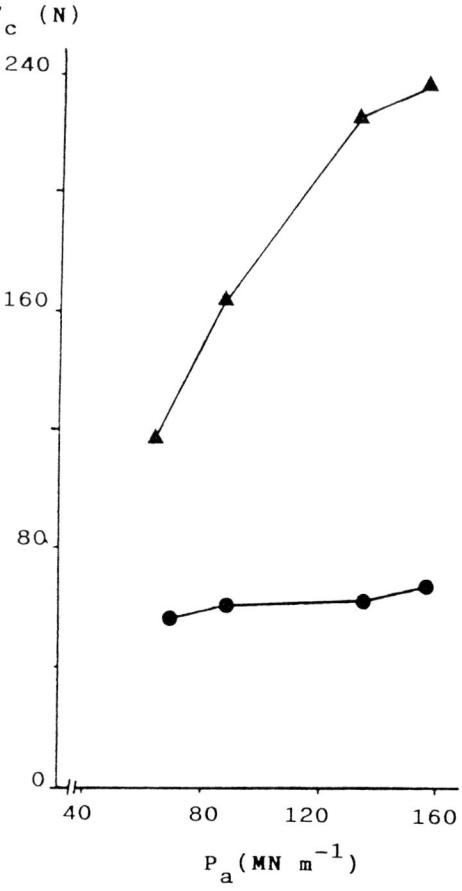

FIG. 13. The effect of the binding agent on the relationship between tablet crushing strength (F_c) and the pressure applied during compression (P_a); (●) sulfadiazine alone; (▲) sulfadiazine and PVP. (Adapted from Ref. 20.)

Very little dust is generated in wet granulation. As consequence, the contamination in the manufacturing plant and the risk for the workers are minimal.

Limitations

For wet granulation of moisture-sensitive drugs organic solvents are used as granulation liquid. However, the industrial use of expensive organic solvents creates problems of inflammability and toxicity. Security considerations demand that the work areas must have a good ventilation system to reduce the toxic effects of the solvents and keep the vapor concentration under explosion limits. Explosion-proof equipment must be used. Removal of the solvents during the drying step must follow the regulations of the Environmental Protection Agency (EPA) that limit the amount of solvent vapors which can be exhausted to the atmosphere and require the installation of a solvent-retrieval system. The drying ovens have to work with high airflow rates, keeping the vapor concentrations in the air always under the explosion limit. Finally, the entire process

Wet Granulation

must be checked, and the facilities must be inspected by security companies. These considerations increase the product price considerably [2,13,37].

The traditional wet granulation is a method that cannot be used for heat-sensitive drugs which would be destroyed during the drying step.

Soluble dyes dissolved in the granulating solution produce a homogeneous colored wet mass, but during drying, as the solvent evaporates, the dyes tend to migrate to the surface of the granules, causing unequal distribution of color. Although some redistribution occurs during subsequent mixing and milling, some color mottling of granulations and tablets may result [2]. This migration is more intense with alcohol or aqueous alcohol solutions. Dye migration is reduced by slow drying at low temperature and constant air circulation. A 5–10% addition of microcrystalline cellulose helps to prevent mottling. The starch paste is, in this sense, an excellent transport medium of dyes since the tendency of the dye to migrate to the surface of the granules during the drying is minimal. The use of insoluble dyes is the main answer to this problem. For this reason, lake dyes dispersed in the granulating liquid by a high-speed mixer are replacing the traditional soluble dyes.

Material migration during the drying step is not only produced by soluble dyes but also with any substance dissolved in the granulating liquid, such as binders or drugs. Figure 14 shows the distribution of PVP binder inside a granule after drying [52].

The active crystalline substance can be dissolved in the granulating liquid during the wet massing when the liquid phase is added to the powder mixture. During the drying of this wet mass, the drug recrystallizes, building solid bridges among the particles. The size of the crystals produced depends on the drying rate; the slower the drying process, the greater the crystal size. If the crystals produced in the recrystallization are larger than originally, the dissolution process should be slower, but if the crystals are smaller, the dissolution rate may increase as a consequence of the wet granulation. In any case, the drug bioavailability may be modified [34].

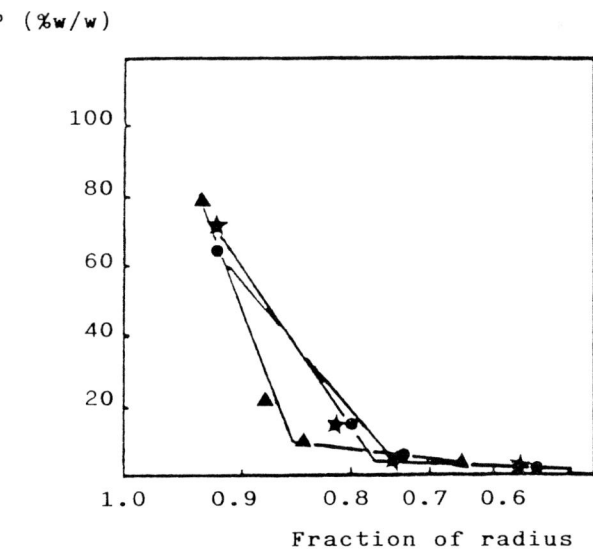

FIG. 14. PVP distribution with depth from the granule surface after: (▲) 1/2 h drying; (★) 3 h drying, and (●) 4 h drying. (Adapted from Ref. 52.)

The dissolution of a water-soluble active substances can be delayed and therefore drug bioavailability reduced. However, this effect can be diminished by the proper choice of the binder and by increasing the granulation porosity.

Any incompatibility among formulation components is increased by the granulation solvent and the binder agent, and by bringing them into close contact [2].

The greatest disadvantages of wet granulation are its complexity and its cost. It is a complex process involving several steps with a great number of parameters to be controlled. It is expensive due to the labor (workers and supervisors), equipment, energy, time (two days), and space requirements [2].

Tablet Manufacture by Wet Granulation

The preparation of granules for tablets by wet granulation is the oldest but still used method, despite the numerous advantages presented today by direct compression. (See the article "Direct Compression Tabletting" by R. F. Shangraw in Vol. 4, pp. 85–106, of this encyclopedia). A comparison of the steps in the manufacture of tablets by both methods is shown in the Table 12. Obviously direct compression is the simpler and less expensive method. However, wet granulation continues to find extensive application for different reasons. Due to its universal use in the past, the method persists with already established products. Some of these products could not be made by direct compression, without at least a change in excipients. However, this change would require a change in proceedings which may necessitate new stability and bioequivalency studies, etc. For this reason, the pharmaceutical industry has been unwilling to eliminate wet granulation. Formulation examples and procedures are given in Tables 13 and 14.

Wet granulation is the process of choice for the production of tablets with high-dosage drugs of poor flow and compressibility properties, of tablets with very powerful drugs that are used at low doses with a minimum of intertablet variation, of uniformely colored tablets, chewable tablets, and some types of sustained-release tablets (2).

Some formulators prefer to use wet granulation to ensure content uniformity in the resulting tablets, as they have more experience with this method.

TABLE 12 Tablet Manufacture by Wet Granulation and Direct Compression

Wet Granulation Steps	Direct Compression Steps
1. Milling of drugs and excipients	1. Milling of drugs and excipients
2. Solid–solid mixing	2. Solid–solid mixing
3. Preparation of binder solution	3. Tablet compression
4. Liquid–solid mixing	
5. Wet screening	
6. Drying	
7. Screening of dry granules	
8. Mixing of granules with additives	
9. Tablet compression	

Wet Granulation

TABLE 13 Wet Granulation Procedure[a] for Magnesium Hydroxide Tablets (Milk of Magnesia Tablets)[b]

Ingredients	Quantity per Tablet	
	mg	% w/w
Magnesium hydroxide (fine powder)	300	68.6
Sucrose, confectioners 6x	60	13.7
Gelatin solution, 5%	q.s.	q.s.
Magnesium stearate	7	1.6
Sodium bicarbonate (fine powder)	30	6.9
Citric acid (fine powder)	40	9.1
Oil of peppermint	0.5	0.1

[a]Mix the magnesium hydroxide and sucrose and moisten with the gelatin solution. Pass through a 12 mesh (1.4 mm) screen and dry at 60°C. Size by passing through a 16 mesh (1 mm) screen. Add the sodium bicarbonate, citric acid, and oil of peppermint and mix well. Finally add the magnesium stearate, mix, and compress using 7/16-in. flat-face bevel-edge punches.
[b]Data from Ref. 2.

Improvements in the Traditional Wet Granulation Method

During recent years some advances have been made to improve the traditional wet granulation method and reduce its cost [59]. These include:

- Development of high precision automatic systems to determine the end point of the granulation process.
- Design of granulation units in which the whole process of solid–solid mix, liquid–solid kneading, and drying can be completed in one unit.
- Design of fluidized-bed granulators by adaptation of a spray nozzle to the fluidized-bed dryers to add the binder. These systems are examples of control granulation to obtain uniform agglomerates. Granulation and drying are carried out simultaneously.

TABLE 14 Wet Granulation Procedure[a] for Aminophylline Tablets[b]

Ingredients	Quantity per Tablet Quantity	
	mg	% w/w
Aminophylline	100	50.8
Tricalcium phosphate	50	25.4
Pregelatinized starch	15	7.6
Water	q.s.	q.s.
Talc	30	15.2
Mineral oil, light	2	1

[a]Mix the aminophylline, tricalcium phosphate, and starch and moisten with water. Granulate by passing the wet mass through a 12 mesh (1.4 mm) screen and dry at 45°C. Pass the dry granulation through a 20 mesh (0.8 mm) screen. Mix with the talc and finally with the mineral oil. Compress using 5/16-in. deep-cut punches for enteric coating.
[b]Data from Ref. 2.

- Development of high speed or shearing mixers which provide efficient and quick solid–solid and solid–liquid blending, reducing time and material handling.
- Development of extrusion techniques as a special wet granulation method using more binder liquid and where the end product exhibits higher bulk density. Specific equipment is used because of different rheologic characteristics of the wet mass caused by higher wetting [60].

Equipment

The most frequently used equipment in wet granulation includes traditional shear mixers, high-speed or high-shear mixer/granulators, double-cone blenders, and fluidized-bed granulators. For specific applications other equipment, like spray dryers and extruders, can be used.

Traditional Equipment

In traditional wet granulation, every step of the process is carried out in a different piece of equipment. Dry powder constituents are mixed in mixers for solid materials. For wet massing, fixed-shell and moving-blade shear mixers, such as sigma blade, planetary mixers (Fig. 15), and conical-screw mixers, are normally used. The mixture of powders is placed in the mixer bowl and granulation liquid is added while the mixer paddle agitates. Later, the wet mass is transferred to a granulator, for example, an oscillating granulator (Fig. 16). The rotor bars of the granulator oscillate and force the wet mass to pass through the sieve screen. The granules are collected on trays and transferred to a drying oven or to a fluidized-bed dryer. The latter provides a faster method and, as it maintains the individual granules separated during drying, reduces the problems of aggregation and intergranular migration of the solute; it also eliminates a screening step after drying. The main disadvantages of the traditional granulation process are the need for several units of the equipment, its long duration, and the high loss of material during the transferences. The main advantages are few batch-to-batch variations in the characteristics of the granulation ingredients and that the final point of the wet-massing step can be often determined by inspection [13,15,36,55].

High-Speed Mixer–Granulators

This equipment can perform both dry and wet massing efficiently and in a short period of time. These granulators are equipped with a stainless steel mixing bowl where the powders are placed, a three-bladed impeller which mixes the dry powders and carries out wet massing, and a three-bladed auxiliary chopper that rotates at high speed (3000 rpm), intimately mixing the dry ingredients and breaking the wet mass to form a bed of fine granular material. The granulation liquid is added directly into the mixer through a port in the lid (Fig. 17).

The granular product is screened to eliminate large aggregates and transferred to a fluidized-bed dryer. Littleford Lodige and Diosnar Mixers are included in this category.

The main advantage of this equipment is that mixing, wet kneading, and granulation can be all carried out in the same unit during a short period of time (6 to 10 min).

Wet Granulation

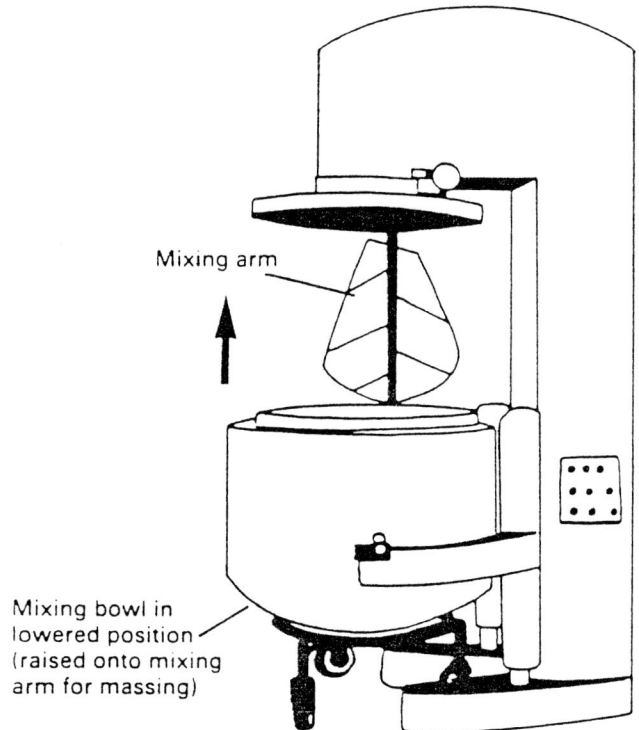

FIG. 15. Schematic of a planetary mixer for wet massing. (From Ref. 15.)

Normally these wet granules are of uniform size from 8 to 14 mesh (1.4–2.4 mm). There is a quick increment in the bulk density of the product due to the powerful compacting forces developed in the high-speed mixers. This is very important for two reasons. First, the quantity of liquid necessary to obtain a wet mass is about two-third or three-fourth parts of that used in traditional mixers. Therefore, when the granulation liquid contains binder, it is necessary to increase its concentration in agreement with the change of

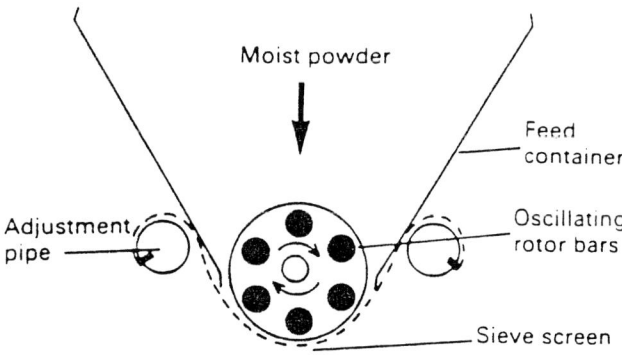

FIG. 16. Schematic of an oscillating granulator. (From Ref. 15.)

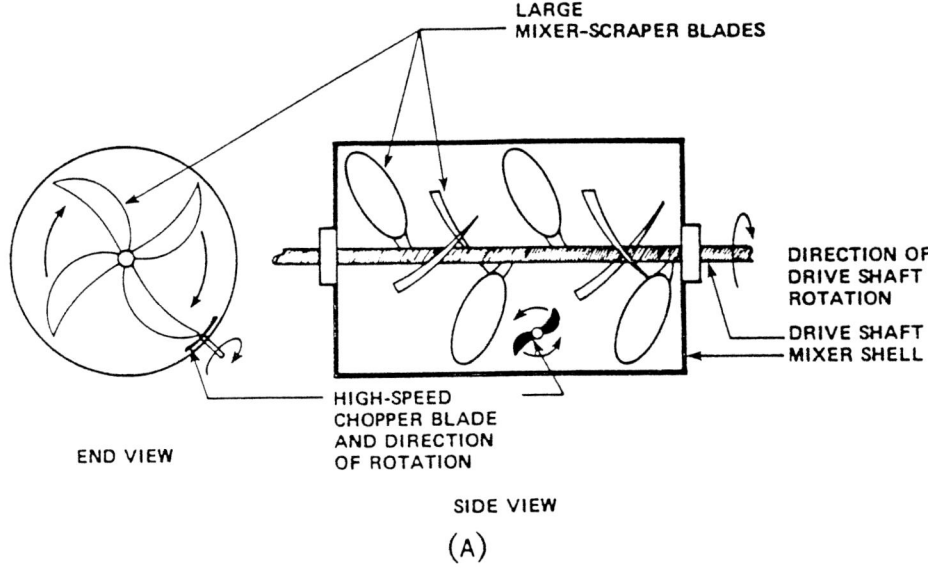

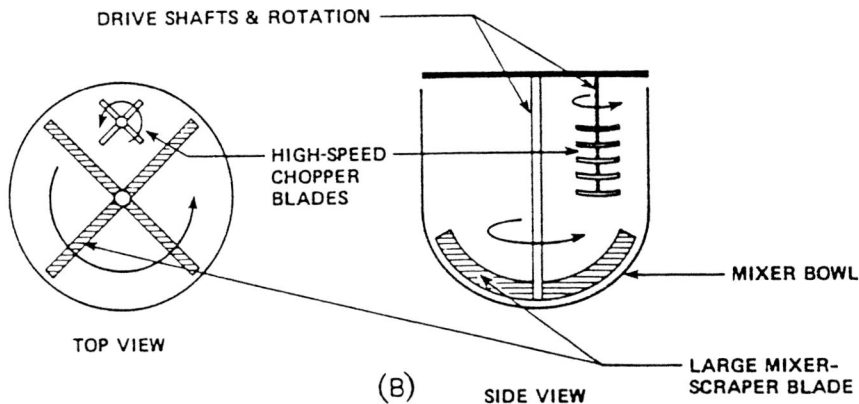

FIG. 17. Schematics of high-speed mixers. (A) Barrel type; (B) bowl type. (From Ref. 36.)

volume mentioned above. Second, the granulation process is so quick and so sensitive to a small variations in the raw material characteristics that it becomes indispensable to join the equipment with a monitoring system which can indicate the end point of the process and thus avoid producing an overmassed system. If dry mixing goes on too long, a reduction of the particle size, which is not wanted, can be happen. This fact may change the characteristics of the final granulation.

Among the disadvantages of this equipment is the possible contamination of the product from the packing gland, where the handle passes through the mixer shell. This has been prevented by using mechanical seals or air-flushed packing glands.

High-speed mixer–granulators are manufactured in ranges from small sizes (0.08 m^3) to production sizes (more than 1000 kg) [13,15,36,27].

Wet Granulation

Double-Cone Mixer-Dryer

Many manufacturers of the double-cone and twin-shell blenders have made several modifications in this equipment so that the steps of powder mixing, wet massing, and drying can be carried out in the same unit (Fig. 18). Included are stirring elements that allow both solid mixing and wet massing; a liquid feeding system which allows the addition of granulation liquid without stopping the mixing; and a vacuum drying system. Normally, the unit is provided with a steam jacket around the mixer shell to increase the granulation temperature.

As in any vacuum drying operation, equipment and drying costs are relatively high and the times are long. The main advantages are the possibility to carry out both wet massing and drying in the same equipment and to use it for granulation with organic solvents. Standard auxiliary equipment is also available to provide complete solvent retrieval [13,15,36].

Fluidized-Bed Granulators

The agglomeration of powder materials and their drying take place simultaneously in the same equipment which is based on the same principle as fluidized-bed dryers. A heated air bed fluidizes and mixes the solid particles. The granulation liquid is pumped through a spray nozzle on the particles causing their agglomeration. The agglomerates are dried by the same heated fluidizing air stream (Fig. 19).

Although this equipment is initially expensive, it reduces the work cost, material loss due to transferences (with the problem of dust generation), and processing time (60 to

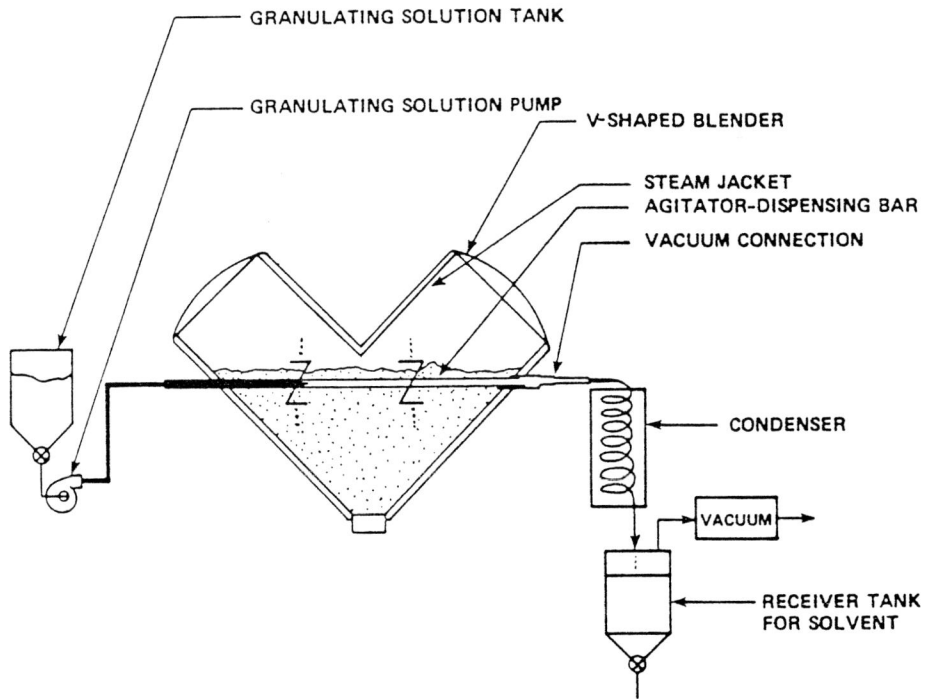

FIG. 18. Schematic of V-shaped blender and processor. (From Ref. 36.)

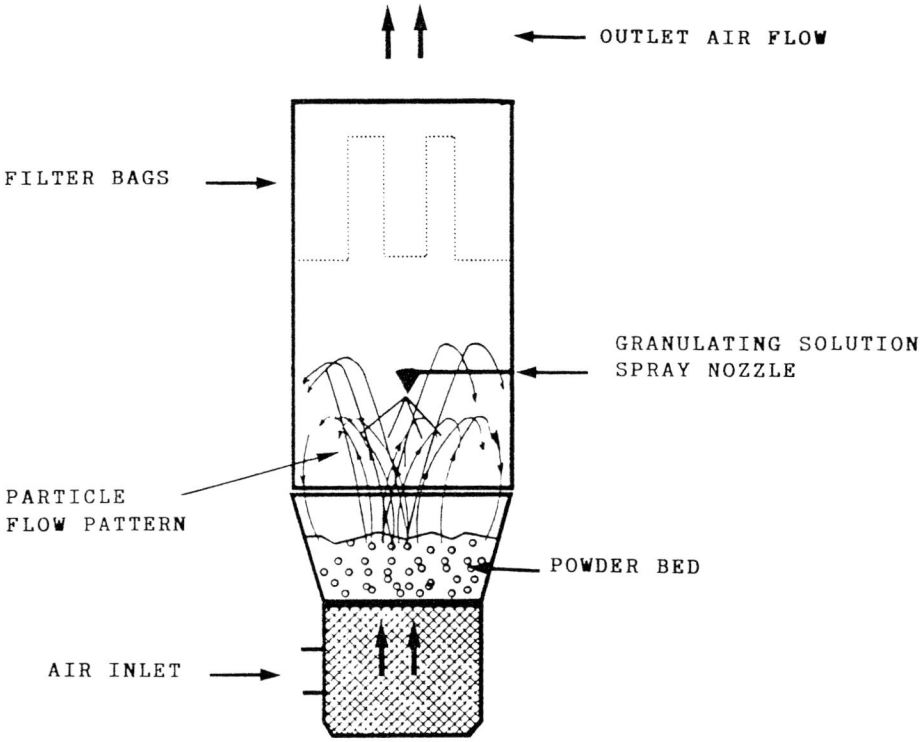

FIG. 19. Schematic of fluidized-bed granulator. (From Ref. 61.)

90 min) because the wet massing and drying are carried out in the same unit, just like in the double-cone mixer-dryer. Other advantages are short exposure time of the product to heat; the possibility of controlling, in a precise way, the level of moisture in the granulations; a solvent-retrieval system; layered granulations; and the possibility to automate the process as soon as the conditions which affect the granulation have been optimized. The optimization parameters of the process require development work not only during the formulation step but also during the scale-up. Many variables affect the quality of the final granulation, such as binder concentration, viscosity, and volatility of the granulation liquid, spraying speed and drop size, speed and temperature of the fluidizing air, and others [15,23,27,61,62].

Spray Dryers

Granules for compression are prepared by spray drying only when other methods cannot be used, because spray drying is very expensive. A suspension of drug and excipients are prepared in the binder solution, which is atomized within the drying chamber of the spray dryer. As granules remain in the drying chamber only for a very short period of time, spray drying is a good wet granulation method for heat-sensitive substances. The resultant granules are free-flowing hollow spheres with high compressibility [13,15,63].

Wet Granulation

Extruders

Spheronization or pelletization equipment, mainly extruders, is used when it is desirable to obtain a spherical and more dense granulation.

The extrusion process is similar to the granulation process in a oscillating granulator, but requires a wetter mass and a stronger screen than that normally used in the oscillating granulator. In extrusion, the wet mass is forced to pass through a perforated plate by means of an auger feed. The formed strings of material are poured on a rotatory plate which turns inside a static cylinder. On rotating, the plate throws the strings to the edges where, on collision with the cylinder wall, they break into spheres. Later, these spheres are transfered to a fluidized bed for drying [15,60,64]. (See the article "Extrusion and Extruders" by K. E. Fielden and J. M. Newton, Vol. 5, pp. 395–442, of this encyclopedia).

Scale-Up Problems

When improving the production process, it should become more efficient with fewer steps, less handling, fewer variables to control, shorter duration of time, and lower costs. Thus, the scale-up of a wet granulation process from laboratory batches to medium-size and industrial-size production scale is a very complex project. It should be kept in mind that there are neither fixed rules nor complex equations that can be applied to the scale-up of a wet granulation process. Normally, the change of the scale is based on empirical schedules and mainly on the experience of those responsible for the project. The difficulty of the project is even greater when economic restrictions do not allow to use the more adequate type and size of the mixer except the one available [30,65,66].

Transfer of materials in the traditional granulation equipments and in the high speed mixer–granulators is the first problem to be considered. Very extensive transfer lines can cause loss of materials which must be taken into account and compensated for. Moreover, this loss of materials produces pollution in the work area. Special locations of the different equipment that takes part in the granulation process must be designed in such a way that the transfer of material from one piece of equipment to another should be carried out directly by gravity. For example, when a high speed mixer is used in production, the mixer unit is lifted up by a pneumatic system, so that the container of the fluidized-bed dryer can be put under it. Obviously, no problem of this type occurs when the whole wet granulation process is carried out in a single unit [28].

Another common problem is connected with viscosity and addition rate of granulating fluid. Sometimes, it may be necessary in the scale-up, that part of the binder should be added as dry powder to avoid working with highly viscous solutions which can clog the pipes. The safety measures needed to work with organic solvents and the solvent-retrieval systems should be considered in the selection and the design of both equipment and manufacturing area.

In general, volume of binder liquid and mixing time are variables in the scale-up in any type of equipment, but the saturation degree of wet mass in the final stage of granulation must be constant. For example, the compactness of the product, due to the larger amount of kneaded mass, increases the density of the wet mass for a same addition of granulating liquid. A 10–20% reduction of the quantity of the granulating liquid

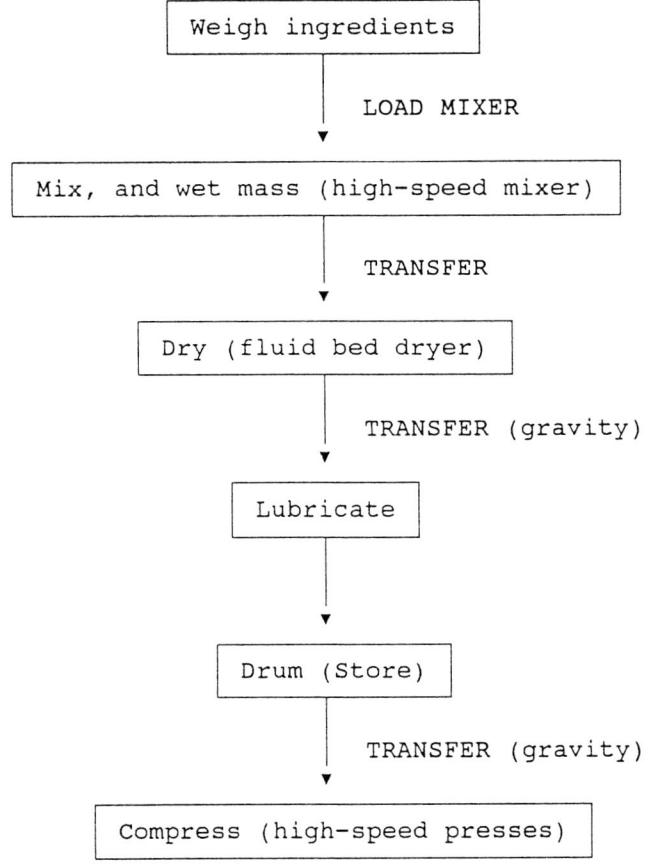

FIG. 20. Systems design of tablet production by wet granulation. (Adapted from Ref. 13.)

is usually necessary to obtain a wet mass with the same characteristics. This adjustment is normally carried out by means of a monitoring system of the wet massing which detects the final point [67,68].

In order that scale-up criteria can be applied in wet granulation procedures, all the equipment, from pilot to industrial scale, should be as similar as possible with regard to shape, diameter/height ratio of the container, and relative volume generated by the paddle in the unit time, and should operate with the same values for the main operating parameters (paddle peripheral speed, spraying specific speed, temperature). Equipment with different geometric shapes does not permit the application of the same scale-up criteria. Generally, scale-up criteria require that pilot experimentation should be carried out in equipment of, at least, 25-L useful capacity [69,70].

The future of the wet granulation method (Fig. 20) in the pharmaceutical industry mainly depends on the improvement of the unitary operations, the possibility of combining the different steps of the process, the improvement of the material-handling techniques, and the design of automated equipment [30].

Bibliography

Ghebre-Sellassie, I., ed., *Pharmaceutical Pelletization Technology*, Vol. 37, Marcel Dekker, Inc., New York, 1989.

Knepper, W. A., ed., *Agglomeration*, John Wiley, New York, 1962.

Lieberman, H. A., and Lachman, L., eds., *Pharmaceutical Dosage Forms: Tablets*, Vols. 1-3, Marcel Dekker, Inc., New York, 1980-1982.

Record, P. C., *J. Powder Bulk Solids Technol.*, 4:33-40 (1980).

Summers, M. P., Granulation. In: *Pharmaceutics. The Science of Dosage Forms Design* (M. E. Aulton, ed.), Churchill Livingstone, New York, 1988, pp. 616-628.

References

1. Suñé-Arbussá, J. M., and Suñé Negré, J. M., Nuevas formas farmacéuticas. In: *Historia General de la Farmacia* (G. Follch, J. M. Suñé, J. L. Valverde, and F. J. Puerto, eds.), Ediciones Sol, S. A., Madrid, 1986, pp. 577-587.
2. Sheth, B. B., Bandelin, F. J., and Shangraw, R. F., Compressed Tablets. In: *Pharmaceutical Dosage Forms, Tablets*, Vol. 1 (H. A. Lieberman and L. Lachman, eds.), Marcel Dekker, Inc., New York, 1980, pp. 109-185.
3. American Pharmaceutical Association and The Royal Pharmaceutical Society of Great Britain, *Handbook of Pharmaceutical Excipients*, The Pharmaceutical Press, London, 1994.
4. Wadke, D. A., and Jacobson, H., Preformulation Testing. In: *Pharmaceutical Dosage Forms*, Vol. 1 (H. A. Lieberman and L. Lachman, eds.), Marcel Dekker, Inc., 1980, pp. 1-60.
5. Torres, A. I., and Camacho, M. A., *Eur. J. Pharm. Biopharm.*, 40(1):41-43 (1994).
6. Wan, L. S., Heng, P. W., and Muhuri, G., *Int. J. Pharm.*, 88(Dec. 8):159-163 (1992).
7. Fonner, D. E., Anderson, N. R., and Banker, G. S., Granulation and Tablet Characteristics. In: *Pharmaceutical Dosage Forms: Tablets*, Vol. 2 (H. A. Lieberman and L. Lachman, eds.), Marcel Dekker, Inc., New York, 1981, pp. 185-267.
8. Torres, A. I., and Camacho, M. A., *Industria Farmacéutica*, Marzo/Abril:85-92 (1991).
9. Carstensen, J. T., Tablets. In: *Pharmaceutical Principles of Solid Dosage Forms* (J. T. Carstensen, ed.), Technomic Publishing Company, Inc., Lancaster, PA, 1993, pp. 63-94.
10. Fiese, E. F., and Hagen, T. A., Preformulation. In: *The Theory and Practice of Industrial Pharmacy*, 3rd ed., (H. A. Lieberman, L. Lachman, and J. L. Kanig, eds.), Lea & Febiger, Inc., Philadelphia, 1986, pp. 171-195.
11. Rubinstein, M. H., Tablets. In: *Pharmaceutics. The Science of Dosage Forms Design* (M. E. Aulton, ed.), Churchill Livingstone, New York, 1988, pp. 304-321.
12. Mohrle, B., Effervescent Tablets. In: *Pharmaceutical Dosage Forms: Tablets,* Vol. 1 (H. A. Lieberman and L. Lachman, eds.), Marcel Dekker, Inc., New York, 1980, pp. 226-257.
13. Banker, G. S., and Anderson, N. R., Tablets. In: *The Theory and Practice of Industrial Pharmacy*, 3rd ed. (H. A. Lieberman, L. Lachman, and J. L. Kanig, eds.), Lea & Febiger, Inc., Philadelphia, 1986, pp. 293-344.
14. Thies, C., Microencapsulation. In: *Encyclopedia of Polymer Science and Engineering* (J. Kroschwitz, ed.), Vol. 9, 2nd ed., John Wiley & Sons, 1987, pp. 724-745.
15. Summers, M. P., Granulation. In: *Pharmaceutics. The Science of Dosage Forms Design* (M. E. Aulton, ed.), Churchill Livingstone, New York, 1988, pp. 616-628.
16. Suñé, J. M., Granulación. In: *Tratado de Farmacia Galénica* (C. Faulí i Trillo, ed.), Luzán 5, S. A de Ediciones, Madrid, 1993, pp. 321-328.

17. Harwood, C. F., and Pilpel, N., *J. Pharm. Sci.,* 57(3):478–481 (1968).
18. Symecko, C. W., Romero, A. J., and Rhodes, C. T., *Drug Dev. Ind. Pharm.,* 19(10):1131–1141 (1993).
19. Rohera, B. D., and Zahir, A., *Drug Dev. Ind. Pharm.,* 19(7):773–792 (1993).
20. Shotton, E., *Boll. Chim. Farm.,* 116:315–333 (1977).
21. Torres, A. I., Gil, M. E., and Gamacho, M. A., *Pharm. Acta Helv.,* 69:101–105 (1994).
22. Salhi, A., Delacourte, A., and Guyot, J. C., *STP Pharma,* 3(1):41–47 (1987).
23. Marshall, K., and Rudnic, E. M., Tablet Dosage Forms. In: *Modern Pharmaceutics,* 2nd ed., revised and expanded (G. S. Banker and C. T. Rhodes, eds.), Marcel Dekker, Inc., New York, 1990, pp. 355–425.
24. Ghebre-Sellassie, I., Mechanism of Pellet Formation and Growth. In: *Pharmaceutical Pelletization Technology,* Vol. 37 (I. Ghebre-Sellassie, ed.), Marcel Dekker, Inc., New York, 1989, pp. 123–143.
25. Rumpf, H., The Strength of Granules and Agglomerates. In: *Agglomeration* (W. A. Knepper, ed.), Interscience Publishers, New York, 1958, pp. 379–419; Rumpf, H., Particle Adhesion. In: *Agglomeration* (W. A. Knepper, ed.), John Wiley, New York, 1962, pp. 97–129.
26. Barlow, C. G., *Chem. Eng.,* 196 (1969).
27. Record, P. C., *J. Powder Bulk Solids Technol.,* 4:33–40 (1980).
28. Worts, O. M., *Rev. Port. Farm.,* 23:438–449 (1973).
29. Newitt, D. M., and Conway-Jones, J. M., *Trans. Instn. Chem. Engrs.,* 36:422–442 (1958).
30. Harder, S., and Van Buskirk, G., Pilot Plant Scale-up Techniques. In: *The Theory and Practice of Industrial Pharmacy,* 3rd ed. (H. A. Lieberman, L. Lachman, and J. L. Kanig, eds.), Lea & Febiger, Inc., Philadelphia, 1986, pp. 681–710.
31. Schubert, H., Tensile Strength and Capillary Pressure of Moist Agglomerates. In: *Agglomeration* (W. A. Knepper, ed.), John Wiley, New York, 1962, pp. 144–155.
32. Adorjan, L. A., Theoretical Prediction of Strength of Moist Particulate Materials. In: *Agglomeration* (W. A. Knepper, ed.), John Wiley, New York, 1962, pp. 130–143.
33. Vázquez, F., Los Comprimidos: una Forma Farmacéutica Clásica en el Umbral del Siglo XXI. In: *III Congreso Internacional de Ciencias Farmacéuticas Proceedings,* Symposium V: Farmacia Industrial (Consejo General de Colegios Oficiales de Farmacéuticos, ed.), 1987, pp. 1129–1167.
34. Marshall, K., Compression and Consolidation of Powdered Solids. In: *The Theory and Practice of Industrial Pharmacy,* 3rd ed. (H. A. Lieberman, L. Lachman and J. L. Kanig, eds.), Lea & Febiger, Inc., Philadelphia, 1986, pp. 66–99.
35. Capes, C. E., Size Enlargement Methods and Equipment. In: *Handbook of Powder Science and Tecnology* (M. E. Fayed and L. Otten, eds.), Van Nostrad Reinhold, New York, 1984, pp. 230–251.
36. Lantz, R. J., and Schwartz, J. B., Mixing. In: *Pharmaceutical Dosage Forms: Tablets,* Vol. 2 (H. A. Lieberman and L. Lachman, eds.), Marcel Dekker, Inc., New York, 1981, pp. 1–53.
37. Armstrong, N. A., Tableting. In: *Pharmaceutics. The Science of Dosage Forms Design* (M. E. Aulton, ed.), Churchill Livingstone, New York, 1988, pp. 647–668.
38. Poole, K. R., Taylor, R. F., and Wall, G. P., *Trans. Instn. Chem. Engrs.,* 42:T305–T315 (1964).
39. Nogueira, L., Correia, A., and Morgado, R., Formas Complementares Dos Pós. In: Téchnica Farmacêutica e Farmácia Galéncia, Vol. I, 4th ed. (L. Nogueira, A. Correia, and R. Morgado, eds.), Fundaçao Calouste Gulbenkien, Lisbon, 1992, pp. 648–948.
40. Zoglio, M. A., Huber, H. E., Koehne, G., Chan, P. L., and Carstensen, J. T., *J. Pharm. Sci.,* 65(8):1205–1207 (1976).

Xenobiotic Metabolism

Introduction

Drug metabolism can be viewed as a series of transformation reactions in which a drug reacts with an enzyme system involved in normal cell metabolism or biosynthesis. These biotransformed chemicals are usually pharmacologically less active and can be more readily excreted. The drug metabolism enzymes consist of a limited number of enzymes, and the major enzyme classes are discussed in this article. Although the biotransformation reactions vary extensively in their chemistry, they do have some common characteristics:

- They are concentrated into major organs of entry (liver, gastrointestinal (GI) tract, lung).
- They are often induced upon exposure to xenobiotic substrates.
- There is a high species variation (i.e., protein sequences) for biotransformation enzymes
- They exhibit a very broad substrate range, often lacking even functional group specificity [1].

Drug metabolism reactions have been classified as Phase I reactions of functionalization and Phase II reactions of conjugation, as outlined in Table 1. Most of the enzyme systems or families involved in xenobiotic metabolism have been shown to consist of subfamilies of enzymes containing many isoenzymes. Classically, isoenzymes are defined as enzymes differing in amino acid sequence, which act on the same substrate(s) to produce the same product(s). Because of the broad substrate reactivity of the enzymes within a family, the term isoenzyme often limited to describe enzymes with extensive protein homology and the term isoform is refers to enzymes within the same subfamily. Currently, a very active area of research in drug metabolism is the purification and characterization of the isoenzymes present within a species and the development of specific substrates and inhibitors of these enzymes. Many excellent texts have been published describing the chemical and biological aspects of drug metabolism [2–5] but due to the rapid discoveries being made in the biochemical, physiological, and genetic aspects of drug metabolism there is a constant need for on-going reviews in this area. However, these texts and articles serve as a valuable resources for understanding the complexity, chemistry, and structural diversity of substrates involved in these reactions. Such detailed structural information cannot be included here.

Phase I Oxidative Metabolism
Cytochrome P450 Enzyme Systems

The most extensively studied oxidative enzyme system consists of the cytochrome P450s, usually abbreviated as CYP450. Many reviews have been written covering its chemis-

TABLE 1 Phase I and Phase II Metabolism Reactions

Phase I, Functionalization Reactions	Phase II, Conjugation Reactions
Oxidation	Glycosylation (primarily glucuronidation)
Reduction	Sulfation
Hydrolysis–hydration	Acetylation
	Methylation
	Coenzyme A (amino acid, chiral inversion, fatty acids)
	Glutathione

try, enzyme mechanism, and structure [6–11], substrate specificity of isoforms [12], and enzyme inhibition [13–16]. The CYP450 consists primarily of two proteins, a heme protein (cytochrome P450) involved in substrate and oxygen binding and a reductase protein (NADPH-cytochrome P450 reductase) that shuttles electrons from NADPH to cytochrome P450. The CYP450 is important in the biosynthesis of numerous endogenous substrates (prostaglandins, fatty acids, steroids, bile acids) and biotransformation of xenobiotic compounds. The CYP450 is present in virtually all tissues with high concentrations in the liver, adrenal medulla, GI mucosal lining, lung, and kidney. Within the cell, the CYP450 exists as a group of membrane-bound enzymes found in the endoplasmic reticulum. They are present in both the microsomal and mitochondrial membrane fractions. The enzyme consists of an apoprotein (45–55 kDa) in which a single iron-heme prosthetic group is embedded. The CYP450s are anchored to the membrane by one or two transmembrane segments at the N-terminus. The portion of the enzyme containing the active site pocket is on the cytosolic side of the membrane, where enzymes may be anchored in a cluster of up to 20 CYP450 for each NADPH-cytochrome P450 reductase [17]. The proteins can be solubilized from the membrane and purified, but many studies are performed with cDNA-expressed human CYP450 isoforms or even crude microsomal preparations.

Cytochrome P450 Oxidation Chemistry

Oxidation occurs by activation of molecular oxygen in which one oxygen is incorporated into the substrate and the second oxygen is reduced to water [6,10,18,19]. The catalytic cycle is depicted in Fig. 1. The active site within the enzymes consists of an iron-heme ligated to the sulfur of a cysteine residue of the apoprotein. The reactive oxene intermediate ($Fe^{+5}=O$) undergoes radical like reactions and is reactive enough to split aliphatic C–H bonds, add to π-bonds comparable to a weak electrophile, or remove single electrons from heteroatoms as shown in Fig. 2. The regioselectivity and stereoselectivity for each isoform of the enzyme is dependent on both electronic and steric components present in the substrate [8]. Based on the mechanism proposed for the reaction intermediate (a radical and/or cationic substrate intermediate followed by radical recombination), the major site(s) of oxidation can usually be predicted, provided the steric constraints imposed by the enzyme active site allows access to that portion of the molecule.

Aliphatic and Alicyclic Hydroxylation. Hydroxylation occurs on aliphatic and alicyclic substituents at the position which best stabilizes the radical intermediate, provid-

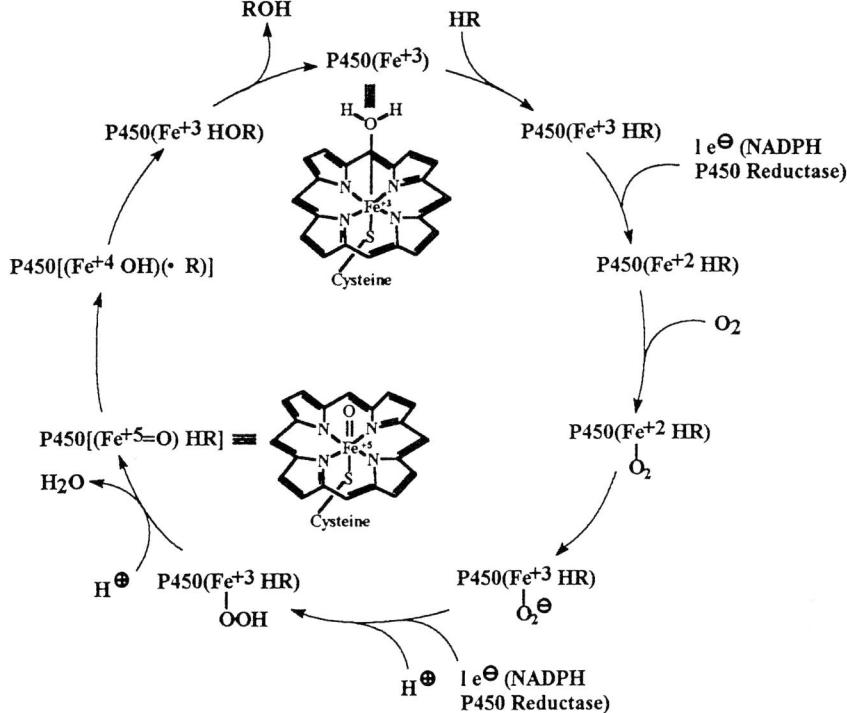

FIG. 1. Catalytic cycle for microsomal CYP450; partial structure of heme complex is shown. (Adapted from Refs. 18 and 19.)

ing there are no steric constraints [7]. Examples include hydroxylation at a benzylic methyl or methylene group, with allylic methylene, or terminal isopropyl substituent present in the molecule. Shown in Fig. 3 are the common reaction products obtained from a molecule that contains an aliphatic side chain. Hydroxylation primarily occurs at the penultimate carbon atom in the chain (ω-1 hydroxylation). However, with the weak steric and electronic constraints imposed by the active site, hydroxylation can occur on the terminal carbon, although usually to a lesser degree. Due to the transient radical intermediate, additional carbon radical transfer can occur, leading to the introduction of a double bond into the substrate (e.g., valproic acid).

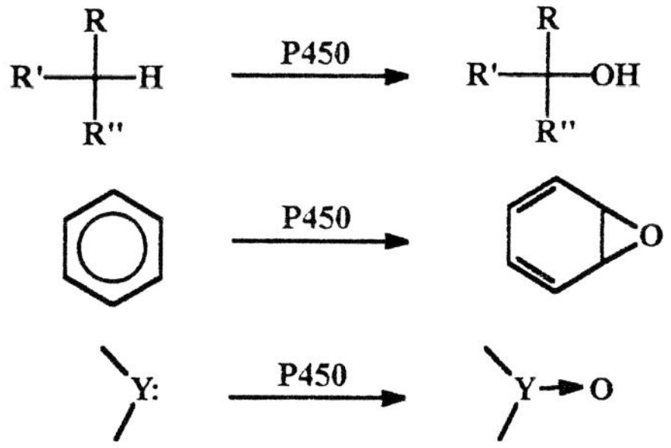

FIG. 2. Oxidation reaction catalyzed by CYP450.

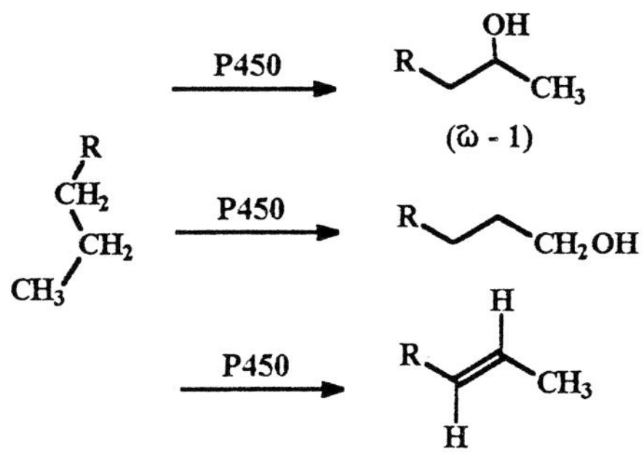

FIG. 3. Products of aliphatic oxidation by CYP450.

Aromatic Hydroxylation. The oxene intermediate adds to π-bonds of an aromatic ring, forming an epoxide on the substrate. The major reaction products obtained when an aromatic ring undergoes epoxidation [6,10,18] are shown in Fig. 4. Depending on the other ring substitutents and the extent to which they destabilize the epoxide, it can rearrange nonenzymatically to phenols or it can be hydrolyzed by epoxide hydrolase to dihydrodiols. The dihydrodiols can be dehydrogenated to catechols or dehydrated to phenols. These phenolic products closely parallel the reaction products of aromatic electrophilic substitution reactions. The electron-donating substituents on the aromatic ring of a substrate usually increase ring hydroxylation at the ortho or para positions, whereas electron-withdrawing substituents reduce or prevent hydroxylation of the ring at the meta position. Steric factors are important, with para hydroxylation usually more likely than ortho hydroxylation. For drugs in which two or more aromatic rings may be substrates for oxidation, the phenol formed continues to follow the pattern predicted by an electrophilic substitution reaction; for example, propranolol is metabolized on the oxygen-substituted ring to 4'-hydroxypropranolol (Fig. 5). When other competitive oxidative pathways are available (i.e., aliphatic oxidation), the quantitative importance of aromatic hydroxylation is often reduced.

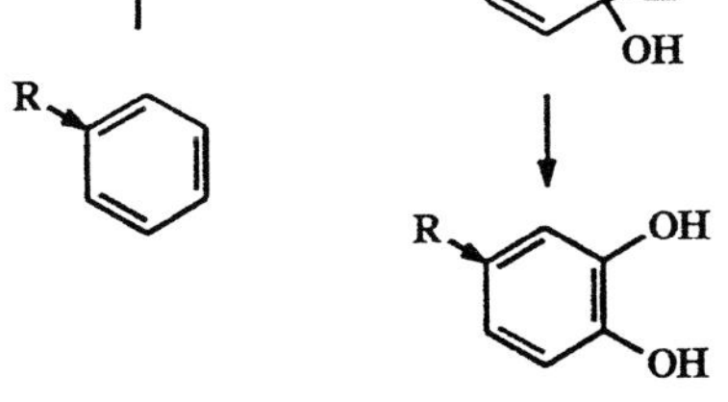

FIG. 4. Products of aromatic oxidation by CYP450.

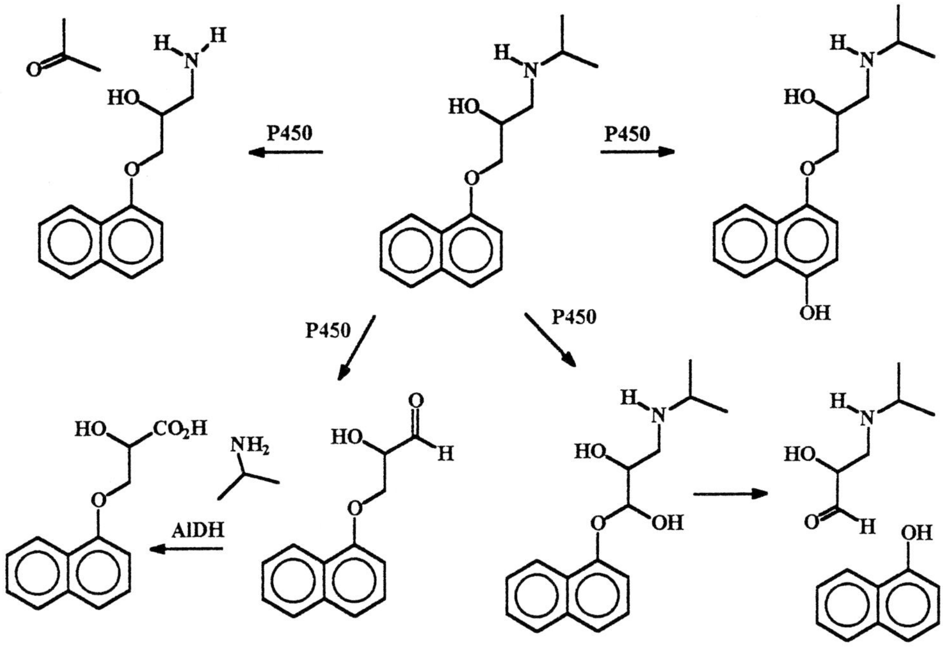

Xenobiotic Metabolism

FIG. 5. Oxidative metabolites of propranolol [19].

N-, O-, and S-Dealkylation. The removal of an alkyl group attached to nitrogen, oxygen, or sulfur is a commonly encountered route of metabolism. The substituents that can be metabolically removed must have a hydrogen atom α to the heteroatom. Some of the substituents commonly lost include methyl, ethyl, isopropyl, benzyl, etc. Oxidation can also occur α to the heteroatom in aliphatic heterocyclic rings accompanied by ring opening. A common mechanism (Fig. 6) has been proposed for N-, O-, and S-dealkylation. Hydroxylation occurs at the carbon atom α to the heteroatom leading to formation of a hemiaminal, hemiacetal, or hemithioacetal. These products rapidly break down to give the amine, alcohol, phenol, or thiol and the alkyl group as the appropriate aldehyde or ketone. A second mechanism has been proposed for N-dealkylation

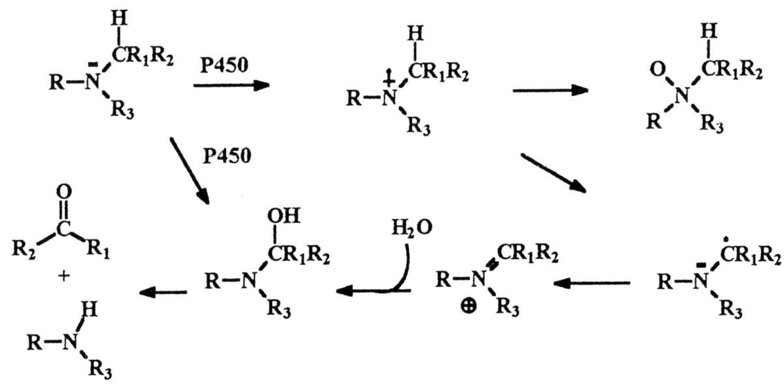

FIG. 6. Oxidative metabolism of nitrogen by CYP450.

in which the electron is abstracted from the nitrogen lone pair electrons to form an amine radical cation followed by loss of a proton to form an iminium ion. This intermediate is hydrated and gives the same products as the first mechanism. The second mechanism (see Fig. 6) is important in the formation of N-oxides by CYP450 from compounds resulting in nitrogen and sulfur oxidation products (disulfides, sulfoxides, and sulfones). During the oxidation of nitrogen, the intermediate amine radical cation can combine with the partially reduced oxene intermediate to form the N-oxide. The N-oxide pathway occurs primarily with tertiary amines and N-heterocycles. In the metabolism of propranolol (Fig. 5) multiple N- and O-dealkylation reactions occur via CYP450.

Induction and Inhibition of CYP450

Many drugs and xenobiotics have been shown to enhance or increase their own metabolism or the metabolism of other compounds, greatly modifying the pharmacological effect of the compound. This phenomenon is called enzyme induction and is defined as an increase in enzyme synthesis after exposure to a chemical over the rate of synthesis of the enzyme in subjects not exposed to the agent. Many drugs and chemicals increase the synthesis of many CYP450 isoforms. These agents have no common structural feature. The mechanism by which induction is initiated is poorly understood, except for the polycyclic hydrocarbons (PAH). The PAHs bind to a specific receptor (Ah receptor) that binds to the nucleus and increases mRNA transcription similar to the way in which steroids bind to their receptors and increase mRNA transcription. Common inducing agents, and the CYP450 isoforms they induce, are phenobarbital (CYP2B), polycyclic hydrocarbons (CYP1A), polychlorinated biphenyls, rifampicin (CYP3A), and dexamethasone (CYP3A) [20,21].

Inhibition of CYP450 is involved in a large number of reported drug interactions. Increasing emphasis is being placed on understanding the importance of a new drug or chemical on this enzyme system prior to their being introduced into humans. Model systems are currently being developed so that interactions with this enzyme system can be accurately predicted at the early stages of drug development. The CYP450s can be inhibited by four mechanisms:

1. Diversion of electrons through the NADPH-cytochrome P450 reductase enzyme (e.g., dipyridium),
2. Competition for the binding site on the apoprotein (e.g., perfluorinated hydrocarbons),
3. Slow reversible binding of lipophilic molecules to the heme iron (e.g., imidazole-based antifungals), and
4. Metabolic inactivation (mechanism-based inhibitor).

The two last mechanism seem to be of primary importance in the inhibition of drug metabolism in clinical situations [13–15].

The slow reversible binding of lipophilic nitrogen to the heme iron can occur with many of the nitrogen-containing heterocycles (imidazoles, pyridines, quinolines, etc.) and anilines attached as substituents to a lipophilic molecule. Whether inhibition occurs with a specific compound is dependent on the substituents adjacent to the nitrogen, that is, if the nitrogen lone pair can complex with the heme iron. If steric hindrance is

Xenobiotic Metabolism

provided around the complexing nitrogen, it cannot act as the sixth ligand to the heme iron and no inhibition is observed (e.g., a 2-substitued or 4,5-disubstituted imidazole), whereas a sterically accessible nitrogen (1- or 4(5)-substituted pyridine) effectively inhibits the enzyme [14].

Metabolic inactivation can occur by reversible binding of the metabolite with the heme iron, or covalent binding of the metabolite to the prosthetic heme or apoprotein [13,15]. Reversible binding can be seen with alkylamine drugs, such as erythromycin, in which the nitrogen can be oxidized to the nitroso metabolite. This metabolite can form a relatively stable complex with the CYP450 in the reduced state and be an effective inhibitor [22].

Nomenclature

With the increasing number of studies on the oxidation of drugs and the broad array of substrates, it became rapidly apparent that multiple forms of CYP450 exist [10-12,23]. The cytochrome P450 is a gene superfamily for which standardized nomenclature has been developed for the classification of the enzymes and genes [24]. The nomenclature is based on the global alignment of the complete amino acid sequence of the CYP450 enzyme protein. Recommendations for naming a P450 gene include:

- The italicized root symbol *CYP* denoting P450,
- An Arabic numeral designating the P450 family, e.g., *CYP*1A1 (two P450s demonstrating >40% amino acid homology represent members of the same family),
- A letter indicating the subfamily, when two or more subfamilies are known to exist within that family, e.g., *CYP*2A, *CYP*2B, etc. (two P450s demonstrating > 59% amino acid homology represent members of the same subfamily), and
- An Arabic numeral representing the individual gene, e.g., *CYP*1A1 (two P450s within the same subfamily demonstrating >70% amino acid homology and expected to exhibit chromosomal linkage). Gene and gene-product data are usually indicated by italic or roman type.

Since the nomenclature system is based on amino acid homology, the terminology gives little insight into the structure of compounds which interact with specific isoforms. In a general sense, CYP1, CYP2, and CYP3 are responsible for xenobiotic metabolism; CYP4 code for fatty acid hydroxylases (palmitic acid, arachidonic acid, prostaglandins); CYP7, CYP11, CYP17, CYP19, CYP21, and CYP27 are involved in steroid and bile acid metabolism (Arabic numerals indicating the site of reaction in the steroid nucleus); CYP51 and above code for plant P450s; and CYP101 and above for the prokaryote P450s (e.g., P450$_{cam}$ is CYP101). Most of the CYP genes in mammalian systems are constituitively expressed, but some are expressed only after induction.

The active oxygenating species is believed to be identical in all of the isoforms, with substrate specificity being dependent on the topographic environment of the binding sites with the isoform. As previously discussed, CYP450s oxidize hydrophobic molecules. Especially with CYP1-3, substrates can bind nonspecifically and multiple orientations of the substrate are possible within the enzyme active site. This "looseness" of fit and the multiple isoenzyme forms enable a broad range of compounds to be oxidized by

CYP450. General rules for predicting compounds that may be metabolized by specific isoforms of human CYP450s have been described [25].

The CYP1 Family. The CYP1A (CYP1A1 and CYP1A2) families are important in the metabolism of aromatic planar compounds. CYP1A1 is detected only after treatment with inducers, e.g., polycyclic aromatic hydrocarbons (PAH) present in cigarette smoke. A unique feature of this P450 is its expression in extrahepatic tissues (lung) upon exposure to PAH with little or no constituitive levels observed in the liver. CYP1A2 is localized in the liver and also induced by PAHs. CYP1A2 is responsible for hydroxylation of arylamines and for the O- or N-dealkylation of aromatic heterocycles (e.g., caffeine). CYP1A2 is selectively inhibited by furafylline, a mechanism-based inhibitor.

The CYP2 Family. The CYP2 family is large and diverse. It is divided into five subfamilies with very little known about the expression and function of the CYP2A and CYP2B subfamily in humans. The CYP2A gene subfamily has been extensively characterized in rats. It has been proposed that expression of the CYP2A1 and 2 may be sex specific. The CYP2B is primarily involved in N- and O-dealkylation reactions, such as O-deethylation of ethylmorphine and N-demethylation of cocaine. The isoenzymes of this subfamily can be induced by phenobarbital and no selective inhibitor is available. The CYP2C subfamily is generally thought to represent a class of constitutively expressed genes. In humans, five isoenzymes from CYP2C8, CYP2C9, CYP2C10, CYP2C18, and CYP2C19 are of primary importance. These isoforms are responsible for the metabolism of a wide range of drugs and xenobiotics. The CYP2C9,10 isoenzymes oxidize a wide variety of compounds, such as warfarin, ibuprofen, phenylbutazone, propranolol, diazepam, tolbutamide, and others. The isoforms are induced by dexamethasone and phenobarbital, and CYP2C9 is selectively inhibited by sulfaphenazole. A number of allelic variants of CYP2C9 exist in humans, but the effects of these variants on metabolism in vivo remain to be determined.

Many protonated amines are metabolized by the enzyme CYP2D6, including β-adrenergic blocking agents (propranolol, timolol), antiarrhythmic agents (lidocaine, mexiletine), antidepressants (imipramine, paroxetine), opioids (codeine, dextromethorphan) and other psychotropic drugs (clozapine, halopreidol). Important inducers of CYP2D have not been identified, but quinidine is a specific inhibitor of this isozyme. The CYP2D exhibits pharmacogenetic polymorphism.

The CYP2E1 catalyzes the oxidation of ethyl alcohol to acetaldehyde. It is the primary enzyme important in the oxidation of low molecular weight compounds, such as general anesthetics (diethyl ether, methoxyflurane), organic solvents (benzene, chloroform), and acetaminophen. It can be induced by ethanol and fasting. Diethyldithiocarbamate is a selective inhibitor of this isoenzyme.

The CYP3 Family. The CYP3A isozymes account for approximately 60% of the total P450 and are a functionally important class involved in the metabolism of a variety of drugs. Four closely related proteins, CYP3A3, CYP3A4, CYP3A5, and CYP3A7, are included in this family. CYP3A5 is expressed polymorphically in 20–25% of adult human livers and CYP3A7 is expressed in fetal liver and uterine tissues. CYP3A4 metabolizes a wide variety of drugs. These include reactions, such as the aromatization of dihydropyridines (nifedipine, felodipine), N-dealkylation (tamoxifen, lidocaine),

N-oxidation (quinidine, dapsone), alkyl hydroxylation (midazolam, valproic acid), and steroid hydroxylation (estradiol, hydrocortisone). The erythromycins are selective inhibitors of this enzyme, especially troleandomycin.

The CYP4A Family. The CYP4A has only a minor role in drug metabolism, appearing to be responsible for the ω-hydroxylation of some fatty acids.

The Flavin Monooxygenase Enzyme System

Another important oxidative enzyme system consists of the flavin monooxygenase (FMO) enzymes. The FMO enzymes provide an alternative pathway for the oxidation of lipohilic molecules containing nitrogen, sulfur, selenium, and phosphorus. Its chemistry [26], enzyme mechanism [27], and structure [28], and the substrate specificity of its isoenzymes [29,30] are reviewed.

The FMO enzymes are found in all mammalian species studied to date. Their natural endogenous substrate and their physiological function has yet to be determined [31]. The FMOs are present in many tissues with high concentrations in the liver, lung, and kidney. Within the cell, they are membrane-bound enzymes found in the microsomal membrane fraction. The FMO enzyme is a polymeric protein, with a monomer of approximately 60 kDa containing one equivalent of flavin-dependent dehydrogenase (FAD). The FMOs are anchored to the membrane by transmembrane segments at the C- and N-terminus. The inducing or inhibiting agents for CYP450 have no effect on the levels or activity of the FMOs. The levels of FMO do seem to be regulated by alterations in plasma hormone levels during development [32] and by nitrogen and sulfur xenobiotic soft nucleophiles present in food [33]. Protonated lipophilic amines can act as allosteric effectors and can stimulate or inhibit catalytic acitivity [27]. FMO proteins have been solubilized and purified, although many studies are currently done with cDNA-expressed human FMO isoforms or crude microsomal preparations [26,34].

The compounds that are substrates for FMOs are soft nucleophiles with an electron-rich center that can be easily oxidized by peracids. The oxidation products indicate that the nucleophilic center is oxidized by an ionic mechanism rather than by the radical mechanism seen for CYP450. The FMO catalytic cycle is shown in Fig. 7. The catalytic center is oriented around the flavin nucleus. The enzyme requires NADPH and oxygen as cosubstrates.

Many compounds that are substrates for FMO are also substrates for CYP450. Figure 8 shows the functional groups containing nitrogen that are substrates for FMO oxidation, such as secondary and tertiary alkyl and arylalkyl amines (acyclic and cyclic), hydroxylamines, and 1,1-hydrazines. The tertiary amines are oxidized to the chemically stable N-oxide, although they can be readily reduced back to the amine by reductase(s). The secondary amines are oxidized to hydroxylamines which can undergo conjugation (primarily seen with alkylarylamines) or be further oxidized by the FMO to nitrones. The nitrones can break down nonenzymatically leading to N-dealkylation. Sulfur is oxidized primarily by FMOs, and shown in Fig. 8 are functional groups that are substrates for FMO oxidation, including thiols (captopril), disulfides, sulfides (cimetidine), sulfoxides (sulindac), thioamides (thiobenzamide), and thiol heterocycles (propylthiouracil) [35].

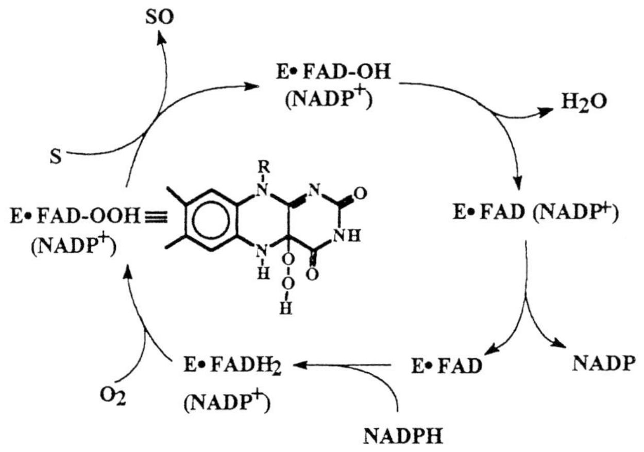

FIG. 7. The FMO catalytic cycle. (From Ref. 1.)

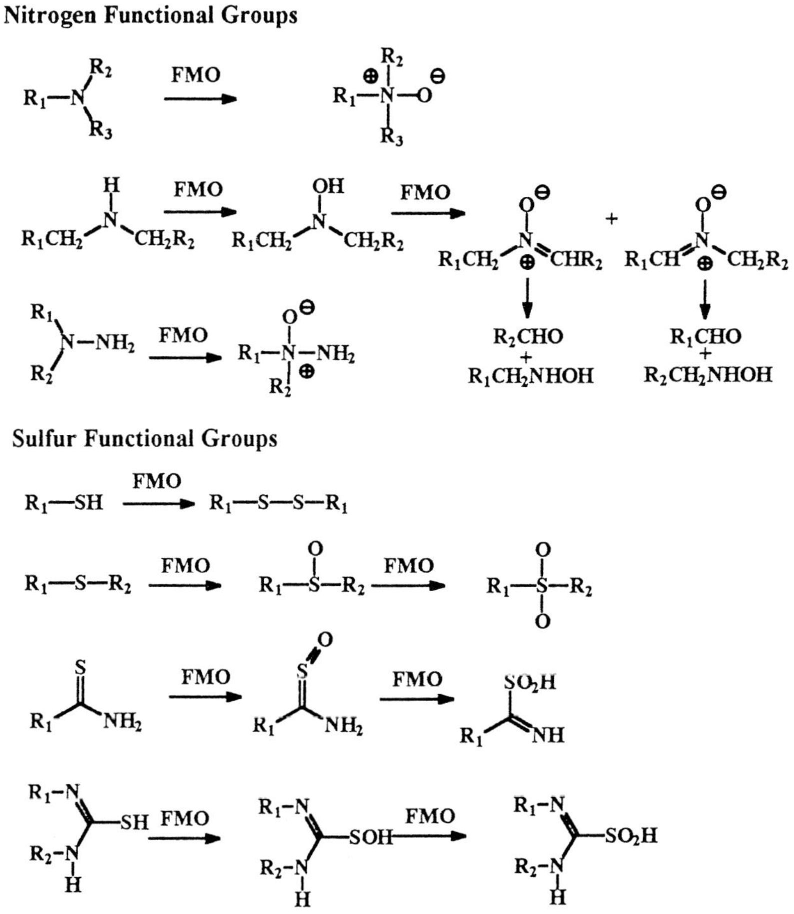

Nitrogen Functional Groups

Sulfur Functional Groups

FIG. 8. Common sulfur and nitrogen oxidation products of FMOs.

Nomenclature

An isozyme classification system based on primary structure has recently been adopted [36]. At this time, four distinct forms of FMO have been detected in the liver of humans: FMO1, FMO3, FMO4, and FMO5 (FMO2 is present in lung of mice and rabbits, but has not yet been characterized in humans) [34]. FMO1 is expressed in fetal liver, but not in adult human liver. FMO3 appears to be the primary FMO expressed in the adult human liver and probably accounts for most of the N- and S-oxidation that occurs in human liver microsomes and in vivo [27].

Alcohol and Aldehyde Dehydrogenases

Alcohol dehydrogenases and related enzymes are important enzymes involved with several protein families. Of primary interest in drug metabolism are the NAD^+-dependent alcohol dehydrogenase (ADH) and aldehyde dehydrogenase (AlDH) [37–39]. These enzymes are located primarily in the liver, but are also present in other organs (stomach, kidney, brain). They have long been of interest because of their involvement in ethanol metabolism. Both ADH and AlDH are polymorphic in humans. Extensive progress has been made in their purification, kinetic characterization, and cloning. The x-ray crystal structures of a human ADH [40] and AlDH [41] have been reported, which made it possible to model potential substrates for these enzymes.

The cytosolic zinc-containing enzyme, ADH, is of primary importance (Fig. 9) in the oxidation of xenobiotics containing alcohols. At present, five classes of human enzyme (I–V) have been characterized including isozymes (α, β, γ). The Class I enzyme is the abundant classical liver enzyme involved in the oxidation of alcohol. The Class III enzyme is a gluthathione-dependent, formaldehyde dehydrogenase protein (the formaldehyde formed by N-demethylation is converted to a S-formylglutathione). The isoenzymes of Class 1 ADH are capable of oxidizing primary (long and short chain, simple and branched, aliphatic and arylalkyl) and secondary alcohols, but not tertiary alcohols. At physiological pH, the ADH oxidation reaction is reversible with formation of the alcohol favored. A comparable, but different enzyme is the aldehyde reductase, a NADPH-dependent enzyme capable of reducing a wide range of aromatic and aliphatic aldehydes to their corresponding alcohols.

The AlDH is a cytosolic, mitochondrial metalloflavoprotein. At present, three classes of human enzymes (I–III) have been characterized. The Class I (cytosolic) and Class II (mitochondrial) AlDH are of major importance in humans for the oxidation of aldehydes to carboxylic acids. The AlDH Class I and Class II enzymes exhibit a broad

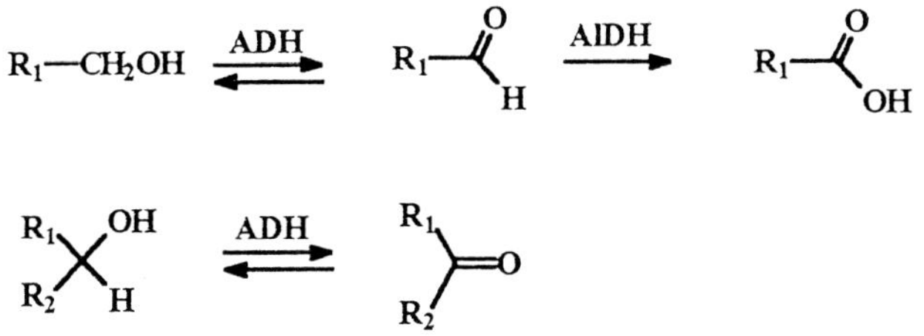

FIG. 9. Oxidation products of ADH and AlDH.

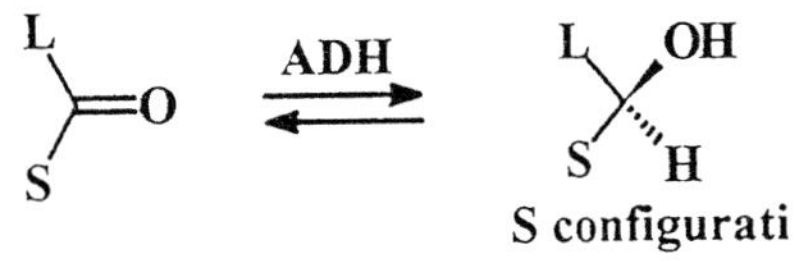

$$\underset{S}{\overset{L}{>}}=O \quad \underset{\longleftarrow}{\overset{ADH}{\longrightarrow}} \quad \underset{S}{\overset{L}{>}}\underset{H}{\overset{OH}{<}}$$

S configurati

FIG. 10. Product stereoselectivity often observed for ketone reductions.

substrate specificity oxidizing alkyl or aryl aldehydes [42]. Class III enzymes have high affinity for γ-aminobutyraldehyde and aldehydes generated from diamines and polyamines.

Compounds that are AlDH inhibitors include disulfiram, alkyl isocyanates, and cyclopropanone. High concentrations of aldehyde due to AlDH inhibition (e.g., disulfiram inhibition of acetaldehyde oxidation) produce facial flushing and a general feeling of malaise.

Reduction to the alcohol is the major metabolic step of ketones and secondary alcohols. As shown in Fig. 10, the formation of the S-carbinol is preferred. Substrate stereoselectivity is also observed, especially in warfarin for both substrate and product [43].

Other Oxidase Enzymes

Other oxidative enzyme have primarily been shown to be involved in the oxidation of endogenous compounds. These include catalase, amine oxidases, xanthine oxidase, aromatase, and an enzyme involved in the β-oxidation of alkyl carboxylic acids. These systems are generally covered under specific drug classes as enzymes for which therapeutic drugs have been developed, such as monoamine oxidase inhibitors or aromatase inhibitors. Therefore, they are not discussed here in greater detail.

Phase I Reductive Metabolism

Reductive enzymes in the liver, kidney, and other tissue are usually considered to be of minor importance in xenobiotic metabolism, but for molecules containing certain functional groups reduction can be an important biotransformation reaction required for their mechanism of action (Table 2). Reduction can occur even in the presence of oxygen which leads to an enzyme-catalyzed oxidation–reduction cycle (redox cycling). Within the mammalian cell these reactions have been observed for both microsomal, mitochondrial, and cytosolic fractions. Compared to the products formed by oxidation, toxicity is often associated with the reduced products since the reduction primarily occurs by one-electron transfer reactions, resulting in highly reactive free-radical intermediates capable of causing undesired cytoxic effects. Often the specific enzyme(s) responsible for the reduction of a drug is difficult to identify because of the relatively low substrate selectivity of flavoprotein enzymes and the ready availability of other reductases. In addition, the activity of the enzyme carrying out the reduction is dependent on the energy status (oxygen tension) of the cell. For example, CYP450s are normally oxidases, but under low oxygen tension or anerobic conditions they can act as reductases. After binding a substrate to the CYP450, the complex undergoes reduction. When this occurs, the oxygen can bind and be reduced or the xenobiotic can end up accepting the elec-

Xenobiotic Metabolism

TABLE 2 Common Reductive Pathways

Compounds to Products,	Reducing Enzyme Systems	References
Quinones and quinoneimines to semiquinone free radicals *Substrates* Mitomycin C, etoposide, adriamycin, N-acetyl-*p*-benzoquinoneimine	NADPH-cytochrome P450 reductase CYP450 (CYP2B1) Xanthine oxidase NADH-cytochrome b_5 reductase Ferrodoxin reductase Mitochondrial NADH dehydrogenase Glutathione reductase	17, 44
Aryl nitro group to nitroanion, niroso, hydronitroxide-free radical, hydroxylamine, or amine *Substrates* Nitrated polycyclic hydrocarbons, nitrofurantoin, nifurimox, nitrazepam	NADPH-cytochrome P450 reductase CYP450 (CYP1A) Xanthine oxidase Mitochondrial NADH dehydrogenase Mitochondrial NAD(P)H nitroreductase DT-diaphorase Aldehyde oxidase	17, 44
Halogenated alkanes to dehalogenated radical intermediates *Substrates* CCl_4, halothane, DDT	CYP450 (CYP2E1, CYP2B)	17
Azo dyes to hydrazo intermediate or arylamines *Substrates* Amaranth, dimethylamino-azobenzene, methyl orange	DT-diaphorase CYP450 Aldehyde oxidase	17, 44
N-Oxide to niroxide radical intermediate or amine *Substrates* (Tirapazine, pyrrolizidine N-oxides, imipramine N-oxide	NADPH-cytochrome P450 reductase CYP450 Xanthine oxidase Aldehyde oxidase Hemaglobin Cytochrome b_5 reductase	45, 46
Sulfoxide to sulfide *Substrates* Sulindac, sulfinpyrazone	Aldehyde oxidase Xanthine oxidase Thioredoxin	47

trons and be reduced. Another complicating factor is that gut microflora can carry out most of these same reductive reactions and actually be responsible for the reduction of the drug [48]. The enzymes associated with the reduction of common functional groups are listed in Table 2.

Phase I Hydrolysis

Enzymes involved in hydrolysis reactions are extensive, including carboxylesterases, carboxyamidases, lipases, phosphatases, sulfatases, carbamidases, phosphoramidases, and glycosidases. Some of the earliest concepts used in drug design were developed to modify drugs that were susceptible to hydrolytic reaction, for example, changing a labile ester in the molecule to an amide to increase its duration of action. All of these hydrolytic enzymes have been extensively studied as systems for modifying drug delivery. Although these enzymes are important in the detoxification of xenobiotics, they are often considered even more important in the metabolic activation of drugs (prodrugs).

Epoxide hydration to form diols is another important hydrolytic pathway previously mentioned. Epoxide hydrase (hydrolase) enzymes are present in both microsomes and cytosol [49]. There are at least two different microsomal enzymes, one catalyzing the hydration of many xenobioitic epoxides and the other the hydrolysis of steroidal 5,6-epoxides. The cytosolic enzyme appears to exhibit specificity toward trans-substituted styrene oxides, and terpenoid, steroid, and fatty ester epoxides. The epoxide hydrolases give trans-dihydrodiols upon hydration of arene oxides (Fig. 4) and epoxides of olefins.

Phase II Metabolism

Phase II or conjugating reactions transfer a hydrophilic groups (polar handle) on the functional groups attached during Phase I metabolism or already existing on a molecules, by conjugating with an endogenous water-soluble molecule (e.g., glucuronic acid), making the metabolite extremely polar and facilitating excretion in bile or urine. For a long time, interest in these pathways was minimal because formation of the conjugate was believed to be associated with termination of the pharmacological effect of the molecule, followed by rapid elimination of the conjugate from the body. In recent years, however, it has been recognized that a better understanding of these enzymes was needed because more and more examples were observed in which the xenobiotic conjugates were found to retain or increase a molecule's original pharmacological activity or exhibit different pharmacological or toxicological effects. Furthermore, formation of the conjugate had a major effect on the pharmacokinetics of a molecule and was often more important than the Phase I enzymes. All of the enzymes involved in Phase II reactions are classified as transferases that utilize an endogenous cofactor. Various conjugation reactions commonly observed in the body are shown in Table 3.

Glucuronic Acid Conjugation

Glucuronidation is a biosynthetic reaction in which the drug is conjugated with glucuronic acid in the presence of uridine diphosphate glucuronic acid (UDPGA) as a cofactor by the enzyme uridine diphosphate glucuronyltransferase (UDPGT). This reaction proceeds according to the general scheme shown in Fig. 11. Conjugation with glucuronic acid is responsible for the deactivation and elimination of a diverse range of xenobiotics and endogenous compounds, involving a wide variety of nucleophilic functional groups. Thus, glucuronidation has been shown to be of importance in the metabolism of drugs and their metabolites, environmental chemicals, carcinogens, steroid hormones, bile acids, and bilirubin. It is beyond the scope, this article to provide a detailed discussion of this important Phase II pathway; good reviews, specifically on glucuronidation, are available. [50–54].

Xenobiotic Metabolism

TABLE 3 Phase II Conjugation Reactions

Conjugation Reaction	Conjugating Agent	Conjugating Enzyme	High-Energy Intermediate	Functional Groups Conjugated
Glucuronidation	Glucuronic acid	Glucuronyltransferase	Uridine diphosphate glucuronic acid	-OH, -COOH, -NH$_2$, -NR$_2$, -SH, -CH
Glucosidation	Glucose	Glucosyltransferase	Uridine diphosphate glucose	-OH, -COOH, -SH, -CO-NH-CO-
Amino acid conjugation	Glycine, glutamine	Amino acid transferase	Coenzyme A thioesters of the amino acid	-COOH
Sulfation	Sulfate	Sulfatase	Adenosine-3'-phosphate-5'-phosphosulfate	-OH, -NH$_2$
Methylation	S-Adenosylmethionine	Methyltransferase	S-Adenosylmethionine	-OH, -NH$_2$
Acetylation	Acetyl CoA	Acetyltransferase	Acetyl CoA	-OH, -NH$_2$
Glutathione conjugation	Glutathione	Glutathione S-transferase	Substrates with epoxides or arene oxides	Electrophilic centers, (arene oxides, epoxides, carbonium ion, aryl halides)

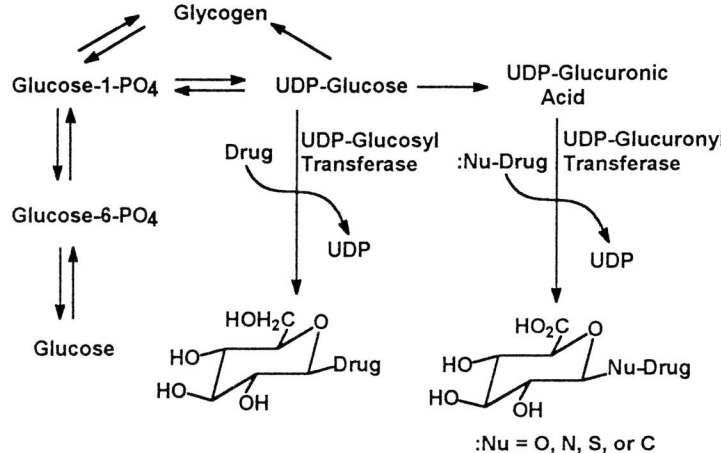

FIG. 11. The glycosylation pathway resulting in conjugation with glucose or glucuronide; Nu = nucleophile.

The versatility of UGTs is mainly due to the fact that they exist as a multigene family. Glucuronidation is quantitatively the most important form of conjugation for drugs and endogenous compounds, particularly those containing alcohols, phenols, hydroxylamines, carboxylic acids, amines, sulfonamides, and thiols. Glucuronidation is not always a detoxification reaction. In some cases, the glucuronide metabolite may be more active or toxic than the parent compound. For example, morphine 6-O-glucuronide is a more potent analgesic than morphine [55]. Toxicity of glucuronide metabolites is illustrated with acyl glucuronides of NSAIDs (nonsteroidal) which bind covalently to proteins in vivo that may produce an immunological response resulting in anaphylactic reaction [56].

The UGTs are located in the endoplasmic reticulum of cells and found in a number of extrahepatic tissues; the highest activity is usually found in the liver. These proteins are extremely labile after membrane perturbation and are dependent upon phospholipids for activity; their molecular weight is between 50 and 60 kDa [50].

Nomenclature

The UGTs are found in almost all mammalian species except the cat and a mutant strain of the GUNN rat. Multiple forms of UGTs are found in humans, most of which are named after an endogenous substrate (e.g., bilirubin UGT) or a class of endogenous substrates (17β- or 3α-hydroxysteroid UGTs). If no endogenous substrate has been identified, the UGT is named for a highly reactive xenobiotic substrate (e.g., *p*-nitrophenol UGT, digitoxigenin monodigitoxoside UGT). However, the trivial names are now being substituted by a new system proposed for the UGT superfamily [57] similar to the P450 nomenclature. The different isozymes of human liver UDP-glucuronyl transferases are: UGT1*1 and UGT1*4 (Bilirubin UGTs), UGT1*02, UGT1*6, UGT2B4, UGT2B7, UGT2B8 (Estriol GT), UGT2B9, UDPGTh-2 (catechol estrogen UGT). The individual UGT isoforms tend to exhibit distinct but overlapping patterns of substrate specificity and regulation.

Xenobiotic Metabolism

Induction and Inhibition of Glucuronidation

Drug glucuronidation, like oxidative metabolism, may be induced or inhibited by the concomitant administration of other agents. A number of drugs have been shown to inhibit glucuronidation in vivo (Table 4), with probenecid being the strongest inhibitor. It is involved in inhibitory interactions for a range of structurally diverse drugs [58–60], including those forming acyl, phenolic, and ether glucuronides. Pretreatment with the anticonvulsant agents phenobarbitone, phenytoin, and carbamezepine [61–63] is known to induce the glucuronidation of a number of drugs (Table 4).

Acyl Group Migration in Acyl Glucuronides

Glucuronidation is a major route of elimination and detoxification of drugs and endogenous compounds possessing a carboxylic acid function. Since the acyl glucuronides are esters, they are susceptible to migration of the acyl group in the glucuronic acid moiety from position 1 to positions 2, 3, and 4 in glucuronic acid (Fig. 12). Acyl migration is the rearrangement of the conjugate by intramolecular trans-esterification at the hydroxyl groups of the glucuronic acid moiety which leads to the formation of β-glucuronidase-resistant glucuronides. [64,65].

Glucoside Conjugation

Since the discovery of a glucosidation pathway in mammals, that is, the glucoside conjugation of 4-nitrophenol by mouse liver microsomes [66], several other glucosides of xenobiotics [67,68] and endogenous substrates [69] have been identified. Glucosides can be formed with or without prior oxidation of a substrate. The glucose molecule can be attached to a nitrogen, oxygen, or sulfur atom of a drug or metabolite, usually in a β-configuration, although in some exceptions an α-configuration is also observed. The structural requirements for glucoside formation are not established. They seem to share

TABLE 4 Drugs That Induce or Inhibit Glucuronidation Pathway

Inducer and Inhibitor	Drugs Affected
Induction	
Carbamazepine, phenobarbitone, phenytoin	Acetaminophen, lamotrigine, chloramphenicol, valproic acid,
Phenobarbitone	Oxazepam, fenoprofen, clofibrin acid,
Oral contraceptive steroids	diflunisal, acetaminophen, salicylic acid
Rifampicin	Temazepam, acetaminophen
Sulfinpyrazone	Acetaminophen
Inhibition	
Probenicid	Carprofen, clofibric acid, ketoprofen, lorazepam, naproxen, acetaminophen, zidovudine, zomepirac
Diflunisal	Indomethacin
Salicylamide	Acetaminophen
Salicylic acid	Salicylic acid
Zomepirac	Salicylic acid

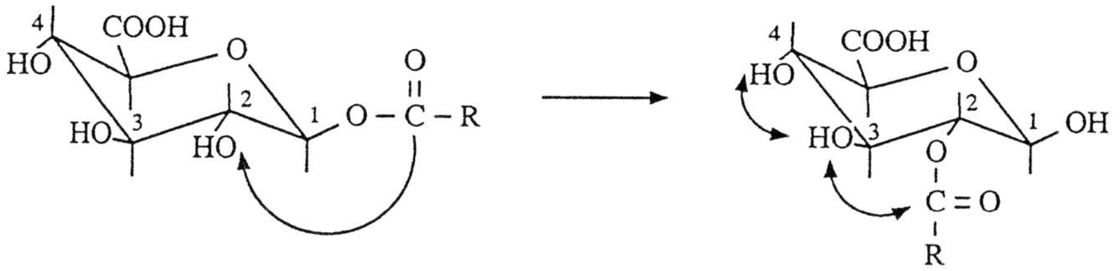

FIG. 12. Migration of the acyl residue within the glucuronic acid molecule of an C1-O-acyl glucuronide, forming positional isomers at C2, C3, and C4. (Adapted from Ref. 65.)

some of the requirements of glucuronidation and acetylation but glucosidation represents a minor pathway, particularly if glucuronidation or acetylation is possible. Urinary elimination of most drug glucosides represents only a minor fraction of drug intake (5% or less) with the exception of barbiturates (up to 30% in humans, Ref. 67).

Glutathione S-Transferase Conjugation

The glutathione S-transferases (GST) are enzymes that catalyze the nucleophilic attack of the sulfur atom of glutathione at electron-deficient centers in the substrate. The GST enzymes are dimeric proteins and the isoforms consist of combinations of different subunits. The enzymes occur abundantly in most tissues and are predominantly found in the cytosol, although presence in microsomal fractions has been reported. The GSTs serve to detoxify mutagens, carcinogens, and other noxious chemical substances. This substrate diversity is handled by a family of GST isoforms, the nomenclature of which varies between species. Excellent reviews providing a detailed description of this family of enzymes can be found in Refs. 70-72.

Many glutathione conjugates are not excreted per se but rather undergo further enzymatic modification of the peptide moiety, resulting in the urinary excretion or biliary excretion of the sulfur-substituted N-acetylcysteines, commonly referred to as mercapturic acids (Fig. 13). Mercapturic acid formation is initiated by glutathione conjugation, followed by removal of the glutamate moiety by glutathionase and subsequent removal of glycine by a peptidase enzyme. These two enzymes are present in both liver and kidney. In the final step, the amino group of cysteine is acetylated by a hepatic N-acetylase, resulting in the formation of the mercapturic acid derivative.

Nomenclature

Human liver GSTs contain isomeric forms which appear to be charged isomers of one another, presumably a result of deamidation. The three major types of human glutathione transferase have been classified as basic, near-neutral, and acidic on the basis of their isoelectric points. The five basic proteins purified from human liver cytosol have been named GST α, β, τ, σ, and ε in the order of increasing isoelectric points [73]. A distinct enzyme with a near-neutral isoelectric point was named GSTμ [74]. A third type, GSTπ, with an acidic isoelectric point, has been isolated from placenta [75]. It is probably identical to the acidic protein first isolated from erythrocytes and designated GSTρ. Acidic transferase from human organs, including lung, kidney and lens also appear to

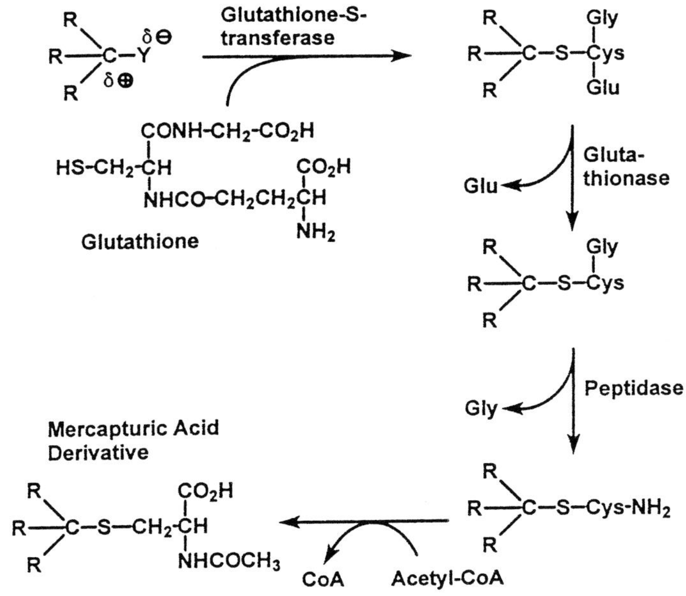

Xenobiotic Metabolism

FIG. 13. Catalytic scheme resulting in the conversion of the glutathione conjugate to a mercapturic acid derivative.

correspond to GSTπ. This placental form is probably the best characterized protein and is used as a reference for comparison. In addition to the cytosolic GSTs, a distinct membrane-bound enzyme has been identified.

Induction of GST Isozymes

Like other drug metabolizing systems, levels of GST activities can be increased substantially with certain drugs, including phenobarbital, 3-methyl cholanthrene, trans-stilbene oxide, benzo(a)pyrene, or 2,3,7,8-tetrachlorodibenzo-*p*-dioxin [76–78]. Most of these compounds increase the activity twofold or more. Dietary constituents can enhance GST activity in the liver and small intestine in mice. Brussel sprouts, cabbage, tea leaves, and green coffee beans increase transferase activity 1.8- to 4.9-fold [79]. Administration of anticarcinogenic antioxidants such as butylated hydroxyanisole (BHA) to mice enhances GST activity of the hepatic cytosol as much as 11-fold [80]. This is of particular significance since GSTs play a role in the metabolism and detoxification of chemical carcinogens.

Acetyl Conjugation

Acetylation reactions are common for primary amine groups (aliphatic and aromatic amines, amino acids, sulfonamides, and hydrazines) and require the cofactor acetyl-CoA which may be obtained from the glycolysis pathway or via direct interaction of acetate and coenzyme A. This takes place mainly in the liver. A detailed description for this pathway can be found in Ref. 81. The conjugation is catalyzed by the enzyme

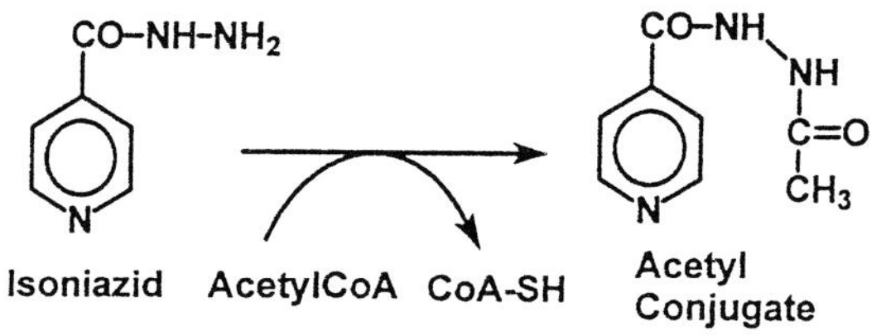

FIG. 14. Conjugation of isoniazid with the acetyl group in the presence of acetylCoA.

N-acetyltransferase, which appears to exist in two forms under different regulatory control. Of the two forms of N-acetyl transferase (NAT1 and NAT2) that have been characterized, NAT2 is a mutant form and not able to carry out the acetylation reaction [81]. The acetylation of substrates such as sulfanilamide and p-amino benzoic acid occurs in the reticuloendothelial cells of the liver, spleen, lungs, and gut, whereas acetylation of compounds like isoniazid and sulfamethazine occurs in hepatocytes. The mechanism of acetyl transfer is shown in Fig. 14.

Sulfate Conjugation

Many drugs are oxidized to a variety of phenols, alcohols, or hydroxylamines which can then serve as excellent substrates for sulfate conjugation, forming the readily excretable sulfate esters [82]. However, inorganic sulfate is relatively inert and needs to be activated by adenosine triphosphate (ATP), as shown in Fig. 15. Phenol sulfotransferase is the most important of the enzymes which catalyze the sulfation of phenolic metabolites [83]. Sulfotransferases are soluble enzymes found in many tissues, including the liver, kidney, gut, and platelets. They catalyze the sulfation of drugs such as acetaminophen, isoprenaline, salicylamide, and steroids. Sulfotransferases exist in multiple enzyme forms [84], with the steroid-sulfating enzymes being distinct from the sulfotransferases responsible for drug conjugation reactions. It should be pointed out that sulfate conjugation reactions are not as widespread or quantitatively as important

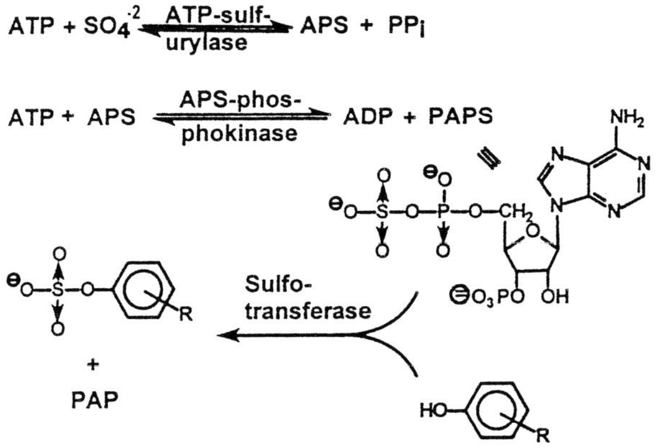

FIG. 15. Metabolic scheme showing the pathway for activation of the sulfate moiety and conjugation of a phenolic group to yield a sulfate conjugate (PP_i = phosphate residue, PAPS = adenosine-3'-phosphate-5'-phosphosulfate).

as glucuronide conjugation reactions, partly because of the limited availability of inorganic sulfate and hence of adenosine-3′-phosphate-5′-phosphosulfate (PAPS). The sulfate metabolite pathway is easily saturated, often seen when a drug is significantly metabolized to phenolic products or when high concentrations of drugs with phenolic groups are reached. However, in spite of saturation, no unacceptable clinical outcomes result, mainly because sulfate conjugation is often a minor pathway and other Phase II conjugation reactions compensate and metabolize the unconjugated drug.

Amino Acid Conjugation

Many classes of drugs including anti-inflammatory, hypolipidemia, diuretic, and analgesic agents have a carboxylic acid moiety in their structure, and as such are susceptible to conjugation with endogenous amino acids prior to excretion [85]. In a manner similar to both glucuronide and sulfate conjugation, amino acid conjugation of free carboxylic acid groups in drugs requires metabolic activation, as shown in Fig. 16.

The drug (Ar-COOH) is activated to its acyl coenzyme A derivative via the coenzyme A (CoASH), prior to amide formation with the amino function of the donating amino acid (NH_2-CH_2-COOH). This conjugation reaction occurs in many species, utilizing a variety of amino acids, and appears to be a complementary pathway to the glucuronidation of carboxyl groups. The conjugation occurs extensively in hepatic mitochondria and therefore has been utilized as a test for liver function. Benzoic acid is conjugated with glycine, resulting in excretion of the benzylglycine conjugate sometimes referred to as hippuric acid. Under conditions of normal liver function, a specified amount of hippuric acid is excreted within a few hours after ingestion. In parenchymal liver disorders, such as hepatitis or cirrhosis, the urinary output of hippuric acid is low (assuming normal renal function) and therefore constitutes a useful indicator of hepatic viability in some cases.

Methyl Conjugation

Methylation reactions occur mainly in endogenous compound metabolism, but some drugs may be methylated by nonspecific methyltransferases found in the lung and by the physiological methyltransferases (e.g., catechol O-methyltransferase found in the liver, kidney, skin, and nerve tissue) [86,87].

The cofactor S-adenosylmethionine (SAM) is required to form methyl conjugates and is produced from L-methionine and ATP (Fig. 17) under the influence of the enzyme L-methionine adenosyltransferase. The nonspecific N'-methyltransferase found in the lung

$$Ar\text{–}CO_2H + ATP + CoA\text{-}SH \xrightarrow{\text{Acyl-CoA Synthetase}} Ar\text{–}CO\text{–}SCoA + AMP + PP_i$$

$$Ar\text{–}CO\text{–}SCoA + H_2N\text{—}CH_2\text{–}CO_2H \xrightarrow{\text{Acyl-CoA:amino acid N-Acyltransferase}} Ar\text{–}CO\text{-}HN\text{–}CH_2\text{–}CO_2H + CoA\text{-}SH$$

FIG. 16. Activation of a carboxylic group of a substrate to be conjugated with glycine.

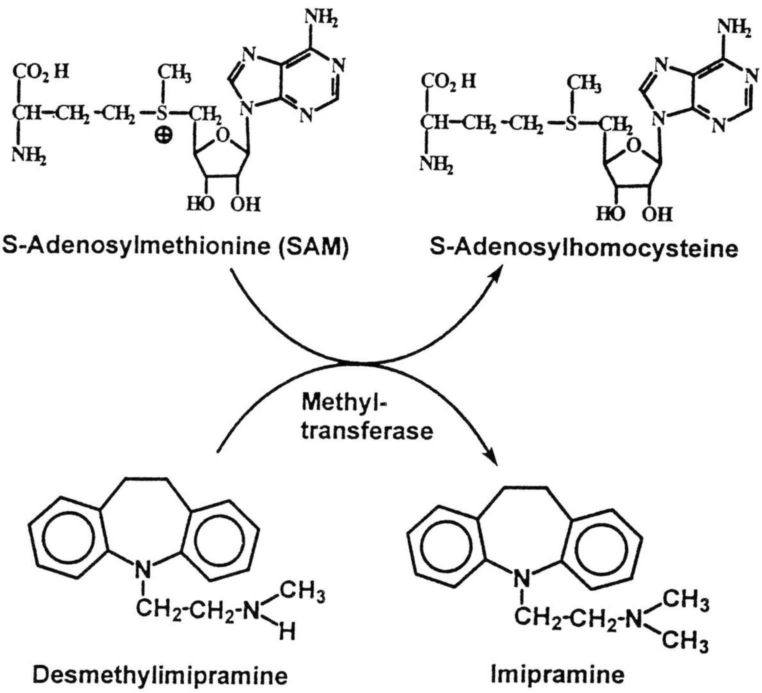

FIG. 17. Methyl conjugation of imipramine which has been previously dealkylated by CYP450.

can reverse the N-demethylation reactions of Phase I metabolism, as shown in Fig. 17. Most of the other methyltransferases are specific for endogenous compounds, except the S-methyltransferase found in the microsomal fraction which methylates many thiols such as thiouracil. In general, unlike other conjugation reactions, methylation leads to a less polar product and thus hinders drug excretion.

Genetic Factors Influencing Xenobiotic Metabolism

Phase I Oxidative Metabolism

CYP2D6 (Debrisoquine Hydroxylase)

This pathway exhibits genetic polymorphism, wherein two subsets of the human population (≈5% of Caucasians and ≈2% of Orientals) are deficient in this enzyme and unable to efficiently carry out this catalytic pathway [88,89]. The CYP2D6 protein mediates the oxidation of a large number of clinically important drugs (bufuralol, propranolol, encainide, etc). It was first isolated via the debrisoquine 4-hydroxylation pathway, hence it is sometimes referred to as debrisoquine hydroxylase. Studies have shown that this polymorphism results from a defective debrisoquine 4-hydroxylase protein. Analysis of human liver samples, where debrisoquine 4-hydroxylation was undetectable, further revealed the presence of mutant alleles of the CYP2D gene that produced defectively spliced RNA transcripts [90].

Other CYP450 isoforms have been suggested to be undergoing genetic polymorphism, such as CYP2C19 (S-mephenytoin hydroxylase, Ref. 91), however none has as much clinical significances the CYP2D6 enzyme.

Phase II Glucuronidation
Gilbert's Syndrome

Bilirubin clearance and bilirubin UDPGT activity are both known to be reduced to some extent in Gilbert's syndrome [92], a mild form of unconjugated hyperbilirubinemia occurring in about 6% of the population.

Crigler-Najjar Syndrome

The Crigler-Najjar syndrome is a much rarer form of unconjugated hyperbilirubinemia [93]. Patients with this disorder may be classified as Type I or II. Type I patients have consistently high plasma concentrations of unconjugated bilirubin due to the complete absence of bilirubin UDPGT. It has been demonstrated that the hepatic glucuronidation of corticosteroids, menthol, 4-methylumbelliferone, 1-naphthol, acetaminophen, salicylic acid, and salicylamide may all be impaired in such patients. The Type II syndrome is characterized by lower concentrations of unconjugated bilirubin in plasma and is generally benign in nature. Bilirubin UDPGT activity is nevertheless markedly reduced or even absent in the livers of such patients.

Acetylation

The NAT2 isoform is an inactive enzyme, predominantly expressed in the population of slow acetylators, whereas the fast acetylators are more abundant in NAT1, the intact enzyme [94]. The polymorphic N-acetyltransferase system carries a number of clinical implications. Many important drugs, such as isoniazid, procainamide, some sulfonamides, hydralazine, and nitrazepam, as well as certain endogenous compounds including serotonin are known to be substrates of this enzyme.

References

1. Ziegler, D.M., *Drug Metab. Disp.*, 19:847-852 (1991).
2. Testa, B., and Jenner, P. In: *Drug Metabolism: Chemical and Biochemical Aspects*, Marcel Dekker, Inc., New York, 1976.
3. Gibson, G.G., and Skett, P. In: *Introduction to Drug Metabolism*, Chapman and Hall, New York, 1986.
4. Testa, B. In: *Burger's Medicinal Chemistry and Drug Discovery*, 5th ed. (M.E. Wolff, ed.), John Wiley &Sons, Inc., 1995, pp. 129-180.
5. Kauffman, F.C., ed., *Conjugation-Deconjugation Reactions in Drug Metabolism and Toxicity*, Vol. 112, Springer-Verlag, New York, 1994.
6. Guengerich, F.P., *Progr. Drug Metab.*, 10:1-54 (1987).
7. Ortiz de Montellano, P.R., *TIPS*, 10:354-359 (1989).

8. Trager, W.F., *Drug Metab. Rev.,* 20:489-496 (1989).
9. Poulos, T.L., *Pharm. Res.,* 5:67-75 (1988).
10. White, R.E., and Coon, M.J., *Ann. Rev. Biochem.,* 49:315-356 (1980).
11. Koymans, L., Den Kelder, G.M.D., Koppele Te, J.M., and Vermeulen, N.P.E., *Drug Metab. Rev.,* 25:325-387 (1993).
12. Spatzenegger, M., and Jaeger, W., *Drug Metab. Rev.,* 27:397-417 (1995).
13. Ortiz de Montellano, P.R., *Progr. Drug Metab.,* 11:99-148 (1988).
14. Murray, M., *Drug Metab. Rev.,* 18:55-81 (1987).
15. Silverman, R.B. In: *Mechanism-Based Enzyme Inactivation: Chemistry and Enzymology,* Vol. II, CRC Press, Boca Raton, FL, 1988, pp. 89-252.
16. Newton, D.J., Wang, R.W., and Lu, A.Y.H., *Drug Metab. Disp.,* 23:154-158 (1995).
17. Goeptar, A.R., Scheerens, H., and Vermeulen, N.P.E., *Crit. Rev. Toxicol.,* 25:25-65 (1995).
18. White, R.E., *Pharmac. Ther.,* 49:21-42 (1991).
19. Walle, T., Walle, U.K., and Olanof, L.S., *Drug Metab. Disp,* 13:204-209 (1985).
20. Williams, D.A., Drug Metabolism. In: *Principles of Medicinal Chemistry,* 4th ed. (W.O. Foye, T.L. Lemke, and D.A. Williams, eds.), Williams and Wilkins, Baltimore, 1995, pp.88-111.
21. Ioannides, C., and Parke, D.V., *Drug Metab. Rev.,* 22:1-85 (1990).
22. Babany, G., Larrey, D., and Pessayre, D., *Progr. Drug Metab.,* 11:61-98 (1988).
23. Gonzalez, F.J., *Pharm. Rev.,* 40:243-288 (1989).
24. Nebert, D.W., et al., *DNA,* 8:1-13 (1989).
25. Smith, D.A., and Jones, B.C., *Biochem. Pharmacol.,* 44:2089-2098 (1992).
26. Ziegler, D.M., *Drug Metab. Rev.,* 19: 1-32 (1988).
27. Poulsen, L.L., and Ziegler, D.M., *Chem.-Biol. Int.,* 96:57-73 (1995).
28. Ziegler, D.M., *Ann. Rev. Pharmacol. Toxicol.,* 33:1979-1999 (1993).
29. Cashman, J.R., Park, S.B., Berkman, C.E., and Cashman, L.E., *Chem.-Biol. Int.,* 96:33-46 (1995).
30. Rettie, A.E., Meier, G.P., and Sadeque, A.J.M., *Chem.-Biol. Int.,* 96:3-15 (1995).
31. Elfarra, A.A., *Chem.-Biol. Int.,* 96:47-55 (1995).
32. Lee, M-Y., et al. *Chem.-Biol. Int.,* 96:75-85 (1995).
33. Ziegler, D.M., *Ann. Rev. Pharmacol. Toxicol.,* 33:179-199 (1993).
34. Phillips, I.R., et al., *Chem.-Biol. Int.,* 96:7-32 (1995).
35. Hodgson, E., and Levi, P.E. In: *The Flavin-Containing Monooxygenase as a Sulfur Oxidase* (J.W. Gorrod, H. Oelschlaeger, and J. Caldwell, eds.), Taylor and Francis, London, 1988, pp.81-88.
36. Lawton, M. P., et al., *Arch. Biochem. Biophys.,* 308:254-257 (1994).
37. Jornvall, H., Danielsson, O., Hjelmqvist, L., Persson, B., and Shafqat, J., *Adv. Exp. Med. Biol.,* 372:281-294 (1995).
38. McMahon, R.E. In: *Metabolic Basis of Detoxification,* Academic Press, Inc., 1982, Orlando, FL, pp. 91–104.
39. Sladek, N.E., Manthey, C.L., Maki, P.A., Zhang, Z., and Landkamer, G.J., *Drug Metab. Rev.,* 20:697-720 (1989).
40. Hurley, T.D., Bosron, W.F., Hamilton, J.A., and Amzel, L.M., *Proc. Natl. Acad. Sci., USA,* 88:8149-8153 (1991).
41. Hurley, T.D., Yang, Z., Bosron, W.F., and Weiner, H. In: *Enzymology and Molecular Biology of Carbonyl Metabolism,* Vol. 4 (H. Weiner, D.W. Crabb, and T.G. Flynn, eds.), Plenum, New York, p. 245.
42. Yin, S-J., Wang, M-F., Han, Ch-L., and Wang, S-L., *Adv. Exp. Med. Biol.,* 372:9-16 (1995).
43. Toon, S., Low, L.K., Gibaldi, M., Trager, W.F., O'Reilly, R.A., Motley, C.H., and Goulart, D.A., *Clin. Pharmacol. Ther.,* 39:15-24 (1986).

44. Kappus, H., *Biochem. Pharmacol.*, 35:1-6 (1986).
45. Patterson, L.H., *Cancer Metastasis Rev.*, 12:119-134 (1993).
46. Barham, H.M., and Stratford, I.J., *Biochem. Pharm.*, 51:829-837 (1996).
47. Lee, S.C., and Renwick, A.G., *Biochem. Pharmacol.*, 49:1557-1565 (1995).
48. Rowland, I.R., *Biochem. Pharmacol.*, 35:27-32 (1986).
49. Guenthner, T.M. In: *Conjugation Reactions in Drug Metabolism* (G.J. Mulder, ed.), Taylor and Francis, London, 1990, pp. 365-404.
50. Clark, D.J., and Burchell, B. In: *Handbook of Experimental Pharmacology*, Vol. 112, *Conjugation-Deconjugation Reactions in Drug Metabolism and Toxicity,* Springer-Verlag, Berlin, 1994, pp 3-43.
51. Miners, J.O., and MacKenzie, P.I., *Pharmacol. Ther.*, 51:347-369 (1991).
52. Tephly, T.R., and Burchell, B., *TIPS Rev.*, 11:276-279 (1990).
53. Tephly, T.R., and Green, M.D., *Drug Metab. Disp.*, 24:356-363 (1996).
54. Mulder, G.J., *Ann. Rev. Pharmacol. Toxicol.*, 32:25-49 (1992).
55. Yoshimura, H., Oguri, K., and Tsukamoto, H., *Biochem. Pharmacol.*, 22:1423-1430 (1973).
56. Smith, P.C., McDonagh., A.F, and Benet, L.Z., *J. Clin. Invest*, 77:934-939 (1986).
57. Burchell, B., Nebert, D.W., Nelson, K.W., et al., *DNA Cell Biol.*, 10:487-494 (1991).
58. Abernethy, D.R., Greenblatt, D.J., Ameer, B., and Shader, R.I., *J. Pharmac. Exp. Ther.*, 234:345-349 (1985).
59. De Miranda, Good, P., Yarchoan, R., Thomas, R.V., Blum, M.R., Myers, C.E., and Broder, S., *Clin. Pharmac. Ther.*, 46:494-500 (1989).
60. Spahn, H., Spahn, I., and Benet, L.Z., *Clin. Pharmac. Ther.*, 40:262-264 (1989).
61. Bock, K.W., Wiltfang, J., Blume, R., Ullrich, D., and Bircher, J., *Eur. J. Clin. Pharmac.*, 31:677–683 (1987).
62. Perucca, E., and Richens, A., *Br. J. Clin. Pharmac.*, 7:201-206 (1979).
63. Prescott, L.F., Crichley, J.A., Balali, M., and Pentland, B., *Br. J. Clin. Pharmac.*, 12:149-153 (1981).
64. Faed, E.M., *Drug Metab. Rev.*, 15:1213-1249 (1984).
65. Spahn, H., and Benet, L.Z., *Drug Metab. Rev.*, 24:5-48 (1992).
66. Gessner, T., and Vollmer, C.A., *Fed. Proc. Fed. Am. Socs. Exp. Biol.*, 28:545 (1969).
67. Tang, B.K., Kalow, W., and Grey, A.A., *Drug Metab. Dispos.*, 1:315-318 (1979).
68. Soine, W.H., Bhargawa, V.O., and Garretson, L.K., *Drug Metab. Dispos.*, 12:792-794 (1984).
69. Tang, B.K., *Pharmacol. Ther.*, 46:53-56 (1990).
70. Mannervik, B., and Danielson, U.H., *CRC Crit. Rev. in Biochem.*, 23:283-337 (1988).
71. Boyer, T.D., and Kenney, W.C., In: *Biochemical and Pharmacology and Toxicology,* John-Wiley and Sons, New York, 1986, pp. 297-361.
72. Harada, S., and Abei, M., In: *Pharmacogenetics of Drug Metabolism*, Pergamon Press, New York, 1992, pp. 249-259.
73. Kamisaka, K., Habig, W.H., Ketley, J.M., Arias, I.H., and Jakoby, W.B., *Eur. J. Biochem.*, 60:153 (1975).
74. Mannervik, B., Alin, C., Guthenberg, C., Jensson, H., Tahir, M.K., Warholm, M., and Jornvall, H., *Proc. Natl. Acad. Sci. U.S.A.*, 82:7202-7209 (1985).
75. Polidoro, G., DiIlio, C., Del Boccio, G., Zulli, P., and Federici, G., *Biochem. Pharmacol.*, 29:1677-1680 (1980).
76. Scotstill, M.E., and Dauterman, W.C., *Drug Chem. Toxicol.*, 5:427-430 (1982).
77. Pickett, C.B., Wells, W., Lu, A.Y.H., and Hales, B.F., *Biochem. Biophys. Res. Commun.*, 99:1002-1006 (1981).
78. Pickett, C.B., Telakowski, C.A., Donohue, A.M., Lu, A.Y.H., and Hales, B.F., *Biochem. Biophys. Res. Commun.*, 104:611 (1982).
79. Sparins, V.L., Vene, P.L., and Wattenberg, L.W., *J. Natl Cancer Inst.*, 68:493-496 (1982).

80. Pearson, W.R., Windle, J.J., Morrow, J.F., Benson, A.M., and Talalay, P., *J. Biol. Chem.*, 258:2052-2057 (1983).
81. Weber, W.W., and Hein, D.W., *Pharmacol. Rev.*, 37:25-79 (1985).
82. Mulder, G.J. In: *Sulfation of Drugs and Related Compounds*, CRC Press, Boca Raton, FL, 1981, pp. 53-82.
83. Anderson, R.J., and Weinshilboum, R.M., *Clin. Chim. Acta*, 103:79-90 (1980).
84. Rein, G., Glover, V., and Sandler, M., *Biochem. Pharmacol.*, 31:1893-1897 (1982).
85. Caldwell, J. In: *Conjugative Reactions in Drug Biotransformation* (Aitio, C.A., ed.), Elsevier, Amsterdam, 1978, pp. 111-122.
86. Williams, R.T. In: *Biogenesis of Natural Compounds* (Benfeld, C.P., ed.), Pergamon Press, Elmsford, NY, 1967, p. 589.
87. Mudd, S.H. In: *Metabolic Conjugation and Metabolic Hydrolysis* (D.H. Snyder, and E. Usdin, eds.) Pergamon Press, Elmsford, NY, 1974, pp 121.
88. Mahgoub, A., Dring, L.G., Idle, J.R., Lancaster, R., and Smith, R.L., *Lancet*, 1977:584-586.
89. Meyer, U.A., Skoda, R.C., and Zanger, U.M., *Pharmacol. Ther.*, 46:297-308 (1990).
90. Gonzalez, F.J., Skoda, R.C., Kimura, S., Umeno, M., Zanger, U.M., Nebert, D.W., Gelboin, H.V., Hardwick, J.P., and Meyer, U.A., *Nature*, 331:442-446 (1988).
91. Goldstein, J.A., Faletto, M.B., Romkes, M., Sullivan, T, Kitareewan, S., et al., *Biochemistry*, 33:1743-1752 (1994).
92. Macklon, A.F., Savage, R.L., and Rawlins, M.D., *Clin. Pharmacokinet.*, 4:223-232. (1979)
93. Schmid, R., and McDonagh, A.F. In: *The Metabolic Basis of Inherited Disease*, McGraw Hill, New York, 1978, pp. 1221-1257.
94. Dupret, J.M., Good, G., Janezic, S.A., and Grant, D.M., *J. Biol. Chem.*, 269:830-835 (1994).

MOHAMADI A. SARKAR
WILLIAM H. SOINE

Zeta Potential

Introduction

Dispersion systems represent an important class of pharmaceutical dosage forms, such as emulsions, suspensions, microspheres, liposomes, and nanoparticles. The medium of these systems is mainly aqueous and the dispersed phase can be solid particles or immiscible liquid droplets. Electrical charges are developed by several mechanisms at the interface between the dispersed phase and the aqueous medium [1]. The two most common mechanisms are the ionization of surface functional groups and the specific adsorption of ions. These electrical charges play an important role in determining the interaction between particles of the dispersed phase and the resultant physical stability of the systems, particularly for those in the colloidal size range. The in vivo fate and therapeutic efficacy of dispersed systems which are used as drug carriers, such as liposomes and microparticles, are both affected by these surface charges. Therefore, the understanding of this electrical phenomenon is essential in developing these systems.

The presence of these surface charges influences an uneven distribution of charges (ions) surrounding the particle and the development of an electrical potential (or an electrical field) between the surface and the electrically neutral bulk-solution phase of the system. The surface potential is not readily measured experimentally; instead, the potential between a stationary fluid layer enveloping the particle and the bulk-solution phase can be determined by measuring the mobility of the particle in an applied electrical field. The potential between the tightly bound surface liquid layer (shear plane) of the particle and the bulk phase of the solution is called zeta potential. It can provide a measure of the net surface charge on the particle and potential distribution at the interface. Zeta potential serves as an important parameter in characterizing the electrostatic interaction between particles in dispersed systems and the properties of the dispersion as affected by this electrical phenomenon.

Theories
Electric Double-Layer Formation and Structure

The separation of charges at the interface between two phases develops an electric double layer consisting of two regions of opposite charges: the surface charge and the counterions in its vicinity [1-3]. The simplest model of the double layer was proposed by Helmholtz in 1879 and consisted of a monolayer of opposite charges in the form of a molecular capacitor. Later, realizing that this model was inadequate to explain all observations associated with the double layer, Gouy in 1910 and Chapman in 1914 proposed a diffuse double- layer model in which the concentration of the counterions is the highest next to the surface but which diminishes with distance from the surface. This diffuse double layer arises as a result of the random thermal motion of the ions in addition to the electrical influence of the surface charge.

The Gouy and Chapman double-layer model can be treated quantitatively with certain assumptions: (a) surface charge is uniform per unit area, (b) ions are point charges, (c) the dielectric constant of the medium is constant, and (d) there is no specific adsorption of ions. The variation of electrical potential with distance from a charged surface is described by the Poisson Eq. (1),

$$\nabla^2 \psi = -\rho_e/\varepsilon \tag{1}$$

where ρ_e is the charge density (charge/volume) and ε is the permittivity. When the potential distribution adjacent to a planar double layer with a positive surface charge is considered, $\nabla^2 \psi$ becomes $d^2 \psi/dx^2$, and Eq. (1) is written as in Eq. (2).

$$d^2 \psi/dx^2 = -\rho_e/\varepsilon \tag{2}$$

Equation (2) cannot be solved because both ψ and ρ_e are unknown. However, the charge density can be expressed as a function of the potential by means of a Boltzmann factor in which the work required to bring an ion to a position with a potential of ψ is given by $z_i e \psi$. The probability of finding an ion at this position is given by the Boltzmann factor, with this work appearing as the exponential energy, as in Eq. (3),

$$n_i/n_{i\infty} = \exp(-z_i e \psi/kT) \tag{3}$$

where n_i is the number of ions of Type I per unit volume near the surface, $n_{i\infty}$ is the concentration in the bulk solution, and z_i is the valence of the ions. The charge density is related to the ion concentration by Eq. (4).

$$\rho_e = \Sigma\, z_i e n_i = \Sigma\, z_i e n_{i\infty} \exp(-z_i e \psi/kT) \tag{4}$$

Combining Eqs. (2) and (4) gives the Poisson-Boltzmann Eq. (5).

$$d^2 \psi/dx^2 = (-e/\varepsilon) \Sigma\, z_i n_{i\infty} \exp(-z_i e \psi/kT) \tag{5}$$

In situations where $z_i e \psi < kT$ ($\psi < 25.7$ mV for 1:1 ions at 25°C), the exponential in Eq. (5) may be expanded as a power series and Eq. (5) can be simplified to Eq. (6),

$$d^2 \psi/dx^2 = \kappa^2 \psi \tag{6}$$

where $\kappa^2 = (e^2 \Sigma\, z_i^2\, n_{i\infty})/\varepsilon kT$. Equation (6) can be further solved to give Eq. (7).

$$\psi = \psi_0 \exp(-\kappa x) \tag{7}$$

This equation satisfies the required boundary conditions that as $\psi \to \psi_0$, $x \to 0$ and as $\psi \to 0$, $x \to \infty$. The simplification of Eq. (5) by taking ψ as small in magnitude is referred to as the Debye-Hückel approximation. The parameter κ is called the Debye parameter and has units of reciprocal length.

The assumptions of Gouy and Chapman in deriving their diffuse double-layer model are not valid under many circumstances. For example, the assumption that ions are point charges (i.e., they have no volume) is contradictory to the fact that the finite size of ions actually limits the inner boundary of the diffuse part of the double layer. The reason is that the center of an ion can only approach the surface to within its hydrated radius without becoming specifically adsorbed. The second major problem with the Gouy and Chapman model is the assumption that rules out specific adsorption of ions.

Zeta Potential

Both these deficiencies are corrected in the Stern model in which the double layer is divided into two parts separated by a plane called the Stern layer. This layer is located at about a hydrated-ion radius from the surface. The Stern model also considers the possibility of specific ion adsorption. Usually, the number of ions in the Stern layer is smaller than that needed to achieve neutralization of the surface charge, and the balance of the neutralization occurs in a Gouy-Chapman layer outside the Stern layer. The potential at the Stern layer, ψ_d, can replace ψ_o in the treatment of the Gouy-Chapman layer. In summary, the potential changes from ψ_o (the surface potential) to ψ_d (the Stern potential) in the Stern layer and decays from ψ_d to zero asymptotically in the diffuse double layer (Fig. 1).

Because of the indefinite end point, the thickness of the diffuse double layer (δ) is arbitrarily assigned the value of the distance over which the potential at the boundary between the Stern and Gouy-Chapman layers drops to $1/e$ (0.37) of its value. The value of δ is approximately equal to the reciprocal of the Debye-Hückel parameter (κ^{-1}). The thickness of the double layer is typically in the range of up to hundreds of nanometers and decreases significantly with counterion valence and concentration. Because the Stern model can accommodate specific adsorption, it is possible, especially with polyvalent or surface-active counterions, for a reversal of charge to take place within the Stern layer. The adsorption of surface-active co-ions could also produce charge intensification.

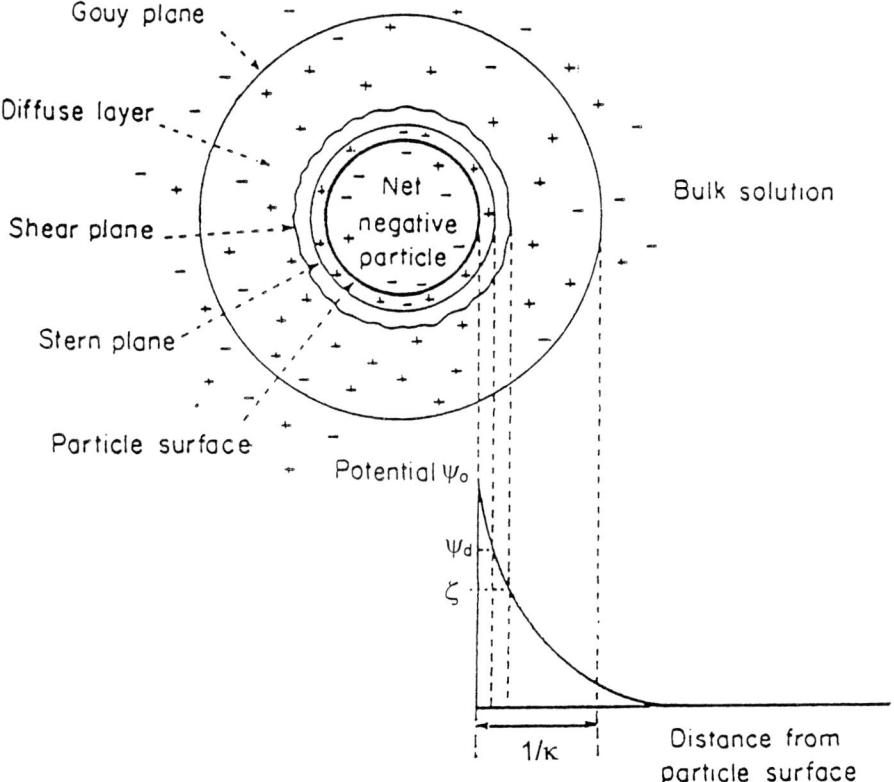

FIG. 1. A schematic representation of the electric double layer around a particle with negative surface charges and electrical potentials surrounding the particle.

Electrokinetic Phenomena and Zeta Potential

The term electrokinetic effect is used to describe phenomena associated with the relative movement of the fluid containing a diffuse electrical double layer with respect to the charged surface of the dispersed phase [4-6]. There are four distinct electrokinetic effects (Table 1), depending on the way in which motion is induced. If the continuous phase (medium) consists of a liquid or gas in which the second phase is dispersed as particles of solid or liquid, the particles can be induced to move by applying an electric field across the system. This is called electrophoresis. However, when the solid remains stationary and the liquid medium moves in response to an applied electric field, it is called electro-osmosis. This occurs when the solid is in the form of a capillary or a porous plug which is filled with the liquid. The applied field acts upon the charges in the liquid, and as they move in response to the field, they carry the liquid along with them.

Streaming potential is another electrokinetic effect which is generated when a liquid is forced through a capillary or porous plug under a pressure gradient. In this case, the excess charges near the wall are carried along by the liquid, and their accumulation downstream causes the build-up of an electric field which drives an electric current back against the direction of the liquid flow. Sedimentation potential is an electrokinetic phenomenon which arises when charged colloidal particles are allowed to settle (or rise) through a fluid under gravity or in a centrifugal field.

In spite of the differences in phenomena, these four electrokinetic effects are all influenced by the potential at the plane of shear between the charged surface and the bulk solution. This potential is called the electrokinetic or zeta potential (ζ). The exact location of the shear plane is another unknown feature of the electric double layer. In addition to the ions in the Stern layer, a certain amount of liquid (water) binds to the charged surface and forms a part of the electrokinetic unit. It is therefore reasonable to suppose than the shear plane is usually located at a small distance further out from the surface that the Stern plane and that ζ is, in general, smaller in magnitude than ψ_d (Fig. 1). Although the assumption of a small difference between ζ and ψ_d can be supported by the bulk of experimental evidence, particularly at lyophobic surfaces, a significant difference between them is found at high potentials and at high electrolyte concentrations. The adsorption of nonionic surfactant results in the surface of shear being located at a relatively large distance from the Stern plane, and ζ is significantly lower than ψ_d. Regardless of these unknown factors concerning zeta potential, the measurement of this parameter can always provide information about the surface charge and the potential of the particles of the dispersed phase.

In theory, zeta potential can be experimentally determined from one of these electrokinetic phenomena. However, electrophoresis has the greatest applicability with respect to zeta-potential determination because the experimental techniques involved in

TABLE 1 The Four Different Types of Electrokinetic Effects

Electrokinetic Effects	Moving Phase	Stationary Phase	Externally Applied Field
Electrophoresis	Dispersed	Medium	Electrical field
Electro-osmosis	Medium	Dispersed	Electrical field
Streaming potential	Medium	Dispersed	Motion of medium
Sedimentation potential	Dispersed	Medium	Gravitational field

Zeta Potential

its measurement are relatively less complicated. Electrophoretic mobility is the electrokinetically determined quantity in electrophoresis. The relationship between electrophoretic mobility and zeta potential is described by various electrophoretic theories. For a spherical particle with a radius R, the shape of the electrical double layer can be described in terms of a dimensionless quantity, κR, which is the ratio of radius to double-layer thickness. When κR is small, a charged particle can be treated as a point charge; when κR is large, the double layer is effectively flat and may be treated as such.

The electrophoresis of large, smooth particles which have a large κR (>100) is described by the Helmholtz-Smoluchowski Eq. (8),

$$U_p = V_p/E = \zeta \varepsilon/\eta \qquad (8)$$

where U_p is the electrophoretic mobility, V_p is the electrophoretic velocity, E is the electric-field strength, ζ is the zeta potential, ε is the permittivity, and η is the viscosity of the medium. When the particles get smaller and/or the double-layer thickness (κ^{-1}) becomes relatively large (i.e., in an aqueous solution with very low electrolyte concentration or in a nonaqueous medium), the particles act like point charges and the Hückel Eq. (9) can be applied ($\kappa R < 0.1$).

$$U_p = V_p/E = \zeta \varepsilon/1.5\eta \qquad (9)$$

Thus, the equations for these two extreme cases differ only by a simple constant. However, many colloidal systems fall between these two limiting cases. Henry was the first to consider the situation corresponding to the intermediate range with the assumptions that the diffuse layer is undistorted by the externally applied field, and that the potentials are assumed to be small (i.e., $ze\psi/kT < 1$). He showed that when the external field was superimposed on the double-layer field around the particle, the elecrophoretical mobility could be written as in Eq. (10).

$$U_p = (\zeta \varepsilon/1.5\eta) f_1 (\kappa R) \qquad (10)$$

The function $f_1 (\kappa R)$ depends on particle shape and, for a sphere, is given for $f_1 (\kappa R) < 1$ by Eq. (11),

$$f_1(\kappa R) = 1 + (\kappa R)^2/16 - 5(\kappa R)^3/48 - (\kappa R)^4/96 + (\kappa R)^5/96$$
$$- [(\kappa R)^4/8 - (\kappa R)^6/96] e^{\kappa R} \int_{\infty}^{\kappa R} (e^{-t}/t) \, dt \qquad (11)$$

and for $kR > 1$ by Eq. (12).

$$f_1 (\kappa R) = 3/2 - 9/2\, \kappa R + 75/2\, (\kappa R)^2 - 330/(\kappa R)^3 \qquad (12)$$

It should be noted that $f_1 (\kappa R)$ varies between 1.0 for small κR, Hückel Eq. (9), and 1.5 for large κR, Smoluchowski Eq. (8). However, when Henry's assumptions are not valid, the situation becomes further complicated. Mutual distortion of the applied electric field and the field of the electrical double layer could affect electrophoretic mobility through abnormal conductance in the vicinity of the charged surface (surface conductance) and through loss of double-layer symmetry.

The effect of surface conductance on electrophoretic behavior can be ignored when κR is small, since the applied electric field is hardly affected by the particle. When κR

is not small, the calculated zeta potentials may be significantly lower. Electrophoretic retardation occurs when ions in the mobile part of the double layer move in a direction opposite to that of the particle under the applied electric field. This creates a local movement of liquid opposing the motion of the particle and results in the double layer being distorted because a finite time (relaxation time) is required for the original symmetry to be restored by diffusion and conduction. The asymmetric mobile part of the double layer exerts an additional retarding force on the particle known as the relaxation effect. Relaxation can be neglected when κR is small or large, but it is significant for intermediate values of κR, especially at high potential and when the counterions have a high charge number and/or low mobilities. Both the surface conductance and relaxation effect can be corrected for with known equations [7].

Method and Instrumentation

Microelectrophoresis

The most common method for determining the zeta potential is the microelectrophoretic procedure in which the movements of individual particles under the influence of a known electric field are followed microscopically. If the Helmholtz/Smouluchowski conditions hold, the zeta potential can be calculated from the electrophoretic velocity of the particle using Eq. (8). However, it is important to realize that the observed electrophoretic migration is the sum of two contributions, one of which is the electro-osmotic flow of the medium through the cell. The glass of the sample cell generally bears negative charges, so that a diffuse layer of cations exists adjacent to them. This sets up an electro-osmotic flow through the cell (with or without particles). This flow has its maximum value at the center, since the layer of fluid adjacent to the walls is stationary. The particles tracked at the center of the cell therefore possess the maximum increment in velocity because of the electro-osmotic flow. Since there is no net liquid flow through the closed cell, a back-pressure builds up which causes fluid flow in the reverse direction in the core of the cell. In the steady state, these flows balance, giving rise to a velocity profile as shown in Fig. 2. Therefore, the tracking of particles at a location where the medium experiences no net flow becomes important in yielding an accurate electrophoretic mobility measurement. A velocity profile has been derived for the liquid contained in a cylindrical electrophoretic cell. The location with zero liquid flow is shown to be 14.6% of the cell diameter inside the surface of the capillary. The location of the surface of zero liquid flow in cells of rectangular cross section has also been determined. For a cell in which the direction of migration is relatively long com-

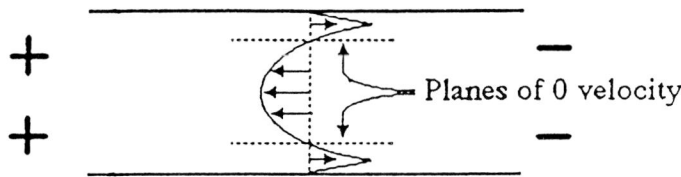

FIG. 2. The velocity profile of fluid flow in an electrophoretic cell.

Zeta Potential

pared to the width of the cell, the surface with zero liquid flow lies 21.1% of the cell depth above the bottom and below the top of the working compartment. Experimentally, particles tracked at these positions of the sample cell display their mobility uncomplicated by the electro-osmotic effect.

The rate of particle migration can be determined by measuring with a stopwatch the time required for a particle to travel between the marks of a calibrated graticule in the microscope eyepiece. Since many particles are usually measured in order to get good statistical results, the measurement of a sample may take 30 min or even longer. As the time of measurement increases, however, the susceptibility to errors also increases. For example, a long measurement time causes convection currents generated by heating the sample, air-bubble formation, settling of particles, and electrode reactions. These potential errors can be avoided if the measurement is taken much more quickly without loss of accuracy. A rotating-prism method employed by the Lazer Zee Meter (Model 501, PenKem, Inc.), allows the operator to measure more than ten particles simultaneously. Data are thereby attained more rapidly and, consequently, with fewer time-dependent errors. Figure 3 shows a diagram of light paths produced by the rotating-prism method [8]. The microscope is focused on the stationary layer of the cell (without fluid flow). Special cylindrical optics compress the laser beam into an illumination sheet of laser light. A vertical adjustment is provided to vary the height so that it coincides with the focal plane of the microscope. A cube prism inside the microscope causes the viewed image to translate at a rate proportional to the prism's speed of rotation. The applied electric field causes the particle to move at an electrophoretic velocity proportional to the mobility and the applied voltage. Adjustment of the potentiometer causes the prism to rotate at a rate proportional to the potentiometer voltage times the applied voltage. When the image velocity caused by prism rotation is equal and opposite to the mean electrophoretic velocity, the cloud of particles appears stationary. The applied voltage is therefore proportional to the mean particle electrophoretic mobility. The mobility value is scaled by an appropriate constant in the digital meter, and the computed zeta potential is displayed on the three-digit readout.

In spite of a major improvement gained from the rotating-prism method, the use of microelectrophoresis in determining zeta potential still has serious limitations. First, this technique cannot be applied to dense dispersions, and the number density of the par-

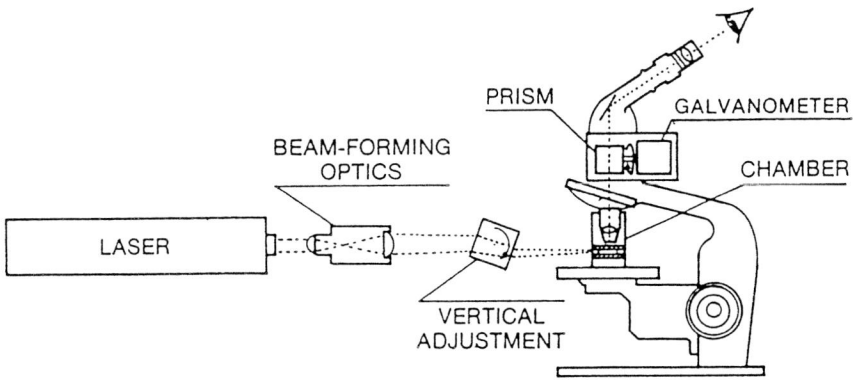

FIG. 3. A diagram of light paths produced by the rotating-prism method of microelectrophoretic measurement.

ticles must be very low. This can sometimes, but not always, be remedied by filtering the sample and diluting a small amount of the original dispersion with a large volume of filtrate. Second, it cannot be applied to particles less than about 0.2 μm in diameter because they are not easily visible in the ultramicrosope, though the particle-size range may be extended by adsorbing the colloidal particles (i.e., protein molecules) on suitable carrier particles. An additional and unsolvable problem with very small particles is the blurring effect imparted by Brownian motion. Furthermore, the microelectrophoretic technique cannot be used to determine mobility distributions or to separate multimodal mobility distributions.

Electrophoretic Light-Scattering

Electrophoretic light-scattering is a technique which determines the electrophoretic velocities by measuring the Doppler shifts of scattered laser light [6,9,10]. The Doppler frequency shift resulting from the laser light and the scatter moving with a relative velocity V_p is given by Eq. (13),

$$\Delta \nu = V_p \, \nu_o / c \qquad (13)$$

where $\Delta \nu$ is the Doppler frequency shift, V_p is the velocity relative to the laser light, and ν_o and c are the frequency and velocity of the laser light, respectively. When the scattered laser light is detected by fixed photodiodes, the Doppler shift in this measurement depends on the scattering angle according to Eq. (14),

$$\Delta \nu = 2 \, n \, V_p \, \sin(\theta/2) / \lambda_o \qquad (14)$$

where θ is the scattering angle, n is the index of refraction of the medium, and λ_o is the wavelength of the laser in a vacuum. From Eq. (14) it should be noted that the Doppler frequency shift is linear with $\sin(\theta/2)$. A combination of Eqs. (13) and (14) gives Eq. (15), an expression for electrophoretic mobility,

$$U_p = \Delta\nu \, \lambda_o / 2 \, n \, E \, \sin(\theta/2) \qquad (15)$$

where U_p is electrophoretic mobility and E is the electric field applied. Since a He-Ne laser light has a frequency of about 6.0×10^{14}, a direct measurement of frequency shifts ranging from zero to several hundred Hz may be problematic because of the difficulty in measuring a small difference between large quantities. However, this can be overcome by using the principle of heterodyning, which measures the difference in frequency resulting from a reference beam and the Doppler-shifted beam.

When the Brownian motion of the particles is negligible, the power spectrum that is generated by the autocorrelation function of the scattered light has very a narrow peak. However, the actual spectral peak has considerable line width attributable to the Brownian motion of the particles and a distribution of electrophoretic mobilities. Line-width broadening (Doppler broadening) caused by Brownian motion follows the following relationship,

$$\text{Line width} = DK^2/\pi \qquad (15a)$$

where D is the diffusion coefficient and K is the scattering vector defined by Eqs. (16) and (17), respectively,

Zeta Potential

$$D = kT/6\pi\eta r \qquad (16)$$

$$K = 4\pi n \sin(\theta/2)/\lambda_o \qquad (17)$$

where k is the Boltzmann constant, T is the absolute temperature, η is the viscosity of the continuous phase, and r is the radius of the particle; the parameters in Eq. (17) are defined as in Eq. (14). Thus, the line-width broadening caused by Brownian motion increases with the scattering angle according to K^2. In addition, the broadening effect as a result of electrophoretic mobility distribution is directly proportional to the breadth of the distribution and increases linearly with the scattering angle, Eqs. (14) and (17).

The separation of these two sources of spectral-peak broadening is critical because, without such a separation, a measurement of electrophoretic mobility at a single angle provides information only about the peak position (Doppler shift). The shape of the peak (Doppler broadening), being attributable to either of the two effects, cannot be interpreted with a single-angle measurement. Simultaneous multiple-angle measurements allow peak shapes to be analyzed to give accurate measurement of the electrophoretic mobility and the subsequent determination of zeta potential according to the Helmholtz-Smoluchowski Eq. (8).

The DELSA 440 (Coulter Scientific Instruments) is a laser-scattering particle electrophoretic analyzer that measures the electrophoretic mobility distribution and zeta-potential distribution [11]. This instrument provides simultaneous measurements of line widths at four different angles so that the motion of the particle can be decomposed with high resolution into components caused by electrophoretic and diffusional motions. Therefore, particle sizing can also be carried out by the same instrument simultaneously with electrophoretic mobility determinations. Figure 4 shows a schematic diagram of the DELSA 440 system. Other commercial electrophoretic analyzers using the laser light-scattering principles are the Zetasizer 3 (Malvern Instruments), ZetaPlus (Brookhaven Instruments), and System 3000 (PenKem, Inc.).

Electrokinetic Sonic Analysis

When a colloidal dispersion is subject to ultrasonic waves, a density difference between the dispersed phase and the continuous phase causes a relative motion between the particles and the surrounding fluid. This relative motion indicates that there is a peri-

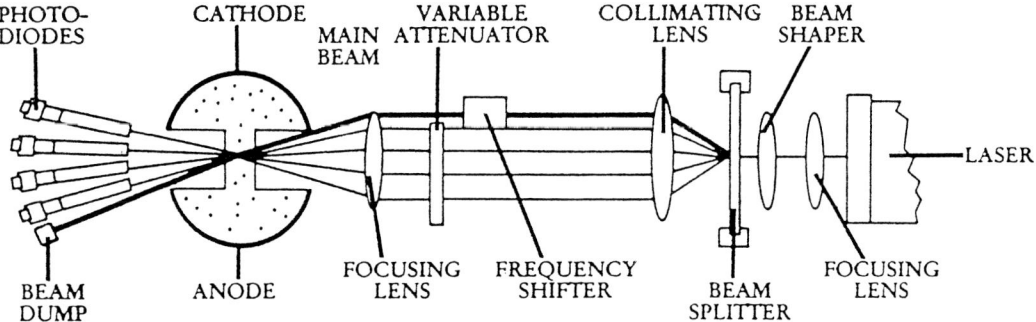

FIG. 4. The DELSA 440 system (Coulter Scientific Instruments).

odic interchange of the charged particle surface and the oppositely charged counterions in the electric double layer. This interchange results in the development of an alternating dipole at the frequency of the applied ultrasound wave. This effect is termed the ultrasound vibration potential (UVP) and is sometimes referred to as the Debye effect because it was first predicted for electrolyte solutions by Debye in 1933. The UVP effect in colloids is also referred to as the colloid vibration potential (CVP). An effect opposite that of CVP is generated when an alternating electric field is applied to a colloidal dispersion, creating an acoustic wave which, by means of a piezoelectric device, may be transduced into an alternating potential of a certain amplitude, depending on the dispersion and the electric double-layer properties. This is called the electrokinetic sonic amplitude (ESA). These two phenomena are both known as electroacoustic effects [6,11,12].

The magnitude of these effects is directly proportional to the electrophoretic mobility of the particles. The mobility determined by electro-acoustic effect is the dynamic or AC mobility of the particle. Equations (18) and (19) describe ESA and CVP in terms of other fundamental properties of the dispersion:

$$\text{ESA}(\omega) = P/E = c\,\Delta\rho\,\phi\,G_f\,U_d(\omega) \tag{18}$$

$$\text{CVP}(\omega) = \Delta\psi/U_o = c\,\Delta\rho\,\phi\,G_f\,U_d(\omega)/K^* \tag{19}$$

where ω is the angular frequency, P is the pressure amplitude of the generated sound wave, E is the amplitude of the applied electric field, c is the velocity of sound in the dispersion, $\Delta\rho$ is the density difference between the particles and the continuous phase, ϕ is the volume fraction of the particles, G_f is the factor of electrode geometry, $\Delta\psi$ is the potential difference measured at the electrode, U_o is the velocity amplitude of the applied sound wave, K^* is the high-frequency conductivity of the suspension, and U_d is the dynamic or high-frequency electrophoretic mobility. In the case of parallel plate-cell geometry, a reciprocal relationship exists between the ESA and CVP, given by Eq. (20).

$$\text{ESA}/K^* = \text{CVP} \tag{20}$$

The ESA measurement offers a distinct advantage over that of the CVP because it is directly proportional to the high-frequency electrophoretic mobility of the particles and not proportional to the high-frequency conductivity of the dispersion. This advantage is particularly helpful for nonaqueous systems because low dielectric-constant organic liquids have a strong capacitive component and their complex conductivity is difficult to measure. Thus, ESA measurements can be applied with increasing electric field strength to attain the higher resolution necessary for the characterization of these systems. Furthermore, CVP measurements are difficult to interpret in high-conducting dispersions because of severe signal-to-noise problems which arise from of the fact that CPV is inversely proportional to conductivity and decreases as conductivity increases. CVP measurement can be further limited as the mobility of most particles is lowered at high conductivities as a result of electric double-layer compression.

The dynamic mobility which is determined by the electro-acoustic effects differs from the low-frequency or DC mobility that is determined by electrophoresis because of the effects of particle inertia which cause particle velocities in an alternate field to become out of phase with the applied field. The higher the frequency, the greater is the phase lag between the particle and the applied field. Dynamic mobility is a function of fre-

Zeta Potential

quency, particle size, particle density, and particle zeta potential. These inertial effects arise in both ESA and CVP measurements. In the case of spherical particles with thin double layers and low zeta potential, Eq. (21) can be applied,

$$U_d = (\varepsilon\,\zeta/\eta)\,G(\alpha) \tag{21}$$

where $G(\alpha)$ is the inertial term. The formula for dynamic mobility is identical to the well-known Helmholtz-Smoluchowski Eq. (8) for dc electrophoretic mobility, except for the $G(\alpha)$ term.

As shown by Eqs. (18) and (19), a linear relationship exists between the ESA or CVP amplitude and the volume fraction of the suspended particles. At relatively high-volume fractions, hydrodynamic and electric double-layer interactions lead to a nonlinear dependence of these two effects on volume fraction. Generally, nonlinear behavior can be expected when the electric double-layer thickness is comparable to the interparticle spacing. In most aqueous systems, where the electric double layer is thin relative to the particle radius, the electro-acoustic signal remains linear with respect to volume fraction up to 10% by volume. At volume fractions that are even higher, particle–particle interactions lead to a reduction in the dynamic mobility.

The commercial systems for zeta-potential determination using these electro-acoustic effects are typified by the AcoustoSizer 8000 (Matek Applied Sciences), consisting of five main components (Fig. 5). The synthesizer produces a continuous sinusoidal voltage which feeds into the gated amplifier. This creates a sinusoidal voltage pulse across the cell which contains the dispersion. The resulting ESA sound waves are converted by a pressure transducer in the cell to an electrical signal, which then passes to the signal-processing electronics. The electronics extract the amplitude and the phase of the ESA signal, storing them in the computer housed in the AcoustoSizer.

A schematic diagram of the measurement cell is shown in Fig. 6. The dispersion is located in the region between the pair of electrodes. The pulse from the gated amplifier is applied across these electrodes, generating the ESA sound waves. Voltage pulses rather than continuous sinusoids are applied to avoid interference by the sound wave emanating from the electrodes. The use of pulsed signals also avoids electrical heating of the suspension and the complications of multiple reflections of the waves at the electrodes and at the ends of the rods. The voltage pulse produced by the sound wave in the transducer on the right passes into the signal-processing electronics, which measures the amplitude and phase of the sinusoidal component of the pulse. These data are passed to the computer where they are stored for subsequent processing.

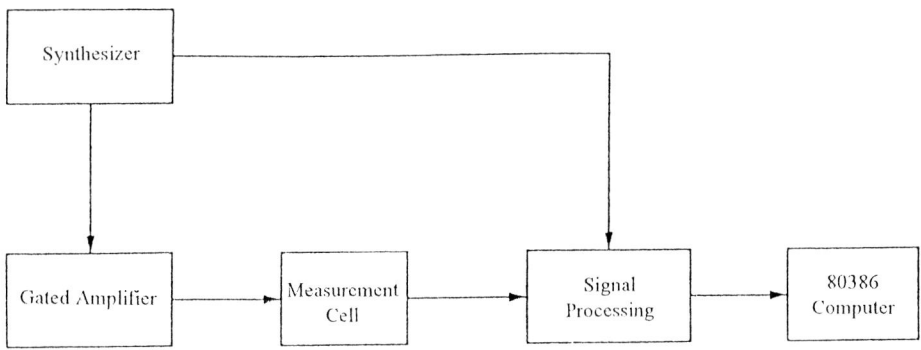

FIG. 5. Block diagram of an AcoustoSizer signal processor.

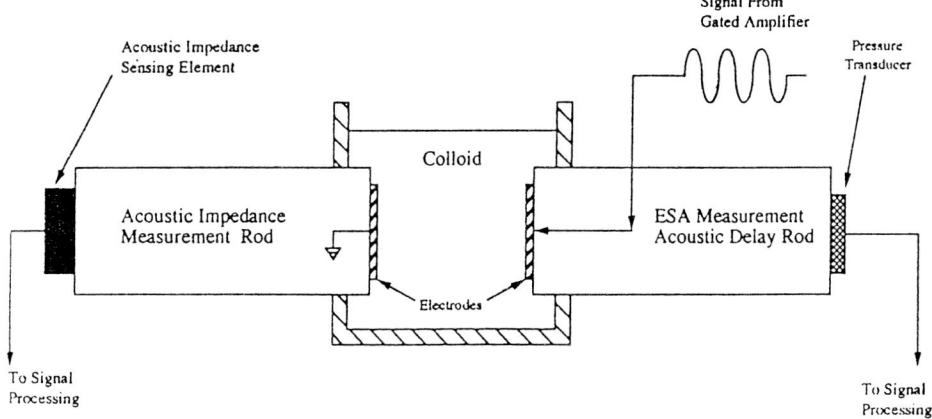

FIG. 6. A schematic diagram of the AcoustoSizer measurement cell.

Since the ESA signal depends on particle motion and also on the acoustic property of the dispersion, the determination of particle motion from the ESA signal requires knowledge of the acoustic impedance of the dispersion. This parameter is measured using sensors associated with the rod on the left immediately after each ESA measurement. The signals from these two rods are stored in the computer and are subsequently converted to a particle-velocity spectrum, from which the zeta potential and size information are determined. The AcoustoPhor 8000 (PenKem, Inc.) is another example of a commercial system which determines the zeta potential and particle size of dispersion with the help of these electro-acoustic effects.

Applications

The practical significance of zeta-potential measurement lies in the fact that strong empirical correlation exists between the measured zeta potential of the system and its properties which are the manifestation of the electrostatic interfacial phenomenon. Since the zeta potential can be conveniently measured, it becomes an ideal parameter for use in routine testing. Zeta-potential control has been successfully applied to various technical fields involving colloidial systems.

Colloid Stability

The physical stability of a colloidal system is determined by the balance between the repulsive and attractive forces which is described quantitatively by the Deryaguin-Landau-Verwey-Overbeek (DLVO) theory. The electrostatic repulsive force is dependent on the degree of double-layer overlap and the attractive force is provided by the van der Waals interaction; the magnitude of both are a function of the separation between the particles. It has long been realized that the zeta potential is a good indicator

Zeta Potential

of the magnitude of the repulsive interaction between colloidal particles. Measurement of zeta potential has therefore been commonly used to assess the stability of colloidal systems [2,4,6].

Electrostatic repulsive energy, V_R, at a given interparticle distance is the work that must be performed to bring the particles to a specific point. Using the Debye-Hückel low-potential approximation and assuming equal spheres, V_R can be described by Eq. (22),

$$V_R = 2\pi\varepsilon a\psi_d^2 \ln(1 + \exp[-\kappa H]) \tag{22}$$

where a is the particle radius and H is the distance of separation between the two particles. For small electric double layers, such that $\exp[-\kappa H] \ll 1$, Eq. (22) can be reduced to Eq. (23).

$$V_R = 2\pi\varepsilon a\psi_d^2 \exp[-\kappa H] \tag{23}$$

When the Debye-Hückel low-potential approximation is not made but the interparticle distance is considered to be sufficiently large, Eqs. (24) and (25) are developed for equal spheres,

$$V_R = (32\pi\varepsilon a k^2 T^2 \gamma^2 / e^2 z^2) \exp[-\kappa H] \tag{24}$$

where z is the counterion charge number and

$$\gamma = (\exp[ze\psi_d/2kT] - 1)/(\exp[ze\psi_d/2kT] + 1) \tag{25}$$

If the Debye-Hückel approximation, $ze\psi_d/kT \ll 1$, is made, Eq. (24) reduces to Eq. (23). All the approximations of V_R show that it decreases in an approximately exponential fashion with increasing H and that its range decreases by increasing κ (i.e., by increasing electrolyte concentration and/or counterion charge number). V_R can be also influenced by other specific factors. Counterion adsorption in the Stern layer may cause a reversal of charge, so that V_R is zero at the reversal-of-charge concentration and positive (repulsion) at both below and above this concentration.

The attractive-force component between particles in a colloidal system is developed by summation of the London dispersion forces between all atom pairs in the particles. Neglecting retardation effects, the expression for the attractive energy V_A between two particles of radius a at a distance of separation H_o, for $a \gg H_o$, is given by Eq. (26),

$$V_A = Aa/12H_o \tag{26}$$

where A is the effective Hamaker constant describing the attraction between the particles and the dispersion medium. The value of V_A calculated from the Eq. (26) is overestimated at large distances ($H_o > 10$ nm) owing to a neglect of the finite time required for propagation of electromagnetic radiation between the particles, the result of which is a weakening of V_A. It is also apparent that V_A decreases as an inverse power of the distance between the particles.

According to the DLVO theory, the total energy of interaction between colloidal particles is given by the sum of the attraction (V_A) and repulsion (V_R) energies, as shown by Eq. (27).

$$V_T = V_R + V_A \tag{27}$$

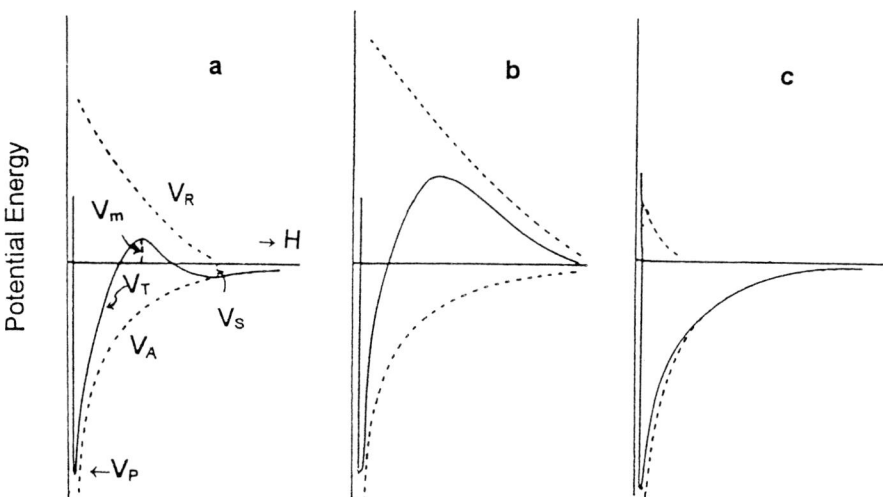

FIG. 7. Variation of the attraction and repulsion energies and the total energy of interaction between two colloidal particles with interparticle distance.

Figure 7a shows the total interaction energy curve for a colloidal system. At very close distances between the particles, the Born repulsion between adjoining electron clouds predominates, and the net interaction is repulsion. However, at slightly greater distances, the van der Waals attraction predominates over the electrostatic repulsion, and the net interaction is strong attraction as shown by the deep potential energy minimum V_p. At even greater distances, the net interaction is moderate attraction (a shallow secondary minimum V_s) because with increasing distance between two particles, electrostatic repulsion weakens more rapidly than the van der Waals attraction energy. At intermediate distances, the electrostatic repulsion predominates and the net interaction becomes repulsion, with an energy barrier, V_m.

The attraction energy arising from van der Waals forces does not vary significantly with changes in the surface potential and electric double-layer properties of the colloidal particles. By contrast, changes in these two parameters have significant impact on the repulsion-energy component of the total interaction energy. Therefore, at greater distances, a further increase in electrostatic repulsion results in a total repulsive net-interaction curve without the secondary minimum (Fig. 7b). However, as the repulsive component of the interaction energy diminishes (i.e., the electrolyte concentration increases), the interaction curve becomes totally attractive and rapid coagulation (controlled by the particle-diffusion rate) of the colloidal particles takes place (Fig. 7c).

An empirical relationship was developed between the zeta potential and the coagulation behavior of a variety of systems. Deryaguin shows that a rapid decrease in stability can be expected when the conditions shown by Eq. (28) are met [6].

$$4\pi\varepsilon\xi^2/\kappa < A \qquad (28)$$

For a given system, A and ε are fixed; therefore, varying the electrolyte (in type and concentration) should produce instability at a particular value of ξ^2/κ. The validity of using zeta potential in describing the coagulation process should come as no surprise

Zeta Potential

because it characterizes the potential of the diffuse part of the electric double layer which is involved in double-layer overlap and which plays an important role in the coagulation process. When the zeta potential is sufficiently high to produce a potential barrier opposing coagulation, the rate of coagulation is slowed by a factor, W, called the stability ratio, defined as the ratio of the total number of particle collisions to the number of collisions forming permanent doublets. Wiese and Healy reported an excellent correlation between the theoretical values for W (calculated from the zeta potential) and the experimental values for TiO_2 and Al_2O_3 sols as a function of pH (Fig. 8) and electrolyte (KNO_3) concentration [13]. Rapid coagulation, whether induced by pH or KNO_3 concentration changes, occurs at a value of $|\zeta| \leq 14 \pm 4$ mV, corresponding to $\zeta^2/\kappa = 6 \times 10^{-4}$ $(mV)^2$ cm.

Pharmaceutical Systems

Most of the pharmaceutical dispersions can be classified as colloidal systems, although this depends upon the size of their dispersed phase. Therefore, in general, the theoretical and empirical relationships between zeta potential and colloid stability are applicable to the physical stability of these pharmaceutical systems. However, the practical aspects of applying zeta potential to these systems may vary because of differences in the chemical composition and physical state of their dispersed and continuous phases. In addition, the practical significance of zeta-potential measurement may be different for products which differ in their clinical requirements such as route of administration and consequent in vivo disposition.

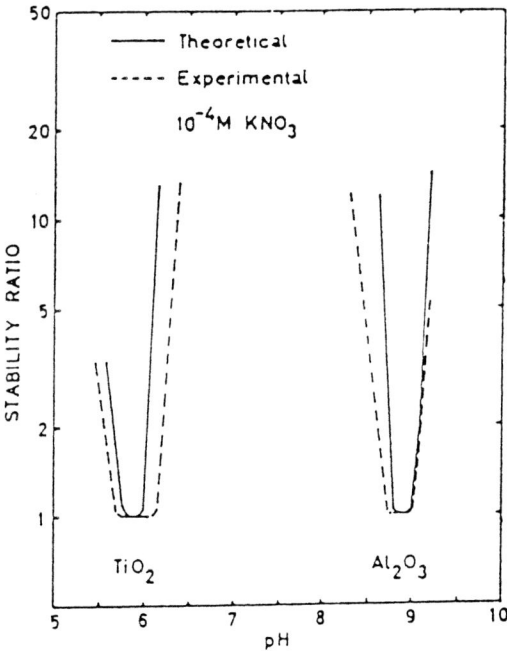

FIG. 8. Comparison of theoretical and experimental stability ratios for TiO_2 (0.05 g/L) and Al_2O_3 (0.15 g/L) colloids in 10^{-4} M KNO_3; theoretical, solid curves; experimental dashed curves.

Emulsions

Emulsions are widely used as vehicles for oral, topical, and parenteral delivery of medications. Although the product attributes of an emulsion dosage form are dependent on the route of administration, a common concern is the physical stability of the system, in particular the coalescence of its dispersed phase and the consequent alteration in its particle-size distribution and phase separation. The stabilization mechanism(s) for an emulsion is mainly dependent on the chemical composition of the surfactant used. Electrostatic stabilization as described by the DLVO theory plays an important role in oil-in-water emulsions (o/w) containing ionic surfactants [14]. For o/w emulsions with low electrolyte content in the aqueous phase, a zeta potential of 30 mV is found to be sufficient to establish an energy maximum (energy barrier) to ensure emulsion stability [14]. For emulsions containing nonionic surfactants (polymers), the principal stabilization mechanism is the repulsion between the adsorbed polymer chains on the surface of the oil globules called steric stabilization [14]. In such a case, zeta-potential measurement may have limited values with respect to emulsion stability.

In the past, injectable emulsions were administered intravenously to provide patients with vegetable oils as a major energy source in nutrition therapy [15]. In recent years, injectable emulsions have been found to be very effective vehicles for the parenteral delivery of water-insoluble drugs [16]. Because of toxicological considerations, surfactants used in the formulation of injectable emulsions have been largely limited to mixtures of phospholipids which are either derived from egg (egg-yolk lecithin) or soybean (soybean lecithin).

The majority of the phospholipids (80–80%) are phosphatidylcholine (PC) and phosphatidylethanolamine (PE), which are uncharged at physiological pH. However, small quantities (2-5%) of acidic components, largely phosphatidylserin (PS) and phosphatidylglycerol (PG), which are ionized at pH 7, confer a surface charge of approximately -40 to -50 mV to the emulsion particles [17]. Therefore, the stability of these emulsions is mainly attributable to electrostatic stabilization. Any factors that alter the surface potential are likely to have an impact on overall emulsion stability. The physical instability of an injectable emulsion as manifested by an increase in particle size ($>$ 5 µm) results in serious clinical consequences such as formation of pulmonary emboli [18]. Therefore, the extent of electrostatic stabilization of an injectable emulsion as measured by its zeta potential has been an important parameter in the characterizing and monitoring of its physical stability [19–24]. Furthermore, the biocompatibility of an injectable emulsion is also related to the net charge on the particle surface as reflected by its zeta potential. Davis and Galloway reported that soybean oil emulsion particles (Intralipid) in plasma exhibit a lower zeta potential, probably a result of the adsorption of albumin or lipoprotein [25]. In general, emulsions with a higher zeta potential (negative) exhibit reduced tendency to aggregate in the presence of blood proteins.

A relative wealth of information relating to the application of zeta potential to injectable emulsions has been documented with respect to the use of total nutrient admixtures (TNA) [26]. These are prepared by mixing the lipid emulsion with other components (i.e., dextrose, amino acids, and electrolytes) in a single container prior to administration. Depending on the composition, the mixtures vary widely in their stability and may show clinically unacceptable coalescence after different periods of storage time.

With regard to the electrostatic stabilization of the emulsion, the electrolytes (monovalent and divalent) added to the mixture are the major destabilizing species. The

Zeta Potential

zeta potential of the emulsion particles is a function of the concentration and type of electrolytes present [17, 27–32]. Two types of emulsion particle-electrolyte (ions) interaction are proposed: nonspecific and specific adsorption [26]. In nonspecific adsorption the ions are bound to the emulsion particle only by electrical double-layer interactions with the charged surface. As the electrolyte concentration is increased, the zeta potential approaches zero asymptotically. As the electrostatic repulsion decreases, a point can be found where the attractive van der Waals force is equal to the repulsive electrostatic force and flocculation of the emulsion occurs (Fig. 9a). This point is called the critical flocculation concentration (CFC).

The DLVO theory predicts that the CFC should vary inversely with the sixth power of the ion charge. The application of CFC alone fails to correlate the TNA stability with electrolytes in the mixtures because divalent ions (calcium and magnesium) adsorbed specifically on the emulsion particles through their complexation with the negatively charged acidic phospholipids. Figure 9b demonstrates the relationship between the concentration of a specifically adsorbed ion and the zeta potential and flocculation rate of an injectable emulsion. The increase in electrolyte concentration causes the particle charge to pass through zero; this is referred to as the point-of-zero charge (PZC). At this point the flocculation rate is at a maximum; a further increase in electrolyte concentration causes a surface-charge reversal of the particles and an increase in zeta potential (opposite sign) as well as a decrease of the flocculation rate from its maximum value.

The effect of pH on the stability of an injectable emulsion can also be followed by measuring its zeta potential (Fig. 10). At pH 7, the ionization of PS and PG imparts a negative surface charge (–30 to –50 mV) to the emulsion particles. As the pH is reduced, this ionization is suppressed until the charge is zero at a pH of 3.2. Further decreases in pH cause the protonation of the phospholipid and a positive surface charge (positive zeta potential). Significant progress has been made in relating the electrokinetic properties of phospholipid-stabilized emulsions to their instability when influenced

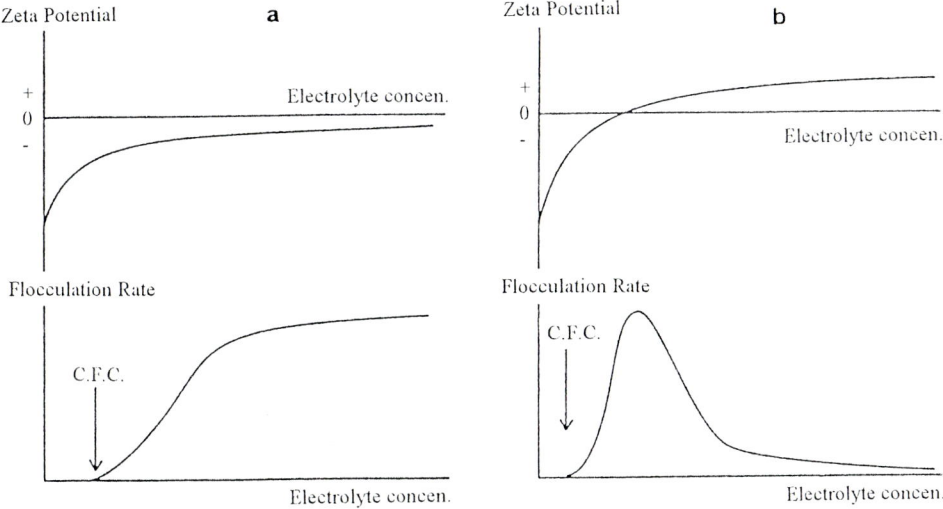

FIG. 9. Zeta potential and flocculation rate of a parenteral emulsion in the presence of (a) a nonspecifically adsorbing electrolyte, and (b) a specifically adsorbing electrolyte.

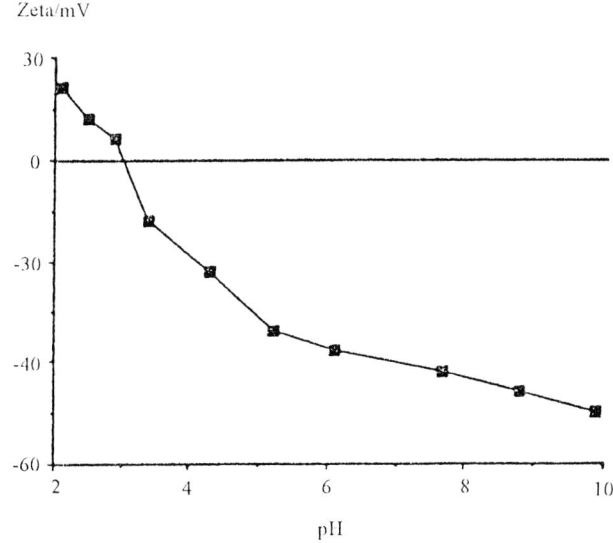

FIG. 10. Zeta potential of a parenteral emulsion as a function of pH.

by other TNA ingredients [33,34]. Washington and co-workers have attempted to develop a model predicting emulsion stability in TNAs using DLVO-based methods in the measurement of the zeta potential of the system [35].

Recently, zeta-potential determination has also been used in the development of positively charged o/w injectable emulsions that enhance the delivery of drug to targeted organs [36–38]. These emulsions are prepared and stabilized by forming a mixture consisting of phospholipids, poloxamer, and stearylamine. The addition of 0.4% stearylamine changes the zeta potential from −14.6 mV to +21.8 mV. The incorporation of drugs does not affect the zeta potential or the mean emulsion particle size. Because of the positive surface charge of the emulsion, the addition of calcium chloride does not result in any adverse effect on the zeta potential and the stability. This may be an advantage of positively charged emulsions because they are not sensitive to the cationic electrolytes generally encountered in the physiological environment.

Suspensions

In pharmaceutical suspensions solid particles are dispersed in a medium or vehicle (usually aqueous). A system with suspended solids below 1 µm is referred to as a colloidal suspension. A coarse suspension contains particle sizes greater than about 1 µm. The practical upper limit for particles in a coarse suspension is approximately 50 to 75 µm. Depending on the affinity or interaction between the dispersed phase and the dispersion medium, a colloidal dispersion can be classified as lyophilic (hydrophilic) or lyophobic (hydrophobic) [39].

The dispersion of hydrophilic particulate solids in water occurs spontaneously and gives rise to a thermodynamically stable system such as colloidal silicone dioxide or microcyrstalline cellulose. Hydrophobic solids are not easily wetted and are not dispersed spontaneously in water, for example, sulfur, clays, and most nonpolar organic compounds. The van der Waals attractive forces between particles cause them to aggregate,

Zeta Potential

since the solvation forces that promote dispersal in water are weak. Therefore, aqueous dispersions of hydrophobic solids can be stabilized only kinetically to resist flocculation and coagulation, which can be defined by referring to the total interaction energy curve (Fig. 7). Flocculation indicates the association of particles in the secondary minimum, whereas coagulation is the aggregation of particles in the primary minimum. Since the attractive forces between particles in a flocculated system are relatively week, they can be redispersed and the process is reversible. In contrast, coagulation is irreversible as attractive forces operating between particles in the primary minimum, are difficult to overcome.

A suspension where the electrostatic repulsion between particles is predominant is called a deflocculated system. For particles with a diameter of 2–5 µm, Brownian movement counteracts sedimentation to a measurable extent at room temperature by keeping the dispersed particles in random motion. This results in a system which is physically stable with respect to sedimentation and flocculation [39]. However, in a deflocculated suspension consisting of larger particles (coarse), gravitational force counteracts Brownian movement and sedimentation occurs [40]. At the bottom of the container, a compact sediment with strong attractive forces between the particles is formed which cannot easily be redispersed. This phenomenon is referred to as caking. The prevention of caking has been one of the main objectives in preparing stable coarse suspensions [40,41]. Although flocculation is referred to as a physical instability of colloids, flocculated suspensions are pharmaceutically acceptable since they are noncaking. In a flocculated suspension, particles attract each other (at the secondary minimum) loosely to form flocs which tend to settle together, creating a distinct boundary between the sediment and the supernatant. Particles in flocs are thereby easily redispersed after settling.

Controlled flocculation is a process by which flocculation of particles in a suspension is purposely produced by adding flocculating agents. One of the most effective methods of controlling flocculation is to reduce the electrostatic repulsive forces between particles [40,41]. Electrolytes have been shown to be effective flocculating agents. Zeta-potential measurement has been a valuable tool in monitoring and evaluating the influence of various electrolytes on the flocculation phenomena in coarse suspensions [42]. The sedimentation volume F, which is the ratio of the volume of sediment (V_u) to the original volume of the suspension (V_o), is a useful parameter in measuring the extent of flocculation. An excellent correlation between the zeta potential, sedimentation volume, and caking was found for a series of bismuth subnitrate suspensions containing various concentrations of potassium monobasic phosphate (Fig. 11) [43]. The addition of the phosphate causes a decrease in the zeta potential of the suspension because of partial neutralization of the positive surface charge on the bismuth subnitrate particles. With the decrease in the zeta potential (positive), the suspension becomes flocculate and noncaking, accompanied by an increase in the sedimentation volume. The continued addition of electrolyte causes the zeta potential to fall to zero and continue in a negative direction. The suspension remains flocculated until the zeta potential becomes sufficiently negative to effect deflocculation which is shown by a decrease in the sedimentation volume and an increase in caking tendency. The use of zeta-potential measurement in monitoring electrolyte-induced controlled flocculation of pharmaceutical suspensions has also been reported for sulfamerazine, griseofulvin, hydrocortisone, nitrofurantoin, zinc insulin, and a variety of suspensions containing inorganic material [44–49].

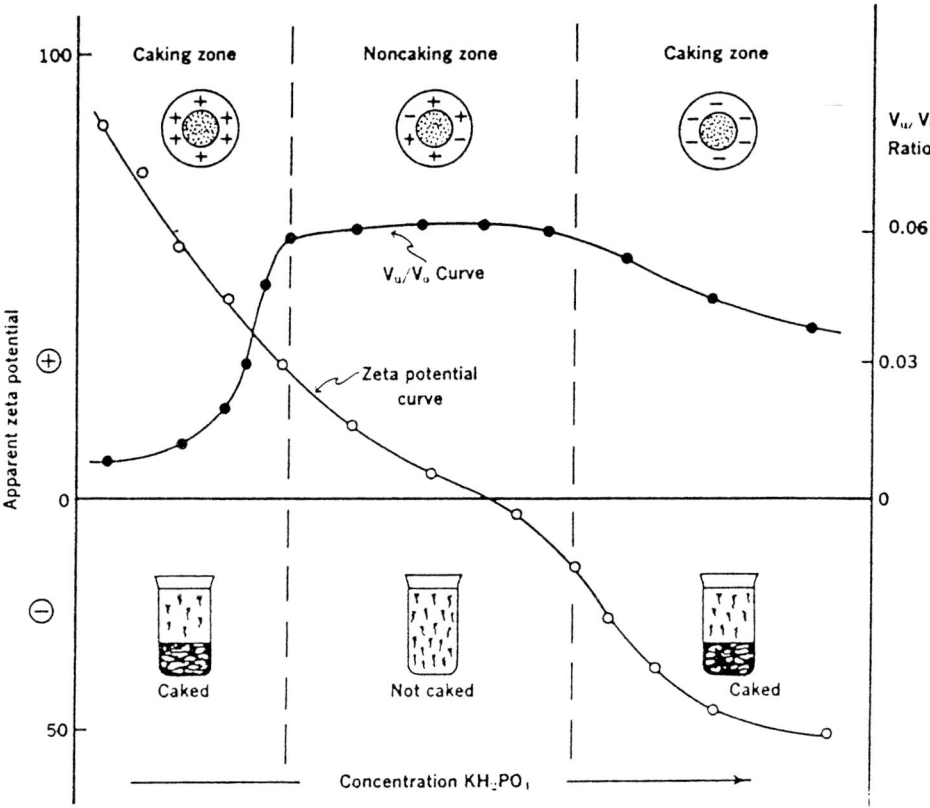

FIG. 11. A caking diagram showing the flocculation of a bismuth subnitrate suspension by means of the flocculating agent potassium monobasic phosphate.

The relationship between the zeta potential and the sedimentation kinetics of the electrolyte-flocculated suspensions was the subject of research by Carstensen et al. [50]. They studied the sedimentation kinetics of suspensions of 25% silica (5 μm) as a function of the zeta potential. The sedimentation of flocculated suspensions was shown to consist of an initial region of a pseudoparabolic nature and a final region of a biexponential character. The rate constant of the initial region was found to be a function of both Stokes and aggregational forces. The two rate-constants of the final phase are dictated by the effect of physical factors on the contraction of the bed of the equilibrium floc aggregate. They showed that the zeta potential has no effect on the first contraction-rate constant, whereas the reciprocal of the second contraction constant is linearly related to the reciprocal of the zeta potential.

In addition to electrolytes, surfactants (ionic and nonionic) can also play an important role in the flocculation–deflocculation of hydrophobic solids. Matthews and Rhodes reported that, in the presence of an anionic surfactant, increasing electrolyte concentration causes coagulation of griseofulvin particles at the primary minimum. The depth of the primary minimum, however, is restricted as a result of steric stabilization of the surfactant film formed on the particles [46]. The resultant coagulated suspension was shown to be redispersible. With the help of a modified DLVO theory, they were able to quantitatively estimate the steric repulsion component of the total interaction energy

Zeta Potential

relationship. Later, Kayes determined the relationship between zeta potential, sedimentation volume, and physical stability for suspensions of betamethasone, griseofulvin, nalidixic acid, and thiabendazole as a function of surfactant (anionic, cationic, and nonionic) concentrations [51,52]. Their results further confirmed that the modified form of the DLVO theory, including the steric repulsion term, is applicable to coarse suspension systems containing surfactants.

Delgado et al. investigated the role of the dispersion medium pH in determining the zeta potential of a nitrofurantoin suspension as affected by adding electrolytes [48]. They found that $AlCl_3$ is more efficient in reducing the negative zeta potential at a pH between 4 and 5. This phenomenon was attributable to the formation of a highly charged hydrolytic species of Al^{3+}. Kim et al. reported that, with the same concentration of NaCl, the zeta potential of zinc insulin suspension is at the maximum in the pH range of 6.6 to 7.2 [49]. Their experimental results indicate that, for this pH range, the greatest adsorption of chloride ions on the zinc insulin particles is responsible for the maximal change in the zeta potential.

The concept of heterocoagulation was applied by Schott to evaluate the effect of adding a colloidal dispersion to a coarse suspension of opposite charge [53]. The charge neutralization of a coarse bismuth subnitrate suspension by a colloidal bentonite dispersion was monitored by determining the zeta potential of the system. Gradual addition of bentonite dispersion first reduced the zeta potential of the bismuth subnitrate particles from +28 mV to zero and then to negative values. Otsuka et al. found that the adsorption of glycyrrhizic acid onto particles of sulfathiazole and graphite affects their zeta potential and the resultant flocculation-deflocculation behavior of the suspensions [54].

The addition of neutral macromolecules to surface-charged particles in suspension was found to alter the sensitivity of the particles to electrolytes. A significant increase in the negative surface charge (zeta potential) was observed when a small amount (0.1%) of a synthetic polymer, Carbopol 934, was present in a nitrofurantoin suspension to which NaCl or $AlCl_3$ was added [48]. Fritz and Riehl reported that the zeta potential of magnesium trisilicate decreases as the concentration of carboxymethylcellulose, hydroxyethylcellulose, or methylhydroxyethylcellulose increases [55]. However, the sedimentation behavior of the suspension cannot be explained solely by the DLVO theory based on the zeta potential data of the system. They concluded that the theory of polymer bridging is a better explanation for the settling characteristics and polymer adsorption onto the drug particles.

Zeta potential has also found an application in relating the surface-charge characteristics of a suspension to properties other than physical stability. Heyd and Dhabhar improved the fluidity of concentrated antacid suspensions by adding a colloidal polyelectrolyte (carrageenan sodium) called a fluidizing agent [56]. As the concentration of this agent increases, the zeta potential of the suspension changes from positive to negative, accompanied by a reduction in viscosity. The mechanism for this viscosity-thinning phenomenon is believed to be the selective adsorption of the negatively charged fluidizing agent onto the positively charged antacid particles. This imparts an electronegative charge (as measured by the zeta potential) onto the antacid particles, decreasing the demand for water.

The influence of the zeta potential on the flow behavior of aluminum hydroxide and magnesium hydroxide suspensions was also observed by Jovanovic and Djuric [57]. They reported that the effect of the additives on the viscosity of the suspensions is dependent on the final zeta potential of the suspensions. Zeta potential measurement was used to study the interaction between water-soluble dye and aluminum hydroxide in forming lake dyes. Desai et al. found that the zeta potential of lake dye varies with the pure-dye content; therefore the knowledge of the zeta potential of a specific lake dye is important when it is used in the formulation and manufacture of color suspensions [58].

In the literature, the use of zeta potential measurement for nonaqueous suspensions is infrequently reported because nonaqueous suspensions only represent a small percentage of all medicated suspension. Su et al. evaluated the flocculation–deflocculation behavior of cefazolin sodium in nonaqueous media and the effect of surfactants as measured by zeta potential along with sedimentation and porosity measurements [59]. A significant difference in zeta potential was observed when the particles were dispersed in peanut oil and ethyl oleate. The addition of lecithin reduced the zeta potential of cefazolin sodium, resulting in a deflocculated state accompanied by a decrease in sedimentation volume. The effect of surfactant excipient on the zeta potential of salbutamol in trichlorofluoroethane (P113) for metered-dose inhalation was determined [60]. Although the zeta potential of the particles is lowered (more negative) by the addition of oleic acid, the overall zeta potential is too low to be effective in providing the system with adequate electrostatic stabilization, particularly in media with low dielectric constant (organic solvents).

Microparticulate drug-delivery systems, including microspheres and nanoparticles, are suspensions when they are administered in a liquid medium. Microspheres are solid particles containing dispersed drug in solution or microcrystalline form, ranging in size from 1 to 1000 μm. Although most microspheres are outside the conventional colloidal size range, in pharmaceutical literature microspheres with sizes up to approximately 15 μm are still considered as colloidal delivery systems [61]. Nanoparticles are similar to microspheres but have particles sizes in the range of 0.01 to 1 μm; therefore, they form colloidal suspensions when dispersed in a liquid medium [62]. Zeta-potential measurement is an important surface-characterization technique which provides information regarding the surface charge of these microparticulate systems. The effect of surface charge (zeta potential) on the physical stability of these systems (i.e., aggregation) can be predicted with the help of the DLVO theory, although steric stabilization plays an important role in systems with surface-adsorbed macromolecules.

When the microparticles are administered intravenously, surface charge is an important parameter affecting the interaction between the microparticles and other biological components of the body and their subsequent in vivo distribution and disposition [63]. Tabata and Ikada reported that phagocytosis of polymer microspheres by macrophages is enhanced as the absolute value of zeta potential increases for both the negatively charged and the positively charged surfaces; the lowest phagocytosis is shown for the surface with a zeta potential of zero [64]. The uptake of charged serum components by nanoparticles (opsonization) in blood is considered to be the first step leading to phagocytosis by liver and spleen macrophages. Müller and co-workers determined the increase in zeta potential of nonparticles in serum as a measure of the extent of opsonization and used the data as selection criteria for IV drug carriers, thus avoiding liver and spleen uptake [65].

Liposomes

Liposomes are phospholipid-based vesicles which have been studied as delivery systems to target drugs to specific sites in the body [66-68]. The surface of a liposome can be

Zeta Potential

neutral or negatively or positively charged, depending on the composition of lipids. For charged liposomes, their surface potential is a critical factor affecting their physical stability and in vivo performance. Instead of their surface potential, zeta-potential measurement is frequently used in the investigation of the behavior of liposomes as influenced by their surface charge. Liposomes in aqueous dispersions have a tendency to aggregate and subsequently fuse on storage. This physical instability potentially limits their application as dosage forms.

Crommelin incorporated charge-inducing components in liposome bilayers to produce electrostatic repulsion between liposomes, thus increasing the shelf life of the dispersion [69]. He investigated the effect of including stearylamine or phosphatidylserin on the zeta potential of liposomes containing phosphatidylcholine and cholesterol. A correlation between the aggregation stability of negatively charge liposomes and the increments in the surface-charge density at both low and high ionic strength was established, whereas the positive liposome dispersions were found to be unstable.

Carrion et al. investigated the effect of incorporating phosphatidic acid on the zeta potential and aggregation of large unilamellar vesicle liposomes of phosphatidylcholine in the presence of neutral electrolytes [70]. Their results show that increasing the concentration of phosphatidic acid in lipid bilayers resulted in high zeta-potential and enhanced physical stability of the liposomes. The destabilizing effect of divalent cations (i.e., calcium ion) on charged liposomes has been well documented and is attributable to the reduced surface potential of the liposomes as the result of cation binding [71–73].

The effect of calcium ions on the aggregation behaviors of neutral liposomes composed of egg phosphatidylcholine and dipalmitophosphatidylcholine was investigated by Mosharraf et al. [74]. Both systems displayed a high negative zeta potential in deionized water, probably the result of adsorption of hydroxyl ions. A reasonable correlation was found in both cases between particle-size increase and zeta potential decrease, suggesting that the mechanism by which the aggregation takes place is related to the surface-charge characteristics. Although it has long been established that liposomes composed of neutral phospholipids acquire negative surface charge via anion adsorption, Makino and his group in Japan found that neutral liposomes exhibit negative zeta potential in buffer solution free of chloride ion [75]. They also reported that changes in the ionic strength and temperature causes the zeta potential of neutral liposomes to reverse sign. They proposed that the reversal of zeta potential is triggered by changes in the direction of the dipole connecting the negative charge of the phosphatidyl group and the positive charge of the choline group in the head group of a lipid molecule.

The effect of sonication conditions (frequency and time) in preparing liposomes as well as storage conditions (temperature and time) on the zeta potential of phosphatidylcholine liposomes was studied by Labhasetwar et al. [76]. They found that an increase in sonication frequency lowered the zeta potential of the liposomes. The zeta-potential of liposomes increases with a higher storage temperature and longer storage time. The breakdown of the phospholipid into free acid was believed to be a contributory factor in the change in zeta potential. Lloyd et al. described the use of zeta potential measurement as a means of investigating the interaction between liposomes and cryoprotectants [77]. Their results show that glycerin reduced the zeta potential of lecithin liposomes, but no change in zeta potential was seen with other sugar cryoprotectants. Glycerin is believed to interact with the phospholipid head group and this effect seems to correlate with its destabilizing effect on liposomes during freezing.

The study of the effect of drug loading on the zeta potential of liposomes provides information regarding the drug–liposome interaction. Lawrence et al. reported that the loading of polymyxin B, a polycationic antibiotic in negatively charged liposomes, results in the decrease of zeta potential, indicating electrostatic attraction between the positive drug and the negative lipid bilayer [78]. The highest drug loading is found in negatively charged liposomes in comparison to positively charged and neutral liposomes which further supports this electrostatic drug-liposome interaction. Beschiaschvili and Seelig investigated the binding of a cyclic somatostatin analogue, a positively charged peptide, to negatively charged multilamellar liposomes [79]. From the binding isotherm and the zeta-potential measurement, they were able to describe a partition equilibrium between the peptide and the negatively charged membrane with a surface-partition constant. They concluded that most of the peptide molecules are embedded in the head-group region with little penetration into the lipid core.

The measurement of the zeta potential of liposomes provides valuable information relating to their in vivo performance because, in addition to size, the surface charge of liposomes is an important determinant of their clearance from the general circulation and their tissue disposition after parenteral administration. Large multilamellar liposomes are cleared from the circulation much more rapidly than small unilamellar liposomes. Among small unilamellar liposomes, however, those with a negative surface charge are cleared rapidly, but positively charged or uncharged liposomes remain in the circulation for longer periods [80]. Rahman and co-workers compared the pharmacological and therapeutic effects of adriamycin entrapped in positively charged and negatively charged liposomes in rats [81]. They found that less cardiotoxicity was associated with the drug entrapped in the positively charged liposomes which exhibited lower in vivo uptake by cardiac tissue. When liposomes are employed to target drugs to lymph nodes, their surface charge has been shown to affect their lymphatic uptake from subcutaneous and intraperitonial injection sites [82]. Patel et al. showed that negatively charged liposomes yield the highest localization in the lymph nodes, followed by positively charged and neutral ones. The drainage of negatively charged liposomes has also shown to be faster than that of positive liposomes after intraperitoneal administration [83].

In recent years, surface modification of liposomes by covalent attachment of polyethylene glycol (PEG) prolongs their circulation and enhances their therapeutic efficacy [84,85]. Woodle et al. used zeta-potential measurement to estimate the thickness of a liposome polymer coating made of PEG conjugated to phosphatidylethanolamine plus zwitterionic lipids [86]. Their data show that the thickness of the hydrodynamic PEG coat as estimated from zeta-potential measurement increases with PEG molecular weight. Results of in vivo studies of blood circulation and hepatosplenic uptake in rats indicate that liposomes with a PEG coat of expanded thickness (molecular weight above 1000 Dalton) exhibited prolonged circulation.

Biomedical Applications

Hematology

The application of basic concepts of zeta potential to cardiovascular diseases was discussed by Riddick [87]. He pointed out that the physical stability of blood is controlled by the zeta potential of its colloidal components. He hypothesized that the intravascular coagulation and the clotting of shed blood are related to the zeta potential of red blood cells as affected by various blood electrolytes during these physiological changes. Sato et al. used electrophoretic mobility measurement to investigate the effect of red blood-cell shape change on the cell membrane as induced by incorporating excess lysolecithin or by hypertonic treatment [88]. They reported that the alteration of electrophoretic mobility of the cell caused by shape change is attributable to redistribution of the surface charge on the cell. Wagaine-Twabwe investigated the effects of pH changes (acidemia or alkalemia) on red blood-cell shape, size, and zeta potential and the viscosity of red blood cells suspended in buffer and plasma [89]. His results showed that the shape of red blood cells changes with increased or reduced zeta potential, depending on the pH of the medium.

Human blood platelets carry a net negative surface charge, which has been shown to be a factor in platelet adhesion and aggregation [90]. Changes in the surface charge would be expected to affect the electrostatic interactions between platelets and alter functional responses [91]. Studies have shown that agents such as adenosine diphosphate and norepinephrine which induce platelet aggregation also change the electrophoretic mobility (zeta potential) of platelets [92,93]. The electrokinetic properties of platelets can be changed by specific surface adsorption of charged macromolecules. Gröttum reported that the addition of dextran sulfate and heparin at low concentrations reduces the electrophoretic mobility of the platelets. When the electrophoretic mobility is reduced to 85% of its normal value, platelet aggregation occurs [94]. Jung and co-workers studied the relationship between platelet electrophoretic mobility and its aggregability in prostate cancer patients undergoing various drug treatments [95]. Their results showed that the platelets of patients on estrogen therapy display higher electrophoretic mobility and reduced aggregability than those of the control group. The platelets from aspirin-treated patients and platelets incubated with aspirin in vitro both exhibited increased electrophoretic mobility.

The role of platelet adhesiveness in intravascular thrombosis has been frequently investigated. Many of the results have been explained in physiological terms, but Dawber and Roberts were the first to investigate platelet adhesiveness based on a physicochemical approach involving the concepts of electrical double layer and zeta potential [96]. They concluded that substances influence platelet adhesiveness by affecting the zeta potential at the platelet surface. They also extended the zeta-potential theory to postulate that thrombus formation at the vascular endothelium–blood interface is attributable to the transient attenuation of the zeta potential of the endothelium and the subsequent adhesion of platelets. Tatsumi et al. measured the zeta potential of platelets from healthy subjects and patients with essential thrombocytosis or polycythemia vera using laser light scattering [97]. Since platelets from healthy controls had a zeta potential lower than those from patients, they indicated that zeta-potential measurement may provide valuable pathophysiological information in various platelet disorders.

Bone Physiology

Bone possesses piezoelectric properties. When external forces are applied to bone, piezoelectricity is responsible for the electrical signal generated, which is called stress-generated potential (SGP) [98]. In addition to the piezoelectric cause, SGP can also be generated when fluid flows past the walls of bone under a pressure gradient developed by stress [99,100]. This electrokinetic phenomenon of steaming potential has generally been accepted as the dominating mechanism for SGPs observed in wet bone upon deformation [101,102]. It has been suggested that this potential plays a role in bone growth, repair, and remodeling by inducing a response at the cellular level [103,104].

Walsh and Guzelsu measured the steaming potential of bone by forcing fluid through intact bone with pressurized nitrogen [105]. The relationship between the applied pressure gradient and developed streaming potential allowed the calculation of the zeta potential. They demonstrated that alterations in the fluid phase (conductivity, viscosity, or dielectric constant) can modify the streaming and zeta potentials and that the electrical double layer may be susceptible to alterations to the fluid phase by mechanical pressure. In a previous study conducted by Berretta and Pollack, the zeta potential of bone particles was determined by an electrophoretic technique [106]. Their results confirm that streaming potentials are the major contributory factor to the stress-generated potentials in fluid-saturated bone. A broad distribution of electrophoretic mobility of the bone particles was also determined. They found that the addition of a buffer caused the zeta potential to change from negative to positive values at ion concentrations exceeding 3.0 M. It is believed that changes in the streaming and zeta potentials of the bones as a result of alterations in the properties of the fluids they contain play an important role in the biofeedback response of bone tissue.

Microbiology

Adherence of microorganisms to the surface of the host is an important step in the infection process [107]. The initial stage of microbial adhesion is considered to be the results of van der Waals and electrostatic interactions as described by the DLVO theory [108]. The total energy–distance curve for such interaction is characterized by the presence of a shallow, secondary minimum at a long distance of separation, an interaction barrier, and a deep, primary interaction minimum at a short distance of separation (Fig. 7a). It is believed that microorganisms are initially captured in a reversible fashion in the secondary minimum and, with time, the bond strengthens and the microorganisms become attached more irreversibly in the primary minimum, overcoming the energy barrier. Zeta-potential measurement is often used to characterize the surface charge of the microorganisms and to calculate the electrostatic repulsion component of the total interaction energy between the microorganism and the adhering substrate [108]. The determination of the electrophoretic mobility and zeta potential of viruses and vaccines has also been reported. Small and Moore measured the electrophoretic mobility of three baculoviruses and determined their isoelectric point [109]. The interaction between the negatively charged viruses and a number of reagents was studied by measuring the change in electrophoretic mobility. The results were discussed in relation to the use of the viruses as biological control agents against insect pests. In order to determine the origins of the surface charge on Tice substrain *Bacillus Calmette-Guerin* (BCG) organisms, Kristensen et al. measured the zeta potential of the organisms after various chemical treatments [110].

Miyake et al. investigated the effect of subinhibitory concentrations of antifungal drugs on zeta potential and the resultant adherence of *C. albicans* to acrylic surfaces [111]. They showed that a negative relationship exists between the microbial adherence and zeta potential. Dealler measured the zeta potential of bacteria in the presence of antibiotics. He showed that the distribution of the zeta potential of *E. coli* and *S. aureus* broadened, and new peaks developed at less negative or more positive zeta potentials with increasing contact time with the antibiotic [112]. Although the cause of these changes in zeta potential is not clear, zeta-potential measurement may be used as a predictive indicator of bacterial antibiotic sensitivity.

Summary

Zeta-potential measurement has long been recognized as an excellent tool for characterizing colloidal systems. Its practical significance stems from the fact that it allows the quantitation of the electrostatic repulsion between particles, which is one of the most important forces governing the behavior and physical stability of colloidal systems. In recent years, the concept of zeta potential has been applied to areas beyond classical colloidal sciences and industrial processes. Pharmaceutical and biological sciences are two new fields to which the application of zeta potential has been extended. The expanding role of zeta potential in these fields is attributable to the advance in modern instrumentation of zeta-potential measurement, the rapid development of colloidal drug-delivery systems, and the emphasis on interdisciplinary basic research. While good correlation has been demonstrated for zeta potential and in vitro properties of colloidal drug-carrier systems, the impact of zeta potential in organ distribution and in vivo clearance of these systems has been the focus of additional research efforts. The determination of zeta potential has provided physicochemical explanations for some interfacial phenomena involving biological systems. Zeta potential has also found new applications in biomedical research, yielding promising results. It is believed that the biomedical application of zeta potential is a new area with great challenges and unlimited potentials.

References

1. Shaw, D.J., *Introduction to Colloid and Surface Chemistry*, 4th ed., Butterworth Heinemann Ltd, Oxford, 1992.
2. Hiemenz, P.C., *Principles of Colloid and Surface Chemistry*, 2nd ed., Marcel Dekker, Inc., New York, 1986.
3. Adamson, A.W., *Physical Chemistry of Surface*, 4th ed., John Wiley & Sons, New York, 1982.
4. Hirtzel, C.S., and Rajagopalan, R., *Colloidal Phenomena, Advanced Topics*, Noyes Publications, Park Ridge, NJ, 1985.
5. Hunter, R.J., *Foundations of Colloid Science*, Vol. II, Clarendon Press, Oxford, 1989.
6. Hunter, R.J., *Zeta Potential in Colloid Science, Principles and Applications*, Academic Press, London, 1981.
7. O'Brien, R.W., and White, L.R., *J. Chem. Soc. Faraday* II, 74:1607 (1978).
8. Goetz, P.J., and Penniman Jr., J.G., *Am. Lab.*, Oct., 1976.
9. Uzgiris, E.E., *Progress in Surface Science*, Vol. X, Pergamon Press, New York, 1981.
10. Oja, T., Bott, S., and Sugrue, S., *Doppler Electrophoretic Light Scattering Analysis Using the Coulter DELSA 440*, Coulter Electronics, Hialeah, FL, 1989.
11. O'Brien, R.W., *J. Fluid Mechanics*, 190:71 (1988).
12. Babchin, A.J., Chow, R.S., and Sawatzky, R.P., *Adv. Coll. Interf. Sci.*, 30:111–151 (1989).

13. Wiese, G.R., and Healy, T. W., *J. Coll. Interf. Sci.*, 51:427–433 (1975).
14. Friberg, S.E., Goldsmith, L.B., and Hilton, M.L., Theory of Emulsion. In: *Pharmaceutical Dosage Forms: Dispersion Systems* (H.A. Liberman, M.M. Rieger, and G. S. Banker, eds.), Vol. 1, Marcel Dekker, Inc., New York, 1988.
15. Wretlind, A., *J. Parenter. Enterol. Nutr.*, 5:230–235 (1981).
16. Davis, S.S., Washington, C., West, P., Illum, L, Liversidge, G., Sternson, L., and Kirsh, R., *Ann. N.Y. Acad. Sci.*, 507:75-88 (1987).
17. Washington, C., Chawla, A., Christy, N., and Davis, S.S., *Int. J. Pharm.*, 54:191-197 (1989).
18. Burnham, W.R., Hansrani, P.K., Knott, C.E., Cook, J.A., and Davis, S.S., *Int. J. Pharm.*, 13:9-22 (1983).
19. Benita, S., Friedman, D., and Weinstock, M., *Int. J. Pharm.*, 30:47-55 (1986).
20. Levy, M.Y., and Benita, S., *Int. J. Pharm.*, 54:103-112 (1989).
21. Ishii, F., Sasaki, I., and Ogata, H., *J. Pharm. Pharmacol.*, 42:513-515 (1990).
22. Rubino, J.T., *J. Parent. Sci. Tech.*, 44:210-215 (1990).
23. Benita, S., and Levy, M.Y., *J. Pharm. Sci.*, 82:1069-1079 (1993).
24. Levy, M.Y., Schutze, W., Fuhrer, C., and Benita, S., *J. Microencaps.*, 11:79-92 (1994).
25. Davis, S.S., and Galloway, M., *J. Pharm. Pharmacol.*, 31:99P (1981).
26. Washington, C., *Int. J. Pharm.*, 66:1-21 (1990).
27. Dawes, W.H., and Groves, M.J., *Int. J. Pharm.*, 1:141-150 (1978).
28. Washington, C., *Int. J. Pharm.*, 58:13-17 (1990).
29. Washington, C., *Int. J. Pharm.*, 64:67-73 (1990).
30. Hall, S.B., Gaskin, P.W., Duffield, J.R., and Williams, D.R., *Int. J. Pharm.*, 70:251-260 (1991).
31. Müller, R.H., and Heinemann, S., *Int. J. Pharm.*, 101:175-189 (1994).
32. Müller, R.H., and Heinemann, S., *Int. J. Pharm.*, 107:121-132 (1994).
33. Washington, C., Athersuch, A., and Kynoch, D.J., *Int. J. Pharm.*, 64:217-222 (1990).
34. Washington, C., Connolly, M.A., Manning, R., and Skerratt, M.C.L., *Int. J. Pharm.*, 77:57–63 (1991).
35. Washington, C., Ferguson, J.A., and Irwin, S.E., *J. Pharm. Sci.*, 82:808-812 (1993).
36. Davis, S.S., Illum, L., Washington, C., and Harper, G., *Int. J. Pharm.*, 82:99-105 (1992).
37. Elbaz, E., Zeevi, A., Klang, S., and Benita, S., *Int. J. Pharm.*, 96:R1-R6 (1993).
38. Klang, S.H., Frucht-Pery, J., Hoffman, A., and Benita, S., *J. Pharm. Pharmacol.*, 46:986-993 (1994).
39. Zografi, G., Schott, H., and Swarbrick J., Dispersion Systems. In: *Remington's Pharmaceutical Sciences* (A.R. Gennaro, ed.), 18th ed., Mack Publishing Company, Easton, PA, 1990.
40. Hiestand, E.N., *J. Pharm. Sci.*, 53:1-18 (1964).
41. Falkiewicz, M.J., Theory of Suspensions. In: *Pharmaceutical Dosage Forms: Dispersion Systems* (H.A. Liberman, M.M. Rieger, and G.S., Banker, eds.), Vol. 1, Marcel Dekker, Inc., New York, 1988.
42. Nash, R.A., and Haeger, B.E., *J. Pharm. Sci.*, 55:829-837 (1966).
43. Martin, A., and Swarbrick, J., *American Pharmacy*, 6th ed., Lippincott, Philadelphia, 1966.
44. Haines, B.A., and Martin, A.N., *J. Pharm. Sci.*, 50:753-756 (1961).
45. Matthews, B.A., and Rhodes, C.T., *J. Pharm. Sci.*, 57:569-573 (1968).
46. Matthews, B.A., and Rhodes, C.T., *J. Pharm. Sci.*, 59:521-525 (1970).
47. Schott, H.,*J. Pharm. Sci.*, 70:486-489 (1981).
48. Delgado, A., Gallardo, V., Salcedo, J., and Gonzalez-Caballero, F., *J. Pharm. Sci.*, 70:82-86 (1990).
49. Kim, Y., Cuff, G.W., and Morris, R.M., *J. Pharm. Sci.*, 84:755-759 (1995).
50. Carstensen, J.T., Stremming, K.P., and Pothisiri, P., *J. Pharm. Sci.*, 61:1999-2000 (1972).

51. Kayes, J.B., *J. Pharm. Pharmacol.*, 29:163-168 (1977).
52. Kayes, J.B., *j. Pharm. Pharmacol.*, 29:199-204 (1977).
53. Schott, H., *J. Pharm. Sci.*, 65:855-861 (1976).
54. Otsuka, A., Yonezawa, Y., and Nakamura, Y., *J. Pharm. Sci.*, 67:151-154 (1978).
55. Fritz, A., and Riehl, J., *Pharm. Ind.*, 51:1150-1156 (1989).
56. Heyd, A., and Dhabhar, D.J., *J. Pharm. Sci.*, 64:1697-1699 (1975).
57. Jovanovic, M., and Djuric, Z., *Pharmazie*, 40:498-499 (1985).
58. Desai, A., White, J.L., Hem, S.L., and Peck, G.E., *Drug Dev. Ind. Pharm.*, 17:1405-1409 (1991).
59. Su, K.S.E., Quay, F., Campanale, K.M., and Stucky, J.F., *J. Pharm. Sci.*, 73:1602-1606 (1984).
60. Clarke, J.G., Wicks, S.R., and Farr, S.J., *Int. J. Pharm.*, 93:221-231 (1993).
61. Burgess, D.J., and Hickey, A. J., Microsphere Technology and Applications. In: *Encyclopedia of Pharmaceutical Technology* (J. Swarbrick and J.C. Boylan, eds.), Vol. 10, Marcel Dekker, Inc., New York, 1994, pp. 1-29.
62. Kreuter, J., Nanoparticles. In: *Encyclopedia of Pharmaceutical Technology* (J. Swarbrick and J.C. Boylan, eds.), Vol. 10, Marcel Dekker, Inc., New York, 1994, pp. 165-190.
63. Wilkins, D.J., and Myers, P.A., *Br. J. Exp. Pathol.*, 47:568-576 (1966).
64. Tabata, Y., and Ikada, Y., *Biomaterials*, 9:356-362 (1988).
65. Müller, R.H., Wallis, K.H., Tröster, S.D., and Kreuter, J., *J. Contr. Rel.*, 20:237-246 (1992).
66. Riaz M., Weiner, N., and Martin, F., Liposomes. In: *Pharmaceutical Dosage Forms: Dispersion Systems* (H.A. Liberman, M.M. Rieger, and G.S. Banker, eds.), Vol. 2, Marcel Dekker, Inc., New York, 1989.
67. Gregoriadis, G., and Florence, A.T., *Drugs*, 45:15-28 (1993).
68. Barenholz, Y., and Crommelin, D.J.A., Liposomes as Pharmaceutical Dosage Forms. In: *Encyclopedia of Pharmaceutical Technology* (J. Swarbrick and J.C. Boylan, eds.), Vol. 9, Marcel Dekker, Inc., New York, 1994, pp. 1-39.
69. Crommelin, D.J.A., *J. Pharm. Sci.*, 73:1559-1563 (1984).
70. Carrion, F.J., De La Maza, A., and Parra, J.L., *J. Coll. Interf. Sci.*, 164:78-87 (1994).
71. Düzgünes, N., Nir, S., Wilschut, J., Bentz, J., Newton, C., Portis, A., and Papahadjopoulos, D., *J. Membr. Biol.*, 59:115-125 (1981).
72. Hope, M.J., Walker, D.C., and Cullis, P.R., *Biochim. Biophys. Res. Commun.*, 110:15-22 (1983).
73. Minami, H., Inque, T., and Shimozawa, R., *J. Coll. Interf. Sci.*, 158:460-465 (1993).
74. Mosharraf, M., Taylor, K.M.G., and Craig, D.Q.M., *J. Drug Target.*, 2:541-545 (1995).
75. Makino, K., Yamada, T., Kimura, M., Oka, T., Ohshima, H., and Kondo, T., *Biophys. Chem.*, 41:175-183 (1991).
76. Labhasetwar, V., Mohan, M.S., and Dorle, A.K., *J. Microencaps.*, 11:663-668 (1994).
77. Lloyd, A.W., Rutt, K.J., and Olliff, C.J., *J. Pharm. Pharmacol.*, 42:143P (1990).
78. Lawrence, S.M., Alpar, H.O., McAllister, S.M., and Brown, M.R.W., *J. Drug Target.*, 1:303-310 (1993).
79. Beschiaschivili, G., and Seelig, J., *Biochemistry*, 29:10995-11000 (1990).
80. Juliano, R.L., Stamp, D., and McCullough, N., *Ann. N.Y. Acad. Sci.*, 308:411-425 (1978).
81. Rahman, A, Kessler, A., More, N., Sikic, B., Rowden, G., Woolley, P. and Schein, P.S., *Cancer Res.*, 40:1532-1537 (1980).
82. Hawley, A.E., Davis, S.S., and Illum, L., *Adv. Drug Del. Rev.*, 17:129-148 (1995).
83. Patel, H.M., Boodle, K.M., and Vaughan-Jones, R., *Biochim. Biophys. Acta*, 801:76-86 (1984).
84. Woodle, M.C., and Lasic, D.D., *Biochim. Biophys. Acta*, 1113:171-193 (1992).
85. Woodle, M.C., *Chem. Phys. Lipids*, 64:249-262 (1993).

86. Woodle, M.C., Newman, M.S., and Cohen, J.A., *J. Drug Target.*, 2:397-403 (1994).
87. Riddick, T.M., *Control of Colloid Stability Through Zeta Potential*, Zeta-Meter, Inc., New York, 1968.
88. Sato, T., Fujii, T., and Kojima, K., *Physiol. Chem. Phys.*, 7:523-527 (1975).
89. Wagaine-Twabwe, D., *J. Physiol.*, 306:13P-14P (1980).
90. Abramson, H.A., *J. Exp. Med.*, 47:677-683 (1928).
91. Mitchell, J.R.A., and Sharp, A.A., *Brit. J. Haematol.*, 10:78-93 (1964).
92. Hampton, J.R., and Mitchell, J.R.A., *Brit. Med. J.*, 1:1074 (1966).
93. Seaman, G.V.F., and Vassar, P.S., *Arch. Biochem. Biophys.*, 117:10-17 (1966).
94. Gröttum, K.A., *Thromb. Diath. Haemorrh.*, 21:450-462 (1969).
95. Jung, S.M., Kinoshita, K., Tanoue, K., Isohisa, I., and Yamazaki, H., *Thromb. Haemostas,* 47:203-209 (1982).
96. Dawber, J.G., and Roberts, J.C., *Thromb. Diath. Haemorrh.*, 19:451-458 (1968)
97. Tatsumi, N., Tsuda, I., Masaoka, M., and Imai, K., *Thromb. Res.*, 65:585-592 (1992).
98. Yasuda, I., *J. Kyoto Med. Soc.*, 4:395-406 (1953).
99. Anderson, J., and Eriksson, C., *Nature*, 218:166-168 (1968).
100. Anderson, J., and Eriksson, C., *Nature*, 227:491-492 (1970).
101. Gross, D., and Williams, W.S., *J. Biomech.*, 15:277-295 (1982).
102. Guzelus, N., and Walsh, W.R., *J. Biomech.*, 23:673-685 (1990).
103. Bassett, C.A.L., Biophysical Principles Affecting Bone Structure. In: *Biochemistry and Physiology of Bone* (G.R. Bourne, ed.), 2nd ed., Vol. 3, Academic Press, New York, 1971.
104. Eriksson, C., Electrical Properties of Bone. In: *Biochemistry and Physiology of Bone* (G.R. Bourne, Ed.), 2nd ed., Vol. 3, Academic Press, New York, 1971.
105. Walsh, W.R., and Guzelsu, N., *Biomaterials*, 14:331-336 (1993).
106. Berretta, D.A., and Pollack, S.R., *J. Orthop. Res.*, 4:337-345 (1986).
107. Ofek, I., and Beachey, E.H., *Bacterial Adherence, Receptors and Recognition*, Series B, Vol. 6, Chapman and Hall, London, 1980.
108. Rutter, P.R., and Vincent, B., The Adnesion of Micro-organisms to Surface: Physico-Chemical Aspects. In: *Microbial Adhesion to Surfaces* (R.C.W. Berkeley, J.M. Lynch, J. Melling, P.R. Rutter, and B. Vincent, eds.), Ellis Horwood Ltd., West Sussex, UK, 1980.
109. Small, D.A., and Moore, N.F., *Appl. Environ. Microbiol.*, 53:598-602 (1987).
110. Kristensen, S., Tian, Y., Klegerman, M.E., and Groves, M.J., *Microbios*, 70:185-198 (1992).
111. Miyake, Y., Tsunoda, T., Minagi, S., Akagawa, Y., Tsuru, H., and Suginaka, H., *FEMS Microbiol. Lett.*, 69:211-214 (1990).
112. Dealler, S.F., *J. Antimicrob. Chemother.*, 28:470-473 (1991).

LUK CHIU LI
YOUQUIN TIAN

INDEX TO VOLUME 16

Abbreviated New Drug Application (ANDA), **XVI**:192, 201
Abrasion transfer, **XVI**:379
Absolute filters, **XVI**:43
Absolute temperature, drying and, **XVI**:51
Acacia, **XVI**:373
4'-Acetamidophenyl 4-guanidinobenzoate, **XVI**:176
Acetaminophen
  Crigler-Najjar syndrome and, **XVI**:425
  cytochrome P450 and, **XVI**:410
  waxes in delivery systems for, **XVI**:339
Acetohexamide, **XVI**:346
Acetylation, **XVI**:421–422, 425
Acetyl conjugation, *see* Acetylation
Acyl glucuronides, **XVI**:419
Acyl group migration, **XVI**:419
Adalat Retard, **XVI**:341
Adenosine triphosphate (ATP), sulfate conjugation and, **XVI**:422
S-Adenosylmethionine (SAM), **XVI**:423
Adenoviruses
  canine, *see* Canine adenovirus
  in vaccines, **XVI**:120, 136, 137
Adhesion forces, in immobile liquid bridges, **XVI**:374
Adjuvants, for vaccines, **XVI**:132–135
Adsorption
  in sterile filtration, **XVI**:100–101
  vapor, *see* Vapor adsorption
Aeromonas, **XVI**:265
Aeromonas hydrophilia, **XVI**:265
Aerosil, **XVI**:338–339
Agitated batch dryers, **XVI**:61
Air-circulation drying, **XVI**:55
Air conditioning, **XVI**:17–22
Air filters, **XVI**:43–45
Air filtration, **XVI**:41–45
Alcohol dehydrogenase, **XVI**:413–414
Aldehyde dehydrogenase, **XVI**:413–414
Alicyclic hydroxylation, **XVI**:404–405
Aliphatic hydroxylation, **XVI**:404–405
Alkyl hydroxylation, **XVI**:411
Alkyloxynol-741, **XVI**:176
Allopurinol, in veterinary pharmacy, **XVI**:264, 265
Alum, vaccines in, **XVI**:133, 134
Aluminum hydroxide
  vaccines in, **XVI**:178
  zeta potential and, **XVI**:449–450
Ambient temperature, water sorption isotherm analysis at, **XVI**:321–325
Amino acid conjugation, **XVI**:423
Aminophylline, **XVI**:341
Amorphous solids, water sorption by, **XVI**:312, 321–328

Ampicillin
  in veterinary pharmacy, **XVI**:255
  water sorption and, **XVI**:318
Amrinone, **XVI**:253
Anemia
  in horses, **XVI**:278
  in pigs, **XVI**:280
Anionic surfactants, in suspensions, **XVI**:449
Anticancer agents, vaginal delivery of, **XVI**:174–175
Antigens
  vaccines and, **XVI**:115
    delivery systems for enhanced response, **XVI**:134–140
    types of, **XVI**:117–129
    vaginal delivery systems and, **XVI**:178–179
    waxes in delivery systems for, **XVI**:343
Antimicrobials, vaginal delivery of, **XVI**:174
Aquatic animals, **XVI**:285–286
Aqueous suspensions, coating with, **XVI**:350–351
Aromatic hydroxylation, **XVI**:406
Arsinamine, **XVI**:255
Arthritis, in dogs, **XVI**:253
Artificial insemination, animal, **XVI**:273
Aspergillus, **XVI**:265
Aspirin, **XVI**:453
  in veterinary pharmacy, **XVI**:253
Atrophic rhinitis, **XVI**:283, 284
Attenuated vaccines, **XVI**:118–119, 135–136
Attractive forces, between solid particles, **XVI**:378
Avicel, **XVI**:338–339
  vaginal delivery of, **XVI**:173
  in wet granulation, **XVI**:368
Azeotropes, **XVI**:16

Bacille Calmette-Guerin (BCG)
  in vaccines, **XVI**:118–119, 124, 136, 137
  zeta potential and, **XVI**:454
Bacillus piliformis, **XVI**:263
Bacillus pumulis, **XVI**:99
Bacillus subtilis, **XVI**:42
  air filtration and, **XVI**:43
Bacillus subtilis var. niger, **XVI**:100
Bacteria
  air filtration and, **XVI**:41–45
  sterilization and, **XVI**:98
  viable nonculturable, **XVI**:228–231
Bacterial vaccines, **XVI**:124–126
Bacteroides, **XVI**:157
Ball growth of granules, **XVI**:379–380
Ball mills, **XVI**:76–78
Batch dryers, **XVI**:57–63
Batched water supplies, **XVI**:244–245

Batch fractionation, **XVI**:14–16
B-cell epitopes, vaccines and, **XVI**:126, 127–128, 129
B cells, vaccines and, **XVI**:124, 127, 137
BCG, *see* Bacille Calmette-Guerin
Beeswax, **XVI**:339, 352–353, 355
   in implants, **XVI**:343
   properties of, **XVI**:335–336
Benzene, **XVI**:410
Benzonatate, **XVI**:344
Benzydamine, **XVI**:179
Betamethasone, in suspensions, **XVI**:449
BET equation, *see* Brunauer, Emmett, and Teller Equation
Bezoic acid, **XVI**:423
Bilirubin, **XVI**:425
Bilirubin UGTs, **XVI**:418
Binders, in wet granulation, **XVI**:369–373
Bioadhesives, in vaginal delivery systems, **XVI**:172–174
Bioprocessing, **XVI**:108–109, 110
Bioreactors, **XVI**:109
Birds, **XVI**:263–265
Blackleg, **XVI**:273, 276
Bleomycin, vaginal delivery of, **XVI**:173
Bloat, **XVI**:270
Boiling
   distillation and, **XVI**:11–13
   evaporation and external pressure in, **XVI**:2–3
   evaporation and heat transfer in, **XVI**:1–2
   evaporation and solute concentration in, **XVI**:2
   evaporation without, **XVI**:8
Boltzmann constant, zeta potential and, **XVI**:437
Bone physiology, zeta potential and, **XVI**:453–454
Bordetella bronchiseptica, **XVI**:254–255, 283, 284
Bordetella pertussis, **XVI**:121, 124, 134
Born repulsion, **XVI**:442
Borrelia bronchiseptica, **XVI**:257
Borrelia burgdorferi, **XVI**:126, 255, 257
Bottom-spray coating, with waxes, **XVI**:348
Botulism, in ferrets, **XVI**:266
Bovine genital campylobacteriosis, **XVI**:273, 275
Bovine herpesvirus-1 (BHV-1), **XVI**:272, 275
Bovine herpesvirus-2 (BHV-2), **XVI**:179
Bovine serum albumin (BSA), **XVI**:343
Bovine trichomoniasis, **XVI**:274
Bovine viral diarrhea (BVD), **XVI**:272, 275
Breakage, **XVI**:379
Bromocriptine, **XVI**:179
Brownian motion
   filtration and, **XVI**:33, 42
   zeta potential and, **XVI**:436, 437
Brucella abortus, **XVI**:274
Brucella suis, **XVI**:283
Brucellosis, **XVI**:274, 283
Brunauer, Emmett, and Teller (BET) Equation, **XVI**:309–311, 312, 322
Budgie fledgling disease, **XVI**:264

Bulk pharmaceuticals, **XVI**:203–206
   impurity profile of, **XVI**:204–206
   physical characteristics of, **XVI**:204
   preformulation studies in, **XVI**:194–195
   process used in manufacture of, **XVI**:204
   terms used for, **XVI**:207
Bull-nose (necrotic rhinitis), **XVI**:283
Butylated hydroxyanisole (BHA), **XVI**:421

Cake filtration, **XVI**:30–31, 40
   compressibility in, **XVI**:34–35
   washing and dewatering in, **XVI**:35–36
Calcitonin, vaginal delivery of, **XVI**:173–174, 177
Calcium salts, **XVI**:366–367
Campylobacter fetus, **XVI**:273, 275
Cancer, vaccines for, **XVI**:115
Candelilla wax, **XVI**:336
Candida albicans
   in birds, **XVI**:265
   in horses, **XVI**:279
   in sheep and goats, **XVI**:269–270
   vaccine for, **XVI**:179
   zeta potential and, **XVI**:454
Canine adenovirus, type 1 (CAV-1), **XVI**:254, 257
Canine adenovirus, type 2 (CAV-2), **XVI**:254, 257
Canine distemper, **XVI**:253–254, 256, 257, 266
Capillary condensation, **XVI**:312–313
Capillary pressure, **XVI**:374–378
Capillary state, **XVI**:375, 376–377
Captopril, flavin monooxygenase system and, **XVI**:411
Carbamezepine, glucuronidation and, **XVI**:419
Carbon-bed operations, **XVI**:240
Carbon beds, **XVI**:302
Carbopol 934, **XVI**:173
Carboxymethyl cellulose, in wet granulation, **XVI**:368
Carboxymethyl starches, in wet granulation, **XVI**:368
Carnauba wax, **XVI**:342, 352–353, 354, 357
   polymers and, **XVI**:341–342
   properties of, **XVI**:336
Castor oil, *see* Hydrogenated castor oil
Castor wax, **XVI**:336, 339, 342
Cationic surfactants, in suspensions, **XVI**:449
Cats, **XVI**:256–260, 261, 268
Cattle, **XVI**:270–274, 275–276
   vaccines for, **XVI**:124, 126, 272, 273
   vaginal delivery systems and, **XVI**:170–172
CD4 cells, vaccines and, **XVI**:127
CD8 cells, vaccines and, **XVI**:123, 126
Cell-mediated immunity, vaccines and, **XVI**:115, 117, 119–121, 123, 126–127, 137
Cellulose
   water sorption and, **XVI**:323–324, 325
   wet granulation and, **XVI**:367, 368, 378
Centrifugal filtration, **XVI**:46–47
Centrifugal sedimentation, **XVI**:47–48

INDEX TO VOLUME 16

Cephalexin monohydrate, XVI:318
Ceresine wax, XVI:353
Cervicovaginal cancer, XVI:174–175
Cetylpyridinium chloride, XVI:342
Chlamydia psittaci, XVI:260, 261, 264
Chloral hydrate, XVI:344
Chlorination, XVI:239
Chloroform, XVI:410
Chlorpheniramine maleate, XVI:339
Chlortetracycline, XVI:264
Cholera, XVI:125
   hog, XVI:280
Cholera toxin, XVI:134, 135, 178
Cholesterol, zeta potential and, XVI:451
Choriomenigitis virus, XVI:137
Chorionic gonadotrophin, XVI:128–129
Ciclopirox, XVI:175
Cimetidine, flavin monooxygenase system and, XVI:411
Circumsporozoite antigen, XVI:126, 127
Cirrhosis, amino acid conjugation and, XVI:423
Cisplatin, vaginal delivery of, XVI:175
Citrobacter freundii, XVI:265
Clarification, XVI:30, 33, 40
Cleaning validation, XVI:202–203
Clindamycin, vaginal delivery of, XVI:174
Closed-circuit grinding, XVI:72
Clostridium botulinum, XVI:266
Clostridium chauvoei, XVI:273, 276
Clostridium perfringens, XVI:269, 271, 275
Clostridium speticum, XVI:273
Clostridium spiroforme, XVI:262
Clostridium tetani, XVI:125, 271, 282, 284
Clostridium welchii, XVI:42
Clotrimazole, XVI:174
Clozapine, XVI:410
Coalescence, XVI:379
Coating, with waxes, XVI:347–352
Coccidiosis, XVI:263, 270, 283
Codeine
   cytochrome P450 and, XVI:410
   water sorption and, XVI:318
Coggins test, XVI:278
Cohesion forces, in immobile liquid bridges, XVI:374
Colchicine, in veterinary pharmacy, XVI:265
Colic, in horses, XVI:277
Coliform mastitis, XVI:124
Colloid mills, XVI:80
Colloid stability, XVI:440–443
Colloid vibration potential (CVP), XVI:438–439
Colonization factor (CFA) I, XVI:125
Colonization factor (CFA) II, XVI:125
Color, wet granulation and, XVI:368–369
Comminution mills, XVI:75–76
Common mucosal immune system (CMIS), XVI:130
Companion animals, XVI:252–268

Complete Freund's adjuvant, vaccines in, XVI:133, 134–135, 139
Compression, solid dosage forms and, XVI:107–108
Concurrent process validation, XVI:187, 188
Concurrent water system validation, XVI:224, 225
Conductivity, of water, XVI:295–297
Conductivity measures, XVI:229–231
Conjunctivitis, in rabbits, XVI:262, 263
Contamination, grinding and, XVI:72
Continous dryers, XVI:63–66
Continuous fractionation, XVI:14–16
Contraceptive sponge, XVI:176
Controlled flocculation, XVI:447
Convective mixing, XVI:90–91
Cooling crystallizers, XVI:28–29
Corn starch, XVI:368
Coronaviruses
   in cats, XVI:261
   in dogs, XVI:254, 256, 257
   in pigs, XVI:284
Corticosteroids
   Crigler-Najjar syndrome and, XVI:425
   in veterinary pharmacy, XVI:277
Cottonseed oil, *see* Hydrogenated cottonseed oil
Creams, vaginal delivery of, XVI:168
Crigler-Najjar syndrome, XVI:425
Critical flocculation concentration (CFC), XVI:445
Critical relative humidity, *see* RH_0
Crushing, XVI:67–69, *see also* Grinding
Crystalline solids, water sorption by, XVI:315–321
Crystallization, XVI:22–30, *see also* Crystallizers
   crystal growth in, XVI:24–25
   defined, XVI:22
   in melts, XVI:23, 24–25
   nucleation and, XVI:23–24, 25, 28
   production of very fine crystals in, XVI:27–28
   production of very large crystals in, XVI:28
   from solutions, XVI:25–26
Crystallizers, XVI:26–27, *see also* Crystallization
   cooling, XVI:28–29
   design and operation of, XVI:26–27
   evaporative, XVI:28
   vacuum, XVI:28, 29–30
Cutaneous ulcerative disease, XVI:265
CYP1, XVI:409, 410
CYP2, XVI:409, 410
CYP2C19 (S-mephenytoin hydroxylase), XVI:425
CYP2D6 (debrisoquine hydroxylase), XVI:424–425
CYP3, XVI:409, 410–411
CYP4A, XVI:411
Cythioate (Proban), XVI:268
Cytochrome P450 enzyme system (CYP450), XVI:403–411, 418
   chemistry of, XVI:404–408
   induction and inhibition of, XVI:408–409
   nomenclature for, XVI:409–411
   reductive metabolism and, XVI:414

Cytomegalovirus, **XVI**:123
Cytotoxic T lymphocytes (CTL), vaccines and, **XVI**:122, 123, 126, 137

Dapsone, cytochrome P450 and, **XVI**:411
Dead zones, **XVI**:94
N-Dealkylation, **XVI**:407–408, 411
O-Dealkylation, **XVI**:407–408
S-Dealkylation, **XVI**:407–408
Debrisoquine hydroxylase (CYP2D6), **XVI**:424–425
Debye-Huckel approximation, **XVI**:430, 441
Deflocculation, **XVI**:449–450
Dehumidification, **XVI**:21–22
Deionization, **XVI**:302
Delayed-type sensitivity (DTH) response, to vaccines, **XVI**:127
Deliquescence
 defined, **XVI**:316
 kinetics of, **XVI**:314, 321
Demixing, **XVI**:90–92
Dental malocclusion, in rabbits, **XVI**:262
Depot effect, **XVI**:133
Depth filters, **XVI**:33–34
Deryaguin-Landau-Verwey-Overbeck (DLVO) theory, **XVI**:440, 441
 emulsions and, **XVI**:444, 445, 446
 in microbiology, **XVI**:454
 suspensions and, **XVI**:448–449, 450
Design qualification (DQ), **XVI**:214
Dew point, **XVI**:18–19
Dexamethasone, cytochrome P450 and, **XVI**:408
Dextromethorphan, cytochrome P450 and, **XVI**:410
Diabetes, in dogs, **XVI**:253
Diazepam, cytochrome P450 and, **XVI**:410
Dibasic calcium phosphate dihydrate, **XVI**:318, 338–339
Diethylcarbamazine, **XVI**:255
Diethyldithiocarbamate, **XVI**:410
Diethyl ether, **XVI**:410
Diethylstilbestrol, **XVI**:253
Differential scanning calorimetry (DSC), of waxes, **XVI**:337, 342, 344, 347, 353, 356
Diffusive mixing, **XVI**:90–91
Diluents, in wet granulation, **XVI**:365–367
Dimethyldioctadecylammonium bromide, **XVI**:178
Dimetridazole, **XVI**:274
Dioctyl sodium succinate, **XVI**:277
Dioctyl sodium sulfosuccinate, **XVI**:342
Dipalmitophosphatidylcholine, **XVI**:451
Diphenhydramine hydrochloride, **XVI**:342
Diphtheria vaccine, **XVI**:124
Dipyridium, **XVI**:408
Dirofilaria immitis, **XVI**:255, 258
Disintegrants, in wet granulation, **XVI**:368
Distemper
 canine, **XVI**:253–254, 256, 257, 266
 feline, **XVI**:259, 261

Distillation, **XVI**:8–17, 303–304
 binary mixtures of immiscible liquids and, **XVI**:8–10
 binary mixtures of miscible liquids and, **XVI**:10–13
 defined, **XVI**:8
 fractionation in, **XVI**:13–16
 molecular, **XVI**:17
 simple (differential), **XVI**:13
 water system validation and, **XVI**:241
Dithiazanine, **XVI**:255
DLVO theory, *see* Deryaguin-Landau-Verwey-Overbeck theory
DNA, vaccines and, **XVI**:123, 128, 137–138
Dobutamine, **XVI**:253
Dogs, **XVI**:252–256, 257–258, 268
Domestic animals, **XVI**:268–285
Double-cone mixer-dryers, **XVI**:395
Drinking (potable) water, **XVI**:299–300
Droplet state, **XVI**:375, 377–378
Drum dryers, **XVI**:66
Dryers, *see also* Drying
 batch, **XVI**:57–63
 continous, **XVI**:63–66
 double-cone, **XVI**:395
 drum, **XVI**:66
 fluidized-bed, *see* Fluidized-bed dryers
 spray, *see* Spray dryers
 tumbling, **XVI**:59
 vacuum tray, **XVI**:58–59
Dry grinding, **XVI**:72
Dry heat sterilization, **XVI**:97
Drying, **XVI**:48–66, *see also* Dryers
 air-circulation, **XVI**:55
 defined, **XVI**:48
 internal mechanism of, **XVI**:53–54
 theory of, **XVI**:49–50
 in wet granulation, **XVI**:386
Duhring's rule, **XVI**:2, 3
Dynafill, **XVI**:344
Dynamic mobility, **XVI**:438–439
Dynasan, **XVI**:336, 344, 346

Eastern equine encephalomyelitis (EEE), **XVI**:277, 281
Edge-runner mills, **XVI**:74–75
Egg yolk lecithin, **XVI**:444
Ehrlichia, **XVI**:279, 282
Electric double-layer formation and structure, **XVI**:429–431
Electrokinetic phenomena, **XVI**:432–434
Electrokinetic sonic amplitude, **XVI**:438–439
Electrokinetic sonic analysis, **XVI**:437–440
Electrolytes
 blood, **XVI**:453
 emulsions and, **XVI**:444–445
 liposomes and, **XVI**:451
 suspensions and, **XVI**:447–448, 449

Electro-osmosis, **XVI**:432, 434, 435
Electrophoresis, zeta potential and, **XVI**:432–433
Electrophoretic light-scattering, **XVI**:436–437
Electrophoretic retardation, **XVI**:434
Electrostatic forces, **XVI**:378
Elutriation, **XVI**:82–84
Emulsions
  hot, **XVI**:350–351
  zeta potential and, **XVI**:444–446
End-runner mills, **XVI**:74–75
Enkephalin, **XVI**:177
Enteritis, **XVI**:266
Enterotoxemia (overeating disease), **XVI**:262, 269, 271, 275
Environmental Protection Agency (EPA)
  water for pharmaceutical use and, **XVI**:299
  water system validation and, **XVI**:231, 233
  wet granulation and, **XVI**:388
Enzymes, vaginal, **XVI**:156–157
Ephedrine hydrochloride, **XVI**:342
Epilepsy, in dogs, **XVI**:253
Epitopes, vaccines and, **XVI**:116, *see also* B-cell epitopes; T-cell epitopes
Epstein-Barr virus (EBV), **XVI**:123
Equilibrium moisture content, **XVI**:49–50
Equilibrium moisture sorption, **XVI**:315
Equine coital exanthema, **XVI**:277
Equine encephalomyelitis, **XVI**:277–278, 281
Equine herpesvirus-1 (EHV-1), **XVI**:278, 282
Equine herpesvirus-3 (EHV-3), **XVI**:277
Equine infectious anemia (swamp fever), **XVI**:278
Equine influenza, **XVI**:278, 281
Equine monocytic ehrlichiosis (Potomac fever), **XVI**:279, 282
Equine viral rhinopneumonitis, **XVI**:278–279, 282
Erysipelas, **XVI**:283, 284
Erysipelothrix rhusiopathiae, **XVI**:283, 284
Erythromycin, cytochrome P450 and, **XVI**:409, 411
Escherichia coli
  vaccines and, **XVI**:124, 125, 126, 179
  water system validation and, **XVI**:233
  zeta potential and, **XVI**:454
Estradiol
  cytochrome P450 and, **XVI**:411
  vaginal delivery of, **XVI**:170, 171
  veterinary applications of, **XVI**:171
Estrogen, 453
  vaginal delivery of, **XVI**:168, 170, 176–177
Estrus cycle, **XVI**:166
Ethylcellulose
  waxes and, **XVI**:341, 351
  wet granulation and, **XVI**:373
Ethylene oxide sterilization, **XVI**:99–100
Ethylmorphine, **XVI**:410
Eudragit L 100, **XVI**:341–342
European Economic Community (EEC)
  vaccines and, **XVI**:140
  water for pharmaceutical use and, **XVI**:300

European Pharmacopeia, on water for pharmaceutical use, **XVI**:300
Evaporation, **XVI**:1–8, *see also* Evaporators
  physical properties of solution and liquids in, **XVI**:2–5
  of water into an air stream, **XVI**:50–51
Evaporative crystallizers, **XVI**:28
Evaporators, **XVI**:5–8, *see also* Evaporation
  film, **XVI**:6–7
  forced-circulation, **XVI**:5–6
  heat transfer to boiling liquids in, **XVI**:1–2
  natural circulation, **XVI**:5
Exotic animals, **XVI**:266
External parasites
  on companion animals, **XVI**:267–268
  on domestic animals, **XVI**:285
External pressure, boiling temperature and, **XVI**:2–3
Extraction, **XVI**:101–106
Extruders, **XVI**:397

Farmer's lung, **XVI**:274
Feather loss, **XVI**:263–264
Feline acquired immune deficiency syndrome, **XVI**:260
Feline calicivirus infection (FCI), **XVI**:260, 261
Feline distemper (panleukopenia), **XVI**:259, 261
Feline infectious anemia (FIA), **XVI**:260
Feline infectious peritonitis, **XVI**:259, 261
Feline leukemia, **XVI**:259–260, 261
Feline lymphosarcoma, **XVI**:259–260
Feline pneumonitis (FPN), **XVI**:260, 261
Feline rhinotracheitis (FVR), **XVI**:260
Felodipine, **XVI**:411
Fenticonazole, **XVI**:174–175
Ferrets, **XVI**:266
Fertility vaccines, **XVI**:128–129
Fibrous media, **XVI**:43
Fick's law, **XVI**:104
Fillers, in wet granulation, **XVI**:365–367
Film evaporators, **XVI**:6–7
Filter aids, **XVI**:34
Filter area, **XVI**:32
Filter integrity, **XVI**:101
Filter media, **XVI**:40–41
Filters
  absolute, **XVI**:43
  air, **XVI**:43–45
  depth, **XVI**:33–34
  gravity, **XVI**:36
  plate-and-frame press, **XVI**:38–39, 40
  vacuum, **XVI**:36–38
Filtration, **XVI**:30–48
  air, **XVI**:41–45
  cake, *see* Cake filtration
  centrifugal, **XVI**:46–47
  clarification, **XVI**:30, 33, 40
  factors affecting rate of, **XVI**:31–32

[Filtration]
  precoat, **XVI**:38
  pressure, **XVI**:38–40
  sterile, **XVI**:100–101
  theories of, **XVI**:31–36
  top feed, **XVI**:38
Fixed media, **XVI**:41
Flavin monooxygenase (FMO) enzyme system, **XVI**:411–413
Flavor, wet granulation and, **XVI**:368–369
Flavor modifiers, wet granulation and, **XVI**:368–369
Fleas, **XVI**:267–268
Flexible media, **XVI**:41
Flocculation
  controlled, **XVI**:447
  emulsions and, **XVI**:445
  slurries and, **XVI**:34
  suspensions and, **XVI**:447–448, 449–450
Fluconazole, vaginal delivery of, **XVI**:174
Fluid energy mills, **XVI**:79–80
Fluidized beds
  dryers, **XVI**:55, 60–61, 392
  granulators, **XVI**:395–396
  wax coatings and, **XVI**:348
  wet granulation and, **XVI**:392, 395–396
Fluorgestone acetate, **XVI**:170–171
Fluorogestone, **XVI**:172
5-Fluorouracil, waxes in delivery systems for, **XVI**:354
FMO1, **XVI**:413
FMO2, **XVI**:413
FMO3, **XVI**:413
FMO4, **XVI**:413
FMO5, **XVI**:413
Foams, vaginal delivery of, **XVI**:168
Food, Drug and Cosmetic (FD&C) Act, **XVI**:204
Food and Drug Administration (FDA)
  process validation and, **XVI**:187, 189, 192–193, 212
  vaccines and, **XVI**:140
  vaginal delivery systems and, **XVI**:168
  water system validation and, **XVI**:211–212, 213, 216–217, 218, 224, 225–226, 227, 229, 233, 241, 242, 245–246, 247, 248
Foot and mouth disease (FMD), **XVI**:269, 271
Foot rot, **XVI**:269–270, 274
Forced-circulation evaporators, **XVI**:5–6
Formal process validation, **XVI**:199–200
Fractionating columns, 13, *see also* Packed columns; Plate columns
Fractionation, **XVI**:13–16
Free crushing, **XVI**:69
Freeze drying, **XVI**:61–63
French mould, **XVI**:264
Freund's adjuvant, *see* Complete Freund's adjuvant; Incomplete Freund's adjuvant
Fungal infections, in reptiles, **XVI**:265–266

Funicular state, **XVI**:375, 376, 384–385
Furafylline, **XVI**:410
Fusobacterium necrophorum, **XVI**:274

GAB equation, *see* Guggenheim, Anderson, and deBoer equation
Gantt charts, **XVI**:190, 191
Gas, in humidification, **XVI**:18
Gastric ulcers, **XVI**:131
Gastroenteritis, transmissible, **XVI**:280, 284
Gelatin, wet granulation and, **XVI**:373
Gelatin capsules
  hard, *see* Hard gelatin capsules
  water sorption and, **XVI**:329–330
Gelucires, **XVI**:341, 344, 345, 346, 347, 352–353
Gentamicin, vaginal delivery of, **XVI**:174
Gilbert's syndrome, **XVI**:425
Glass transition temperature, water sorption and, **XVI**:326, 327, 329
Glucoside conjugation, **XVI**:419–420
Glucuronic acid conjugation, *see* Glucuronidation
Glucuronidation, **XVI**:416–419, 425
Glutathione S-transferase (GST), **XVI**:127–128
Glutathione S-transferase (GST) conjugation, **XVI**:420–421
Glycerides, **XVI**:337
Glycerol monostearate, **XVI**:342, 353, 357
Goats, **XVI**:268–270, 271
Good Manufacturing Practices (GMPs)
  process validation and, **XVI**:187, 188, 196, 204
  vaccines and, **XVI**:140
  water system validation and, **XVI**:213, 219, 242–243
Gordon-Taylor-Kelly-Bueche equation, **XVI**:327
Gout
  in birds, **XVI**:264
  in reptiles, **XVI**:265
Gouy-Chapman layer, **XVI**:431
Granular beds, **XVI**:43
Granulating solvents, **XVI**:369
Granulation
  melt, **XVI**:339
  solid dosage forms and, **XVI**:107
  wet, *see* Wet granulation
Gravity filters, **XVI**:36
Grinding, **XVI**:67–80, *see also* Mills
  closed-circuit, **XVI**:72
  dry, **XVI**:72
  dust hazards in, **XVI**:73
  efficiency of, **XVI**:69–71
  equipment in, **XVI**:73–80
  fundamental aspects of, **XVI**:67–69
  open-circuit, **XVI**:72
  structural changes in, **XVI**:73
  wet, **XVI**:72
Griseofulvin
  in suspensions, **XVI**:447, 449
  wet granulation and, **XVI**:370

Group-B Streptococcus polysaccharide vaccines, **XVI**:125
Guaifenesin, **XVI**:351
Guggenheim and deBoer equation, **XVI**:311–312
Guggenheim, Anderson, and deBoer (GAB) equation, **XVI**:312, 322–323

Haemobartonella felis, **XVI**:260
Haemophilus influenzae type B vaccines, **XVI**:124
Hairballs, **XVI**:256
Halopreidol, **XVI**:410
Hammer mills, **XVI**:75–76
Haptens, **XVI**:115
Hard gelatin capsules, waxes in, **XVI**:337, 343–347
Heartworm, **XVI**:255–256, 258, 266
Heat, effect on solutions in evaporation, **XVI**:4–5
Heat exhaustion, in rabbits, **XVI**:262
Heat transfer, to boiling liquids in evaporation, **XVI**:1–2
Height equivalent of a theoretical plate (HETP), **XVI**:15
Helicobacter felis, **XVI**:128
Helicobacter pylori, **XVI**:128, 131
Helmholtz-Smoluchowski equation, **XVI**:433, 434, 437, 439
Helminth vaccines, **XVI**:126–128
Helper T cells, vaccines and, **XVI**:122, 124, 134
Hemagglutinin (HA), **XVI**:122–123
Hematology, zeta potential and, **XVI**:452–453
Hepatitis
 amino acid conjugation and, **XVI**:423
 in dogs, **XVI**:254, 256, 257
Hepatitis B surface antigen, **XVI**:138
Hepatitis B virus vaccines, **XVI**:121, 143
Herpesviruses
 bovine, *see* Bovine herpesvirus
 equine, *see* Equine herpesvirus
 feline, **XVI**:261
 in vaccines, **XVI**:119, 123
High-speed mixer-granulators, **XVI**:392–394
Hippuric acid, **XVI**:423
HIV, *see* Human immunodeficiency virus
Hog cholera, **XVI**:280
Horses, **XVI**:274–280, 281–282
Hot air ovens, **XVI**:57–58
Hot emulsions, coating with, **XVI**:350–351
Hot melts, **XVI**:348–350
Huckel equation, **XVI**:433
Human immunodeficiency virus (HIV), **XVI**:260
 spermicides and, **XVI**:176
 vaccine development for, **XVI**:123, 178
Human simian virus 1 (HSV), **XVI**:178
Humidification, **XVI**:17–22
 hygrometry of, **XVI**:18–21
Humidity, *see* Relative humidity
Humoral immunity, vaccines and, **XVI**:115, 119–121

Hutch burn, **XVI**:262
Hydrates, water sorption onto, **XVI**:318–319
Hydrocortisone
 cytochrome P450 and, **XVI**:411
 in suspensions, **XVI**:447
Hydrogenated castor oil, **XVI**:340–341, 355
Hydrogenated cottonseed oil, **XVI**:336, 357–358
Hydrogenated palm oil, **XVI**:336
Hydrogenated soybean oil, **XVI**:336
Hydrogenated vegetable oils, **XVI**:336
Hydrolysis, xenobiotic metabolism and, **XVI**:415–416
Hydrophilic-lipophilic balance (HLB), of waxes, **XVI**:344, 346, 354, 358
Hydrophilic solids, **XVI**:446
Hydrophobic solids, **XVI**:446–447
Hydroxypropyl methylcellulose (HPMC)
 water sorption and, **XVI**:327
 wet granulation and, **XVI**:373
Hygrometry, **XVI**:18–21

Ibuprofen
 cytochrome P450 and, **XVI**:410
 waxes in delivery systems for, **XVI**:344, 346, 352–353
Imidazole, cytochrome P450 and, **XVI**:408, 409
Imipramine, cytochrome P450 and, **XVI**:410
Immersion, leaching by, **XVI**:103
Immiscible liquids, binary mixtures in distillation, **XVI**:8–10
Immobile liquid bridges, adhesion and cohesion forces in, **XVI**:374
Immunoglobulin A (IgA), vaccines and, **XVI**:122, 125, 178, 179
Immunoglobulin E (IgE), vaccines and, **XVI**:127
Immunoglobulin G (IgG), vaccines and, **XVI**:122, 124, 125, 178
Immunoglobulin M (IgM), vaccines and, **XVI**:122, 124
Immunostimulation, **XVI**:133, 134
Impurities
 in bulk pharmaceuticals, **XVI**:204–206
 water system validation and, **XVI**:233–238
Inactivated microorganism vaccines, **XVI**:117–118
Incomplete Freund's adjuvant, vaccines in, **XVI**:132, 133, 134–135
Indomethacin, waxes in delivery systems for, **XVI**:346
Infectious agent vaccines, **XVI**:122–128
Infectious bovine rhinotracheitis (IBR), **XVI**:272, 275
Infectious keratitis (pinkeye), **XVI**:272–273, 275
Infectious myxomatosis, **XVI**:262
Infectious pustular vulvovaginitis, **XVI**:275
Influenza
 equine, **XVI**:278, 281
 in ferrets, **XVI**:266
Influenza vaccines, **XVI**:122, 137, 139, 266

Installation qualification (IQ)
  process validation and, **XVI**:190
  water system validation and, **XVI**:214, 217–219, 305
Insulin, *see also* Zinc insulin
  microparticle delivery systems for, **XVI**:139
  vaginal delivery of, **XVI**:177
  waxes in delivery systems for, **XVI**:343
Interfacial forces, in mobile liquid films, **XVI**:374–378
Interferon gamma (IFN-γ), vaccines and, **XVI**:122, 127, 133
Interleukin-1 (IL-1), vaccines and, **XVI**:133, 134
Interleukin-2 (IL-2), vaccines and, **XVI**:122, 133
Interleukin-4 (IL-4), vaccines and, **XVI**:127
Interleukin-6 (IL-6), vaccines and, **XVI**:133
Internal parasites
  in companion animals, **XVI**:267
  in domestic animals, **XVI**:283–285
International Organization for Standardization (ISO), on bulk pharmaceuticals, **XVI**:205–206
Ion-exchange resins, **XVI**:238, 241, 247
Ionic surfactants, suspensions and, **XVI**:448–449
Ipratropium bromide, **XVI**:318
Ipronidazole, **XVI**:274
Iron regulated outer member proteins (IROMPs), **XVI**:126
Iscoms, **XVI**:133
Isoniazid, **XVI**:422
ISO 9000 Series, **XVI**:205–206
Ivermectin, **XVI**:255–256

Japanese encephalitis virus (JE), **XVI**:277
Japanese synthetic wax, **XVI**:355
Jellies, vaginal delivery of, **XVI**:168

Kaopectate, **XVI**:256, 269
Kelvin equation, **XVI**:312
Kennel cough, **XVI**:254–255, 256, 257, 258
Ketoconazole, **XVI**:265
Ketoprofen, 344
Ketosis, **XVI**:268, 270–272
Kick's law, **XVI**:70, 71
Kinetics of deliquescence, **XVI**:314, 321
Krystal crystallizers, **XVI**:28

Lactobacillus, **XVI**:157
Lactose, in wet granulation, **XVI**:366
Lanolin, **XVI**:335
Laplace's law, **XVI**:375
Layering, **XVI**:380
Leaching, **XVI**:101–106
Lecithin
  egg yolk, **XVI**:444
  soybean, **XVI**:444
  zeta potential and, **XVI**:444, 450, 451
Legionella pneumophilia, **XVI**:239
Leptospirosis, **XVI**:255, 256, 257
Leuprolide, **XVI**:177–178
Levonorgestrel, **XVI**:170
Lidocaine, cytochrome P450 and, **XVI**:410, 411
Limping syndrome, **XVI**:260
Lipid-polysaccharide subunit vaccines, **XVI**:121, 134, 135
Liposomes
  vaccines and, **XVI**:133, 135
  zeta potential and, **XVI**:450–452
Liquid entrainment, **XVI**:7–8
Liquids
  heat transfer to boiling in evaporation, **XVI**:1–2
  immiscible, **XVI**:8–10
  in leaching, **XVI**:105–106
  miscible, **XVI**:10–13
  mixing of, **XVI**:94–97
  mixing of solids and, **XVI**:95–97
  physical properties in evaporation, **XVI**:2–5
  separation of in distillation, **XVI**:16
Listeria monocytogenes, **XVI**:121, 128
Loose media, **XVI**:41
Lubritab, **XVI**:336
Lufenuron (Program), **XVI**:267–268
Luteinizing hormone-releasing hormone (LHRH), **XVI**:128–129
  vaginal delivery of, **XVI**:177–178
Lutrol-F68, **XVI**:344
Lyme disease, **XVI**:255, 256, 257
Lyphophilization, *see* Freeze drying

Magnesium hydroxide, zeta potential and, **XVI**:449–450
Major histocompatiblity complex (MHC), vaccines and, **XVI**:115, 116
Major histocompatiblity complex (MHC) type 1, vaccines and, **XVI**:120, 126, 137
Major histocompatiblity complex (MHC) type 2, vaccines and, **XVI**:120, 127
Malaria, **XVI**:126
Mannitol, **XVI**:366
Marc, **XVI**:102
Matrix-type drug delivery systems, waxes in, **XVI**:338
Maximum boiling mixtures, **XVI**:11–12
Measles vaccines, **XVI**:118, 123
Medroxyprogesterone acetate (MPA), **XVI**:169–170, 171
Melt-dispersion techniques, **XVI**:352–355
Melt granulation, **XVI**:339
Melting point, of waxes, **XVI**:337, 344, 346, 349–350, 354
Melts
  crystallization in, **XVI**:23, 24–25
  hot, **XVI**:348–350
Menopause, **XVI**:158–159, 168
Menthol, **XVI**:425
Meperidine, **XVI**:277

S-Mephenytoin hydroxylase (CYP2C19), **XVI**:425
Mercapturic acid, **XVI**:420
-Metarhizium, **XVI**:265
Metazoan vaccines, *see* Helminth vaccines
Methotrexate, vaginal delivery of, **XVI**:176
Methoxcyflurane, **XVI**:410
Methylcellulose, wet granulation and, **XVI**:372, 373
Methyl conjugation (methylation), **XVI**:423–424
S-Methyltransferase, **XVI**:424
4-Methylumbelliferone, **XVI**:425
Metronidazole
   vaginal delivery of, **XVI**:174
   in veterinary pharmacy, **XVI**:274
Mexiletine, **XVI**:410
Microbiological water system validation, **XVI**:225–227, 228
Microbiology, zeta potential and, **XVI**:454–455
Microcrystalline cellulose, in wet granulation, **XVI**:367
Microcrystalline wax, **XVI**:336
Microelectrophoresis, **XVI**:434–436
Microencapsulation, with waxes, **XVI**:352–358
Microorganisms, in water, **XVI**:237–238, 299
Microparticles
   vaccines and, **XVI**:133, 139–140
   wax, **XVI**:352–358
Micropolyspora faeni, **XVI**:274
Midazolam, **XVI**:411
Mifepristone (RU486), **XVI**:176
Milling, in wet granulation, **XVI**:380
Mills
   ball, **XVI**:76–78
   colloid, **XVI**:80
   comminution, **XVI**:75–76
   edge-runner, **XVI**:74–75
   end-runner, **XVI**:74–75
   fluid energy, **XVI**:79–80
   hammer, **XVI**:75–76
   operation of, **XVI**:71–73
   pin, **XVI**:76
   roller, **XVI**:80
   vibratory, **XVI**:78–79
Milrinone, **XVI**:253
Mineral oil, **XVI**:277
Minimum boiling mixtures, **XVI**:11–13
Miscella, **XVI**:102
Miscible liquids, binary mixtures in distillation, **XVI**:10–13
Misoprostol, **XVI**:176
Mixers, **XVI**:93, *see also* Mixing
   double-cone, **XVI**:395
   high-speed, **XVI**:392–394
   paddle, **XVI**:93, 95
   propeller, **XVI**:95
   ribbon, **XVI**:91, 93
   trough, **XVI**:93
   tumbler, **XVI**:91, 93
   turbines, **XVI**:96

Mixing, **XVI**:84–97, *see also* Mixers
   convective, **XVI**:90–91
   defined, **XVI**:84
   diffusive, **XVI**:90–91
   negative, **XVI**:84
   neutral, **XVI**:84
   positive, **XVI**:84
   scale of scrutiny in, **XVI**:85
   shear, **XVI**:90–91
   in wet granulation, **XVI**:380
Mobile liquid films, **XVI**:374–378
Modified vaginal pessaries, **XVI**:172
Moist dermatitis (wet dewlap), **XVI**:262
Moist heat sterilization, **XVI**:97–98
Moisture content, **XVI**:49
   equilibrium, **XVI**:49–50
Moniliasis, **XVI**:265
Monophosphoryl lipid-A, **XVI**:133, 178
Moraxella bovis, **XVI**:272, 275
Morphine sulfate dihydrate, **XVI**:318
Mosquitoes, **XVI**:126, 277–278
Mucoid enteropathy, **XVI**:263
Mucor, **XVI**:265
Mucosal administration, of vaccines, **XVI**:129–132
Mucosal-associated lymphoid tissue (MALT), **XVI**:130
Multimedia deep-bed filters, **XVI**:239–240
Municipally treated feedwater, **XVI**:244
Muramyl dipeptide, **XVI**:133, 178
Mussel adhesive protein (MAP), **XVI**:139
Mycobacterium bovis, **XVI**:124
Mycobacterium leprae, **XVI**:138
Mycobacterium tuberculosis
   BCG strain of, *see* Bacille Calmette-Guerin
   vaccines and, **XVI**:118–119, 124, 138
Mycoplasma, **XVI**:260
Mycoplasma bovoculi, **XVI**:272
Mycoplasma hypopneumoniae, **XVI**:132

Nalidixic acid, **XVI**:449
1-Naphtol, **XVI**:425
National Formulary (NF)
   on bulk pharmaceuticals, **XVI**:203
   on waxes, **XVI**:335
Natural circulation evaporators, **XVI**:5
Necrotic enteritis, **XVI**:283
Necrotic rhinitis (bull-nose), **XVI**:283
Negative mixing, **XVI**:84
Neisseria gonorrhoeae, **XVI**:125
Neisseria meningitidis, **XVI**:124
Neuraminidase (NA), **XVI**:122–123
Neutral mixing, **XVI**:84
Neutral Protamine Hagedorn (NPH), **XVI**:253
New Drug Application (NDA), **XVI**:192, 201
Newtonian flow, of waxes, **XVI**:344
Nicotinic acid, **XVI**:344
Nifedipine
   cytochrome P450 and, **XVI**:411
   waxes in delivery systems for, **XVI**:341

Nitrofurantoin
   in suspensions, **XVI**:447, 449
   waxes in delivery systems for, **XVI**:338
Non-compendial water, **XVI**:300–301
Nonhydrates, water sorption onto, **XVI**:316–318
Nonionic surfactants, suspensions and, **XVI**:448–449
Nonliving microparticulate vaccine delivery
    systems, **XVI**:138–140
Nonoxynol-9, **XVI**:168, 176
Nonporous solids, **XVI**:51–53
Non-purgeable organic carbon (NPOC), **XVI**:297
Nonsteroidal anti-inflammatory drugs (NSAIDs),
    glucuronidation and, **XVI**:418
Norethhindrone, **XVI**:165
Norgestrel, **XVI**:170
Norwalk virus capsid proteins, **XVI**:138
Nucleation, **XVI**:23–24, 25, 28, 378
Nystatin, in veterinary pharmacy, **XVI**:265

Octoxynol, **XVI**:168, 176
Oil/water (o/w) emulsions
   of waxes, **XVI**:350–351
   zeta potential and, **XVI**:444
Open-circuit grinding, **XVI**:72
Operational qualification (OQ)
   process validation and, **XVI**:190
   water system validation and, **XVI**:214, 220, 306
Oral administration, of vaccines, **XVI**:130–132
Organic solvents, **XVI**:369
Organic wax solutions, coating with, **XVI**:350–351
Oslo crystallizers, **XVI**:28, 29, 30
Outer member proteins (OMPs), **XVI**:126
Out-of-specifications (OOS), **XVI**:201–202
Overeating disease (enterotoxemia), **XVI**:262, 269,
    271, 275
Over-the-counter (OTC) drugs
   vaginal delivery of, **XVI**:168
   in veterinary pharmacy, **XVI**:251–252
N-Oxidation, **XVI**:411, 413
S-Oxidation, **XVI**:413
Oxidative metabolism, **XVI**:403–414, 424–425
   cytochrome P450 in, *see* Cytochrome P450
     enzyme system
   flavin monooxygenase system in, **XVI**:411–413
Oxytetracycline, in veterinary pharmacy, **XVI**:263
Ozone, **XVI**:239

Pacheco's disease, **XVI**:264, 265
Packed columns, **XVI**:13–14, 15
Packed crushing, **XVI**:69
Paddle mixers, **XVI**:93, 95
Paeciolmyces, **XVI**:265
Palm oil, *see* Hydrogenated palm oil
Panleukopenia (feline distemper), **XVI**:259, 261
Paraffin wax, **XVI**:336, 341, 352–353
Parainfluenza viruses, in dogs, **XVI**:254, 258
Paramethadione, **XVI**:344
Paramyxoviruses, **XVI**:123

Parasites, *see* External parasites; Internal parasites
Parenteral administration
   unit process applications in, **XVI**:106–107
   of vaccines, **XVI**:129, 132
Paroxetine, **XVI**:410
Particles
   attractive forces between solid, **XVI**:378
   importance of fine, **XVI**:66–67
   retention in depth filters, **XVI**:33–34
   size and distribution of solid in leaching, **XVI**:104–
    105
Parvoviruses
   in cats, **XVI**:261
   in dogs, **XVI**:254, 256, 258
Pasteurella, **XVI**:273
Pasteurella haemolytica, **XVI**:126, 276
Pasteurella multocida, **XVI**:263, 276, 283, 284
Pasteurellosis, **XVI**:263, 276
Pendular state, **XVI**:375–376
Penicillin, in veterinary pharmacy, **XVI**:263, 273
Penicillum, **XVI**:265
Pentazocine, **XVI**:277
Peptides, vaginal delivery of, **XVI**:177–178
Percolation, **XVI**:102–103
Performance qualification (PQ)
   process validation and, **XVI**:190
   water system validation and, **XVI**:221–222, 306
Permeability, vaginal absorption and, **XVI**:160–
    164, 166
Permeability coefficient
   filtration and, **XVI**:32
   vaginal absorption and, **XVI**:160–163
PERT charts, **XVI**:190
Pertussis vaccines, **XVI**:124
Pessaries, **XVI**:170–172, 175
Petroleum wax, **XVI**:336
pH
   emulsions and, **XVI**:445
   of feline urine, **XVI**:259
   suspensions and, **XVI**:449
   vaginal, **XVI**:156, 168
   vaginal absorption and, **XVI**:162
   water conductivity and, **XVI**:296–297
   water system validation and, **XVI**:229–231, 238
   waxes and, **XVI**:337, 342, 352, 354
   zeta potential and, **XVI**:444, 453
Pharmacokinetics, of vaginal absorption, **XVI**:164–
    165
Phenobarbital, cytochrome P450 and, **XVI**:408
Phenobarbitone, glucuronidation and, **XVI**:419
Phenols, **XVI**:256
Phenylbutazone
   cytochrome P450 and, **XVI**:410
   in veterinary pharmacy, **XVI**:253, 277
Phenylpropanolamine, **XVI**:253
Phenytoin
   glucuronidation and, **XVI**:419
   in veterinary pharmacy, **XVI**:253

Phosphatidic acid, zeta potential and, **XVI**:451
Phosphatidylcholine (PC), zeta potential and, **XVI**:444, 451
Phosphatidylethanolamine (PE), zeta potential and, **XVI**:444, 452
Phosphatidylglycerol (PG), zeta potential and, **XVI**:444, 445
Phosphatidylserine (PS), zeta potential and, **XVI**:444, 445, 451
Picornaviruses, **XVI**:269, 271
Pigs, **XVI**:125, 280–283, 284
Pinkeye (infectious keratitis), **XVI**:272–273, 275
Pin mills, **XVI**:76
Plasmodium, **XVI**:118
Plasmodium falciparum, **XVI**:126–127
Plasticizers, water as, **XVI**:326–328
Plate-and-frame press filters, **XVI**:38–39, 40
Plate columns, **XVI**:13, 14
Pneumonia
  in cattle, **XVI**:273
  in pigs, **XVI**:280
  in rabbits, **XVI**:263
  in sheep, **XVI**:269
Point of zero change (PZC), **XVI**:445
Poisson equation, **XVI**:430
Polio vaccines, **XVI**:118, 120, 136, 179
Polyacrylamides, wet granulation and, **XVI**:373
Polyacrylic acid, in vaginal delivery systems, **XVI**:173
Polychorinated biphenyls, **XVI**:408
Polycyclic aromatic hydrocarbons (PAH), cytochrome P450 and, **XVI**:408, 410
Polyethylene glycol (PEG)
  liposomes and, **XVI**:452
  zeta potential and, **XVI**:452
Polyethylene glycol (PEG) 10,000, **XVI**:344
Polyethylene glycol (PEG) 20,000, **XVI**:344–346
Polyethylene oxide, **XVI**:172
Poly-(lactide-*co*-glycolide) (PLG), **XVI**:138–139
Polymers, waxes and, **XVI**:341–342
Polymethyl methacrylate, water sorption and, **XVI**:325, 327
Polymyxin B
  in liposomes, **XVI**:452
  zeta potential and, **XVI**:452
Polyoxyethylene 23 lauryl ether, **XVI**:342
Polysaccharides
  vaccines and, **XVI**:124
  in wet granulation, **XVI**:366
Polytetrafluoroethylene (PTFE), in water systems, **XVI**:304
Polyvinyl alcohol, waxes and, **XVI**:352
Polyvinylidene fluoride (PVDF), in water systems, **XVI**:304
Polyvinyloxazolidones, **XVI**:373
Polyvinylpyrrolidone (PVP)
  water sorption and, **XVI**:325–327
  in wet granulation, **XVI**:368, 372, 373, 378, 382, 387, 389

Porous media, **XVI**:31
Porous solids, **XVI**:54–55
Portectaid, **XVI**:176
Positive mixing, **XVI**:84
Potassium bromide, **XVI**:253
Potassium chloride, **XVI**:339, 351
Potomac fever (equine monocytic ehrlichiosis), **XVI**:279, 282
Powders, in wet granulation, **XVI**:380, 381–385
Poxvirus avium, **XVI**:264
Poxviruses
  in birds, **XVI**:264, 265
  in vaccines, **XVI**:137
Pre-approval Inspection Program, **XVI**:192–193
Precirol, **XVI**:339, 342, 346, 347, 352–353
Precoat filtration, **XVI**:38
Preformulation studies, **XVI**:194–195
Pregnancy, vaccines during, **XVI**:125
Premarket validation, *see* Prospective process validation
Pressure filtration, **XVI**:38–40
PRID vaginal insert, **XVI**:171
Primidone, **XVI**:253
Proban (cythioate), **XVI**:268
Procaine hydrochloride, **XVI**:342
Process and instrumentation drawings (P&IDs), **XVI**:219
Process development: pilot laboratory (clinical), **XVI**:196–198
Process qualification (PQ), **XVI**:214
Process validation, **XVI**:187–207, 212
  change control in, **XVI**:200–201
  cleaning, **XVI**:202–203
  concurrent, **XVI**:187, 188
  formal, **XVI**:199–200
  master plan in, **XVI**:190
  out-of-specifications in, **XVI**:201–202
  pilot production in, **XVI**:198–199
  pilot scale-up and technical transfer in, **XVI**:193
  pre-approval inspection in, **XVI**:192–193
  preformulation studies in, **XVI**:194–195
  process development: pilot laboratory (clinical) in, **XVI**:196–198
  product design and development in, **XVI**:195–196
  prospective, **XVI**:187–189
  protocol and reports in, **XVI**:192
  retrospective, **XVI**:187, 188
  revalidation, **XVI**:187, 189
  terms used in, **XVI**:207
  validation commitee in, **XVI**:189
Product design and development, **XVI**:195–196
Product development, **XVI**:99
Progesterone
  vaginal delivery of, **XVI**:171, 176–177
  veterinary applications of, **XVI**:171
Progestins, vaginal delivery of, **XVI**:170
Program (lufenuron), **XVI**:267–268

Promazine, **XVI**:277
Propeller mixers, **XVI**:95
Propranolol
   cytochrome P450 and, **XVI**:410
   waxes in delivery systems for, **XVI**:347
Propylthiouracil, **XVI**:411
Prospective process validation, **XVI**:187–189
Prospective water system validation, **XVI**:224
Prostaglandin E_1 (PGE_1), vaginal delivery of, **XVI**:175–176
Prostaglandin E_2 (PGE_2), vaginal delivery of, **XVI**:175
Prostaglandins, vaginal delivery of, **XVI**:170, 175–176
Proteins, vaginal delivery of, **XVI**:177–178
Protein subunit vaccines, **XVI**:120–121
Protozoan vaccines, **XVI**:126–128
Pseudomonas, **XVI**:265
Pseudomonas aeruginosa, **XVI**:227
Pseudophedrine hydrochloride, **XVI**:354–355
Psittacosis, **XVI**:264
Purgeable organic carbon (POC), **XVI**:297
Purified Water systems, validation for, **XVI**:224, 226, 227, 228–229, 237–238

Quillaja saponaria, **XVI**:133
Quinidine
   cytochrome P450 and, **XVI**:411
   water sorption and, **XVI**:318
   waxes in delivery systems for, **XVI**:346

Rabbits, **XVI**:125, 260–263
Rabies
   in cats, **XVI**:260, 261
   in cattle, **XVI**:272, 276
   in dogs, **XVI**:253, 254, 256, 258
   in ferrets, **XVI**:266
   in horses, **XVI**:279, 282
   in pigs, **XVI**:284
   in rabbits, **XVI**:262
   in sheep and goats, **XVI**:271
   in wolves, **XVI**:286
Radiation, in sterilization, **XVI**:98–99
Random mixtures, **XVI**:86–88
Raoult's law, **XVI**:11
Recombinant vaccines, **XVI**:136–138
Rectal administration, of vaccines, **XVI**:131
Rectification, *see* Fractionation
Reductive metabolism, **XVI**:414–415
Relative humidity, *see also* RH_0
   control of, **XVI**:313–314
   measurement of, **XVI**:314
   water sorption by crystalline solids and, **XVI**:315–316
Relaxin, **XVI**:177
Remoxipride, **XVI**:356
Replens, **XVI**:174
Reptiles, **XVI**:265–266

Respiratory syncytial virus (RSV), in vaccines, **XVI**:120–121
Retrospective process validation, **XVI**:187, 188
Retrospective water system validation, **XVI**:224, 225
Revalidation, **XVI**:187, 189
Reverse osmosis, water systems and, **XVI**:232, 238, 241, 244, 246, 247, 303
RH_0, **XVI**:319–320
   kinetics of deliquescence above, **XVI**:321
   measurement of, **XVI**:314
   measurement of moisture uptake, **XVI**:314
   water sorption by crystalline solids and, **XVI**:315–316
   water sorption onto hydrates below, **XVI**:318
   water sorption onto nonhydrates below, **XVI**:316–318
Rhabdomyosarcoma, **XVI**:175
Rhinotracheitis, **XVI**:261
Ribbon mixers, **XVI**:91, 93
Rifampicin, cytochrome P450 and, **XVI**:408
Rigid media, **XVI**:41
Rittinger's law, **XVI**:69–70
Roller mills, **XVI**:80
Rotary drums, **XVI**:36–38
RU486 (mifepristone), **XVI**:176

Sabin polio vaccines, **XVI**:118
Saccharomyces cerevesiae, **XVI**:136
Salbutamol, **XVI**:450
Salicylamide, **XVI**:425
Salicylic acid, Crigler-Najjar syndrome and, **XVI**:425
Salmonella, vaccines and, **XVI**:118, 136, 137
Salmonella typhi, vaccines and, **XVI**:119, 127
Salmonella typhimurium, vaccines and, **XVI**:119, 124
Scale-forming elements, **XVI**:236–237
Scale of scrutiny, **XVI**:85
Scale rot (ulcerative dermatitis), **XVI**:265
Scanning electron microscopy, of waxes, **XVI**:351, 354
Schiff-base compound, vaccines in, **XVI**:133
Schistosoma, **XVI**:136
Schistosoma mansoni, **XVI**:121
Schistosomiasis, **XVI**:126, 127
Scours, **XVI**:269
Screening, **XVI**:81–82
   in sterile filtration, **XVI**:100–101
   wet, **XVI**:385
Sedimentation
   centrifugal, **XVI**:47–48
   description of, **XVI**:82–84
   suspensions and, **XVI**:447–448, 449
Sedimentation potential, **XVI**:432
Sendai virus vaccines, **XVI**:121
Septicemia, **XVI**:124
Serratia, **XVI**:265

Serratia marcescens, **XVI**:44
Sharks, **XVI**:285
Shear mixing, **XVI**:90–91
Sheep, **XVI**:170–172, 268–270, 271
Shipping fever, **XVI**:276, 279
Sieving, **XVI**:81–82
Simple (differential) distillation, **XVI**:13
Size classification/separation, **XVI**:80–84
Size reduction, **XVI**:66–80, *see also* Grinding
   in wet granulation, **XVI**:386
Slurries, **XVI**:34, 37, 38
Smallpox vaccines, **XVI**:118
Smoluchowski equation, **XVI**:433
Sodium carboxymethylcellulose (CMC), **XVI**:373
Sodium chloride
   water sorption and, **XVI**:328
   waxes and, **XVI**:339
Sodium lauryl sulfate, **XVI**:351
Sodium nitroprusside, **XVI**:253
Sodium salicylate, **XVI**:328
Sodium stearate, **XVI**:342
Softisan 154, **XVI**:336
Solid bridges, **XVI**:378
Solid dosage forms, **XVI**:107–108
Solid particles
   attractive forces between, **XVI**:378
   size and distribution in leaching, **XVI**:104–105
Solids
   amorphous, *see* Amorphous solids
   crystalline, *see* Crystalline solid
   hydrophilic, **XVI**:446
   hydrophobic, **XVI**:446–447
   in leaching, **XVI**:105–106
   mixing of, **XVI**:85–93
   mixing of liquids and, **XVI**:95–97
   moving over a hot surface, **XVI**:57
   nonporous, **XVI**:51–53
   porous, **XVI**:54–55
   total suspended, **XVI**:233–236
   water sorption by processed, **XVI**:328–329
   water transfer between components via headspace, **XVI**:329–330
Solubility, temperature and in evaporation, **XVI**:3–4
Solutions
   crystallization from, **XVI**:25–26
   physical properties in evaporation, **XVI**:2–5
Solvent coating, **XVI**:351
Solvents
   granulating, **XVI**:369
   in leaching, **XVI**:103–104
   organic, **XVI**:369
Sorption-desorption moisture transfer (SDMT), **XVI**:329–330
Soybean lecithin, **XVI**:444
Soybean oil, *see* Hydrogenated soybean oil
Spermaceti, **XVI**:339, 342
Spermicides, **XVI**:176

Spontaneous nucleation, **XVI**:24, 25, 28
Spray congealing, **XVI**:355–358
Spray dryers, **XVI**:55
   properties and applications of, **XVI**:63–65
   in wet granulation, **XVI**:396
Spray drying, wax microparticles prepared by, **XVI**:355–358
Staphylococcus albus, **XVI**:42
Staphylococcus aureus, **XVI**:454
Staphylococcus epidermidis, **XVI**:157
Staphylococcus equi, **XVI**:282
Starches
   water sorption and, **XVI**:323–324
   in wet granulation, **XVI**:368, 372–373, 378
Steam, **XVI**:301
Stearic acid, **XVI**:357
Stearyl alcohol, **XVI**:353, 357
Stearylamine, **XVI**:451
Sterile filtration, **XVI**:100–101
Sterilization, **XVI**:97–101
   damage resistance in, **XVI**:98–99
   dry heat, **XVI**:97
   ethylene oxide, **XVI**:99–100
   moist heat, **XVI**:97–98
   product development and, **XVI**:99
   thermal, **XVI**:97–98
Stern layer, **XVI**:431, 432
Stern plane, **XVI**:431, 432
Steroid hydroxylation, **XVI**:411
Steroids
   vaginal delivery of, **XVI**:162–163, 176–177
   in veterinary pharmacy, **XVI**:253
Sterotex, **XVI**:336
Stokes's equations
   elutriation and, **XVI**:82
   evaporation and, **XVI**:8
   filtration and, **XVI**:47
Stomatitis, **XVI**:265
Strangles, **XVI**:279, 282
Streaming potential, **XVI**:432
Streptococcal meningitis, **XVI**:125
Streptococcus equi, **XVI**:279
Streptococcus gordonii, **XVI**:137
Streptococcus pneumoniae, **XVI**:121
Streptococcus pyogenes, **XVI**:116
Streptomycin, in veterinary pharmacy, **XVI**:255, 263, 273
Stress, in grinding and crushing, **XVI**:67–69
Stress-generated potential (SGP), **XVI**:453
Sublimation coating, **XVI**:351
Subunit vaccines, **XVI**:119–121, 137
Sulfaethylthiadiazole, **XVI**:355
Sulfamerazine, **XVI**:447
Sulfamethazine
   acetyl conjugation of, **XVI**:422
   waxes and, **XVI**:355
Sulfamethoxazole, **XVI**:353–354
Sulfate conjugation, **XVI**:422–423

Sulindac, **XVI**:411
Suppositories, waxes in delivery systems for, **XVI**:337, 344, 347
Surface areas, from water sorption studies, **XVI**:326
Surfactants
  suspensions and, **XVI**:448–449
  waxes and, **XVI**:342, 351, 354, 355–356
Suspensions, zeta potential and, **XVI**:446–450
Sustained-release effects, of vaccines, **XVI**:133–134
Swamp fever (equine infectious anemia), **XVI**:278
Swine, *see* Pigs

Tablets, manufacture by wet granulation, **XVI**:390–392
Tamoxifen, cytochrome P450 and, **XVI**:411
Tangential-spray coating, **XVI**:348–349
T-cell epitopes, vaccines and, **XVI**:126, 127–128
Temperature, *see also* Absolute temperature; Ambient temperature; Boiling; Glass transition temperature
  crystallization and, **XVI**:26
  drying and, **XVI**:57–58, 64
  freeze drying and, **XVI**:62, 63
  grinding and, **XVI**:72–73
  leaching and, **XVI**:105
  solubility and in evaporation, **XVI**:3–4
  viscosity and in evaporation, **XVI**:3
  water conductivity and, **XVI**:295
  water sorption isotherm analysis as a function of, **XVI**:325–326
  water system maintenance and, **XVI**:304
  waxes and, **XVI**:339, 344, 349, 354, 356
Testosterone, urinary incontinence in dogs and, **XVI**:253
Tetanus, **XVI**:269
  in cattle, **XVI**:274, 275
  in horses, **XVI**:279, 282
  in sheep and goats, **XVI**:271
  in swine, **XVI**:284
Tetanus toxoid
  in vaccines, **XVI**:124, 125
  in veterinary pharmacy, **XVI**:269, 279
Tetracycline, in veterinary pharmacy, **XVI**:255, 265, 279
Theophylline, waxes in delivery systems for, **XVI**:346, 347, 357–358
Therapeutic vaccines, **XVI**:128
Thermal sterilization, **XVI**:97–98
Thiabendazole, **XVI**:449
Thiobenzamide, **XVI**:411
Thiouracil, **XVI**:424
Thrush, in horses, **XVI**:279–280
Ticks, **XVI**:267
Timolol, **XVI**:410
Togavirus, **XVI**:275
Tolazoline hydrochloride, **XVI**:342
Tolbutamide, **XVI**:410

Top-feed filtration, **XVI**:38
Top-spray techniques, **XVI**:348
Total organic carbon (TOC), water concentration of, **XVI**:231, 232, 237, 243–244, 297–299
Total suspended solids, **XVI**:233–236
Tragacanth, **XVI**:373
Tranexamic acid, **XVI**:179
Tranquilizers, in veterinary pharmacy, **XVI**:286
Transition, in granule formation, **XVI**:378–379
Transmissible gastroenteritis (TGE), **XVI**:280, 284
Trepomena pallidum, **XVI**:120
Trichomonas foetis, **XVI**:274
Tripelenamine hydrochloride, **XVI**:342
Troleandomycin, **XVI**:411
Trough mixers, **XVI**:93
Trypanosoma rhodesiense, **XVI**:121
Trypanosomes, **XVI**:127
Tuberculosis vaccines, **XVI**:124
Tumbler mixers, **XVI**:91, 93
Tumbling dryers, **XVI**:59
Tumor necrosis factor (TNF), **XVI**:123
Turbines, **XVI**:96
Tyzzer's disease, **XVI**:263

Ulcerative dermatitis (scale rot), **XVI**:265
Ultrafiltration, **XVI**:303
Ultrasound vibration potential (UVP), **XVI**:438
Ultraviolet (UV) radiation, water system validation and, **XVI**:239, 247
United States Pharmacopeia (USP)
  on bulk pharmaceuticals, **XVI**:203
  on water for pharmaceutical use, **XVI**:293, 296, 300, 301
  on water system validation, **XVI**:224, 225, 233, 242–243
Unit processes, **XVI**:1–110, *see also* Crystallization; Distillation; Drying; Evaporation; Extraction; Filtration; Humidification; Leaching; Mixing; Size reduction; Sterilization
Uridine diphosphate glucuronic acid (UDPGA), **XVI**:416–418
Uridine diphosphate glucuronyltransferase (UDPGT), **XVI**:416–418
Urinary calculi, in cats, **XVI**:259
Urinary incontinence, in dogs, **XVI**:253

Vaccines, **XVI**:115–143
  adenovirus, **XVI**:120, 136, 137
  adjuvants for, **XVI**:132–135
  attenuated, **XVI**:118–119, 135–136
  bacterial, **XVI**:124–126
  clinical trials of, **XVI**:140–142
  delivery systems for enhanced response, **XVI**:134–140
  design of, **XVI**:115–117
  fertility, **XVI**:128–129
  Haemophilus influenzae type B, **XVI**:124

[Vaccines]
   helminth, **XVI**:126–128
   hepatitis B virus, **XVI**:121
   herpesvirus, **XVI**:119, 123
   inactivated microorganism, **XVI**:117–118
   infectious agent, **XVI**:122–128
   influenza, **XVI**:122, 137, 139, 266
   measles, **XVI**:118, 123
   nonliving microparticulate delivery systems for, **XVI**:138–140
   polio, **XVI**:118, 120, 136, 179
   production of, **XVI**:142–143
   protozoan, **XVI**:126–128
   recombinant, **XVI**:136–138
   routes of administration, **XVI**:129–135
   smallpox, **XVI**:118
   subunit, **XVI**:119–121, 137
   therapeutic, **XVI**:128
   tuberculosis, **XVI**:124
   vaccinia virus, **XVI**:120, 123, 137
   vaginal delivery of, **XVI**:131, 178–179
   in veterinary pharmacy, **XVI**:142, 179
     for birds, **XVI**:265
     for cats, **XVI**:259, 260, 261
     for cattle, **XVI**:124, 126, 272, 273
     for dogs, **XVI**:254, 255, 257–258
     for ferrets, **XVI**:266
     for goats, **XVI**:271
     for horses, **XVI**:275–276, 278, 279
     for pigs, **XVI**:125, 280, 281–282, 283, 284
     for rabbits, **XVI**:125, 262
     for sheep, **XVI**:269, 271
     for wolves, **XVI**:286
   viral, **XVI**:122–123
   whole organism, **XVI**:117–119
Vaccinia virus vaccines, **XVI**:120, 123, 137
Vacuum crystallizers, **XVI**:28, 29–30
Vacuum filters, 36–38
Vacuum tray dryers, **XVI**:58–59
Vagina, **XVI**:153–159
   cellular structure of, **XVI**:154–156
   fluids and enzymes of, **XVI**:156–157
   general anatomy of, **XVI**:153–157
   physiology and dynamics of, 157–158
Vaginal absorption, **XVI**:159–166
Vaginal delivery, **XVI**:153–179
   drug candidates for, **XVI**:174–179
   human applications of, **XVI**:166–170
   types of systems for, **XVI**:166–174
   of vaccines, **XVI**:131, 178–179
   veterinary applications of, **XVI**:170–172
Vaginal rings, **XVI**:168–170, 177
Validation, *see* Process validation; Water system validation
Validation committee, **XVI**:189
Validation master plan
   in process validation, **XVI**:190
   in water system validation, **XVI**:216–217

Valproic acid, **XVI**:411
van der Waals forces
   emulsions and, **XVI**:445
   in microbiology, **XVI**:454
   suspensions and, **XVI**:446
   wet granulation and, **XVI**:378
   zeta potential and, **XVI**:442, 445, 446
Vapor
   in humidification, **XVI**:18
   removal of in evaporation, **XVI**:7–8
Vapor adsorption, *see also* Water sorption
   by amorphous solids, **XVI**:312
   capillary condensation and, **XVI**:312–313
   models describing, **XVI**:309–313
Vapor pressure, **XVI**:10–11
Variang surface glycoprotein (VSG), **XVI**:127
Vegetable oil, *see* Hydrogenated vegetable oil
Venezuelan equine encephalomyelitis (VEE), **XVI**:277, 281
Veterinary pharmacy, **XVI**:251–287
   for aquatic animals, **XVI**:285–286
   for birds, **XVI**:263–265
   for cats, **XVI**:256–260, 261, 268
   for cattle, *see* Cattle
   for dogs, **XVI**:252–256, 257–258, 268
   for exotics, **XVI**:266
   for ferrets, **XVI**:266
   for goats, **XVI**:268–270
   history of, **XVI**:251
   for horses, **XVI**:274–280, 281–282
   for pigs (swine), **XVI**:125, 280–283, 284
   for rabbits, **XVI**:125, 260–263
   for reptiles, **XVI**:265–266
   for sheep, **XVI**:170–172, 268–270, 271
   vaccines in, *see* Vaccines, in veterinary pharmacy
   vaginal delivery systems in, **XVI**:170–172
   for zoo animals, **XVI**:285–286
Viable nonculturable bacteria, **XVI**:228–231
Vibratory mills, **XVI**:78–79
Vibrio cholerae, **XVI**:125, 134, 138
Viral vaccines, **XVI**:122–123
Viruses, sterilization and, **XVI**:98
Viscerotropic velogenic Newcastle disease (VVND), **XVI**:264
Viscosity
   evaporation and, **XVI**:3
   filtration and, **XVI**:32
   of suspensions, **XVI**:449
   of waxes, **XVI**:337, 346
Vitamin A, in veterinary pharmacy, **XVI**:265
Vitamin C, in veterinary pharmacy, **XVI**:265
Vitamin K, in veterinary pharmacy, **XVI**:256–259
Volatility, **XVI**:16
Vulvovaginal candidiasis, vaginal delivery systems for, **XVI**:174, 175

Warfarin
   cats and, **XVI**:256–259
   cytochrome P450 and, **XVI**:410

Water, **XVI**:293–306
  capillary state in, **XVI**:375, 376–377
  conductivity of, **XVI**:295–297
  drinking (potable), **XVI**:299–300
  droplet state in, **XVI**:375, 377–378
  funicular state in, **XVI**:375, 376, 384–385
  monographs on, **XVI**:293
  non-compendial, **XVI**:300–301
  pendular state in, **XVI**:375–376
  pharmacopeial history of, **XVI**:293
  as a plasticizer, **XVI**:326–328
  purified, **XVI**:300
  transfer between solid components via headspace, **XVI**:329–330
  in wet granulation, **XVI**:369
Water Conductivity Test Method, **XVI**:296–297
Water For Injection (WFI) systems
  attributes of, **XVI**:300
  distillation and, **XVI**:303–304
  validation for, **XVI**:224, 226–227, 228–229, 237–238
Water/oil (w/o) emulsions, **XVI**:336
Water/oil/water solvent evaporation method, **XVI**:354
Water softeners, **XVI**:240
Water sorption, **XVI**:307–330, *see also* Vapor adsorption
  by amorphous solids, **XVI**:321–328
  by crystalline solids, **XVI**:315–321
  by solids subjected to processing, **XVI**:328–329
  specific surface areas calculated from, **XVI**:326
Water sorption isotherms, **XVI**:308–309
  analysis at ambient temperature, **XVI**:321–325
  as a function of temperature, **XVI**:325–326
Water systems
  design of, **XVI**:301–304
  sanitary designs for, **XVI**:304
Water system validation, **XVI**:211–248, 305–306
  activities following, **XVI**:246
  alert and action levels in, **XVI**:228–229
  audit in, **XVI**:246–248
  of batched water supplies, **XVI**:244–245
  concurrent, **XVI**:224, 225
  conductivity measures in, **XVI**:229–231
  documentation and information in, **XVI**:212–214
  equipment design and, **XVI**:214–216
  final reports in, **XVI**:222–224
  impurities in, **XVI**:233–238
  instruments and controls in, **XVI**:219–220
  life cycle of, **XVI**:305
  maintenance of, **XVI**:306
  microbiological, **XVI**:225–227, 228
  of municipally treated feedwater, **XVI**:244
  principal unit purification processes in, **XVI**:240–241
  prospective, **XVI**:224
  purification unit processes in, **XVI**:238–239
  retrospective, **XVI**:224, 225

[Water system validation]
  sequence of, **XVI**:214–224
  source-water testing in, **XVI**:231
  specific processes in, **XVI**:243–244
  steps in, **XVI**:214
  viable nonculturable bacteria in, **XVI**:228–231
Wax beads, **XVI**:338–339
Waxes, **XVI**:335–338
  characterization of, **XVI**:336–338
  coating with, **XVI**:347–352
  in hard gelatin capsules, **XVI**:337, 343–347
  in matrix-type drug delivery systems, **XVI**:338
  microencapsulation with, **XVI**:352–358
Wax granules, **XVI**:338–339
Wax implants, **XVI**:343
Wax matrix tablets, **XVI**:340–342
Western equine encephalomyelitis (WEE), **XVI**:277, 281
Wet-bulb depression, **XVI**:18–21, 50–51
Wet dewlap (moist dermatitis), **XVI**:262
Wet granulation, **XVI**:363–398
  advantages of, **XVI**:387–388
  binders in, **XVI**:369–373
  color, flavor, and flavor modifiers in, **XVI**:368–369
  diluents or fillers in, **XVI**:365–367
  disintegrants in, **XVI**:368
  drug substance in, **XVI**:365
  drying in, **XVI**:386
  equipment in, **XVI**:392–397
  granulating solvents in, **XVI**:369
  limitations of, **XVI**:388–390
  mechanism of granule formation in, **XVI**:378–380
  particle-bonding mechanisms in, **XVI**:374–378
  scale-up problems in, **XVI**:397–398
  sizing in, **XVI**:386
  steps in, **XVI**:380–386
  tablet manufacture by, **XVI**:390–392
  wet screening in, **XVI**:385
Wet grinding, **XVI**:72
Wet massing, **XVI**:381–385
Wet screening, **XVI**:385
White wax USP, **XVI**:355–356
Whole organism vaccines, **XVI**:117–119
Whooping cough vaccines, **XVI**:124
Wolves, **XVI**:286
World Health Organization (WHO)
  process validation and, **XVI**:192
  vaccines and, **XVI**:140
Worst-case analysis, **XVI**:197
Wurster bottom-spray coating, **XVI**:348

Xenobiotic metabolism, **XVI**:403–425
  alcohol and aldehyde dehydrogenases in, **XVI**:413–414
  genetic factors influencing, **XVI**:424–425
  hydrolysis in, **XVI**:415–416
  oxidative, **XVI**:403–414